SKELETAL NUCLEAR MEDICINE

SKELETAL NUCLEAR MEDICINE

B. David Collier, Jr., M.D.
Professor of Radiology
Medical College of Wisconsin
Director of Nuclear Medicine
Froedtert Memorial Lutheran Hospital
Clement J. Zablocki Veterans Affairs Medical Center
Milwaukee, Wisconsin

Ignac Fogelman, B.Sc., M.D., F.R.C.P.
Reader in Nuclear Medicine
United Medical and Dental Schools
Consultant Physician
Department of Nuclear Medicine
Guy's Hospital
London, England

Leonard Rosenthall, M.S., M.D.
Professor of Radiology
McGill University
Director of Nuclear Medicine
Senior Radiologist
The Montreal General Hospital
Montreal, Quebec, Canada

*with **662** illustrations*

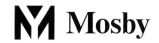

St. Louis Baltimore Boston Carlsbad Chicago Naples New York Philadelphia Portland
London Madrid Mexico City Singapore Sydney Tokyo Toronto Wiesbaden

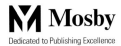
Mosby

Dedicated to Publishing Excellence

A Times Mirror Company

Publisher: Anne S. Patterson
Executive Editor: Robert A. Hurley
Managing Editor: Elizabeth Corra
Associate Developmental Editor: Mia Cariño
Project Manager: Linda Clarke
Senior Production Editor: Allan S. Kleinberg
Manufacturing Manager: Bill Winneberger
Designer: Carolyn O'Brien
Composition Specialist: Steve Cavanaugh

Composition by Mosby Electronic Publishing
Printing/binding by Maple-Vail—York
Printed in the United States of America

Mosby–Year Book, Inc.
11830 Westline Industrial Drive
St. Louis, Missouri 63146

Library of Congress Cataloging-in-Publication Data
Skeletal nuclear medicine / [edited by] B. David Collier, Jr., Ignac
  Fogelman, Leonard Rosenthall.
      p. cm.
    Includes bibliographical references and index.
    ISBN 0-8151-3273-5
    1. Bones--Radionuclide imaging. I. Collier, David.
  II. Fogelman, Ignac, 1948- . III. Rosenthall, Leonard.
    [DNLM: 1. Bone Diseases--diagnosis. 2. Bone and Bones-
  -radionuclide imaging. 3. Neoplasm Metastasis--diagnosis. WE 225
  S627 1996]
  RC930.5.S54 1996
  616.7'107575--dc20
  DNLM/DLC
  for Library of Congress   96-13282
                                                     CIP

96 97 98 99 00 / 9 8 7 6 5 4 3 2 1

Glen M. Blake, Ph.D.
Honorary Senior Lecturer
United Medical and Dental Schools
Consultant Physicist
Guy's Hospital
London, England

Robert J. Boudreau, Ph.D., M.D.
Professor of Radiology
University of Minnesota
Director, Division of Nuclear Medicine
Department of Radiology
University of Minnesota Hospital and Clinic
Minneapolis, Minnesota

Manuel L. Brown, M.D.
Professor of Radiology
University of Pittsburgh Medical Center
Pittsburgh, Pennsylvania

Guillermo F. Carrera, M.D.
Professor of Radiology and Orthopaedic Surgery
Medical College of Wisconsin
Chief, Diagnostic Radiology
Froedtert Memorial Lutheran Hospital
Milwaukee, Wisconsin

B. David Collier, Jr., M.D.
Professor of Radiology
Medical College of Wisconsin
Director of Nuclear Medicine
Froedtert Memorial Lutheran Hospital
Clement J. Zablocki Veterans Affairs Medical Center
Milwaukee, Wisconsin

David B. Coupland, M.D., B.Sc., F.R.C.P.
Assistant Professor
University of British Columbia
Nuclear Medicine Radiology Consultant
Vancouver Hospital and Health Sciences Centre
Vancouver, British Columbia, Canada

Douglas F. Eggli, M.D.
Associate Professor of Radiology
Pennsylvania State University
Chief, Division of Nuclear Medicine
The Milton S. Hershey Medical Center
Hershey, Pennsylvania

Ignac Fogelman, M.D., F.R.C.P.
Reader in Nuclear Medicine
United Medical and Dental Schools
Consultant Physician
Department of Nuclear Medicine
Guy's Hospital
London, England

Charles A. Forscher, M.D.
Staff Physician
Cedars-Sinai Comprehensive Cancer Center
Clinical Consultant
University of California, Los Angeles, Medical Center
Los Angeles, California

Henry W. Gray, M.D., F.R.C.P.
Honorary Clinical Senior Lecturer
University of Glasgow
Consultant Physician in Medicine and Nuclear Medicine
The Royal Infirmary University NHS Trust
Glasgow, Scotland

Harry J. Griffiths, D.M.R.D., F.R.C.P.
Professor of Radiology and Orthopaedics
Director of Radiology Residency Program
University of Minnesota School of Medicine
Director of Outpatient Radiology
University of Minnesota Hospital and Clinic
Minneapolis, Minnesota

H. Theodore Harcke, M.D., F.A.C.R.
Professor of Radiology and Pediatrics
Thomas Jefferson Medical College
Philadelphia, Pennsylvania;
Attending Radiologist
Chief of Imaging Research
Alfred I. duPont Institute
Wilmington, Delaware

Randall A. Hawkins, M.D., Ph.D.
Professor of Radiology
Chief, Nuclear Medicine Program
Vice Chairman, Department of Radiology
University of California, San Francisco
San Francisco, California

Robert S. Hellman, M.D.
Associate Professor of Radiology
Medical College of Wisconsin
Froedtert Memorial Lutheran Hospital
Clement J. Zablocki Veterans Affairs Hospital
Milwaukee, Wisconsin

Carl K. Hoh, M.D.
Assistant Professor
University of California, Los Angeles, School of Medicine
Nuclear Medicine Clinic
UCLA Medical Center
Los Angeles, California

Lawrence E. Holder, M.D., F.A.C.R., F.A.C.N.P.
Professor of Radiology
University of Maryland School of Medicine
Director, Division of Nuclear Medicine
University of Maryland Medical Systems
Baltimore, Maryland

Ali T. Isitman, M.D.
Professor of Radiology-Nuclear Medicine
Medical College of Wisconsin
Milwaukee, Wisconsin

Arnold F. Jacobson, M.D., Ph.D.
Associate Professor of Radiology
University of Washington School of Medicine
Chief, Nuclear Medicine Section
Department of Veterans Affairs Medical Center
Seattle, Washington

Arthur Z. Krasnow, M.D.
Associate Professor of Radiology
Medical College of Wisconsin
Froedtert Memorial Lutheran Hospital
Milwaukee, Wisconsin

Brian C. Lentle, M.D., F.R.C.P.
Professor and Head, Department of Radiology
University of British Columbia
Vancouver Hospital and Health Sciences Centre
Vancouver, British Columbia, Canada

Gerald A. Mandell, M.D., F.A.C.R., F.A.A.P.
Professor of Radiology
Thomas Jefferson Medical College
Adjunct Professor of Radiology
University of Pennsylvania School of Medicine
Philadelphia, Pennsylvania;
Chief of Nuclear Medicine
Alfred I. duPont Institute
Wilmington, Delaware

Robert E. O'Mara, M.D.
Professor, Department of Radiology
University of Rochester School of Medicine and
    Dentistry
Chief, Division of Nuclear Medicine
Strong Memorial Hospital
Rochester, New York

Kutlan Ozker, Ph.D.
Associate Professor of Radiology
Medical College of Wisconsin
Froedtert Memorial Lutheran Hospital
Milwaukee, Wisconsin

David W. Palmer, Ph.D.
Associate Professor of Radiology
Medical College of Wisconsin
Milwaukee, Wisconsin

Gerald Rosen, M.D.
Medical Director
Cedars-Sinai Comprehensive Cancer Center
Associate Professor of Medicine
University of California, Los Angeles, Medical Center
Los Angeles, California

Leonard Rosenthall, M.S., M.D.
Professor of Radiology
McGill University
Director, Nuclear Medicine
Senior Radiologist
The Montreal General Hospital
Montreal, Quebec, Canada

Paul J. Ryan, M.A., M.Sc., M.R.C.P.
Consultant Physician
Medway Hospital
Kent, United Kingdom
Honorary Senior Lecturer
Nuclear Medicine Department
Guy's Hospital
London, England

Donald S. Schauwecker, Ph.D., M.D.
Professor of Radiology
Indiana University School of Medicine
Chief of Nuclear Medicine
Wishard Memorial Hospital
Indianapolis, Indiana

Leanne L. Seeger, M.D.
Associate Professor and Chief, Musculoskeletal
    Radiology
Department of Radiological Sciences
University of California, Los Angeles
Los Angeles, California

Edward B. Silberstein, M.D.
Professor of Medicine and Radiology
University of Cincinnati Medical Center
Associate Director, E.L. Saenger Radioisotope Laboratory
University of Cincinnati Hospital
Cincinnati, Ohio

Gopal Subramanian, Ph.D.
Professor of Radiology
Division of Nuclear Medicine, Department of Radiology
State University of New York Health Science Center
Syracuse, New York

James R. Swinghammer, B.S, C.N.M.T.
Clement J. Zablocki Veterans Affairs Medical Center
Milwaukee, Wisconsin

Mark Tulchinsky, M.D., F.A.C.P.
Assistant Professor, Radiology and Medicine
Pennsylvania State University
Associate Chief, Division of Nuclear Medicine
The Milton S. Hershey Medical Center
Hershey, Pennsylvania

Alan D. Waxman, M.D.
Clinical Professor of Radiology
University of Southern California School of Medicine
Director, Department of Nuclear Medicine
Cedars-Sinai Medical Center
Los Angeles, California

Daniel F. Worsley, B.Sc.(Hons), M.D.
Instructor
University of British Columbia
Vancouver Hospital and Health Sciences Centre
Vancouver, British Columbia, Canada

The radionuclide bone scan with its ability to image osteoblastic activity is the greatest diagnostic triumph of nuclear medicine. Today it is a widely available, accurate, and cost-effective examination that has improved the medical or surgical treatment of countless patients. There have been many recent developments in the field, and the indications for bone scanning continue to expand. The editors and contributing authors of *Skeletal Nuclear Medicine* have prepared this volume for those nuclear medicine physicians and radiologists who wish to update their bone scanning knowledge and improve the quality of their bone scan examinations.

Skeletal Nuclear Medicine focuses on the practical aspects of bone scanning and closely related skeletal procedures. Each chapter presents a state-of-the-art review of an important clinical topic in skeletal nuclear medicine. For example, Chapter 6, "Bone Scanning in Metastatic Disease," comprehensively reviews the topic but is also organized so that the reader interested in a specific subtopic such as prostate carcinoma can easily locate the pertinent material within the chapter.

For an in-depth study of all of skeletal nuclear medicine, the reader will be interested in the logical scientific progression of topics from the beginning to the end of the book. The initial chapter by Dr. O'Mara on the history of bone scanning renews our appreciation of the decades of scientific advancement in this area. Chapter 2 by Dr. Subramanian, "Radiopharmaceuticals for Bone Scanning," then offers invaluable background material for the many clinically oriented chapters that follow. For physicians learning to interpret abnormal studies, Drs. Eggli and Tulchinsky's Chapter 3, "Normal Planar Bone Scan," presents requisite information about the normal examination and normal variants. The SPECT bone scanning technique is covered in detail in Chapter 4, and the value of correlating bone scanning with conventional radiography, CT, and MRI is appreciated in Dr. Carrera's Chapter 5, "A Multi-Modality Approach to Bone Imaging." By first reading these five chapters, the physician who is beginning to study bone scanning will be prepared to understand the topics addressed in the sixteen clinical chapters that follow.

Chapter 6, "Bone Scanning in Metastatic Disease" by Dr. Jacobson, explores the advances of radiologic imaging in identifying metastases. Coverage of essential clinical material then continues in Chapters 7 and 8: "Primary Bone Tumors" by Drs. Waxman, Seeger, Forscher, and Rosen, and "Radionuclide Imaging of Bone Marrow" by Drs. Lentle, Worsley, and Coupland. Chapters 9 and 10 authoritatively discuss bone scanning in metabolic bone disease and Paget's disease. In Chapter 11, "The Role of Nuclear Medicine in Osteomyelitis," Dr. Schauwecker describes his successful approach to the imaging of bone and soft tissue infection. Arthritis and allied disorders are reviewed in Chapter 12, while skeletal nuclear medicine applications in orthopedics and sports medicine are examined in Chapters 13 and 14: "Orthopedic Imaging in Trauma and Sports Medicine" and "Selected Topics in Orthopedic Bone Scanning," by Drs. Holder and Brown. These are followed by Drs. Boudreau and Griffith's Chapter 15, "Bone Infarcts and Osteonecrosis," a highly detailed Chapter 16, "Pediatric Bone Scanning" by Drs. Mandell and Harcke, and Drs. Gray and Krasnow's Chapter 17, "Soft Tissue Uptake of Bone Agents." Finally, Chapter 18, "Deceptions in Nuclear Medicine Imaging of Bone" by Dr. Krasnow and colleagues describes common pitfalls and technical artifacts in bone scanning.

Doctors Hawkins and Hoh's Chapter 19, "PET Bone Imaging," discusses novel imaging techniques which will hopefully become standard in the practice of skeletal nuclear medicine in future years. Chapter 20, "Bone Mineral Analysis," describes techniques that are currently in common use in many nuclear medicine and radiology practices. With the introduction of more specific and effective treatments for osteoporosis, the clinical value of bone mineral analysis will dramatically increase. Finally, Dr. Silberstein's concluding Chapter 21, "Treatment of the Pain of Bone Metastases," will introduce many physicians who have not yet performed their first radionuclide treatment of painful bone metastases to this important therapeutic procedure.

Presently, in the late 1990's, many physicians are taking an increasingly practical and pragmatic approach toward the practice of nuclear medicine and radiology. For these readers, the chapters in *Skeletal Nuclear Medicine* supplement purely scientific and clinical material with appropriate information on practice management. Recommendations for equipment purchases, procedure protocols, department management, and in some cases even billing for skeletal nuclear medicine examinations are all discussed. The editors feel that in the modern era important lessons for the nuclear medicine physician-in-training include not only basic science and clinical knowledge but the essentials of successful practice management.

As the editors of this volume, it was a great pleasure to review and edit the outstanding chapters submitted by the various contributing authors. We hope that you share our enthusiasm for *Skeletal Nuclear Medicine*!

B. David Collier, Jr., M.D.
Ignac Fogelman, B.Sc., M.D., F.R.C.P.
Leonard Rosenthall, M.S., M.D.

ACKNOWLEDGMENTS

We thank the contributing authors for their outstanding manuscripts and for working as a team to make *Skeletal Nuclear Medicine* a cohesive, well-written volume. A seemingly endless series of telephone calls, chapter outlines, and manuscript drafts is evidence of their dedication to the project.

The support of colleagues and staff at all the institutions supplying chapters for *Skeletal Nuclear Medicine* is gratefully acknowledged. The editors in particular wish to thank secretaries Arline Pluer and Shevon Wilson for their contribution to the development of the book.

The editors also extend their appreciation to Anne Patterson and her very capable staff at Mosby–Year Book, Inc., including Maura Leib, Allan Kleinberg, Steve Cavanaugh, Elizabeth Corra, and Mia Cariño for their highly professional assistance in producing *Skeletal Nuclear Medicine*.

B. David Collier, Jr., M.D.
Ignac Fogelman, B.Sc., M.D., F.R.C.P.
Leonard Rosenthall, M.S., M.D.

CONTENTS

Color plates follow page 178

SKELETAL NUCLEAR MEDICINE

A SHORT HISTORY OF BONE SCANNING

Robert E. O'Mara

EARLY HISTORY

Since the early part of this century, it has been known that many radioactive substances will concentrate in the osseous system and may well lead to bone necrosis, osteomyelitis, and osteogenic sarcoma formation. Blum and others reported on the localization of radium, mesothorium, and radiothorium in the mandible (radium jaw), and the development of tumors and radiation osteitis.[4,13] Indeed, radium chloride was used in small doses in the treatment of patients with arthritis and gout, as well as thorium dioxide in radiographic studies. The initial organized study of radionuclide uptake in bone is best traced to the reports of Chiewicz and Hevesy in 1935, who used P-32 to study metabolism in rats.[6] Others were using isotopes of calcium to study bone metabolism in animals and, in the early 1950s, humans.

In that time frame many other isotopes were being used to study deposition in both the organic and inorganic components of bone. Radioactive cerium and radioactive gallium were found to deposit in the osteoid tissues, whereas radioactive sulfur labeled chondroitin sulfate targeted the nonmineral phase of bone. In 1942 Treadwell et al demonstrated similarities between the handling of strontium-89 and calcium with autoradiograms of human bone cancer.[23] The results of Pecher's studies of strontium-89 treatment of metastatic bone cancer were reported posthumously the same year.[18] In the late 1940s and 1950s, Dudley and others broke similar ground by demonstrating radioactive gallium uptake at the site of osteogenesis and that such increased uptake may be seen before radiographic changes in both neoplastic and benign disease.[8,15]

Metabolic studies with probe techniques continued to develop especially with the introduction of strontium-85 for human use by Spencer et al and Van Dilla and Arnold in 1956.[20,24] The application of this radionuclide was extended to both benign and malignant conditions. Bauer reported on the uptake of strontium-85 in bony disease even before radiographic changes.[2] In 1961, Gynning et al related increased strontium uptake at the site of metastatic breast carcinoma, with over 40% of such activity patterns being found before the radiographic stigmata of disease (Fig. 1-1).[11] During this time, two major developments occurred—the first of which was a change in emphasis. Early investigators were interested primarily in exploring the therapeutic applications of radionuclides to tumors of bone, both benign and malignant. Later, interest focused on the diagnostic use of these bone-seeking test agents. The second development was improvement in the instrumentation to detect and quantify bone uptake and distribution. Initial measurements were made with probes, ranging from hand-held Geiger-Mulller tube counting to mechanized, collimated probe systems (Fig. 1-1). In 1961 Fleming et al introduced the first strontium-85 photoscans of bone abnormalities (Fig. 1-2).[9]

DEVELOPMENTS SINCE THE 1960s

A major stride in bone imaging came with the introduction of fluorine-18 in 1962 by Blau et al and strontium-87m in 1963 by Myers and Olejar (Figs. 1-3 and 1-4).[3,16] Scintiscanning with strontium-87m was reported by Charkes et al.[5] The advantages of fluorine-18 are a shorter half-life and the ability to do total-body bone scanning in a reasonable period of time. Strontium-87m was obtained from a yttrium-87/strontium-87m generator system, had a short half-life and a photon emission better suited to scanning than that of either strontium-85 or fluorine-18.[14] These two agents paved the way for clinical studies of benign diseases of bone.

Before 1962 nuclear physicians were limited to use of strontium-85 when imaging patients with proven primary malignancy for possible bone metastases. Doses of strontium-85 up to 150 µCi were administered, and following a 2- to 5-day wait, with intervening bowel ablutions to clear the gut of radioactivity, the patient was imaged with a rectilinear scanner fitted with either a single 3- or 5-inch scintillation crystal. Because of the low photon flux, it could take from 2 to 2 1/2 hours to scan the lower lumbar spine and pelvis, although Simpson and Orange demonstrated the feasibility of total-body scanning with an 8-inch scintillation crystal.[19] The later introduction of a rectilinear scanner with dual opposed detectors facilitated faster imaging. The advent of fluorine-18 and strontium-87m permitted total-body scanning in 30 to 60 minutes because of the greater flux afforded by the permissible given doses (Figs. 1-3 and 1-4). The skeleton had the semblance of a skeleton on the images produced by these radiotracers and provided landmarks for lesion localization. Fluorine-18 was also used with early positron camera systems.[25]

During the mid to late 1960s considerable effort was directed toward the development of tumor-specific bone-scanning agents and more effective routine bone imaging agents. Research groups around the world studied virtually every isotope that had even the slightest tendency to localize in any of the constituents of bone. Still the mainstays remained the strontiums and fluorine-18. Numerous papers appeared on the clinical utility of fluorine-18 and studies comparing strontium-85, strontium-87m, and fluorine-18.[5,10,21]

Whitley and associates presented the first evidence

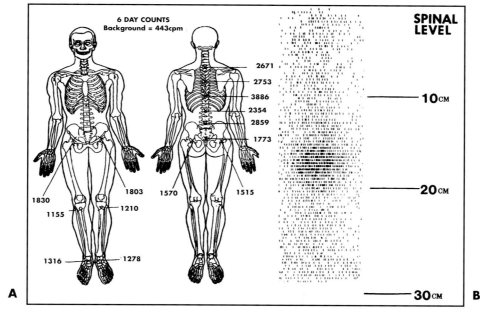

Fig. 1–1. A 53-year-old woman with metastatic carcinoma of the breast. **A,** Sr-85 probe counts over the spine, hips, knees, and ankles 6 days after intravenous injection of 100 µCi of the test agent and intervening enemas to clear the bowel of radioactivity. A relatively high count rate is registered 20 cm below the spine of C7. **B,** A scan of the area was performed with a Baird-Atomic rectilinear scanner equipped with a single probe containing a 3-inch scintillation crystal and convergent collimator, and a count rate tapping mechanism for the readout. It visualized the metastatic lesion in the lower thoracic spine as a focus of increased tap mark density. Scanning time for this small field was about 1 hour owing to the overall low count rate of Sr-85 and small crystal size that was commercially available in 1962. *(Courtesy of L. Rosenthall, M.D.)*

of potential use of the technetium-99m label to visualize bone.[26] However, it was not until 1971 when Subramanian and McAfee, building on the earlier experience with radiophosphate complexes for therapy, developed the first technetium-99m polyphosphate complex for successful bone imaging (Fig. 1-4).[12,22] The advantages of this compound were obvious: Tc-99m was widely available, it had a suitable 140 keV energy for gamma camera imaging, a favorably short 6-hour half-life, and in clinical practice a high photon flux for the higher permissible doses given to facilitate rapid total-body imaging in benign and malignant conditions with a low radiation burden. After the introduction of the polyphosphate complex, other agents were investigated—both inorganic and organic phosphates—for greater stability and higher bone accretion. The most popular agents used presently are the technetium-99m labeled diphosphonates, such as methylene diphosphonate (MDP). They have gained widespread acceptance as a result of extensive experience and the educational efforts of the initial clinical users of these products.[17]

As noted earlier, advances in instrument development are major catalysts to clinical acceptance of nuclear medicine procedures. During the progression from hand-held Geiger-Muller tube counting systems to mechanized counting systems to rectilinear photoscanning systems, there was dramatic improvement in the visualization of the functional changes in bone affected by benign or malignant disease. However, the most important innovation was the gamma-ray scintillation camera developed by Anger.[1] Fortunately the commercial version of this instrument was introduced just as technetium-99m labeled bone-seeking agents appeared on the market. They were an excellent match because their physical characteristics complemented each other. Some nuclear medicine practitioners were quick to give up the rectilinear scanner in favor of the gamma camera, whereas others were more reluctant because of prevailing debates on the resolution capabilities of the two devices. Further improvements in gamma camera resolution overcame this resistance. Small stationary camera systems quickly gave way to larger fields of view (LFOV), moveable systems suitable for imaging the entire body, with or without having to put it together in pieces with a "zipper." Today LFOV camera devices can perform total-body

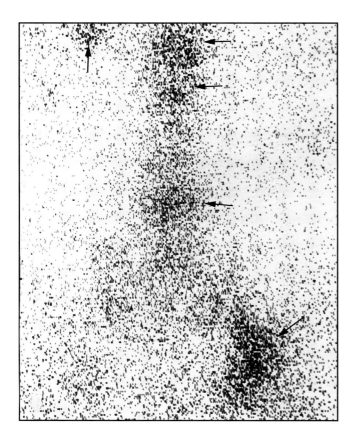

Fig. 1-2. Posterior Sr-85 photoscan of the lower thoracic and lumbosacral spine obtained 48 hours after injection in a 65-year-old woman. Lesions were seen in ribs, spine, and right pelvis (*arrows*). The scan was produced in 1966 with a Nuclear-Chicago 3-inch crystal rectilinear photoscanner.

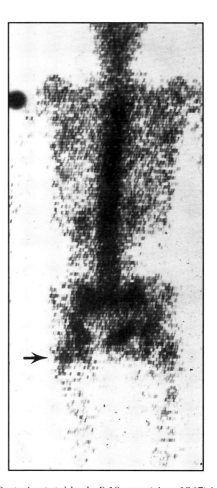

Fig. 1-3. Posterior total-body F-18 scan (circa 1967) in a patient with an osteoid osteoma in the left femoral neck (*arrow*). It took 40 minutes to obtain with an Ohio-Nuclear rectilinear scanner fitted with dual opposed 5-inch scintillation crystal probes.

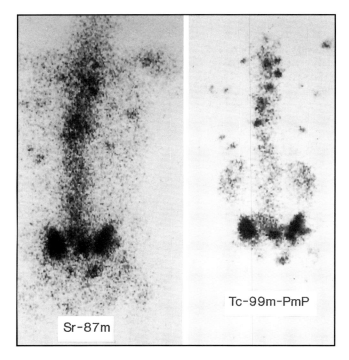

Fig. 1–4. A crossover comparison of Sr-87m and Tc-99m labeled polymetaphosphate (circa 1972) in a patient with metastatic breast carcinoma. The polymetaphosphate was a commercial kit manufactured by New England Nuclear and consisted of a mixture of short-chained polyphosphates. Total-body photoscans were obtained with the Ohio-Nuclear dual opposed 5-inch scintillation crystal rectilinear scanner. Note that more lesions are seen with Tc-99m-polymetaphosphate (PmP) than with Sr-87m; also note the presence of a higher background with Sr-87m. *(Courtesy of L. Rosenthall, M.D.)*

imaging either in a single pass or as multiple spot views in a matter of minutes. Equipment vendors introduced rotating gamma camera SPECT (single photon emission computed tomography) systems in the early 1980s. It was soon demonstrated convincingly by Collier et al that skeletal SPECT imaging provided better sensitivity than planar imaging, particularly in areas of the spine and joints.[7] Progressive developments in the 1990s have given us high-resolution, multidetector SPECT systems with remarkable improvements in computers, software, and digital displays.

FUTURE PROGRESS

As we enter the 21st century, how will bone scanning develop? Much will depend on radiopharmaceutical innovations, such as tumor-specific bone imaging agents. Currently bone scanning remains a highly sensitive, but nonspecific modality, which for clinical application relies heavily on pattern recognition to render an element of specificity. Nonetheless, the rapidity of progress in the 30 years since true radionuclide imaging of the skeleton was introduced bodes well for the near future of this procedure, which today is one of the most commonly per-

formed studies in the nuclear medicine laboratory. The many current uses of radionuclide functional imaging of the skeleton, and how they interact with other imaging modalities, such as computed tomography and magnetic resonance imaging, are the subject of this textbook.

REFERENCES

1. Anger HO: Scintillation cameras. *Rev Sci Instrum* 1958; 29:27.
2. Bauer GCH, Wendeberg B: External counting of Ca^{47} and Sr^{85} in studies of localized lesions in man. *J Bone Joint Surg Br* 1959; 41B:558.
3. Blau M, Negler W, Bender MA: Fluorine-18: A new isotope for bone scanning. *J Nucl Med* 1962; 3:332.
4. Blum T: Osteomyelitis of the mandible and maxilla. *J Am Dent Assoc* 1924; 11:802.
5. Charkes ND, Sklaroff TM, Bierly J: Detection of metastatic cancer to bone by scintiscanning with strontium-87m. *Am J Roentgenol* 1964; 91:1121.
6. Chiewicz O, Hevesy G: Radioactive indications in the study of phosphorus metabolism in rats. *Nature* 1935; 13:754.
7. Collier BD, Hillman RS Jr, Krasnow AZ: Bone SPECT. *Semin Nucl Med* 1987; 17:247.
8. Dudley HC, Maddox GE: Deposition of radiogallium (Ga^{72}) in skeletal tissues. *J Pharmacol Exp Ther* 1949; 96:244.

9. Fleming WH, McIlraith JD, King ER: Photoscanning of bone lesions utilizing strontium-85. *Radiol* 1961; 77:635.

10. French RJ, McCready VR: The use of 18F for bone scanning. *Br J Radiol* 1967; 40:655.

11. Gynning I et al: Localization with Sr-85 of spinal metastases in mammary cancer and changes in uptake after hormone and roentgen therapy. *Acta Radiol* 1961; 55:119.

12. Kaplan E et al: Therapy with polyphosphate. *J Nucl Med* 1960; 1:1.

13. Martland HA, Humphries RE: Osteogenic sarcoma in dial painters using luminous paint. *Arch Pathol* 1929; 7:406.

14. Mecklenburg RI: Clinical value of generator-produced strontium-87m. *J Nucl Med* 1964; 5:929.

15. Mulry WC, Dudley HC: Studies of radiogallium as a diagnostic agent in bone tumors. *J Lab Clin Med* 1951; 37:239.

16. Myers WG, Olejar M: Radiostrontium-87m in studies of healing bone fracture. *J Nucl Med* 1963; 4:202.

17. O'Mara RE: Review of new bone scan agents. *Semin Nucl Med* 1972; 2:38.

18. Pecher C: Biological investigation with radioactive calcium and strontium: Preliminary report on the use of radioactive strontium in the treatment of metastatic bone cancer. *Univ Cal Berk Pub Pharmacol* 1942; 2:117.

19. Simpson WJ, Orange RP: Total body scanning with strontium-85 in the diagnosis of metastatic bone disease. *Can Med Assoc J* 1965; 93:1237.

20. Spencer H, et al: Strontium-85 metabolism in man and effect of calcium on strontium excretion. *Proc Soc Exp Biol Med* 1956; 91:55.

21. Spencer R et al: Bone scanning with [85]Sr, [87m]Sr and [18]F. *Br J Radiol* 1967; 40:641.

22. Subramanian G, McAfee JG: A new complex of ^{99m}Tc for skeletal imaging. *Radiol* 1971; 99:192.

23. Treadwell A, et al: Metabolic studies on neoplasm of bone with the aid of radioactive strontium. *Am J Med Sci* 1942; 204:521.

24. Van Dilla MA, Arnold JS: Strontium-85 tracer studies in humans. *Int J Radiat Isot* 1956; 1:129.

25. Van Dyke D et al: Bone blood flow shown with F-18 and the positron camera. *Am J Physiol* 1965; 209:65.

26. Whitley JE et al: Tc[99m] in the visualization of neoplasm outside the brain. *Am J Roentgenol* 1966; 96:706.

CHAPTER 2

RADIOPHARMACEUTICALS FOR BONE SCANNING

Gopal Subramanian

Bone scanning is one of the most widely used imaging studies in nuclear medicine. This procedure has found excellent clinical utility over a period of more than three decades. During this time a wide variety of radiopharmaceuticals have been in clinical use for bone imaging. They include anionic fluoride ion (F-18), cationic calcium analogs (Sr-85, Sr-87m, Ba-131, Ba-135m), rare earth complexes (Sm-153, Dy-157, Er-171, HEDTA [hydroxy ethylene diamine tetra acetic acid] chelates), and Tc-99m labeled phosphate and phosphonate complexes. This chapter reviews these developments in detail.

EARLY BONE SCANNING AGENTS

The first radionuclide investigation of the skeleton can be traced back to Chiecwitz and Hevesy,[11] who found in 1935 that P-32 (beta emitter) was deposited in bones of adult rats. In 1942 Treadwell[74] demonstrated by autoradiography the deposition of Sr-89 (beta emitter) in active osteogenic sarcoma. This work illustrated that strontium behaved biologically similar to calcium in bone localization. In 1961 Fleming[16] introduced bone scanning with Sr-85 by demonstrating the localization of Sr-85 in normal bone with increased concentration in abnormal sites of the skeleton. Because of its long physical (65 days) and biologic half-life (similar to that of bone mineral), only a very small quantity (100 to 150 μCi) of Sr-85 can be safely administered to patients. Even though the bone images were of poor quality, they nevertheless provided clinically useful information. Also in 1961 Myers[39] produced Sr-87m in a cyclotron. Sr-87m is a short-lived analog of Sr-85 and can be made available from a Y-87/Sr-87m radioisotope generator.[36] Y-87 has a half-life of 80 hours and therefore can be shipped to distant sites. Sr-87m with a short half-life (2.8 hours) and reasonable photon energy (388 keV) was used in bone imaging when Y-87/Sr-87m generators became commercially available. Sr-87m offered several advantages over Sr-85. Its much shorter half-life and lower gamma energy (511 keV vs. 388 keV) were more suitable than Sr-85 for external imaging of the bone. However, the images obtained with Sr-87m were not completely satisfactory because its plasma clearance was relatively slow and the resultant concentration in the soft tissues partially obscured the bone.

In 1961 Blau et al[5] introduced fluorine-18 for use in bone scanning. This was the agent of choice for many years thereafter. This radionuclide may be administered orally or intravenously. The blood clearance of radioactivity is very rapid, with up to 50% to 60% of injected activity accumulated in the normal skeleton and the remainder of activity excreted by the kidneys in the urine. F-18 proved superior to Sr-85 because of its faster blood clearance and lower soft-tissue concentration. Scanning can be performed within 2 hours after intravenous injection. Nevertheless, F-18 has had its drawbacks. This nuclide has to be produced daily in a cyclotron or a nuclear reactor and should be used within a short time because of its short half-life (110 minutes). Hence, availability of F-18 in locations where cyclotrons are not situated is still a problem. So the search continued for new bone imaging agents.

Barium radionuclides Ba-131 and Ba-135m[59,60] have been experimentally used for bone imaging. Barium is an analog of divalent calcium and its biologic behavior resembled that of strontium after intravenous administration. Ba-135m possessed better characteristics than Ba-131 (268 keV gamma energy and 29-hour half-life). In experimental animals more than 50% of injected dose localized in the skeleton. Ba-135m also cleared from blood much faster than Sr-85. Of all the alkaline earth elements barium-135m was perhaps the best agent for bone imaging.

So far we have dealt with anionic (F-18 fluoride) and divalent cationic radionuclides (Sr-85, Sr-87m, Ba-131, Ba-135m) for skeletal imaging. In 1953 Newman and Newman[40] discussed the possibility that anionic metal complexes could concentrate in bone. The first set of these complexes was derived from trivalent cationic lanthanons. Durbin et al[76] and later Jowsey[27] demonstrated in experimental animals that citrate complexes of lanthanons, particularly the heavier atoms, localized primarily in the skeleton. The lighter lanthanides are more basic, have larger ionic radii, localize primarily in liver, are excreted in feces, and show some localization in bone. The heavier members of this group are more acidic, have smaller ionic radii, and localize predominantly in the bone; the remaining activity is excreted in the urine. Of these lanthanides, radionuclides Sm-153, Er-171, and Dy-157 have been complexed with HEDTA and were used in clinical studies.[43] Another radionuclide, thulium-167, was evaluated only in experimental animals. The physical properties of these radionuclides and other bone imaging agents are summarized in Table 2-1.

The radionuclides samarium-153 and erbium-171 can be produced in a nuclear reactor, whereas dysprosium-157 and thulium-167 require a cyclotron for their production. Although the lanthanide chelates of high stability constant (e.g., diethylene triamine penta acetic acid [DTPA]) are excreted predominantly in the urine with minimal localization in the skeleton, the chelates of intermediate stability (e.g., HEDTA) allow bone localization to occur. These agents were evaluated first in experimental animals[42,64] and later in patients.[43] Of this group of rare earths, Dy-157 seemed to be the best agent because of its short half-life (8.2 hours) and monoenergetic gamma energy of 326 keV with 91% external photon yield. However, its limited availability from cyclotrons prevented its clinical use.

More recently the radionuclide Sm-153 has been

TABLE 2-1
Physical Properties of Radionuclides Evaluated for Skeletal Imaging

Radionuclide	Half-Life	Gamma Energy (keV)	External Photon Yield (%)	Beta Energy (EβMeV)	Recommended Dose (mCi)	Radiation Estimates (Skeleton)	Dose (rad) (Red Marrow)
Flourine-18	1.85 hr	511	194	0.25	5	0.75	0.2
Strontium-87m	2.7 hr	388	78	0.082	10	0.71	0.21
Erbium-171 (HEDTA)	7.5 hr	296	91	0.38	4	3.0	0.76
		308					
Dysprosium-157 (HEDTA)	8 hr	326	91	0.014	10	1.27	0.55
Barium-135m	28.7 hr	268	16	0.200	3	4.08	0.87
Samarium-153 (HEDTA)	47 hr	103	28	0.290	1	3.3	0.85
Thulium-167 (HEDTA)	9.6 days	208	49	0.126	0.5	3.45	0.91
Barium-131	11.7 days	124	28	0.043	0.3	4.28	1.35
		215	19				
		373	13				
		496	48				
Strontium-85	65 days	512	99	0.015	0.15	3.89	1.35
Technetium-99m	6 hr	140	90	0.015	15	0.57	0.37

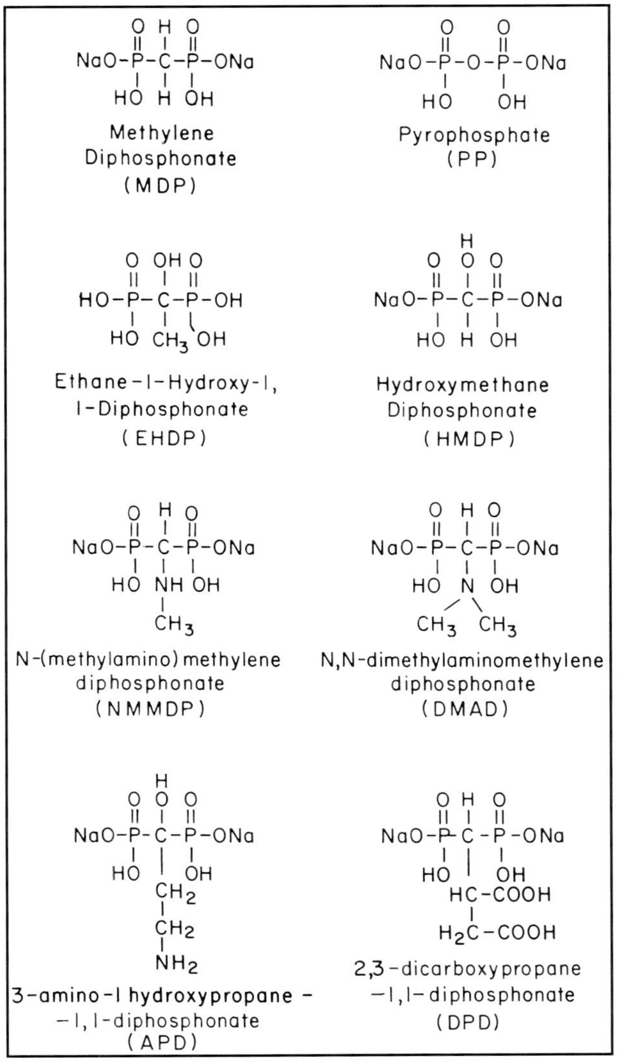

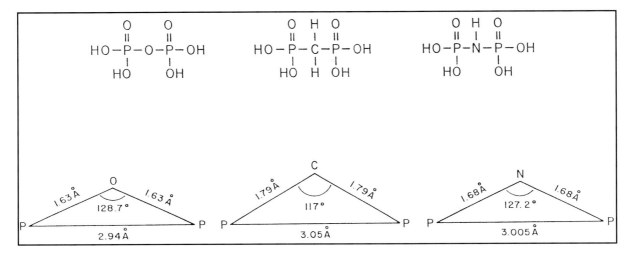

$$NaO-\overset{\overset{O}{\|}}{P}-\overset{\overset{H}{|}}{C}-\overset{\overset{O}{\|}}{P}-ONa$$
$$\underset{HO}{|}\ \underset{H}{|}\ \underset{OH}{|}$$

Methylene
Diphosphonate
(MDP)

$$NaO-\overset{\overset{O}{\|}}{P}-O-\overset{\overset{O}{\|}}{P}-ONa$$
$$\underset{HO}{|}\quad\underset{OH}{|}$$

Pyrophosphate
(PP)

$$HO-\overset{\overset{O}{\|}}{P}-\overset{\overset{OH}{|}}{C}-\overset{\overset{O}{\|}}{P}-OH$$
$$\underset{HO}{|}\ \underset{CH_3}{|}\ \underset{OH}{|}$$

Ethane-1-Hydroxy-1,
1-Diphosphonate
(EHDP)

$$NaO-\overset{\overset{O}{\|}}{P}-\overset{\overset{H}{|}}{C}-\overset{\overset{O}{\|}}{P}-ONa$$
$$\underset{HO}{|}\ \underset{H}{|}\ \underset{OH}{|}$$

Hydroxymethane
Diphosphonate
(HMDP)

$$NaO-\overset{\overset{O}{\|}}{P}-\overset{\overset{H}{|}}{C}-\overset{\overset{O}{\|}}{P}-ONa$$
$$\underset{HO}{|}\ \underset{NH}{|}\ \underset{OH}{|}$$
$$\underset{CH_3}{|}$$

N-(methylamino)methylene
diphosphonate
(NMMDP)

$$NaO-\overset{\overset{O}{\|}}{P}-\overset{\overset{H}{|}}{C}-\overset{\overset{O}{\|}}{P}-ONa$$
$$\underset{HO}{|}\ \underset{N}{|}\ \underset{OH}{|}$$
$$\underset{CH_3}{}\ \underset{CH_3}{}$$

N,N-dimethylaminomethylene
diphosphonate
(DMAD)

$$NaO-\overset{\overset{O}{\|}}{P}-\overset{\overset{H}{|}}{C}-\overset{\overset{O}{\|}}{P}-ONa$$
$$\underset{HO}{|}\ \underset{CH_2}{|}\ \underset{OH}{|}$$
$$\underset{CH_2}{|}$$
$$\underset{NH_2}{|}$$

3-amino-1 hydroxypropane-
-1,1-diphosphonate
(APD)

$$NaO-\overset{\overset{O}{\|}}{P}-\overset{\overset{H}{|}}{C}-\overset{\overset{O}{\|}}{P}-ONa$$
$$\underset{HO}{|}\ \underset{HC-COOH}{|}\ \underset{OH}{|}$$
$$\underset{H_2C-COOH}{}$$

2,3-dicarboxypropane
-1,1-diphosphonate
(DPD)

Fig. 2-1. Structural formula of diphosphonates evaluated for possible use in bone scanning. Pyrophosphate (PP) is included for structural comparison.

incorporated with EDTMP (phosphonate analog of ethylene diamine tetra acetic acid [EDTA] described in the following material) for use as a palliative agent in patients with extensive skeletal metastases.[21] All these radiopharmaceuticals have been superseded by the introduction of Tc-99m agents described as follows.

Tc-99m LABELED BONE IMAGING AGENTS

Tc-99m—with its easy availability from Mo-99/Tc-99m generators in every nuclear medicine facility and excellent physical properties—is eminently suitable for any imaging study including the skeleton. In 1971 this possibility became a reality when Subramanian and McAfee[61] reported a new complex of Tc-99m using tripolyphosphate as a chelate. Phosphates in different chemical forms dominate the living world[81] and are ubiquitously present predominantly in the bone. When sodium tripolyphosphate was labeled with Tc-99m using stannous tin as a reductant for pertechnetate, a water-soluble phosphate chelate was formed and localized in the skeleton of experimental animals. This should have been anticipated because as long ago as 1961 Fleish and Neuman[15] reported that polyphosphates were potent inhibitors of both crystallization of calcium phosphate and dissolution of hydroxyapatite crystals in vitro. Also, Kaplan et al[29] demonstrated that P-32 labeled condensed phosphate (polyphosphate) initially localized in the metastasic lesions in the bone. Since then a variety of Tc-99m labeled phosphate containing compounds have been evaluated for possible use in skeletal imaging. These included (1) linear phosphates, (2) cyclic phosphates, (3) fluorophosphates, (4) beta glycerophosphate, (5) diphosphonates, (6) triphosphonates, and (7) tetraphosphonates. These phosphate compounds and methods for labeling them with Tc-99m are well described in the literature.* The chemical formulas for important compounds are shown

*References 4,12,45,47,62,63,65,66,68,75,79,82.

$$HO-\overset{\overset{O}{\|}}{\underset{\underset{HO}{|}}{P}}-O-\overset{\overset{O}{\|}}{\underset{\underset{OH}{|}}{P}}-OH$$

$$HO-\overset{\overset{O}{\|}}{\underset{\underset{HO}{|}}{P}}-\overset{\overset{H}{|}}{\underset{\underset{H}{|}}{C}}-\overset{\overset{O}{\|}}{\underset{\underset{OH}{|}}{P}}-OH$$

$$HO-\overset{\overset{O}{\|}}{\underset{\underset{HO}{|}}{P}}-\overset{\overset{H}{|}}{N}-\overset{\overset{O}{\|}}{\underset{\underset{OH}{|}}{P}}-OH$$

P — 1.63 Å — O (128.7°) — 1.63 Å — P 2.94 Å

P — 1.79 Å — C (117°) — 1.79 Å — P 3.05 Å

P — 1.68 Å — N (127.2°) — 1.68 Å — P 3.005 Å

Fig. 2-2. Structural formulas of pyrophosphate, methylene diphosphonate, and imido diphosphate are shown with their interatomic distances.

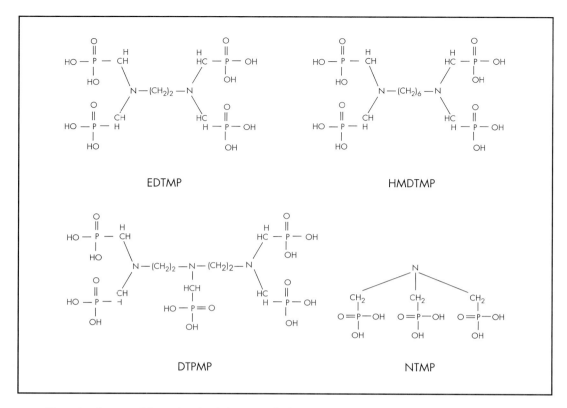

Fig. 2–3.   Structural formula of polyfunctional phosphonates suitable for labeling with Tc-99m and trivalent cations such as Sm-153, In-111. Typically they all contain P—C—N—C—P linkages. Note the similarity of EDTMP to EDTA and DTPMP to DTPA.

in Figs. 2-1 to 2-3. Basically all these agents can be classified into distinctive groups that have different structure in between the phosphorus atoms[12,62]: (1) P—O—P, (2) P—C—P, (3) P—C—C—P,[4] (4) P—N—P, and (5) P—C—N—C—P. The first is the polyphosphate group, the least member of which is pyrophosphate,[47] containing only two phosphorus atoms. The class of compounds having a carbon between the phosphorus atoms have the strongest chemical bonding.[4,45,75] The structural similarity of P—O—P, P—C—P and P—N—P compounds are shown in Fig. 2-2. This demonstrates that the interatomic distance between P—P bond is similar for all three compounds, which could account for their similarity in bone localization.

In Fig. 2-3, the structural formulas for polyfunctional phosphonates containing P—C—N—C—P structure are shown. These agents have been labeled with Tc-99m and also with trivalent cationic radionuclides In-113m, In-111, and Sm-153.[12,21,68] None of these agents are optimal for diagnostic imaging of the skeleton.

The phosphonate compounds shown in Fig. 2-1 have been labeled with Tc-99m, and the pure compounds were evaluated in experimental animals. The results of whole blood clearance of these agents in rabbits studied individually with Sr-85 as an internal control are shown in Fig. 2-4. The differences in blood clearances can be partly explained by the different degree of plasma protein binding of these agents. Also the rate of extraction

of these compounds by the skeleton may vary. Blood clearance studies in rabbits shown in Fig. 2-4 clearly demonstrate that Tc-99m DPD has the fastest blood clearance followed by HMDP (also known as HDP [hydroxy dimethyl pyrimidine]) and methylene diphosphate [MDP], the three most important bone imaging agents. It is worth noting that Tc-99m pyrophosphate readily diffuses into the red cells and presumably binds to the hemoglobin. This is the basis for the development of in vivo labeling of red cells using Tc-99m pyrophosphate.

Blood and urinary clearance studies of Tc-99m diphosphonates and phosphates were performed in human volunteers.[67] Blood clearance data in normal adult male volunteers up to 24 hours following intravenous injection are shown in Fig. 2-5. The same six volunteers were injected with three of the Tc-99m agents, and the polyphosphate data were obtained from 10 adults. The most rapid blood clearace was seen with MDP; its blood clearance curve up to 4 hours postinjection was identical with that of F-18.[38] The differences in blood clearance are probably due to the varying degree of transient plasma protein binding of these agents. The cumulative urinary clearance of the four Tc-99m agents are shown in Fig. 2-6. The urinary excretion (up to 24 hours) of the diphosphonates are similar. The F-18 excretion in the urine is lower than the phosphate compounds because the bone uptake of F-18 is considerably higher than

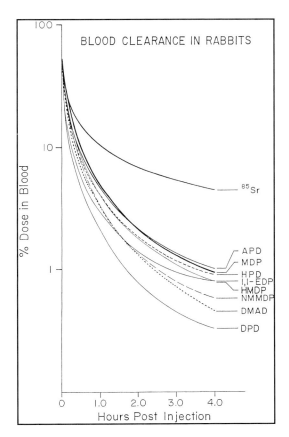

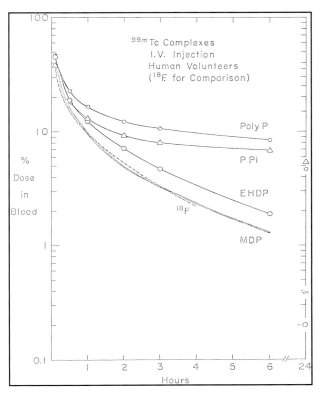

Fig. 2-4. Blood clearance of Tc-99m phosphonate complexes shown in Fig. 2-1. Each compound was studied in six animals. HPD refers to hydroxy propylene diphosphonate not shown in Fig. 2-1. (*Data from SUNY HSC files.*)

Fig. 2-5. Blood clearance of Tc-99m MDP in humans compared with three other Tc-99m complexes and F-18 (corrected for physical decay). Blood volume was assumed to be 7% of the body weight. PPi indicates pyrophosphate and PolyP denotes polyphosphate. (*From Subramanian G, McAfee JG, Blair RJ, et al: Technetium-99m methylene diphosphonate—a superior agent for skeletal imaging: Comparison with other technetium complexes. J Nucl Med 1975; 16:744; reprinted by permission of the Society of Nuclear Medicine.*)

other agents. The urinary excretion of Sr-85 is low because a major fraction of this radionuclide is excreted in the feces.

A number of comparative clinical evaluations of Tc-99m MDP, Tc-99m HMDP (HDP), and Tc-99m DPD have been reported.* Pauwels et al were among the first to perform comparative studies of these three agents in 20 patients with bone metastases. They concluded that lesion-to-normal-bone ratio in this patient group was significantly higher for MDP than for DPD. No other significant differences between the three radiopharmaceuticals were noted. Bergqvist et al [3] reported similar results in 24 patients, 12 each with prostatic and breast carcinoma. Godart et al[20] studied 20 patients with both MDP and DPD and concluded that Tc-99m MDP showed slightly better lesion-to-bone ratios in the group of patients with skeletal metastases. Lanto et al[32] also studied 12 patients with metastatic disease and concluded that there is no real practical difference between the above agents in detecting metastatic disease. They reported that in this small group of patients the metastatic-lesion-to-normal-bone concentration ratios for Tc-99m MDP and Tc-99m DPD ranged from 2.6 to 3.0, whereas the normal-bone-to-soft-tissue ratios were 8.5 to 9.5 for these agents. More

*References 3,7,8,20,30,32,34,37,38,44,50,52,58,67,69.

recently Kassamali et al[30] reported that bone-to-soft-tissue ratios decreased in elderly patients as a function of age, irrespective of which of the above three diphosphonates is used.

From these studies it can be stated that any one of the preceding three agents—MDP, HMDP, or DPD—can be used for skeletal imaging (DPD is not available in the United States). In normal patients it is known that initial Tc-99m MDP localization in the normal skeleton is lower than both DPD and HMDP (35% vs. 50% to 60%). The lesion localization of DPD and HMDP are also higher than that for MDP. Hence, the lesion-to-normal-bone ratio remains similar for all three agents at scanning time. The blood plasma clearance of DPD is faster than both MDP and HMDP, but this advantage is minimal when scanning is performed 2 to 3 hours after administration of the agents. Because MDP localizes less in the bone, its radiation dose to normal tissue is slightly lower than both DPD and HMDP. Nevertheless all three agents are quite suitable and acceptable for clinical use in skeletal imaging.

Rosenthall et al[52] compared Tc-99m DMAD and Tc-99m-MDP in patients and found that Tc-99m DMAD localized in bone lesions as well as MDP but its concentration in the normal skeleton was lower than MDP. This resulted in higher lesion-to-normal-bone ratios for DMAD, and a higher lesion detection rate than MPD in a clinical crossover study.

MECHANISM OF LOCALIZATION OF BONE IMAGING AGENTS

Bone is a heterogeneous calcified connective tissue consisting of about two-thirds mineral and one-third collagen, extracellular matrix, and a variety of bone-lining cells.[49] The mineral part of the bone is made up of amorphous calcium carbonate, calcium phosphate, and crystalline hydroxyapatite. The mineral phase functions as an amphoteric ion exchanger. The bone cells include (1) osteoblasts (bone-forming cells), (2) osteocytes (cells that have become surrounded by the mineralized matrix) and (3) osteoclasts (bone-resorbing cells). Of these cells it is the osteoblast, under the influence of local and systemic factors, that is primarily responsible for the synthesis of extracellular matrix—which later becomes mineralized during bone formation, remodeling, and focal turnover.[2] In disease states the function of osteoblasts is severely altered, and there is uncontrolled change of the mineralization process.[1] In bone imaging we attempt to "image" this change in osteoblastic and/or osteoclastic activity by using radiotracers that

localize in these sites of increased mineralization activity. A variety of physicochemical factors control the localization of bone-seeking radiopharmaceuticals. Reviews on this subject by Fogelman[17] and Pauwels[46] are available.

Skeletal uptake of bone-scanning radiopharmaceuticals depend on several important factors. These include (1) blood flow, (2) molecular size and net electric charge on the molecule, (3) metabolic process in the various parts of bone (i.e., kinetics of calcium, phosphate transfer), (4) increased bone surface area, (5) increased capillary permeability, and (6) local pH (enzyme concentration, alkaline and acid phosphatase). In discussing mechanisms of skeletal uptake we assume that the radiopharmaceutical is pure and in vivo breakdown in the vascular pool is minimal. However, polyphosphates (pyrophosphate) with their P—O—P linkages are subject to enzymatic hydrolysis. Pyrophosphate is known to break down into orthophosphate (P-32 studies) by this process. Diphosphonates with P—C—P linkages are very stable and resistive to hydrolysis by enzymes. The variations in blood clearance of these Tc-99m phosphate agents can be attributed to their relative plasma protein binding. In almost all cases the activity in the plasma 2 to 3 hours after intravenous administration is less than 2% of the injected dose. Therefore blood clearance differences of current Tc-99m agents are not significant. The least protein-bound bone-seeking radiopharmaceutical F-18 ion (sodium fluoride) is also small in size. Therefore F-18 fluoride is extracted by bone almost quantitatively. On the other hand, anionic complexes such as Tc-99m phosphate agents, rare earth chelates, are comparatively large in size and molecular configuration and therefore extracted by bone to a lesser extent than the F-18 fluoride ion. Since the introduction of Tc-99m bone agents, several studies have concentrated on the mechanism of their skeletal uptake. The major topics included (1) blood flow (vascularity), (2) uptake in mineral part of bone, (3) localization in the immature collagen, and (4) enzymatic influence. We examine these factors in the following sections.

Influence of Blood Flow

The radiopharmaceutical has to be delivered to the bone surface by vascular supply for the uptake to occur. In normal bone there is an increase in the bone uptake in areas of high blood flow. Knowledge about quantitative blood flow to various regions of a bone is very useful in diagnosing skeletal disesase.[9,10] Quantitation of blood flow is a problem in humans because it involves injection of nondiffusible tracers (microspheres) into arteries supplying blood to the bones. Several reports* have outlined different methods for measuring regional and local blood flow in both humans and animals. Okubu et al[41] measured blood flow in adult dogs using radioactive microspheres of 15 ± 5 µm labeled with both Sr-85 and Ce-141. They injected the microspheres suspended in 20% dex-

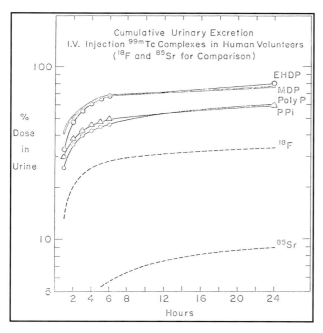

Fig. 2-6. Urinary excretion of Tc-99m MDP in humans compared with three other Tc-99m complexes, F-18, and Sr-85 (corrected for physical decay). PPi indicates pyrophosphate and PolyP denotes polyphosphate. *(From Subramanian G, McAfee JG, Blair RJ, et al: Technetium-99m methylene diphosphonate—a superior agent for skeletal imaging: Comparison with other technetium complexes. J Nucl Med 1975; 16:744; reprinted by permission of the Society of Nuclear Medicine.)*

*References 19,35,44,55,73,78.

tran into the femoral artery of the dog using a catheter and sampled the blood. The animals were then sacrificed and the whole femur and the tibia were assayed for radioactive content. The quantitative blood flow to various parts of both the femur and the tibia are shown in Table 2-2 and Fig. 2-7.

In normal bone the localization pattern of bone-seeking agents closely parallels the blood flow, but in abnormal bone this correlation may not exist. The results of several studies indicate that increased blood flow can get increased quantity of bone agents to the site but the actual uptake is controlled by local disease conditions. Even in Paget's disease the finding that local increase in blood flow results in increased lesion uptake can be disputed. After a study of several patients with Paget's disease, Heistad et al[23] concluded that the actual blood flow increase in Paget's disease areas does not necessarily mean the blood actually goes to the skeleton. They claimed that the increase in blood flow in pagetic extremities is primarily the result of cutaneous vasodilation. From these reports it can be said that blood flow to the bone lesions is an important factor in delivering the radiotracer to the bone, but local conditions and skeletal metabolism play a more important role in skeletal lesion uptake.[17,19]

Localization in the Mineral Phase of the Bone

The mineral phase of the bone functions as an amphoteric ion exchanger. Cations similar in ionic dimension to calcium (Sr, Ba) substitute for calcium ions in the physiochemical exchange at the solid-liquid interface between bone crystals and interstitial fluid and accumulate in the mineral phase. The anionic element F-18 fluoride, unlike cations, substitutes for hydroxyl or bicarbonate ions in the mineral phase. Other anionic species such as rare earth chelates (e.g., Sm-153 HEDTA, Sm-153 ENTMP) and Tc-99m phosphates and phosphonates are larger in ionic size and molecular configuration. Their extent of localization in bone lesions may also be controlled by the available capillary permeability at the interface of bone matrix and interstitial fluid. The exact kinetics of transfer may vary from compound to compound.

For Tc-99m labeled phosphates and phosphonates, it is well documented that these agents become adsorbed on the hydroxyapatite matrix of the bone. Experiments conducted both in vitro and in vivo confirmed this fact. The in vivo uptake may be associated with only newly forming bone. A variety of reports* substantiate this aspect of bone localization of Tc-99m agents. Gross autoradiographs of animal bones following intravenous administration of bone agents reveal a nonuniform distribution of radioactivity. In adult bones activity appears in a thin layer along the endosteum and periosteum and also in the spongiosa of the metaphysis. Only a very low diffused localization is present in the compact bone of the cortex. This concentration pattern parallels that of blood flow. In a growing animal a very high localized concentration appears at the metaphyseal ends of the long bones immediately adjacent to the epiphyseal cartilage. Most microautoradiograph studies suggest that diphosphonates localize in the mineral phase of bone at

*References 6,14,22,25,26,28,33,54,72,77.

TABLE 2-2
Blood Flow Rates through Various Regions of Rabbit Femur and Tibia*

Femur Samples	Blood Flow Rate (ml/min/100 g) Mean ± SE	n	Tibia Samples	Blood Flow Rate (ml/min/100 g) Mean ± SE	n
Head	11.5 ± 1.5	14	Proximal ephiphysis	10.6 ± 1.6	14
Neck	20.8 ± 2.4	14	Proximal metaphysis I	15.5 ± 3.2	12
Trochanter	9.9 ± 1.6	14	Proximal metaphysis II	14.4 ± 4.0	14
Proximal metaphysis I	19.3 ±2.6	14	Cortex	3.0 ± 0.8	14
Proximal metaphysis II	21.7 ± 2.6	14	Distal metaphysis	12.0 ± 3.9	14
Marrow	48.7 ± 8.2	12	Distal epiphysis	9.4 ± 2.2	11
Cortex	7.0 ± 1.1	14			
Distal metaphysis I	19.8 ± 2.7	14			
Distal metaphysis II	15.6 ± 2.1	14			
Condyle	8.9 ± 1.3	13			

From Okubo M, Kinoshita T, Yokimura T, et al: Experimental study of measurement of regional bone blood flow in the adult mongrel dog using radioactive micropsheres. *Clin Orthop Rel Res* 1978; 138:263; with permission.

*Please refer to Fig. 2-7 for the diagrammatic representation of sample sites.

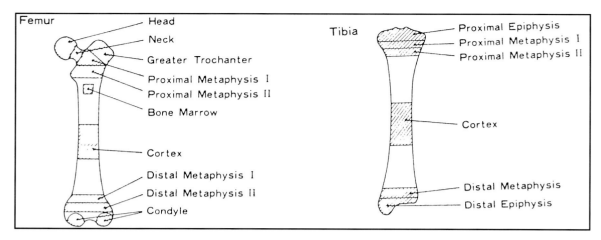

Fig. 2–7. Diagram of the tissue samples. Cortical bone in the middle third of the femur and the tibia were samples of compact bone alone without periosteal and endosteal tissue. Bone marrow was taken from the proximal metaphysis of the femur just below the lesser trochanter as a sample mainly composed of cancellous bone. Other samples were composed of both cancellous and compact bone. *(From Okubo M, Kinoshita T, Yokimura T, et al: Experimental study of measurement of regional bone blood flow in the adult mongrel dog using radioactive microspheres.* Clin Orthop Rel Res *1978; 138:263; with permission.)*

active sites of bone formation or resorption, particularly at the osteoid mineral interfaces. Einhorn et al[14] performed microautoradiography of specimens of normal bone and bone reparative tissue of rabbits. Rabbits underwent operations in which two 1.5-mm drill holes were created in the femur. Seven days after surgery, the operated animals and normal animals were injected with Tc-99m MDP and sacrificed at 2 hours postinjection. Samples from normal and abnormal bones were studied by microautoradiography. Some of their results are shown in Figs. 2-8 and 2-9. These results demonstrate that Tc-99m localized along the mineralization fronts. Also osteocytic lacunae showed the presence of Tc-99m at their borders. The isotope was occasionally found in the substance of the osteoid but was absent from the cytoplasm and nuclei of the osteoblasts and osteocytes. In more recent in vitro experiments Kanishi[28] used fetal mice calvaria, osteoblast-like cells, collagen sponges, and hydroxyapatite powder to study the Tc-99m MDP accumulation mechanisms in bone. He concluded that Tc-99m MDP accumulation in bone is due to both chemisorption of the diphosphonate onto the surface of the hydroxyapatite and incorporation into the crystalline structure of hydroxyapatite. No uptake in the collagen sponges was observed in these in vitro tests.

The binding sites for diphosphonates on the mineral matrix of the bone can be saturated by administration of large quantities of diphosphonates. Hommeyer et al[25] performed a Tc-99m MDP bone scan in a 65-year-old patient who underwent ethane-1-hydroxy-1,1-diphosphate [EHDP] (cold) therapy for acute hypercalcemia associated with metastatic disease. The patient received an intravenous infusion of 500 mg of EHDP over 12 to 36 hours before bone scanning, and there was no visible skeletal uptake of Tc-99m MDP on the scan. This result also augments the theory that diphosphonates act as carriers for the Tc-99m isotope for its localization in the

bone, and the reduced technetium has to compete for the same sites on the bones as the diphosphonates. Lausten and Christensen[33] performed autoradiographic studies to determine the distribution of Tc-99m MDP in nontraumatic necrotic femoral heads and compared that with the histology of the similar adjacent segment. The highest uptake was seen at the provisional calcification areas with enchondral ossification in the demarcation zone. The uneven distribution of Tc-99m was found to be mainly due to the remodeling process. This study also demonstrated that Tc-99m bone agents localized in the mineral phase of bone and was a major part of the mechanism of localization.

Localization in the Immature Collagen

In 1973 Tilden et al[70] reported that Tc-99m polyphosphate localized in areas of bone which appeared more immature than the surrounding bone. Rosenthall and colleagues[31,51,80] reported similar findings. In an experiment using P-32 pyrophosphate, C-14 diphosphonate and Tc-99m labeled polyphosphate, pyrophosphate and EHDP in rats with induced rickets, they demonstrated that Tc-99m compounds localized in both inorganic and organic matrices (collagen), whereas the P-32 and C-14 activity was associated with only the mineral phase. Weigman et al[80] found that bone uptake of Tc-99m pyrophosphate was related to hydroxyproline concentration in blood and urine of uremic patients. In hyperparathyroidism the increased localization of bone agents may be related to excess of immature collagen characteristic of osteomalacia.[51,80] Also de Groeff et al[13] reported that in uremic patients with renal osteodystrophy, the defective mineralization results in increased quantities of immature collagen and amorphous calcium phosphate, thus indicating the possibility that Tc-99m diphosphonates may localize in immature collagen.

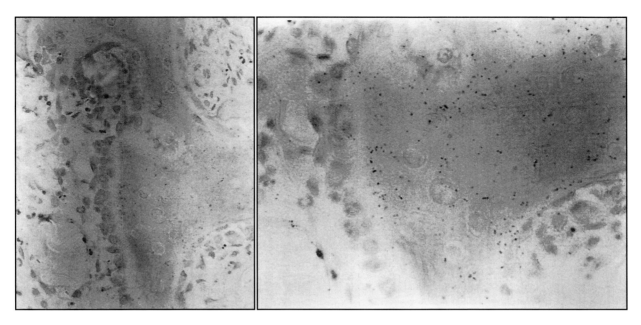

Fig. 2-8. *Left,* Microautoradiograph shows the location of Tc-99m MDP in a bone spicule from reparative callus. The surfaces are lined by osteoblasts that are actively producing osteoid. Note that exposed silver grains are located along the mineralization front and are conspicuously absent from the marrow. Silver grains are not seen with any consistency in either the osteoblasts or in osteoid. (Magnification X160.) *Right,* Higher-power microautoradiograph of the bone spicule shown on left. (Magnification X320.) *(From Einhorn TA, Vigorita VJ, Aairon A: Localization of technetium-99m methylene diphosphonate in bone using microautoradiography.* J Orthop Res *1986; 4:180; with permission.)*

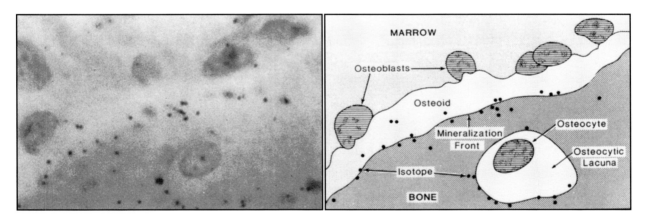

Fig. 2-9. *Left,* High-power microautoradiograph showing localization of Tc-99m MDP to the mineralization front of bone as well as to the border of an osteocytic lacuna. This indicates the uptake of isotope at the osteoid mineralized bone interface. (Magnification X512.) *Right,* Schematic representation of the histology viewed in the microautoradiograph shown on the left. *(From Einhorn TA, Vigorita VJ, Aairon A: Localization of technetium-99m methylene diphosphonate in bone using microautoradiography.* J Orthop Res *1986; 4:180; with permission.)*

Uptake by Enzymatic Inhibition

There is some evidence presented in the literature that the localization of Tc-99m bone seekers may also depend on enzymes (alkaline, acid phosphatases) present at abnormal sites of the skeleton. Zimmer et al[83] reported that EHDP (labeled with Tc-99m or by itself) inactivates alkaline and acid phosphatases. By this mechanism Tc-99m EHDP is localized at sites of increased enzyme concentration. Also acid phosphatases in metastatic lesions impart locally lower pH levels (6.8 to 7.0). Whether this decreased pH in lesions containing acid phosphatases plays any role in increased bone uptake is not yet known. Fogelman[17] disputes this finding, attesting that in Paget's disease, when the serum levels of both acid and alkaline phosphatase are very high, the blood clearance of Tc-99m agents is not altered.[26] Therefore it is highly unlikely that phosphatase enzymes have any substantial role in bone uptake of Tc-99m agents.

In summary, the localization of Tc-99m bone imaging agents is definitely related to blood flow in normal bone. In the abnormal skeleton, newly forming (remodeling) bone absorbs these agents and eventually mineralizes them. Since the formation of hydroxyapatite and collagen are closely related, both the newly forming inorganic matrix and the immature collagen may play substantial roles in trapping Tc-99m bone imaging agents. (See Chapter 9.)

PHYSICOCHEMICAL PROPERTIES OF Tc-99m LABELED DIPHOSPHONATES

Tc-99m—with a short half-life of 6 hours and 140-keV gamma energy with 90% external photon yield—is ideally suitable for bone scanning. It is easily available from a Mo-99/Tc-99m generator and eluted as pertechnetate ion $^{99m}TcO_4^-$. Tc-99m pertechnetate may contain undesirable impurities such as oxidizing agents (from Mo-99 solution and locally produced in the generator column due to intense radiation) and too much Tc-99 from the decay of Tc-99m. These two impurities in Tc-99m pertechnetate may interfere with the preparation of any Tc-99m labeled compounds including bone agents. Typically any Tc-99m labeled bone imaging agent may contain the following impurities: (1) free pertechnetate, (2) colloids, and (3) hydrolyzed and reduced technetium. Therefore quality control of each preparation is important. Instant thin-layer chromatography (ITLC) is used for these quality-control tests. Gelman ITLC SG medium and saline eluant are used to separate colloids and hydrolyzed Tc-99m from Tc-99m bone agents. Whatman No. 1 paper and acetone or 85% methanol can be used for separating pertechnetate from all other components. Typically the Tc-99m bone agent has a purity of greater than 95% at the time of use. The shelf life of Tc-99m labeled bone agents after labeling can be as long as 6 hours. Bone imaging agents are usually available as freeze-dried kits (10-ml vial with 5 to 25 mg of diphosphonate and 100 µg to 1.0 mg $SnCl_2$ $2H_2O$) containing stabilizing agents (antioxidants—e.g., ascorbic acid or gentisic acid). These reducing agents prevent oxidation of stannous tin in the preparation and protect against oxidation due to the presence of air into the multidose vial. Care should be taken not to inject too much air into the multidose vial containing Tc-99m labeled bone agents during withdrawal of individual doses. A single kit vial can be used to label up to 500 mCi of technetium-99m.

The chemistry as applied to the skeletal imaging agent is rather complex and is not well understood. Tc-99m in pertechnetate ion has to be reduced from its +7 valence state to +4 valency by stannous tin ion. This reaction is instantaneous, and the reduced Tc-99m ion in +4 state complexes with the phosphate or phosphonate. Published reports confirm this labeling mechanism.[53,71]

Russell and Cash[53] state that at physiologic pH, the Tc-99m in Tc-99m bone agents is in the +4 valence state and at slightly alkaline pH +5 valence state is predominant. Because the diphosphonates have an open structure, many investigators believe that Tc-99m diphosphonates contain at least two molecules of diphosphonates to one atom of Tc-99m (polynuclear complex). These molecular configurations can influence in vivo protein binding.

The acute intravenous toxicity of diphosphonates is relatively low. The LD_{50} for EHDP and MDP in rodents is similar (45 to 50 mg/kg).[67] Because of their low toxicity and their avidity to the bone, several diphosphonates are now being proposed for therapeutic purposes for the treatment of osteoporosis.[48,56] Over the past 20 years several hundreds of thousands of bone scans have been performed worldwide, and the current Tc-99m labeled agents are considered very safe from a chemical toxicity point of view.

The sensitivity of bone scanning is outstanding with the current Tc-99m phosphonates. Even though the specificity of these bone imaging agents is low, it is unlikely any new bone imaging agents will be developed in the near fututre to improve specificity without considerable research and development.

REFERENCES

1. Anderson HC: Biology of disease: Mechanism of mineral formation in bone. *Lab Invest* 1989; 60:320.
2. Barres DM: Clsoe encounters with an osteoclast. *Science* 1987; 236:914.
3. Bergqvist L, Brismar J, Cederquist E, et al: Clinical comparison of bone scintigraphy with Tc-99m DPD, Tc-99m HDP and Tc-99m MDP. *Acta Radiol* 1984; 25:217.
4. Bevan JA, Tofe AJ, Benedict JJ, et al: Tc-99m HMDP (Hydroxymethylene phosphonate): A new radiopharmaceutical for skeletal and acute myocardial imaging. II— Comparison of Tc-99m HMDP with other technetium labeled bone imaging agents in a canine model. *J Nucl Med* 1980; 21:967.
5. Blau M, Nagler W, Bender MA: Fluorine-18: A new isotope for bone scanning. *J Nucl Med* 1962; 3:332.
6. Budd RS, Hodgson GS, Hare WSC, et al: The relation of radionuclide uptake by bone to the rate of calcium mineralization. I—Experimental studies using Ca-45, P-32 and Tc-99m MDP. *Br J Radiol* 1989; 62:314.
7. Buell U, Kirsch CM, Kleinhans E, Jager B: Comparison of Tc-99m MDP, HMDP and DPD with respect to bone to soft tissue ratios. *J Nucl Med* 1983; 24:1201.
8. Buell U, Kleinhand E, Zork-Bopp E, et al: A comparison of bone imaging with Tc-99m DPD and Tc-99m MDP: Concise communication. *J Nucl Med* 1982; 23:214.
9. Charkes ND: Mechanisms of skeletal tracer uptake. *J Nucl Med* 1979; 20:794.
10. Charkes ND: Skeletal blood flow: Implication for bone scan interpretation. *J Nucl Med* 1980; 21:91.
11. Chiecwitz O, Hevesy G: Radioactive indicators in the study of phosphorus metabolism in rats. *Nature* 1935; 136:754.
12. Davis MA, Jones AG: Comparison of Tc-99m labeled phosphate and phosponate agents for skeletal imaging. *Semin Nucl Med* 1976; 6:9.
13. De Groeff P, Te Velde J, Pauwels EKJ, et al: Increased bone tracer uptake in renal osteodystrophy. *Eur J Nucl Med* 1980;

14. Einhorn TA, Vigorita VJ, Aairon A: Localization of technetium-99m methylene diphosphonate in bone using microautoradiography. *J Orthop Res* 1986; 4:180.

15. Fleish H, Neuman WF: Mechanisms of calcification: Role of collagen polyphosphates and phosphatase. *Am J Physiol* 1961; 200:1296.

16. Fleming WH, McIraith JD, King ER: Photoscanning of bone lesions utilizing strontium-85. *Radiology* 1961; 77:635.

17. Fogelman I. Skeletal uptake of diphosphonate: A review. *Eur J Nucl Med* 1980; 5:473.

18. Freeman LM, and Blaufox M (eds): Radionuclide studies of the osseons structures. *Semin Nucl Med* 1972; 3:1.

19. Genant HK, Bautovich GJ, Singh M, et al: Bone seeking radionuclides: An in vivo study of factors affecting skeletal uptake. *Radiology* 1974; 113:373.

20. Godart G, Durez M, Bevilacqua M: Technetium-99m MDP vs. technetium-99m dicarboxy propane disphosphonate: A clinical comparison in various pathologic conditions. *Clin Nucl Med* 1982; 11:92.

21. Goeckler WF, Edwards B, Volkert WA, et al: Skeletal localization of Sm-153 chelates: Potential therapeutic bone agents. *J Nucl Med* 1987; 28:495.

22. Guillemart A, Besnard JC, Le Pape A, et al: Skeletal uptake of pyrophosphate labled with Technetium-95m and Technetium 96, as evaluated by autoradiography.

23. Heistad DD, Abboud FM, Schmid PG, et al: Regulation of blood flow in Paget's disease of bone. *J Clin Invest* 1975; 55:69.

24. Hommeyer SH, Varney DM, Early JF: Skeletal nonvisualization in a bone scan secondary to intravenous etidronate therapy. *J Nucl Med* 1992; 35:748.

25. Hommeyer SH, Varney DM, Feary J: Skeletal nonvisualization in a bone scan secondary to intravenous etidronate therapy. *J Nucl Med* 1992; 33:749.

26. Jones AG, Francis MD, Davis MA: Bone scanning: Radionuclide reaction mechanisms. *Semin Nucl Med* 1976; 6:3.

27. Jowsey J, Rowland RE, Marshall JH, et al: The deposition of the rare earths in bone radiation research. 1958; 8:490.

28. Kanishi D: Tc-99m MDP accumulation mechanism in bone. *Oral Surg Oral Med Oral Pathol* 1993; 75:239.

29. Kaplan E, Gordon I, Kotlowski BR, et al: Therapy of carcinoma of the prostate metastatic to bone with P-32 labeled condensed phosphate. *J Nucl Med* 1960; 1:1.

30. Kassamali H, Hosain F, Spencer RP, et al: Nuclear medicine studies of aging VIII. Bone to soft tissue ratio of Tc-99m labeled MDP and HMDP vs. age. *Int J Radiat Appl Instrum B* 1989; 16:473.

31. Kaye M, Silverton S, Rosenthall L: Technetium-99m pyrophosphate: Studies in vivo and in vitro. *J Nucl Med* 1975; 16:40.

32. Lanto T, Vorne M, Mokka R, et al: Tc-99m MDP and Tc-99m DPD in pathological bone lesions. A visual and quantitative comparison. *Acta Radiol* 1987; 28:631.

33. Lausten GS, Christensen S: Distribution of 99m-Tc-phosphate compounds in osteonecrotic femoral heads. *Acta Orthop Scand* 1989; 60:49.

34. Littlefield JL, Rudd TG: Tc-99m hydroxymethylene diphosphonate and Tc-99m methylene diphosphonate: Biological and clinical comparison: Concise communication. *J Nucl Med* 1983; 24:463.

35. McElfresh EC, Kelly PJ: Simultaneous determination of blood flow in cortical bone, marrow, and muscle in canine hind leg by femoral artery catheterization. *Calcit Tissue Res* 1974; 14:301.

36. Meckelnburgh RL: Clinical value of generator produced Sr-87m. *J Nucl Med* 1964; 5:929.

37. Mele M, Conte E, Fratello A: Computer analysis of Tc-99m DPD and Tc-99m MDP kinetics in human: Concise communication. *J Nucl Med* 1983; 24:334.

38. Moon NK, Dworkin HJ, La Fleuer PD: The clinical use of sodium fluoride F-18 in bone photoscanning. *JAMA* 1968; 204:974.

39. Myers WG: Radiostrontium 87-m. *J Nucl Med* 1960; 1:124 (abstract).

40. Newman WF, Newman MW: The nature of the mineral phase of the bone. *Chem Rev* 1953; 53:1.

41. Okubo M, Kinoshita T, Yokimura T, et al: Experimental study of measurement of regional bone blood flow in the adult mongrel dog using radioactive microspheres. *Clin Orthop Rel Res* 1978; 138:263.

42. O'Mara RE, McAfee JG, Subramanian G: Rare earth nuclides as potential agents for skeletal imaging. *J Nucl Med* 1969; 10:49.

43. O'Mara RE, Subramanian G: Experimental agents for skeletal imaging. *Semin Nucl Med* 1972; 2:38.

44. Pauwels EKJ, Blom J, Camps JAJ, et al: Comparison between the diagnostic efficacy of 99mTc-MDP, 99mTc-DPD and 99mTc-HDP for the detection of bone metastases. *Eur J Nucl Med* 1983; 8:118.

45. Pauwels EKJ, Camps JAJ, Blom J, et al: Clinical evaluation of a technetium-99m bone imaging agent based on the vicinal diphosphonate 1,2-diphosphonoethylene glycol (DPEG). *Nucl Med Commun* 1985; 6:739.

46. Pauwels EKJ: Radiopharmacology of bone seeking radiopharmaceuticals and scintigraphic imaging techniques. In EKJ Pauwels, HH Schutte, WK Taconis (eds): *Bone Scintigraphy.* Leiden University Press, 1981, p 3.

47. Peres R, Cohen Y, Henry R, et al: A new radiopharmaceutical for Tc-99m bone scanning.

48. Regisuster SY, DeRoisy R, Denis D, et al: Prevention of postmenopausal bone loss by tiludronate. *Lancet* 1989; 1469.

49. Robey PG: The biochemistry of bone. *Endocrinol Metab Clin North Am* 1989; 18:859.

50. Rosenthall L, Arzoumanian A, Damtew B, et al: A crossover study of Tc-99m labeled HMDP and MDP in patients. *Clin Nuc Med* 1981; 6:353.

51. Rosenthall L, Kaye M: Observations on the mechanism of Tc-99m labeled phosphate complex uptake in metabolic bone disease. *Semin Nucl Med* 1976; 6:59.

52. Rosenthall L, Stern J, Arzoumanian A: A clinical comparison of MDP and DMAD. *Clin Nucl Med* 1982; 7:403.

53. Russel CD, Cash AG: Oxidation state of technetium in bone scanning agents as determined at carrier concentration by amperometric titration. *Int J Appl Radiat Isotop* 1975; 30:485.

54. Schumichen C, Rempfle H, Wagner M, et al: The short-term fixation of radiopharmaceuticals in bone. *Eur J Nucl Med* 1979; 4:423.

55. Shim SS, Coff DH, Patterson FP: An indirect method of bone blood flow measurement based on the bone clearance of a circulating bone seeking radioisotope. *J Bone Joint Surg Am* 1967; 49a:693.

56. Shinoda H, Adamek G, Felix R, et al: Structure activity relationship of various bisphosphonates. *Calcif Tissue Int* 1983; 35:87.

57. Sietsema WK, Ebetino FA, Salvagno AM, et al: Antiresorptive dose response relationships across three generations of biphosphonates. *Drugs Exp Clin Res* 1989; XV:389.

58. Simon TR, Carrasquillo JA, Fejka R, et al: A clinical comparison of bone imaging agents. *Int J Radiat Appl Instrum B* 1990; 17:793.

59. Spencer RP, Lange RC, Treves S: Ba-131: An intermediate lived radionuclide for bone scanning. *J Nucl Med* 1970; 11:95.

60. Subramanian G: Ba-135m: Preliminary evaluation of a new radionuclide for skeletal imaging. *J Nucl Med* 1970; 1:649.

61. Subramanian G, McAfee JG: A new complex of Tc-99m for skeletal imaging. *Radiology* 1971; 99:192.

62. Subramanian G, McAfee JG, et al: Radiopharmaceuticals for bone and bone marrow imaging. *Proceedings: IAEA International Symposium on Medical Radionuclide Imaging*, Los Angeles, 2:83, 1977.

63. Subramanian G, McAfee JG, Bell EG, et al: Tc-99m labeled polyphosphate as a skeletal imaging agent. *Radiology* 1972; 102:701.

64. Subramanian G, McAfee JG, Blair RJ, et al: Dysprosium-157 HEDTA for skeletal imaging. *J Nucl Med* 1971; 12:558.

65. Subramanian G, McAfee JG, Blair RJ, et al: Tc-99m EHDP: A potential radiopharmaceutical for skeletal imaging. *J Nucl Med* 1971; 13:947.

66. Subramanian G, McAfee JG, Blair RJ, et al: Tc-99m labeled stannous imidodiphosphate: A new radiodiagnostic agent for bone scanning: Comparison with other Tc-99m complexes. *J Nucl Med* 1975; 16:1137.

67. Subramanian G, McAfee JG, Blair RJ, et al: Technetium-99m methylene diphosphonate: A superior agent for skeletal imaging: Comparison with other technetium complexes. *J Nucl Med* 1975; 16:744.

68. Subramanian G, McAfee JG, Rosensteich M, et al: Indium-113m-labeled polyfunctional phosphonates as bone imaging agents. *J Nucl Med* 1975; 16:1080.

69. Subramanian G, McAfee JG, Thomas FD, et al: New diphosphonate complexes for skeletal imaging: Comparison with methylene diphosphonate. *Radiology* 1983; 149:823.

70. Tilden RL, Jackson J, Ennecking WF, et al: Tc-99m polyphosphate: Histological localization in human femurs by autoradiography. *J Nucl Med* 1973; 14:576.

71. Tji TG, Vink HA, Gelsema WJ, et al: Determination of the oxidation state of Tc in Tc-99(Sn)EHDP, Tc-99 Sn MDP and Tc-99m(Sn) MDP complexes: Characterization of Tc (III), Tc (IV) and Tc (V) EHDP complexes. *Int J Radiat Appl Instrum A* 1990; 41:17.

72. Tote AJ, Francis MD: Optimization of the ratio of stannous tin: Ethane 1-hydroxy-1,1-diphosphonate for bone scanning with Tc-99m pertechnetate. *J Nucl Med* 1974; 15:69.

73. Tothill P: Bone blood flow measurement: Review. *J Biomed Eng* 1984; 6:251.

74. Treadwell A, Low-Beer VL, et al: Metabolic studies on neoplasm of bone with the aid of radioactive strontium. *Am J Med Sci* 1942; 204:521.

75. Unterspann S: Experimental examination on the suitability of organo-amino-methane-*bis*-phosphonic acids for bone scintigraphy by means of Tc-99m in animals. *Eur J Nucl Med* 1976; 1:151.

76. USAEC Report ORINS. 1956; 12:171.

77. Van Langerelde A, Driessen OMJ, Pauwels EKJ, et al: Aspects of Tc-99m binding from an ethane-1-hydroxy-1,1-diphosphonate Tc-99m complex to bone. *Eur J Nucl Med* 1977; 2:47.

78. Vattimo A, Martini G, Pisani M: Bone uptake of Tc-99m MDP in man: Its relationship with local blood flow. *J Nucl Med Allied Sci* 1982; 26:173.

79. Wang TST, Hosain P, Spencer RP, et al: Synthesis, radio technetium labeling and comparison of biologic behaviour of longer-chained analogs of methylene diphosphonate. *J Nucl Med* 1978; 19:1151.

80. Weigman T, Rosenthall L, Kaye M: Technetium-99m pyrophosphate bone scans in hyperparathyroidism. *J Nucl Med* 1977; 18:231.

81. Westheimer FH: Why nature chose phosphates. *Science* 1987; 235:1173.

82. Yano Y, McRae J, VanDyke DC, et al: Tc-99m labeled stannous ethane 1-hydroxy-1,1-diphosphonate: A new bone scanning agent. *J Nucl Med* 1973; 14:73.

83. Zimmer AM, Isitman AT, Holmes RA: Enzymatic inhibition of diphosphonate: A proposed mechanism of tissue uptake. *J Nucl Med* 1975; 16:352.

IN THIS CHAPTER

CHAPTER 3

NORMAL PLANAR BONE SCAN

Douglas F. Eggli

Mark Tulchinsky

Bone imaging is one of the most versatile and time-proven nuclear medicine procedures. It comprises the largest single segment of many clinical practices, accounting for as much as a quarter to a third of studies performed in a typical clinical practice. Bone imaging is also one of the oldest imaging procedures performed in nuclear medicine, dating back to the early 1960s. Despite the evolution of imaging technology over the last 30 years, bone imaging remains a cornerstone of nuclear medicine practice. Accurate interpretation of this important examination requires a thorough understanding of the normal planar bone scan.

BONE ANATOMY AND PHYSIOLOGY

The skeleton is a dynamic active organ system that is undergoing continuous change in response to environmental demands. Inorganic hydroxyapatite crystals composed of calcium salts are deposited on an organic matrix that is composed primarily of collagen and mucopolysaccharides. Bone is approximately 65% mineral, 35% organic matrix, and less than 1% cellular elements. Approximately 90% of the organic matrix is made up of collagen fibers. Bone mineral exists in a state of equilibrium with plasma, exchanging freely and rapidly between compartments. The skeleton is a critical component of normal calcium balance, containing 99% of the body's calcium reserves. At least 70% of the plasma calcium concentration is maintained by exchange with the skeleton.[33] Normal bone health depends on the balance between resorption of bone and the deposition of bone. Bone continuously repairs and strengthens itself.

Bone has an outer compact surface (cortical bone) and an inner spongy trabecular structure (cancellous bone). The spaces between the trabeculae are filled with bone marrow and fat. This architecture results in a bone structure that is both lightweight and strong. The trabecular pattern is not random but responds to gravity, stress, and weight-bearing activities. The trabeculae are oriented along lines of stress to provide maximum strength. When osteoporosis is present, the critical structural trabeculae are preserved at the expense of non–weight-bearing trabeculae. Bone is surrounded by a thick fibrous sheath, the periosteum. Arterioles and capillaries originating in the periosteum penetrate the bone and enter the Haversian system and the medullary spaces. Along with the infrequent nutrient artery, the periosteum provides the major vascular supply to bone. In addition to its nutrient function, the periosteum also participates in bone formation. The periosteum contains an inner layer of osteogenic cells. In infants and children the periosteum has two distinct layers, is thicker, and is more loosely attached. As bone matures, the periosteum thins, the cell layers merge, and the periosteum becomes firmly adherent to bone. Although a distinct endosteal membrane exists in the fetus, it disappears with time. There is no distinct endosteal tissue layer in the mature bone.

On a cellular level there are five types of bone cells: osteoprogenitor cells, osteoblasts, osteocytes, osteoclasts, and bone-lining cells.[33,36] Osteoprogenitor cells are the undifferentiated stromal cells that can become osteoblasts when stimulated. They are spindle-shaped cells with oval nuclei and minimal cytoplasm, located at the surface of bone. They are found in abundance in growing or repairing bone. Osteoblasts are the bone-forming elements. They lay down the collagen and mucopolysaccharide matrix of bone. Osteoblasts decrease in both size and number at skeletal maturity. Osteoblasts become osteocytes when they are trapped and isolated by the expanding bone matrix, which they produce. The osteocyte is a mature cell that has lost the capacity to divide. An osteocyte can perform both resorptive and synthetic functions but only on a limited basis. It can only perform these activities locally within its own structural unit, the lamella. Its primary function is to perform matrix maintenance activities. Osteoclasts are multinucleated giant cells that resorb bone. They are derived from a hematopoietic stem cell, rather than a cell of bone origin. Hematopoietic stem cells are also the precursors of the monocyte cell line. Blood monocytes also have bone resorptive capability.[6] They have the same organelles and enzyme systems as osteoclasts and additionally secrete an osteoclastic stimulating factor. Bone resorption by-products are chemotactic for monocytes. Osteoclasts are known to secrete lytic enzymes. Osteoclastic villi also secrete acids, including lactic acid and citric acid, which are released from mitochondria. The secreted acids dissolve the inorganic calcium salts.[15] The cellular process of bone resorption is not fully understood and has to some extent been inferred from anatomic specimens. The crystalline component of bone has to be dissolved before the matrix can be enzymatically digested. Bone-lining cells line the surface of mature bone. Their actual function is unclear, but morphologically they resemble inactive osteoblasts and are thought to be the equivalent of osteoprogenitor cells in mature bone. They appear to be involved in the maintenance and nutrition of embedded osteocytes. Cytoplasmic projections from bone-lining cells extend into canalicular channels and communicate with cytoplasmic processes of nearby osteocytes.[36]

Normally bone metabolism and remodeling is a balanced process, with matching amounts of bone being resorbed and laid down. Physiologic processes that either stimulate or suppress metabolic activity in bone usually affect both resorption and accretion equally. The process of bone remodeling, the resorption followed by formation of new bone, occurs on the surface of bone. The trabecular component of bone comprises about 20% of bone by volume but has about 60% of the surface area.[33] Because cancellous or trabecular bone has the largest surface area, that is where the largest changes occur. During the resorptive process, bone crystal is first dissolved and then collagen is broken down by osteoclastic collagenase enzyme. The reverse process occurs during bone apposition. First the organic matrix is synthesized by osteoblasts, then mineralization follows.

Collagen fibers are organized in an overlapping pattern that creates holes or gaps in the matrix. These gaps are the earliest sites of hydroxyapatite crystal deposition. Local tissue factors promote crystal deposition and growth on the matrix. The osteoblast is the primary source of these local factors. It provides a locally increased pH and, by the production of alkaline phosphatase, provides an increased phosphate ion concentration. These effects combine to reduce the solubility of calcium salts and favor crystallization.

Creation of bone matrix and its mineralization does not occur simultaneously. Through a complex process the matrix must be modified in preparation for mineralization.[20] The process takes about 10 days and creates the osteoid seam seen microscopically. The seam represents the time gap between matrix production and mineralization.

Newly deposited bone is not in its final form. Cortical bone is subsequently remodeled into osteons, which are comprised of the concentric lamella of a Haversian system. The osteons strengthen bone by creating a twisted cable effect so that the bone has a synergistic strength greater than its individual fibers. The mechanics are analogous to the increased strength of a steel cable composed of twisted steel fibers compared with a steel rod of the same diameter. In the medullary space, trabecular bone is reinforced along lines of stress, while non–weight-bearing trabeculae are eliminated.

Bone remodeling is a complex process regulated both locally and systemically. Parathyroid hormone (PTH), 1,25-dihydroxycholecalciferol (active form of vitamin D_3), and to a lesser extent, calcitonin, play active roles in this process. PTH enhances calcium mobilization from the skeleton by stimulating both osteoclastic and osteocytic bone resorption. PTH has a biphasic effect on osteoblasts, initially decreasing osteoblastic activity and causing cells to retract and decrease in size. This exposes bone surface for osteoclastic resorption. A delayed PTH effect stimulates osteoblastic bone formation at about the same time that the kidney and gut effects have made more calcium available for bone formation.

Vitamin D acts directly on osteoblasts, which have vitamin D receptors. It stimulates the synthesis of a critical matrix protein containing gamma-carboxyglutamic acid, stimulates bone-specific alkaline phosphatase release, and stimulates collagen synthesis. Vitamin D may also be involved in the process of osteoblast maturation. On the balancing side, vitamin D stimulates bone resorption through its effect on blood monocytes.

The role of calcitonin in the maintenance of calcium homeostasis is less well defined. It inhibits bone resorption and promotes bone growth. Calcitonin has no direct effect on the osteoblast but rather reduces bone resorption by deactivating osteoclasts. It also interferes with calcium migration from bone to interstitial fluid.

PHYSIOLOGY OF NORMAL BONE IMAGING

Bone physiology and radiopharmaceuticals for bone imaging are often mentioned in this textbook. To the reader particularly interested in these topics, Chapters 2 and 9 will be useful.

Two radiopharmaceuticals are currently approved by the United States Food and Drug Administration (FDA) for bone imaging. Both are organophosphate compounds chelated to technetium-99m, technetium-99m-hydroxymethylene diphosphonate (HDP or HMDP), and technetium-99m-methylene diphosphonate (MDP). At 3 and 4 hours after injection, HDP (also known as oxidronate) has slightly better blood clearance.[3] For HDP, blood level is approximately 10% of injected dose at 1 hour and falls to 3% by 4 hours after injection. Skeletal retention is approximately 50% at 24 hours.[8] HDP also demonstrates approximately 20% higher bone uptake than MDP (also known as medronate).[11] Clinically both radiopharmaceuticals behave in a similar fashion and produce similar quality studies. The physician interpreting the study would not be able to determine which radiopharmaceutical was used.[26,35,40]

Radiopharmaceutical localization in bone depends on both blood flow and metabolic activity. The radiopharmaceutical distributes rapidly in extracellular water. It must be able to diffuse from blood to the bone surface. As blood flow to bone increases, so does the uptake of diphosphonate compounds. At low levels of incremental blood flow, the process is linear but falls off as blood flow increases to several multiples of baseline. This suggests that radiopharmaceutical uptake is diffusion limited at high blood flow.[21] As a general rule, hyperemia causes increased bone uptake.

For bone lesions to be seen as different from normal bone, the radiopharmaceutical must have a higher affinity for sites of abnormal bone than for normal bone. This appears to be related to the deposition of amorphous calcium phosphate at sites of bone pathology.[12,13] The diphosphonates have a higher binding affinity for amorphous calcium phosphate than for calcium in the normal hydroxyapatite crystal. Bone accumulation occurs by the process of chemisorption. The process is poorly understood and is probably related to electrostatic attraction to the crystalline matrix of bone. The soft tissues are cleared by renal excretion.

Bone imaging is typically performed when background is adequately cleared to permit bone visualization, but before radioactive decay has significantly reduced radioactivity in bone. Peak activity is present in bone about 1 hour after injection.[28] Peak contrast (target-to-background ratio) between bone and soft tissue does not develop until about 6 hours after injection. Since soft-tissue clearance is substantially complete between 3 and 4 hours after injection, imaging can begin at that time.

The standard adult dose for either approved radiopharmaceutical is 740 MBq (20 mCi). Pediatric doses vary depending on practitioners. We use a dose of 9.25 MBq/kg (250 µCi/kg) with a minimum dose of 74 MBq (2 mCi). At lesser doses, high-resolution images with adequate information density cannot be obtained in a reasonable time. Radiation dosimetry in children is similar to adult dosimetry, with the exception of bone surface doses, which are higher in children (Table 3-1). Dosimetry in infants weighing less than 8 kg will also be higher because of the minimum dose requirement for adequate images. Although most radiopharmaceuticals used in the routine clinical practice of pediatric nuclear medicine do not have FDA-approved pediatric indications, HDP is specifically approved for use in children.

Both HDP and MDP are available as lyophilized kits and are prepared by adding sterile and pyrogen-free Tc-99m-pertechnetate. The addition of antioxidants such as

TABLE 3-1
Pediatric Dosimetry for ^{99m}Tc-HDP (rads)

Tissue	Newborn	1-Yr-Old	5-Yr-Old	10-Yr-Old	15-Yr-Old	Adult
Weight (kg)	3.5	12.1	20.3	33.5	55.0	70.0
Kidneys	0.50	0.30	0.29	0.32	0.37	0.44
Ovaries	0.25	0.18	0.17	0.19	0.21	0.24
Red marrow	1.82	0.93	0.76	0.72	0.71	0.96
Bone surface	17.47	8.15	5.66	5.61	5.60	6.44
Testes	0.20	0.14	0.13	0.14	0.15	0.16
Bladder wall	1.90	1.24	1.12	1.25	1.37	1.55
Total body	0.30	0.19	0.19	0.19	0.21	0.25

Based on pediatric doses recommended in the Osteoscan-HDP technical product data bulletin, Mallinckrodt.

ascorbic acid or gentisic acid to the kit provides additional stability to the radiopharmaceutical and prevents the formation of free pertechnetate over time. Antioxidants allow the kits to be formulated with low tin concentrations.

IMAGING STRATEGY

There are a number of ways to perform a bone imaging study. The method chosen is typically influenced by the clinical diagnosis to be evaluated. Bone imaging techniques include three-phase, four-phase, limited studies, whole-body scanning, and whole-body spots. The three-phase examination includes a radionuclide angiogram or flow study performed dynamically over the site of interest. The second phase is the soft-tissue phase or blood pool. The third phase is the bone or static phase. Three-phase examinations are typically performed to evaluate trauma, inflammatory disease, and primary bone tumors (Box 3-1). Some soft-tissue neoplasms such as sarcomas may also benefit from a three-phase study. A three-phase study characterizes the vascularity of a process as well as metabolic activity. Knowledge of the flow and blood pool activity may help to date traumatic lesions and evaluate healing. Flow and blood pool images may also help to define the activity of an inflammatory lesion such as an arthropathy.

The fourth phase of a multiphase study is a delayed bone phase image, usually obtained 18 to 24 hours after the initial injection. The fourth phase is often employed to better visualize bone when initial soft-tissue clearance is reduced. This commonly occurs in the lower extremities and in the presence of peripheral vascular disease or venous insufficiency.[1] Evaluation of the diabetic foot is an example of a clinical condition that often requires the fourth phase to adequately evaluate bone. Soft-tissue clearance in the lower extremities of diabetic patients is often very poor at 3 hours after injection. The fourth phase is also employed to evaluate the changing metabolic pattern in a lesion. Diagnosis may be aided by knowing whether an abnormal focus has persistent or relatively increasing bone tracer accumulation over time versus decreasing activity by the fourth phase, when compared with adjacent normal bone.

When the likelihood of diffuse skeletal involvement is remote, a limited study may be appropriate. High-resolution spot images are usually obtained in limited studies, and the site of interest is usually evaluated in multiple projections. Conditions that lend themselves to a limited study are also often many of the same conditions that benefit from flow and blood pool imaging. As a consequence, flow and blood pool images often accompany limited studies. Skeletal pain is frequently poorly localized by patients. When obtaining a limited study, it is wise to consider imaging locations from which pain may be referred. We routinely image at least one field of view both proximal and distal to a painful site.

Whole-body imaging, whether using a scanning technique or whole-body spots, is most commonly performed to evaluate bone metastasis and somewhat less commonly to evaluate metabolic bone disease. Whenever a disease process is spread hematogenously, the entire skeleton should be evaluated. Although adult osteomyelitis can be adequately evaluated with a limited study, osteomyelitis in a pediatric patient is a hematogenously spread process and requires whole-body imaging.

A study performed with spot images will always be a higher-resolution study than one performed using the same collimator but with a scanning technique. As a result, scanning studies should be limited to systems with high-resolution detectors and preferably large rectangular field-of-view detectors, which can obtain a complete image in a single pass. It is unlikely that a 10-year-old gamma camera will produce a scanning study with adequate resolution, but with proper collimation this older camera may produce a diagnostic spot imaging study. The primary factors degrading a scanned study are distance from the patient and low count-density secondary to inappropriately short scan times.

BOX 3-1   A Protocol for Digital Three-Phase Planar Bone Scan

Dose
- 20 mCi MDP or HDP (adult)
- 250 µCi/kg with a minimum does of 2 mCi (pediatric)

Acquisition
1. Flow study and blood pool images
- Low-energy all-purpose collimator
- 20% energy window centered at 140 keV
- 128×128 matrix for flow study
- 1 sec/frame for 60 seconds
- 256×256 matrix for blood pool images
- 60-sec blood pool images
2. 2- to 3-hour delayed images
- Low-energy high-resolution collimator
- 256×256 matrix
- Image statistics: 150- to 1000-k counts depending on body part
- For limited studies in patients with localized pain, acquire at least one view to include major joints proximal and distal to the painful site

Display on Film
- Reformat flow study at 3-5 sec/frame for filming
- Nonlinear gray scale, which simulates the nonlinear response of analog techniques
- Film delayed bone scan images using nine-on-one format

THE MODERN GAMMA CAMERA

Most new gamma cameras are digital integrated systems. Unlike older analog systems a photographic imaging intensity does not have to be selected before image acquisition. The operator only has to define matrix size and termination parameters. All other parameters are display or postprocessing parameters. With a digital system, images are never lost because of an inappropriately selected intensity. The acquired image is neither too light nor too dark. It is information stored in a digital matrix, which can be displayed to suit the preferences of the physician interpreting the study. The presentation format can be composed after all images are acquired.

The final display product from an analog system must be determined before acquisition of the first image. The order in which the images are to be presented, the photographic intensity, the image display size and orientation, in addition to termination parameters, must all be determined in advance. If an error is made, the image must be repeated. Off-peak imaging is also a potential problem for analog systems. A digital camera can have an imaging protocol that will automatically peak the camera for the correct isotope, so that when a bone imaging protocol is selected, the camera is automatically peaked with an appropriate window at 140 keV.

Analog images have been considered the gold standard by which digital images are judged. The film generated from digital images has been criticized for looking "pixely" (appearing as a collection of square dots). This is a result of the combination of an inadequate image matrix size and an overly large display format on film. Often the image formatter is the weak link in the system. After purchasing an expensive camera system, an effort is made to save money by purchasing an image output device with limited versatility. An analog image subjected to the same mistreatment will be equally unpleasant to look at. A 256-matrix image photographed using a nine-on-one format will look analog, will save film, and will be of approximately the same size as most spot images obtained using analog output devices. The response of an analog imaging system on film is not linear, whereas the unmodified output of a digital camera is linear. This also contributes to the nonanalog appearance of digital images. Most digital camera vendors now provide a series of black-and-white display gamma maps that will simulate the nonlinear analog film response. Gamma maps, which will allow contrasts to be adjusted to the preferences of the interpreting physician, are available or can be developed on most systems.[34]

IMAGING TECHNIQUE

Early nuclear medicine computers had limited storage capacity. As a result, images were stored on the minimum matrix necessary for a diagnostic study. Current integrated systems may have storage capacities of a gigabyte or more. As a result, larger matrices for image acquisition can be used. Matrix size should be matched not only to the nominal resolution of the system but also to the spot size used for photography. A 128 word mode image, although matching the system resolution of most gamma cameras, will have an obvious pixely appearance when photographed in a nine-on-one format, whereas a 256

word mode image will appear analog. Using a matrix that somewhat overmatches the system resolution in order to match the image formatter spot size will improve the perceived image quality. Enlarging the matrix further will only either make the image appear noisy or require an increase in imaging time. Most static blood pool or bone phase spot images should be obtained on a 256 word mode matrix. If byte mode is used, only 8-bit data can be obtained in any one pixel (255 counts per pixel). Most systems drop the least significant digit at pixel overflow in byte mode and continue counting. This will result in the loss of low-level activity from the image. Again, the large storage capacity of most integrated camera systems eliminates the need to use byte mode acquisition for static images.

Dynamic flow images should be acquired with a general all-purpose collimator, using a 128 matrix. Flow images are displayed at framing rates of between 2 and 5 seconds per frame, typically using a sixteen-on-one format. The actual framing rate for the display depends on the body part to be imaged. With an analog system the data must be acquired at the desired display framing rate. Since the framing rate that will produce the best image may not be known in advance, the technologist must use an average that will work in most cases. With a digital system, data can be acquired at a faster rate than the desired display. It is better to overframe than to underframe the data acquisition. The data can be reformatted into the most appropriate framing rate for display purposes. We typically acquire flow studies at 1 second per frame for 60 frames and display at between 3 to 5 seconds per frame, depending on bolus quality. The digital acquisition permits optimization of the final display.

Collimation limits the system resolution of most new gamma cameras. Since maximum anatomic resolution is desirable for static bone images, high-resolution collimators should be routinely employed. Static images can be acquired for either time or statistics. When whole-body spot images are obtained, we acquire a posterior thoracic spine image for 1 million counts and then acquire all other images for the same time. For limited studies, specific total counts can be obtained for various anatomic sites. General useful ranges are indicated in Table 3-2. If there is doubt about the adequacy of the counting statistics for a limited study, a posterior thoracic spine image can be obtained for statistics and the limited spot images can then be obtained for same time as the spine image. Because bone activity is not distributed homogeneously, information density as a termination parameter is less useful and may produce unpredictable results.

For a whole-body scanning camera, a 256 × 1024 matrix will produce a study of similar quality to spot images on a 256 matrix. The study is terminated at a specified scan length, based on the patient's height. The quality of the study is determined by the collimator used and the scan speed. A high-resolution collimator is essential for high-quality images. The temptation to scan too fast and reduce the total imaging time will result in a suboptimal image. The scan speed should be chosen to match the count statistics available in a spot image. This

TABLE 3-2
Planar Spot Image Acquisition Parameters

Projection	Image Statistics (counts)
T-Spine, L-spine, anterior chest, anterior abdomen, anterior and posterior pelvis	750-1000 k
Skulls (all four views)	450-500 k
Femurs, humeri	500-600 k
Knees	350-400 k
Forearms, lower legs	200-250 k
Hands, feet	150-200 k

can be determined for an individual system by displaying a posterior whole-body image and using the region-of-interest tool to determine the count statistics in an equivalent posterior thoracic spine image and then adjusting the scan speed so that total counts in the posterior chest of the scanned image match the total counts desired in a spot image. Scan speeds of 10 to 12 min/m or 8.3 to 10 cm/min will produce the desired result when using high-resolution collimation.

Neutral anatomic positioning is critical to the quality of the final product. Lower extremities should be turned in fifteen to twenty degrees. This guarantees neutral anatomic position at the hips with visualization of both greater and lesser trochanters as well as the complete femoral neck. Proper visualization of the fibulae and the ankle mortise also require this positioning. Normal whole-body scans and whole-body spot images are illustrated in Figs. 3-1 and 3-2.

One pitfall of whole-body scanning is bladder filling. If the patient followed oral hydration instructions given at the time of bone tracer injection, the bladder may refill during imaging, even when the patient voids before starting the scan. Whether you start scanning at the head or feet, the bladder is at least 10 minutes away from the field of view. Significant bladder refilling may occur during this time. If the full bladder obscures bony structures, postvoid spot images of the pelvis should be obtained.

PATIENT FACTORS AFFECTING IMAGE QUALITY

Controlling technical factors alone will not guarantee a high-quality bone image. The patient both directly and indirectly contributes. Anything that interferes with the delivery of isotope to bone, its active accumulation on the surface of bone, or clearance of activity from the soft tissues will affect image quality. Several common patient factors affecting bone image quality are listed in Box 3-2.

BOX 3-2   Patient Factors Influencing Image Quality

1. State of hydration
2. Vascular insufficiency
   Venous
   Arterial
3. Renal failure
4. Age
5. Patient size
   Attenuation
   Scatter
6. Medications
   Aluminum in antacids
   Chemotherapy
   Steroids
   Antibiotics
   Nonsteroidal antiinflammatory drugs
   Iron
   Phosphorus ions
   Dextroxe
   Radiographic contrast agents
7. Altered metabolic states
   Hypercalcemia

Probably the most common problem in clinical practice is state of hydration. Patients should be orally hydrated for bone scintigraphy. Oral hydration should occur between injection and delayed imaging. Adequacy of hydration depends on patient cooperation. Clinical practice varies, but the CRC Manual recommends having the patient drink at least two large glasses of water.[24] The patient chooses whether or not to drink the fluid, when to drink it, and how much to drink. Patients with voiding or bladder problems may choose not to follow the hydration instructions. Some patients don't cooperate because frequent voiding between injection and imaging is inconvenient. The importance of hydration in obtaining a diagnostic-quality study should be fully explained to the patient. Patients who understand and are interested in the outcome of the study are more likely to cooperate with oral hydration than patients who are simply told to drink a lot of fluid.

Vascular insufficiency, particularly venous insufficiency, is probably the next most common problem in bone imaging. Soft-tissue activity clears most slowly in the lower extremities, particularly in older patients. Bones of the lower extremities are sometimes poorly seen at 3 hours after injection. The problem, however, is not limited to older people and may be seen in young people undergoing lower extremity imaging for stress fractures. The best way to avoid the problem is for the patient to be up walking around so that the muscles of the legs will aid in blood return. Sitting quietly in the waiting room with the legs dependent and with the patient compressing venous return is probably the best way to ensure venous stasis and poor soft-tissue clearance. If the patient has limited ability to ambulate, simply elevating the feet will improve lower extremity drainage.

Since soft-tissue activity is cleared from the body by

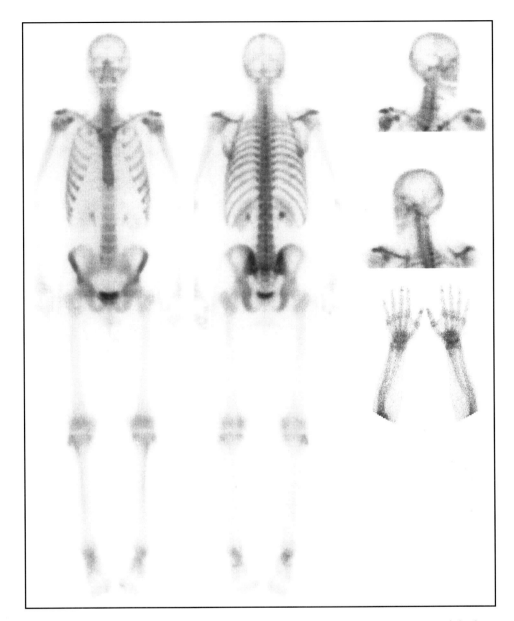

Fig. 3-1. Normal adult anterior and posterior whole-body bone images. Spot views of the lateral skull and forearms complete the sequence. The forearms are spotted because distance and position limit visualization on the whole-body scan.

renal excretion, renal dysfunction will reduce the quality of bone images. This is particularly a problem for patients on dialysis who require bone imaging. Since, as previously discussed, bone activity peaks at about 1 hour after injection, dialysis after reaching peak bone accumulation will improve the quality of bone images. We typically time bone imaging to coincide with routine dialysis in these patients. A recirculating dialysis unit, however, may cause significant tag breakdown with resultant free pertechnetate and subsequent thyroid and gastric activity.[9] It is therefore important to know what kind of dialysis unit will be used before attempting to employ this strategy.

The age of the patient has been shown to be inversely correlated with the quality of bone images.[43] It is unclear whether this is an independent factor or whether this might be a function of increasing venous insufficiency and decreasing renal function that accompany aging. Patient size also plays a role in image quality. Larger patients have both increased Compton scatter and increased attenuation; both of these factors degrade image quality compared with a thin person.

Several medications and treatments have been reported to have an impact on bone and soft-tissue activity. Chemotherapeutic agents,[18] steroids,[31,39] iron,[30,42] phosphorus ions,[37] vitamin D_3,[5] and even dextrose infused intravenously just after bone tracer injection[38] have all been reported to cause decreased bone accumulation of tracer. Hypercalcemia has also been reported to cause decreased bone uptake,[29] an effect we have seen many times.

Radiation therapy has a delayed effect on bone image quality. In the subacute phase, between 45 days and 3 months following radiation therapy, a radiation-induced osteitis may result in increased activity in the distribution of the radiation port.[22,23] As a late sequela, usually 6 months to a year or more after therapy, radiation fibrosis is present. This results in diffusely decreased uptake of the bone tracer within the radiation port.[2,17] Radiation defects are not seen in patients receiving less than 2000

rad (20 Gy) and are seen in 60% of patients receiving more than 4500 rad (45 Gy). On a rare occasion the increased activity associated with radiation may persist for years. Biopsy of such a lesion will show only evidence of radiation fibrosis. The mechanism of this persistently increased bone tracer is not understood.

In the soft tissues we have frequently seen uptake at intramuscular injection sites. Muscular activity at the injection site disappears over time. This has been reported with meperidine (Demerol)[14] and iron[4,42] injections. The soft-tissue activity is probably related to the injection itself rather than the substance injected.

Increased kidney activity has been seen following

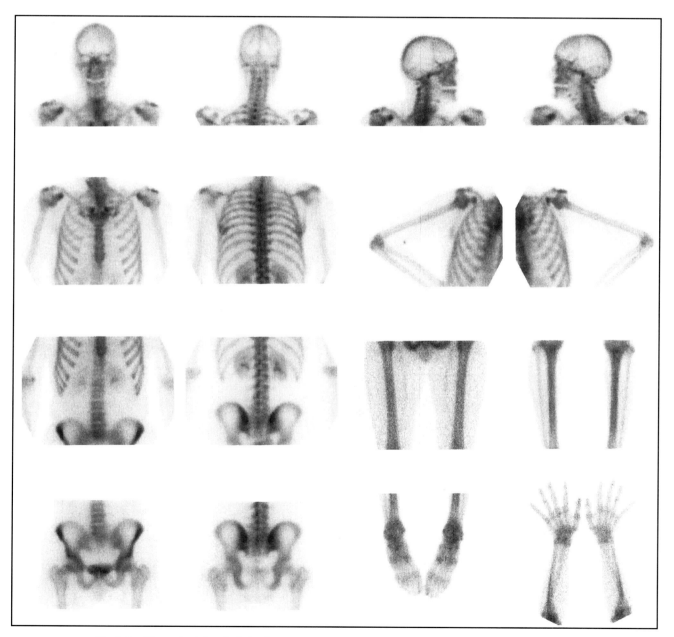

Fig. 3-2. Normal adult whole-body spot images. A rectangular field-of-view camera with a spot size of approximately 20 × 15 in. was used. Sixteen individual spots were required to cover the whole body in this 6-ft, 4-in. patient.

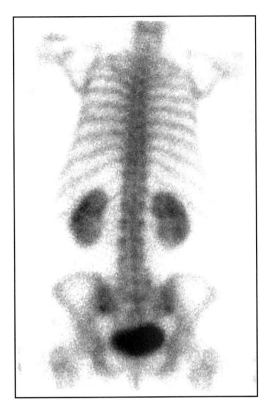

Fig. 3-3. Increased renal parenchymal activity. The posterior spine image is from a patient being evaluated for low back pain. The patient has normal renal function and no known renal disease but is taking nonsteroidal antiinflammatory drugs for her low back pain. The increased kidney activity is within the renal parenchyma and is not excreted activity within the collecting systems. Kidney activity will return to normal when the medication is discontinued.

chemotherapy[27] (within 1 week), antibiotics, nonsteroidal antiinflammatory drugs, and intravenous radiographic contrast agents.[7] These effects are usually transient and are seen only when bone scans are performed during or shortly after completion of the course of drug therapy (Fig. 3-3). The aluminum in antacids has a dose-related effect.[19,25] At blood levels below 10 μg/ml, no effect is seen. Over 20 μg/ml, increased kidney activity is seen. Over 40 μg/ml, liver deposition of the diphosphonates will occur.

Radiographic contrast material administered orally rather than intravenously does not directly affect bone image quality. It can, however, produce attenuation artifacts that project over bone and may simulate a photon-deficient defect or alternatively may obscure a lesion. This is particularly a problem following gastrointestinal (GI) fluoroscopy with barium. Even the dilute radiographic contrast material used to opacify the bowel for computed tomography (CT) may on rare occasions produce attenuation artifacts when concentrated in the colon as a result of water reabsorption. Bone scans should be performed before examinations using barium GI contrast agents. Otherwise, the patient must wait for several days for the barium to clear.

NORMAL VARIANTS

One of the keys to the interpretation of bone imaging studies is an in-depth understanding of normal variants and artifacts. Artifacts are discussed in detail in Chapter 18. Normal variants that could possibly simulate disease exist throughout the skeleton and the soft tissues. Soft-tissue uptake is discussed in detail in Chapter 17. A thorough knowledge of normal anatomy as depicted on bone scans is essential.

The skull is often a source of confusion. Bone scan

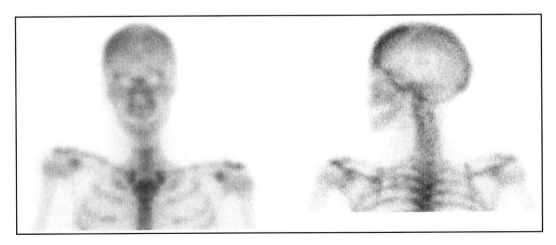

Fig. 3-4. Hyperostosis frontalis interna, most often seen in women, is a benign thickening of the frontal bone of the skull. It has a characteristic appearance both radiographically and scintigraphically. On the anterior view of the skull, it is seen as a diffuse increase in bone tracer accumulation, often sparing the midline. It has been described as having a butterfly pattern. Less commonly, as shown here, the pattern is better demonstrated on the lateral view of the skull as distinctly increased frontal activity.

activity within the skull is not uniform. The activity may appear irregular and patchy. Hyperostosis frontalis interna (Fig. 3-4) is commonly seen in the skull of females and is manifest on an anterior view as areas of increased bone tracer symmetrically located on either side of the sagittal suture. In addition many small benign skull lesions of unknown etiology (Fig. 3-5) are present in the skull, commonly associated with the sutures.[16] On the lateral view of the skull, a pseudolesion created by the confluence of the greater and lesser sphenoid wings may be present (Fig. 3-6).

The sternum may have many different appearances on bone scans. The xiphoid tip (Fig. 3-7) has a variable appearance, and the distal sternum may have a duckbill shape with a photon-deficient center (Fig. 3-8). Costochondral calcification may be seen prominently on the anterior view of the chest (Fig. 3-9). The pattern is variable but becomes more pronounced with age. Soft-tissue activity in the breasts (Fig. 3-10) is related to functional ductal tissue and may obscure ribs or simulate a chest wall lesion. Symmetric breast uptake has been reported in males with prostate cancer treated with sex steroids.[32] In the humerus the deltoid tubercle (Fig. 3-11) may appear prominent. Proper positioning will demonstrate the focus to be cortical in location. The deltoid tubercle is not necessarily symmetric from side to side. Its appearance depends on musculoskeletal use. Ribs may appear irregular in the midportion posteriorly as a result of the pull of the interosseous muscles[10] (Fig. 3-12). With a dose infiltration at an injection site in the arm, normal nodes in the lymphatic drainage pathway may be seen (Fig. 3-13). This occurs if there is an intradermal component to the dose infiltrate.

Since the excretory pathway for bone imaging agents is renal excretion, kidneys should be faintly visualized on the normal bone scan. Anomalies of renal position may be detectable. The three-phase bone scan is sensitive for renal functional abnormality, particularly blood pool images, but lacks specificity. Many renal abnormalities result in either abnormal parenchymal retention, hydronephrosis and stasis, or abnormal soft-tissue clearance.

In the pelvis the bladder may obscure the anterior portions of the pelvic ring and the lower sacrum. The first intervention is to have the patient void again and reimage the pelvis. For the sacrum, posterior oblique views or a lateral view will project the sacrum free from the more anterior bladder. To see the symphysis pubis, a specialized view with the patient sitting on the detector (Fig. 3-14), a "tail-on-detector" view, may be obtained. This view, however, superimposes the superior pubic ramus on the inferior pubic ramus and ischium. Side-to-side asymmetries can be seen, but localization may be difficult. In some patients the bladder has to be drained by catheter to adequately visualize the bony pelvis.

In the lower extremities the patella and the tibial tubercles may occasionally be the site of pseudolesions

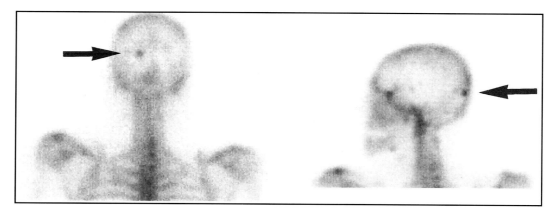

Fig. 3-5. Hot spots in the skull. A small focal lesion is seen in the left occipital bone adjacent to the lambdoid suture on both the posterior and left lateral views of the skull (*arrows*). Such benign lesions are of unknown etiology and are considered to be normal variants.

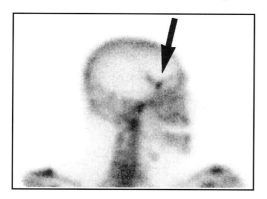

Fig. 3-6. Sphenoid confluence. The confluence of the greater and lesser wings of the sphenoid creates a pseudolesion just behind the orbit on the lateral view of the skull (*arrow*).

(Fig. 3-15). This can be easily recognized as a pseudo-lesion on either a medial or lateral view of the knee. Since the cause of the pseudolesions is usually related to degenerative changes, findings are commonly asymmetric.

THE GROWING SKELETON

The principles of successful pediatric bone imaging are the same as those for adult imaging: obtain high-resolution, motion-free images in neutral anatomic position. These basic requirements are even more critical in small children because of the reduced radiopharmaceutical doses employed for bone imaging. Young children with normal kidneys clear their soft tissues faster than adults. A delay of 1.5 hours is usually adequate for bone phase images. Growth centers have extremely high tracer accumulation compared with adjacent bone and must be resolved as thin, well-demarcated lines.

A blurred growth plate is suggestive of metaphyseal disease. Neutral anatomic position is absolutely critical for optimal visualization of growth plates. Small children may have to be held in the correct position by a parent, the technologist, or a physician. The lazy "shoot 'em as they lie" technique will usually produce a nondiagnostic study. This can be particularly troublesome around the knees. Infants prefer to lie with legs abducted and externally rotated. This is made worse by disposable diapers, which are bulky and tend to exaggerate this natural tendency and prevent straightening of the legs. An abducted, flexed position will blur every growth plate from the femoral head to the ankles. Often the diaper has to be removed to facilitate positioning of lower extremities.

The shoulder is a special case for which neutral anatomic position will not resolve the growth plate. In neutral anatomic position the shoulder growth plate is oblique rather than perpendicular to the face of the camera and therefore will appear blurred. The projections demonstrated in Fig. 3-16 show the growth-oriented

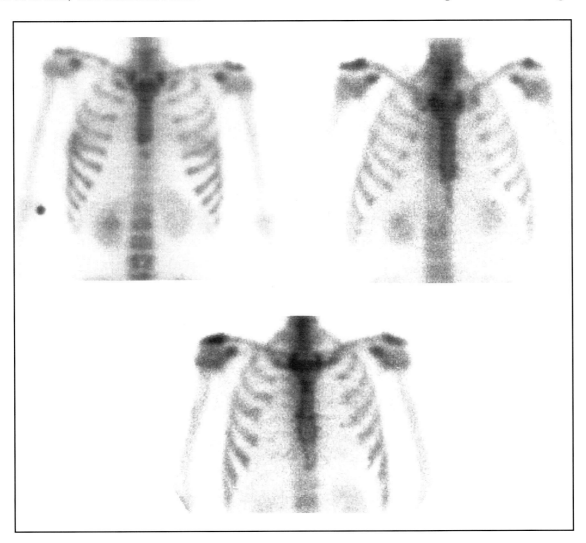

Fig. 3-7. The xiphoid tip has a variable appearance. Three patients who demonstrate the range of variability are illustrated.

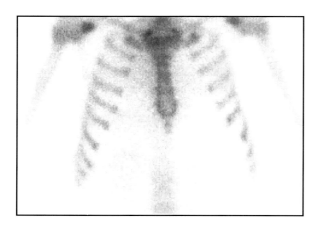

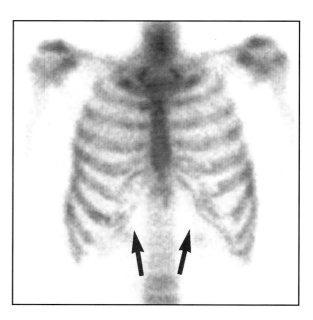

Fig. 3-8.   The hollow sternum. The sternum may be "duckbill" shaped with prominent central thinning and may have a fairly photon-deficient center. This may be prominent enough to simulate a "cold" lesion.

Fig. 3-9.   An anterior view of the chest demonstrates prominent bone tracer uptake in calcified costochondral cartilages (*arrows*).

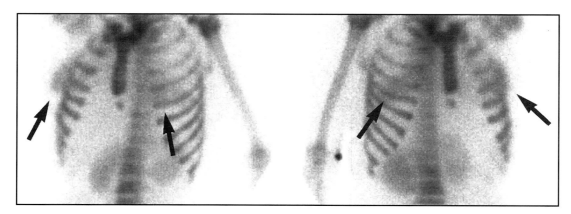

Fig. 3-10.   Normal breast uptake. Bilateral anterior oblique views of the chest demonstrate focal collections of increased soft-tissue activity (*arrows*). This activity is located in functioning ductal breast tissue. This activity tends to be more prominent in younger women and may vary with phase of the menstrual cycle.

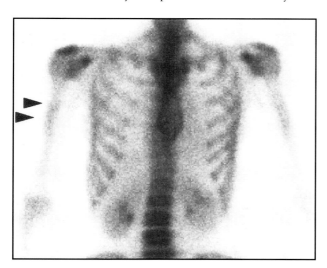

Figure 3-11.   The insertion of the deltoid muscle onto the proximal humerus occurs at a bony prominence known as the deltoid tubercle (*arrowheads*). The normal muscular pull at the site of attachment may be responsible for the increased bone tracer accumulation at this location.

plates correctly relative to the face of the camera. The skeletal anatomy is clearly depicted. Costochondral growth centers commonly shine through on a posterior view of the chest. All four oblique views of the chest are routinely obtained in children as long as rib growth center activity is still present. The hips may also present special problems in children. Magnified views of the hips, such as pinholes, may be necessary to resolve growth plate and femoral head activity. Frog-leg pinhole views of the hips may provide additional information about the femoral heads (Fig. 3-17).

Visually, growth plate activity is of similar intensity from side to side and in the larger growth centers throughout the body. Activity in the growth plates is to some extent a function of age. A single growth center

with either increased or decreased activity should suggest a problem requiring further evaluation. A growth plate in an infant or young child may appear metabolically active before the corresponding ossification center appears radiographically. Similarly, a growth plate may appear metabolically active on a bone scan after the growth plate has closed radiographically. All growth plates potentially visualized on the routine bone scan appear by the age of 5 years.[41] The main growth plates of the humeri, radii, ulnae, and femurs all appear within the first year of life. The proximal fibula appears 2 years earlier and the greater trochanter 1 year earlier in females than in males.[41] Growth plate activity decreases slowly over the period of metabolic closure. The distal femoral and proximal tibial growth plates are commonly seen in

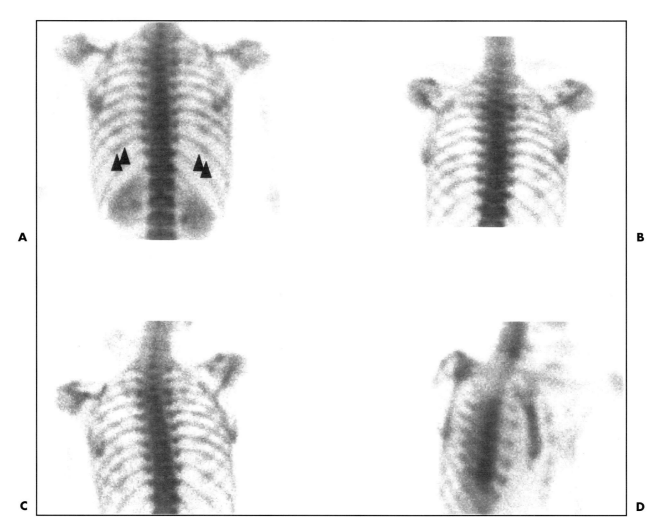

Fig. 3-12. Stippled ribs and scapular positioning. The pull of the interosseous muscles of the chest wall may create increased bone tracer in the midportion of the ribs posteriorly (*arrowheads*). The phenomenon tends to occur bilaterally and in multiple adjacent ribs. The figure also demonstrates the technique for projecting the scapulae off of the ribs. **A,** Posterior chest with scapulae superimposed over ribs. **B,** Arms crossed with hands on opposite shoulders does not bring the scapulae off the ribs. **C,** Bringing the right elbow to the midline projects the scapula off the ribs. This view is best for viewing the ribs. The scapula is seen on end. This image is obtained with a straight posterior projection. **D,** To visualize the scapula to best advantage, the patient is positioned in the same way as in **C,** but the image is obtained from an anterior oblique projection.

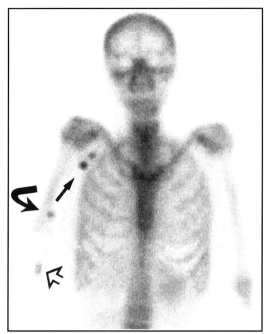

Fig. 3-13. Normal lymph nodes may accumulate bone tracer if the dose is infiltrated with an intradermal component. Both epitrochlear (*curved arrow*) and axillary (*straight arrow*) nodes are seen. The dose infiltrate in the antecubital fossa is partially visualized through lead shielding (*open arrow*).

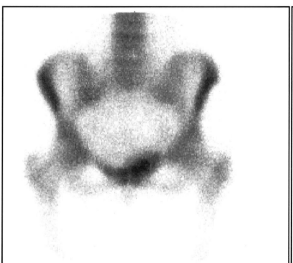

A

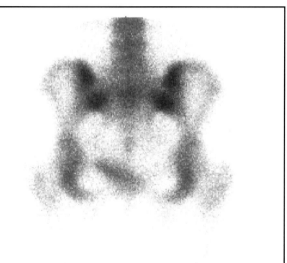

B

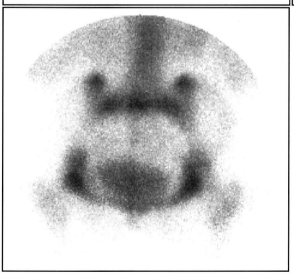

C

Fig. 3-14. TOD (tail-on-the-detector) view. **A** and **B,** In anterior and posterior views of the pelvis, the postvoid bladder obscures the symphysis pubis, particularly on the left. **C,** With the patient sitting on the detector, the bladder is projected off the anterior pelvic ring bones. The pubic rami, however, are superimposed on the ischia. If the ischial rami are free of abnormality on the anterior view, any asymmetry can be presumed secondary to a pubic ramus lesion.

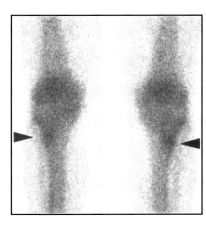

Fig. 3–15. An anterior view of the knees demonstrates bilaterally prominent tibial tubercles (*arrowheads*), creating pseudolesions in the proximal tibias. Like the increased activity at the deltoid tubercles, the increased activity is created by the pull of the quadriceps insertion.

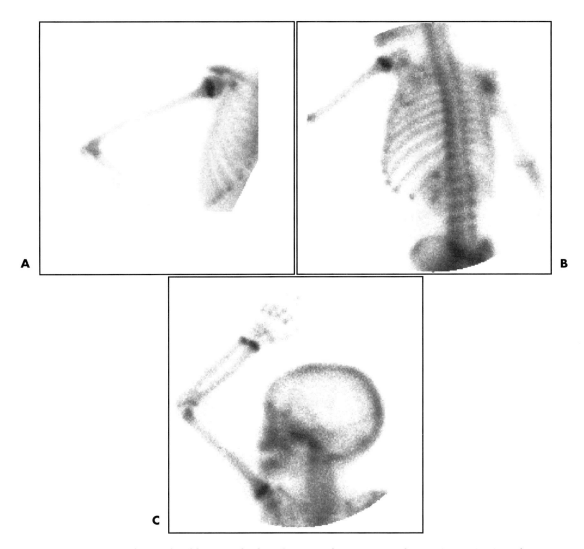

Fig. 3–16. Pediatric shoulder growth plate. In a straight anterior and posterior projection, the shoulder growth plate will be blurred, because it is oblique to the face of the camera. The proximal humeral growth plate must be positioned perpendicular to the camera for clear visualization. Any of the three views demonstrated will resolve this growth plate. **A,** Anterior oblique position with hand on hip, thumb toward back. The arm is in contact with the face of the camera. **B,** Posterior oblique view with the arm extended. **C,** Straight posterior view with the arm flexed over the skull and thumb toward skull. This view also includes both elbow and wrist.

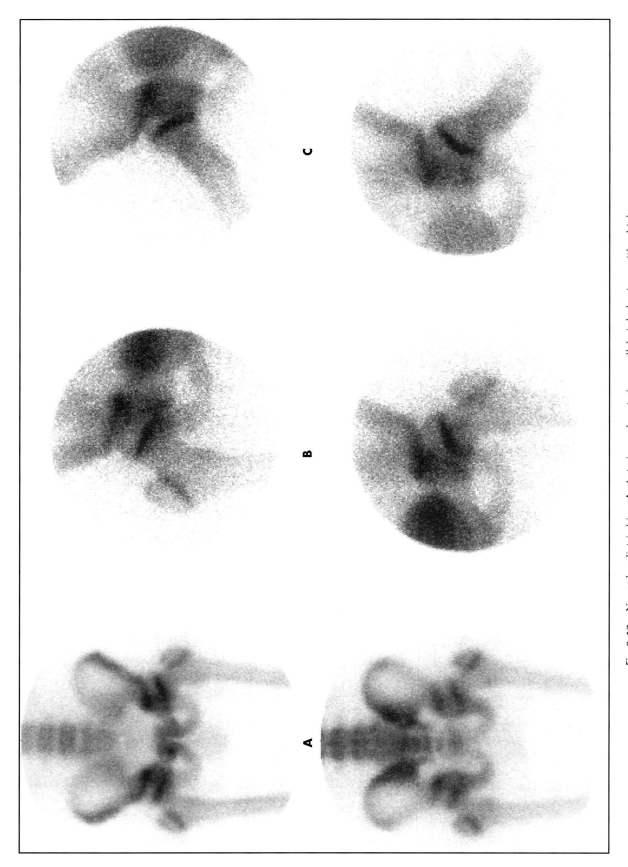

Fig. 3-17. Normal pediatric hips. **A,** Anterior and posterior parallel pinhole views with a high-resolution collimator. **B,** Anterior pinhole views of both hips. **C,** Frog-leg lateral views of both hips.

the late teenage years and into the midtwenties. The scintigraphic appearance and disappearance of growth plate activity cannot be used to evaluate bone age. Most growth plates develop metabolic activity too early and maintain increased activity too long after radiographic closure. No significantly discriminating changes, which would permit reliable evaluation of bone age, occur between the ages of 4 to 5 years and the late teenage years. The normal pediatric skeleton is demonstrated in Figs. 3-18 and 3-19.

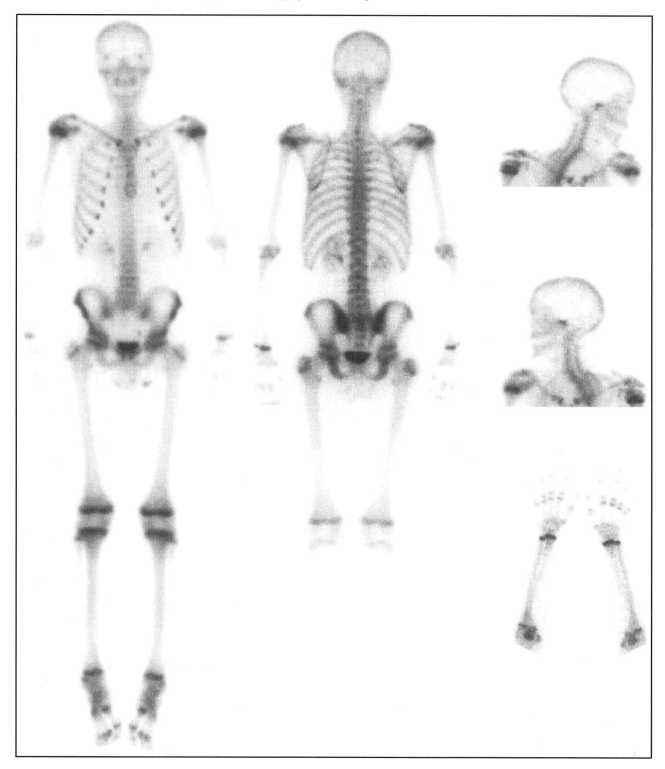

Fig. 3-18. Normal pediatric whole-body scan. This study was performed on an 11-year-old. Under the age of 7 years, pediatric bone studies are usually done with whole-body spots.

OPTIMIZATION FOR EFFICIENCY

In the current health care environment, clinical practice has to be optimized to deliver the best-quality care for the lowest unit cost. As health care dollars shrink further, so must the cost per unit of service delivered. Capital equipment and personnel are the two most expensive items in the budget of a nuclear medicine department. Radiopharmaceuticals are typically third. Capital equipment must be carefully chosen to enhance efficiency. All other things being equal, the practice that best utilizes its equipment and human resources will be most successful. For many years there was a trend toward multipurpose gamma cameras that could do every type of nuclear medicine study but were not optimized for any particular study. This has provided flexibility. If one camera was out of service, any other camera could pick up the work load. That kind of flexibility has had a price: reduced efficiency. With the more recent arrival of multidetector cameras and flexible detector geometries, greater

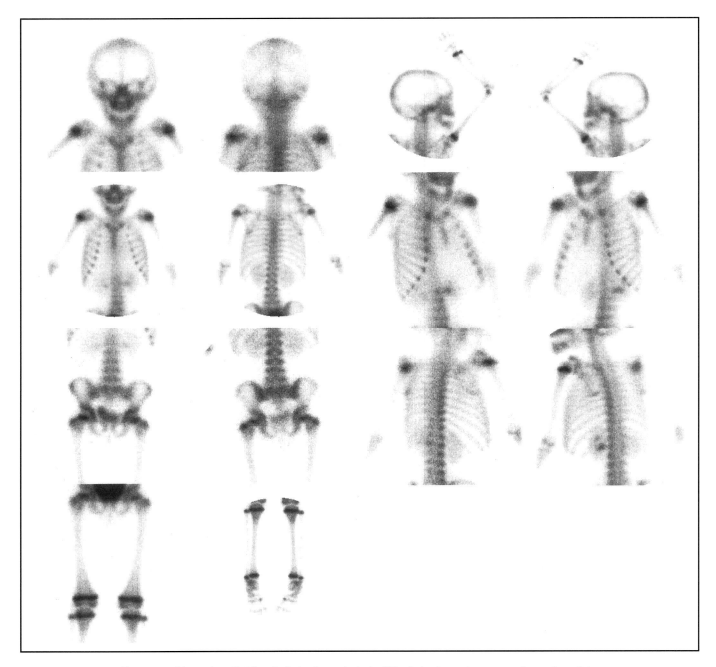

Fig. 3-19.   Normal pediatric whole-body spot study. Whole-body spots were performed on this 3-year-old patient. All four oblique views of the chest were obtained because of costochondral growth center activity.

specialization became available. This has permitted optimization of individual studies but at the cost of reduced flexibility. If such a specialized camera goes down, other specialized equipment may not be able to accommodate the work load.

The goal is to find the right combination of specialization and flexibility. The critical question to ask is, "If the study for which I purchased this optimized camera disappears tomorrow, never to be done again, what else can I do with this camera?" If the answer is nothing or very little, you may be taking an unnecessary risk. If the answer is "lots of things," you may have found the right combination of optimization and flexibility. Optimization also depends on volume. The larger the volume of a specific study type, the more efficiency there is to be gained with specialized equipment.

For bone imaging the answer to the optimization question often is a dual-detector system with a large rectangular field of view. The heads should be 180 degrees opposed to permit simultaneous anterior and posterior imaging in either whole-body scan mode or as simultaneous spot images. This allows imaging time to be cut in half with no loss of image quality. Three-headed cameras generally do not improve efficiency for planar bone imaging. Most bone imaging is comprised of anterior and posterior views. A triple-headed camera would produce either an anterior image and two posterior obliques or a posterior view with two anterior obliques. Even for bone single photon emission computed tomography (SPECT), some three-headed systems do not improve efficiency over a two-headed system because the vertical field of view of many three-headed cameras is shorter than that of two-headed cameras. As a result, two serial three-head acquisitions are required to image the same vertical territory as would be seen in one dual-headed acquisition.

Total imaging time, however, is only one component of total throughput. As imaging time becomes shorter on multiple-headed systems, patient handling time takes a proportionately larger portion of total throughput time. The imaging table is an often overlooked feature of the system that may further improve total patient throughput. The vast majority of bone imaging patients are either fully or partially ambulatory. An integrated imaging table that facilitates the loading and unloading of these patients will improve total throughput. If the imaging table can drop low enough for a wheelchair patient to stand with assistance, pivot 90 degrees, and sit down on the table, loading time will be reduced. If the patient has to be assisted to step onto a table, more assistance and time will be required, reducing throughput. Further, a table (or gantry) that can be manually slid into approximate imaging position is much more efficient than a table (or gantry) that must be driven into imaging position from the patient loading position. Even under the best of circumstances, such patient handling may represent up to one third of the total study time.

The combination of reduced imaging time and reduced patient handling time will increase patient throughput without increasing total capital equipment or personnel costs. Furthermore, image quality is preserved. The ability to reduce cost per unit service delivered while maintaining the quality of the service often makes the difference between success and failure in an increasingly competitive marketplace.

REFERENCES:

1. Alazraki N et al: Value of a 24 hour image (four phase bone scan) in assessing osteomyelitis in patients with peripheral vascular disease. *J Nucl Med* 1985; 26:711.
2. Bell EG, McAfee JG, Constable WC: Local radiation damage to bone and marrow demonstrated by radioisotopic imaging. *Radiology* 1969; 92:1083.
3. Bevan JA et al: Tc-99m HMDP (hydroxymethylene diphosphonate): A radiopharmaceutical for skeletal and acute myocardial infarct imaging. I—Synthesis and distribution in animals. *J Nucl Med* 1980; 21:961.
4. Byun HH, Rodman SG, Chung KE: Soft tissue concentration of ^{99m}Tc-phosphates associated with injections of iron dextran complex. *J Nucl Med* 1976; 17:374.
5. Carr EA Jr, Carroll M, Montes M: Effect of vitamin D_3, other drugs altering serum calcium or phosphorus concentrations, and desoxycorticosterone on the distribution of Tc-99m pyrophosphate between target and non target tissues. *J Nucl Med* 1981; 22:526.
6. Coccia PF: Cells that resorb bone. *N Engl J Med* 1984; 310:456.
7. Crawford JA, Gumerman LW: Alterations of body distribution of ^{99m}Tc pyrophosphate by radiographic contrast material. *Clin Nucl Med* 1978; 3:305.
8. Davis MA, Jones AG: Comparison of ^{99m}Tc-labeled phosphate and pyrophosphate agents for skeletal imaging. *Semin Nucl Med* 1976; 6:19.
9. deGraff P et al: Scintigraphic detection of gastric calcification in dialysis patients. *J Nucl Med* 1980; 21:197.
10. Fink-Bennett D, Johnson J: Stippled ribs: A potential pitfall in bone scan interpretation. *J Nucl Med* 1986; 27:216.
11. Fogelman I, et al: A comparison of skeletal uptake of three diphosphonates by whole-body retention: Concise communication. *J Nucl Med* 1981; 22:880.
12. Francis MD et al: Imaging the skeletal system. In Sorenson JA (ed): *Radiopharmaceuticals II*, Society of Nuclear Medicine, New York, 1979, p 603.
13. Francis MD et al: Comparative evaluation of three diphosphonates: In vitro adsorption (C-14 labeled) and in vivo osteogenic uptake (Tc-99m complexed). *J Nucl Med* 1980; 21:1185.
14. Go RT et al: Etiology of soft tissue localization in radionuclide bone image. 28th Annual Meeting of the Society of Nuclear Medicine, Las Vegas, Nevada, 1981.
15. Guyton AC: Parathyroid hormone, calcitonin, calcium and phosphate metabolism, vitamin D, bone, and teeth. In Guyton AC (ed): *Textbook of Medical Physiology*, ed 8, WB Saunders, Philadelphia, 1991, p 868.
16. Harbert J, Desai R: Small calvarial bone scan foci—normal variations. *J Nucl Med* 1985; 26:1144.
17. Hattner RS, Hartmeyer J, Wara WM: Characterization of radiation-induced photogenic abnormalities on bone scan. *Radiology* 1982; 145:161.
18. Hladik WB III, Nigg KK, Rhodes BA: Drug-induced changes in the biologic distribution of radiopharmaceuticals. *Semin Nucl Med* 1982; 12:184.
19. Jaresko GS et al: Effect of circulating aluminum on the biodistribution of Tc-99m-Sn-diphosphonate in rats. *J Nucl Med Technol* 1980; 8:160.

20. Jee WSS: The skeletal tissues. In Weiss L, Lansing L (eds): *Histology: Cell and Tissue Biology*, Elsevier Biomedical, New York, 1983.
21. Jones AG, Francis MD, Davis MA: Bone scanning: Radionuclide reaction mechanisms. *Semin Nucl Med* 1976; 6:3.
22. King MA, Casaret GW, Weber DA: A study of irradiated bone: I—Histologic and physiologic changes. *J Nucl Med* 1979; 20:1142.
23. King MA et al: A study of irradiated bone. Part II—Changes in Tc-99m pyrophosphate bone imaging. *J Nucl Med* 1980; 21:22.
24. Kline RC: Bone scanning. In Carey RE Jr, Kline RC, Keyes JW Jr (eds): *Manual of Nuclear Medicine Procedures*, ed 4, CRC Press, Boca Raton, 1983, p 1.
25. Lentle BC et al: Iatrogenic alterations in radionuclide biodistributions. *Semin Nucl Med* 1979; 9:131.
26. Littlefield JL, Rudd TG: Tc-99m hydroxymethylene diphosphonate (HMDP) versus Tc-99m methylene diphosphonate (MDP): Biological and clinical comparison. *Clin Nucl Med* 1980; 5:S28.
27. Lutrin CL, McDougall IR, Goris ML: Intense concentration of technetium-99m pyrophosphate in the kidneys of children treated with chemotherapeutic drugs for malignant disease. *Radiology* 1978; 128:165.
28. Makler PT Jr, Charkes ND: Studies of skeletal tracer kinetics: IV—Optimum time delay for Tc-99m(Sn) methylene diphosphonate bone imaging. *J Nucl Med* 1980; 21:641.
29. McRae J et al: Chemistry of ^{99m}Tc tracers: II—In vitro conversion of tagged HEDP and pyrophosphate (bone seekers) into gluconate (renal agent). Effects of Ca and Fe(II) on in vivo distribution. *J Nucl Med* 1976; 17:208.
30. Parker JA et al: Reduced uptake of bone-seeking radiopharmaceuticals related to iron excess. *Clin Nucl Med* 1976; 1:267.
31. Powell ML: Bone imaging. In Matin P (ed): *Handbook of Clinical Nuclear Medicine*, Medical Examination Publishing, Flushing, NY, 1977.
32. Ram Singh PS, Pujara S, Logic JR: ^{99m}Tc-pyrophosphate uptake in drug induced gynecomastia. *Clin Nucl Med* 1977; 2:206.
33. Resnick D, Manolagas SC, Niwayama G: Histiogenesis, anatomy, and physiology of bone. In Resnick D, Niwayama G (eds): *Diagnosis of Bone and Joint Disorders*, ed 2, vol 4, WB Saunders, Philadelphia, 1988, p 1940.
34. Rogers WL, Keyes JW Jr: Techniques for precise recording of gray-scale images from computerized scintigraphic displays. *J Nucl Med* 1981; 22:283.
35. Rosenthal L, et al: A crossover study comparing Tc-99m-labeled HMDP and MDP in patients. *Clin Nucl Med* 1981; 6:353.
36. Ross MH, Reith EJ, Romrell LJ: Bone. In Ross MH, Reith EJ, Romrell LJ (eds): *Histology: A Text and Atlas*, ed 2, Williams and Wilkins, Baltimore, 1989, p 141.
37. Saha GB, Herzberg DL, Boyd CM: Unusual in vivo distribution of ^{99m}Tc-diphosphonate. *Clin Nucl Med* 1977; 2:303.
38. Sampson CB: A study of paediatric radiopharmaceuticals in America. *Br J Pharm Pract* 1980; 2:17.
39. Scott SM et al: Technetium-99m imaging of bone trauma: Reduced sensitivity caused by hydrocortisone in rabbits. *Am J Roentgenol* 1987; 148:1175.
40. Silberstein EB: A radiopharmaceutical and clinical comparison of Tc-99m-Sn-hydroxymethylene diphosphonate with Tc-99m-Sn-hydroxyethylidene diphosphonate. *Radiology* 1980; 136:747.
41. Spencer RP et al: Role of bone scans in assessment of skeletal age. *Int J Nucl Med Biol* 1981; 8:33.
42. Van Antwerp JD et al: Bone scan abnormality produced by interaction of Tc-99m diphosphonate with iron dextran (Imferon). *J Nucl Med* 1975; 18:577.
43. Wilson MA: The effect of age on the quality of bone scans using Tc-99m pyrophosphate. *Radiology* 1981; 139:703.

CHAPTER 4

SPECT BONE SCANNING

B. David Collier, Jr.

Arthur Z. Krasnow

Robert S. Hellman

In many nuclear medicine practices, single photon emission computed tomography (SPECT) bone scanning is a frequently performed, high-volume examination. The widespread availability of SPECT scanners is certainly one of the factors responsible for this adoption of bone SPECT. During the same week, SPECT scanners may perform both bone and cardiac SPECT in addition to less frequently requested tomographic examinations such as brain and tumor SPECT studies. These multiple potential uses for SPECT instrumentation have reinforced one another, leading to both high-quality medical imaging and cost-effective utilization of equipment.

Technetium-99m methylene diphosphonate (Tc-99m-MDP) and other similar compounds have proven to be almost ideal radiopharmaceuticals for bone SPECT. High count rates and favorable target-to-background ratio allow for high-quality bone SPECT imaging even when using a single detector rotating gamma camera, and the general availability and relatively low cost of Tc-99m-MDP has also favored the adoption of bone SPECT. More recently introduced multidetector systems allow for superior bone SPECT image quality and/or shorter examination times.

During the day-to-day operation of most well-staffed and well-equipped nuclear medicine departments, adding yet another bone SPECT study to the daily schedule is both convenient and cost effective. However, adequate technical and professional reimbursement for SPECT bone scanning must be available. As is discussed later in this chapter, at many locations in the United States, a SPECT examination is reimbursed at a higher rate than planar bone scanning.

Bone SPECT often yields unique diagnostic information not available on planar images. Based on reports in the scientific literature and the experience at institutions that we have visited, it appears that bone SPECT of the lumbosacral is the most frequently requested examination. However, our personal list of favorite bone SPECT indications and applications (Box 4-1) shows that the technique has been applied to a great variety of skeletal pathology. This list is based largely on experiences in adult populations. Pediatric applications of bone SPECT are covered in greater detail in Chapter 16. Unfortunately, with the aging of the population in North America, Europe, and Japan, the prevalence of these adult skeletal diseases will increase with a corresponding increase in the need for high-quality SPECT bone scanning.

POTENTIAL DIAGNOSTIC ADVANTAGES OF BONE SPECT

When compared with planar imaging, SPECT offers both improved image contrast and more accurate localization of lesions. On a planar image all overlapped layers of activity are superimposed, thereby obscuring some lesions. SPECT—by sectioning through the layers of activity within the patient's body—can remove activity that originates from in front of and behind the tomographic plane of medical interest. By removing such unwanted underlying and overlying activity, SPECT improves image contrast or target-to-background ratio.

SPECT also allows for more accurate localization of skeletal lesions within large and/or anatomically complex bony structures. For example, consider the advantages of SPECT when imaging the femoral head. In the hip the acetabulum extends around and behind the femoral head. Therefore on planar images, a photon-deficient zone of osteonecrosis within the femoral head may be obscured by activity originating in the underlying acetabulum. The problem of detecting this photon-deficient lesion is further compounded by underlying and overlying soft-tissue activity. Using SPECT, however, it is possible to separate the femoral head from underlying and overlying activity (Fig. 4-1). For this reason, SPECT improves detection of a photon-deficient lesion due to osteonecrosis of the femoral head.[16,30,38,41,57] Furthermore, when examining large and complex skeletal structures, the very complete three-dimensional information available with SPECT may yield important additional anatomic information. SPECT images of the spine, base of skull and facial bones, hips, and knees often allow observers to visualize separately bony structures that would overlap on planar images. For example, articular facet and vertebral body osteoarthritis may occur at the same level in the lumbar spine. When imaged with planar techniques, the vertebral body and articular facet lesions often are superimposed. Using SPECT, however, these bone scan abnormalities can easily be separated so that accurate localization and more precise diagnoses are possible (Fig. 4-2).

When choosing whether to use SPECT or planar techniques, the improvements in image contrast and spatial information available with SPECT must be weighed against the potential for superior spatial resolution with optimal planar bone-scanning techniques. For single-detector high resolution bone SPECT techniques (Box 4-2), spatial resolution in the lumbosacral spine is no better than 14-mm full width at half maximum (FWHM). In addition, in clinical practice, optimized multi-detector SPECT systems can produce lumbosacral spine bone SPECT studies with a FWHM no better than 12 mm. This is to be compared with a 7- to 8-mm FWHM resolution (at a depth ≤ 5 cm using high-resolution collimation) for a state-of-the-art planar bone scan. Thus when evaluating relatively small and superficial bony structures such as the hands and feet, high-resolution planar techniques may provide all necessary diagnostic information. SPECT makes an important contribution to the bone scan evaluation of large and anatomically complex structures such as the spine, hips, and knees. SPECT may also be essential for evaluating smaller bony structures that one wants to separate from adjacent skeletal activity. For example, SPECT can isolate temporomandibular joint (TMJ) uptake from activity originating in other bony structures of the face and the skull.

TECHNIQUES FOR BONE SPECT

SPECT supplements but does not replace planar bone imaging. Therefore when reviewing requests for bone

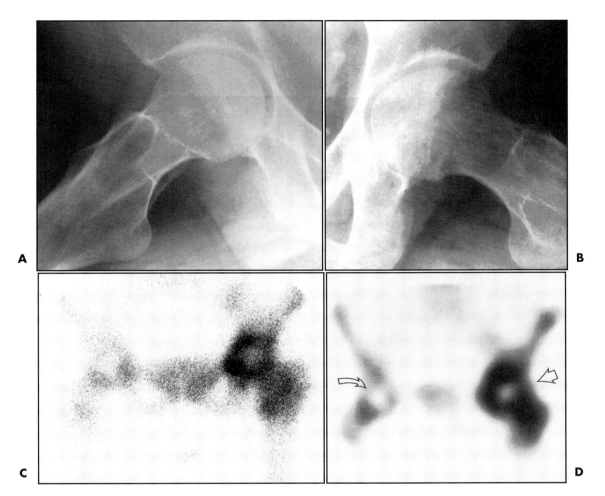

Fig. 4–1. Osteonecrosis of the left and right femoral heads. A 42-year-old female undergoing treatment with prednisone for chronic active hepatitis had experienced left hip pain for the past 4 months. Radiograph of the asymptomatic right hip (**A**) is normal. Left hip radiograph (**B**) shows sclerosis and flattening of the left femoral head. Anterior view planar image (**C**) shows increased activity over the proximal femur and acetabulum without convincing evidence of a photon-deficient defect in the left femoral head. Coronal SPECT image (**D**) through both femoral heads clearly demonstrates a central photon-deficient defect surrounded by increased activity within the left femoral head (*straight arrow*). In addition, a photon-deficient defect is seen with asymptomatic right femoral head (*curved arrow*). The patient eventually developed painful end-stage osteonecrosis of both femoral heads treated with bilateral hip arthroplasties. *(From Collier BD, Carrera GF, Johnson RP, et al: Detection of femoral head avascular necrosis in adults by SPECT. J Nucl Med 1985; 26:979; with permission.)*

scanning, nuclear medicine physicians specify not only SPECT but also appropriate planar views. In addition, some patients complaining of bone or joint pain may benefit from a flow study and a blood pool image.

Positioning for Bone SPECT

The protocols at our institution for bone SPECT (Boxes 4-2 and 4-3) require that the patient lie supine and immobile on the imaging table for nearly 30 minutes. Patients with musculoskeletal pain frequently find it difficult to remain motionless on the narrow imaging table for this length of time. For this reason, patient motion artifacts are the most frequently encountered technical difficulty. This unwanted motion, however, can be minimized by instructing the patient in the importance of remaining motionless and in addition by paying careful attention to patient comfort. Securing arms and legs with light straps often helps, and the addition of a pillow under the knees may relieve low back pain.

The importance of symmetric skeletal positioning for optimal SPECT bone scanning cannot be overemphasized. Strict adherence to proper positioning (e.g., having both knees equally extended and in a neutral position during bone SPECT) results in images for which any left-to-right asymmetry is due to skeletal pathology. Other special considerations for bone SPECT examinations are listed in Box 4-4.

Data Acquisition and Processing for Bone SPECT

Box 4-2 lists bone SPECT protocols for single-detector rotating gamma cameras. Note that for the lumbar spine and skull, high-resolution collimation and slightly longer imaging times are appropriate. For the hips, low-energy all-purpose collimation and the shorter imaging time of 20 seconds per projection is preferred. SPECT images of the hips may suffer from an artifact created by filling of the bladder with isotope labeled urine, and the shorter acquisition time helps to suppress this artifact. In addition, all-purpose rather than high-resolution collimation for SPECT images of the knees has proven to be adequate.

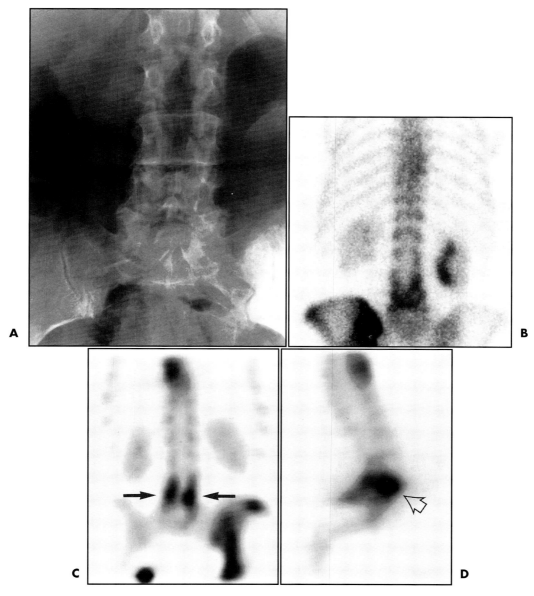

Fig. 4-2. Articular facet and vertebral body osteoarthritis. A 73-year-old female with renewed back pain following L2 and L3 laminectomies. Radiograph (**A**) shows laminectomy sites, osteoarthritic changes particularly at the L4/L5 articular facets, and Paget's disease involving the left side of the pelvis. Posterior view planar image (**B**) shows increased activity in the lower lumbar spine. Note as well the increased activity over the left side of the pelvis typical of Paget's disease along with the L2 and L3 laminectomy defects. Coronal SPECT image (**C**) through the plane of the articular facets shows increased uptake bilaterally at the L4/L5 articular facets located just above the top of the sacroiliac joints (*arrows*). Midline sagittal SPECT image (**D**) shows increased vertebral body activity in the lower lumbar spine at the L4/L5 level (*open arrow*). On the posterior planar image, the activity arising in the vertebral bodies and the articular facets is superimposed. SPECT, however, can be used to localize such findings to specific anatomic sites.

Data acquisition should be performed only with a system that has successfully passed appropriate quality-control tests (Box 4-5). The optional use of noncircular camera/table body contouring orbital motion as a method of improving spatial resolution is of value with SPECT of the lumbosacral spine. In addition, for processing of lumbosacral spine studies, distance-weighted backprojection (also called linear-weighted backprojection) is useful. This technique improves SPECT image quality by emphasizing an object when it is closer to the camera on particular projection images. The technique is of value in the lumbosacral spine.[42,78] For most bone SPECT studies performed on a single-detector rotating gamma camera, a Hanning filter with a cutoff frequency of 0.8 cycles per centimeter is appropriate. However, for studies of the spine, particularly when imaging young adults or thin patients, a "sharper" Hanning filter with a cutoff frequency up to 1.2 cycles per centimeter will improve resolution with little increase in unwanted noise.

Box 4-3 gives a bone SPECT protocol for a three-detector SPECT system (PRISM 3000XP, Picker International Inc.) at one of the hospitals at the Medical College of Wisconsin. Because of the greater sensitivity of the multidetector systems, it is possible to acquire a study comparable to what may be obtained with a single-detector rotating gamma camera in a much shorter time. Alternately, using high-resolution collimation and greater count-densities, it is possible to acquire superior images. The Medical College of Wisconsin protocol is tailored toward the latter approach.

While the basic protocols for a bone SPECT shown in Boxes 4-2 and 4-3 have been used for over 95% of the examinations performed at our institution, other techniques to improve image quality or to facilitate SPECT bone scanning include cone-beam, fan-beam, or long-bore collimators; data acquisition over 180 degrees rather than a full 360 degrees; three-dimensional displays; quantitation; scatter correction; special reconstruction filters; increased angular sampling with thinner slices; and asymmetric Tc-99m energy windows.* Be aware, however, that making such changes in the bone SPECT protocols shown in Boxes 4-2 and 4-3 may necessitate other modifications in quality-control, acquisition, or processing methods that are not obvious to the unexperienced user.

*References 20,23,34,45,82,106,111.

BOX 4-2   Protocols for Bone SPECT Using a Single-Detector Rotating Gamma Camera

Dose
- 25-30 mCi Tc-99m methylene diphosphonate; for patients weighing over 325 lb, a 35-mCi dose will improve image quality

Data Acquisitions
- Hips, knees
  Low-energy all-purpose collimator
  20 sec/projection; 64 projections over 360 degrees
- Lumbar spine, skull
  Low-energy high-resolution collimator
  25 sec/projection; 64 projections over 360 degrees
- 64 × 64 matrix for 400-mm circular camera (1 pixel = 6 mm)
- 128 × 128 matrix for 500-mm circular camera (1 pixel = 4 mm)
- 128 × 128 or similar matrix for large rectangular cameras
- Noncircular camera/table orbital motion for body contouring (optional)

Processing (in sequential order)
- Uniformity correction
- Hanning filter (cutoff frequency of 0.8-1.2 cycles/cm)
- Filtered backprojection with ramp filter; for the spine use distance-weighted backprojection
- No attenuation correction
- Transaxial, coronal, sagittal images
  6 mm (1-pixel slice thickness) for 400-mm camera
  8 mm (2-pixel slice thickness) for 500-mm camera
  Approximately 8-mm thick images for large rectangular cameras
- Oblique images of hips (optional)

Display
- Linear gray scale: skull, spine, knees
- Log or other nonlinear gray scale: osteonecrosis of the hips
- 3D Display (optional)

BOX 4-3   Protocol for High-Resolution Bone SPECT of the Spine Using a Three-Headed SPECT System

Dose
- 25-30 mCi Tc-99m methylene diphosphonate; for patients weighing over 325 pounds, a 35-mCi dose will improve image quality

Data Acquisitions
- Low-energy high-resolution collimator
- 128 × 128 matrix (1 pixel = 3.6 mm)
- Body-contouring orbit
- 45 sec/projection; 120 projections over 360 degrees

Processing (in sequential order)
- Filtered backprojection with ramp filter and linear weighting
- 3D Low-pass filter (order of 8, frequency of 0.4)
- No attenuation correction
- Transaxial, coronal, and sagittal 3.6-mm (1 pixel thick) images

Display
- Linear gray scale
- 3D Display (optional)

BOX 4-4   Solutions to Common Technical Problems

Patient Motion
- Keep the patient comfortable
- Instruct the patient not to move or talk
- Secure knees and feet in a neutral position for hip and knee SPECT
- Secure head in comfortable hyperextension for TMJ SPECT

Bladder Filling Artifacts
- Empty bladder before starting data acquisition
- Start data acquisition in the lateral position, then rotate camera anteriorly
- Bladder catheterization
- Pixel truncation to "remove" artifact (optional)

Low count studies
- Recommended count rates
  Skull: 1.5-k counts/sec
  Spine: 2.5-k counts/sec
  Knees: 1.5-k counts/sec
  Pelvis: 2.5-k counts/sec
- Increase acquisition time as necessary

Positioning
- Check postioning over all 360 degrees of camera rotation
- Strive for left-to-right symmetry
- Skull: hyperextend neck and place pillows under the shoulders
- Lumbar spine: Elevate knees to relieve back pain and reduce lumbar curvature
- Knees: Place a 5-7.5-cm pad between the knees and secure the knees in neutral position; particularly for obese patients be sure that both knees are in the field of view for all projections

BOX 4-5   Gamma Camera Quality Control for Planar and SPECT Bone Scanning

Daily
Extrinsic flood for uniformity check
- 3.0 million counts, 400-mm field-of-view camera
- 4.5 million counts, 500-mm field-of-view camera

Weekly
Update energy correction per manufacturer recommendation
Intrinsic flood for uniformity check
- 3.0 million counts, 400-mm field-of-view camera
- 4.5 million counts, 500-mm field-of-view camera
Update tomographic center of rotation
Update high count extrinsic flood for uniformity correction:
- 30 million counts for 64 × 64 matrix
- 100 million counts for 128 × 128 matrix

Monthly
Image bar phantom for check of planar resolution
Image tomographic phantom (optional)

SCHEDULING, SUPERVISING, AND MANAGING BONE SPECT

Efficient operation of the nuclear medicine department is important if one is to provide high-quality SPECT bone examinations at a reasonable price. When setting up the daily work schedule, the availability of medical personnel, equipment, and other resources needs to be taken into account. Because this will vary from one department to another, it is not possible to describe a single, universally applicable approach to the scheduling of bone SPECT. Rather, we will describe the current approach at our institutions in the hope that readers are able to extract useful information.

In 1993 at the Medical College of Wisconsin, 958 adult SPECT bone scans were performed at the principal teaching hospitals; approximately two thirds of the scans were studies of the lumbosacral spine. This is predominantly an outpatient examination, with outpatients outnumbering inpatients by 9 to 1. Many referring physicians are familiar with bone SPECT and request the examination by name. In other instances, on reviewing the request for bone scanning, nuclear medicine physicians may decide that SPECT should be part of the examination. The recommendation of our nuclear medicine physicians is always to perform SPECT as part of the adult bone scan of the lumbosacral spine, hips, knees, and TMJ or skull base except when patients are being imaged for possible bone metastases, osteomyelitis, fracture, or loosening of an orthopedic prosthesis. When scheduling an examination, the nuclear medicine physician also may choose to include flow study and blood pool imaging or whole-body bone scan images as part of the examination. These initial views will be reviewed by the attending nuclear medicine physician before the patient leaves the department. There are instances when SPECT will not be obtained as part of the initial views but will be an "add-on" to the examination. For example, the patient with prostate cancer and low back pain who has normal planar images will be asked to remain in the department for SPECT of the lumbosacral spine.

In 1981, when one of our hospitals first acquired a single-detector rotating gamma camera SPECT system, bone SPECT examinations had to be scheduled around other SPECT studies. With growth in SPECT imaging, SPECT facilities have expanded so that currently six of eight stationary imaging systems are SPECT-capable. Two of these current systems are single-detector rotating gamma cameras, which are preferred instruments for bone SPECT. However, planar bone scanning and other examinations are also performed on these gamma cameras. In scheduling for the typical adult outpatient who will undergo three- or four-view planar and SPECT imaging of the lumbosacral spine, we reserve 90 minutes of gamma camera time. This includes 10 minutes for setup, approximately 30 minutes for SPECT data acquisition, and 40 minutes for planar imaging. Those institutions using multidetec-

TABLE 4-1 Relative Value Units for Bone Scan Procedures			
Bone Scan Procedure	Current Procedural Terminology Code	Relative Value Units (Technical)	Relative Value Units (Professional)
Multiple areas	78305	11.0	4.5
Whole body	78306	12.5	4.5
SPECT	78320	17.1	5.8

tor SPECT systems may choose to shorten the approximately 30-minute SPECT acquisition time. Physician review of each case and additional views as necessary may also add to the time of the examination. Each bone SPECT patient is made secure and comfortable on the table before starting the bone SPECT data acquisition; during data acquisition the nuclear medicine technologist is able to perform other duties. We have found that under normal circumstances a single technologist can simultaneously operate two SPECT systems.

In today's competitive environment, efficient operating procedures with diligent cost controls are not enough. To be successful the nuclear medicine department also must generate sufficient revenues. Bone SPECT usually is a profitable examination. At most sites in the United States, bone SPECT is both billed and reimbursed at higher technical and professional fees than other bone scan procedures. Table 4-1 identifies bone scan procedures by CPT code, the Current Procedural Terminology System of the American Medical Association, and lists the Relative Value Units for each of these bone scan procedures. Relative Value Units for Physicians is an accurate and comprehensive Relative Value System in use throughout the United States. In establishing the system, physicians across the country were asked to evaluate procedures that they frequently perform using the following five criteria: time, skill, severity of illness, risk to patient, and risk to physician (medicolegal). The system is periodically updated to accommodate such changes as new CPT coding and new technologies. Note that the Relative Value Units for both the technical and professional component of a bone scan procedure are greater for SPECT than for either a planar whole-body bone scan or a more limited planar bone scan covering multiple areas of the skeleton. To determine dollar fees for these procedures, a billing service multiplies the Relative Value Units by the Conversion Factor for the nuclear medicine practice. At the Medical College of Wisconsin, the current appropriate Conversion Factor is close to $30.00. Multiplication of the Relative Value Units by this Conversion Factor yields a technical fee of $513.00 and a professional fee of $174.00. Thus Table 4-1 points to the incremental increase in billings and revenues when a SPECT rather than a planar bone scan is performed. However, the total impact of bone SPECT on departmental revenues is much greater. This is because SPECT increases the clinical appli-

cations of bone scanning and thus the volume of referrals. For example, there are large patient populations with low back pain for whom bone scanning is an appropriate examination only if SPECT is included as part of the study.

COMMON TECHNICAL PITFALLS

The following four technical pitfalls are the most commonly encountered problems: (1) patient motion (Fig. 4-3), (2) significant bladder filling during SPECT of the pelvis, (3) low count study, and (4) bony structures moving in and out of the field of view. Most of these common technical problems can be avoided or minimized (Box 4-4). The bladder filling artifact, however, cannot always be eliminated simply by having the patient void before beginning the study. Approximately 20% of studies still will have "hot" or "cold" streak artifacts extending outside of the bladder and obscuring the hips and other pelvic structures (see Chapter 18, Fig. 18-9). A number of techniques have been proposed for manipulating the data so as to reduce the effect of this artifact. Of course, the artifact could be prevented by bladder catheterization with continuous urinary drainage. However, bladder catheterization often is not acceptable. Gillan, Khouris, and Bunker have all independently developed computer processing techniques to minimize bladder filling artifacts.[14,36,55] O'Connor compared the methods of Bunker and Gillan in three different settings using a phantom of the pelvis.[79] Both techniques improve visualization of the phantoms but neither one fully removes the artifacts or fully restored counts to their true values. However, the pixel truncation method of Bunker was thought to cause minimal distortion. At our institution we used a pixel truncation method and have found it to be valuable.

CLINICAL APPLICATIONS OF BONE SPECT
Spine and Sacroiliac Joints

Many physicians recommend that SPECT be included as part of the routine bone scan for patients with low back pain. Bone SPECT has a diagnostic advantage when

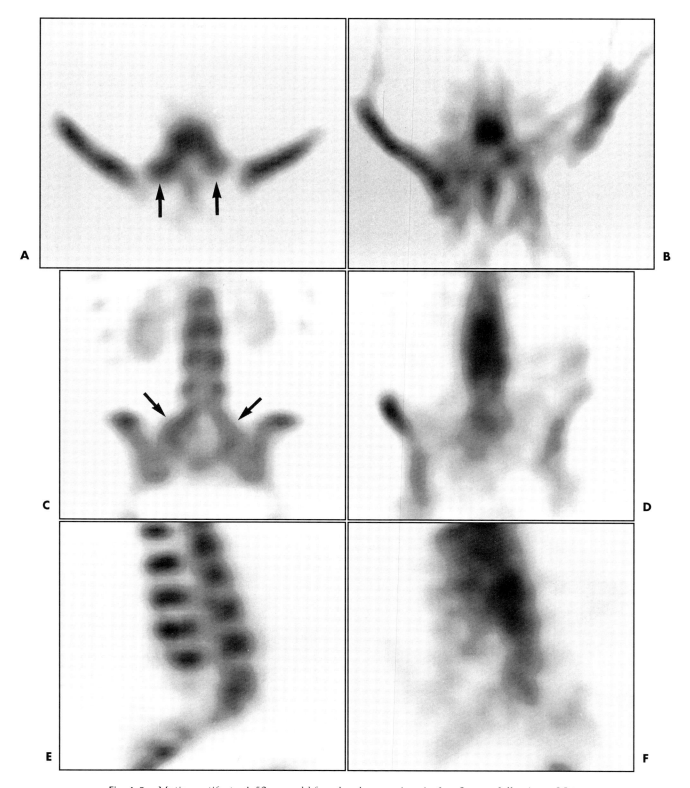

Fig. 4-3. Motion artifacts. A 52-year-old female who now is pain-free 2 years following a L5 to S1 spinal fusion. Lumbosacral spine bone SPECT studies were acquired first without motion and then with motion. Matched pairs of transaxial (**A** and **B**), coronal (**C** and **D**), and sagittal (**E** and **F**) images demonstrate the degradation in image quality produced by patient motion. Bony fusion mass appears normal (*arrows*).

the tomographic technique is used to study a variety of pathologies including (1) spondylolysis, spondylolisthesis, and stress fractures; (2) articular facet osteoarthritis (facet syndrome); (3) degenerative disk disease; (4) sacroiliitis; (5) postoperative evaluation of the patient with failed low back surgery; (6) primary bone tumors; (7) bone metastases; (8) osteomyelitis and diskitis; and (9) fractures.

Given the reported advantages of SPECT relative to planar imaging in demonstrating such a wide range of pathology of the spine and sacroiliac joint (SIJ), it is not surprising that physicians reporting their experience in patients referred to them with low back pain have found SPECT to be superior to planar imaging. For example, working independently Anees (150 consecutive patients), Gates (100 consecutive patients), and Ryan (70 consecutive patients) found that between 13% and 24% of the patients had abnormalities demonstrated only on the SPECT studies.[4,35,90] In addition, when analyzing abnormalities rather than patient studies, these same investigators found that between 21% and 39% of abnormalities were demonstrated only by SPECT. These earlier results were confirmed in a larger although selected series of 1390 patients with chronic low back pain reported by Kanmaz in 1992.[52] Patients with a history of tumor, infection, or inflammatory arthritis were excluded by Kanmaz. Osteoarthritis, articular facet arthritis, fracture/trauma, continued pain following spinal surgery, spondylolysis, spondylolisthesis, and idiopathic low back pain were common diagnoses for patients in this series. Examinations were normal for 384 patients with one site of abnormal increased uptake for 400 patients, two abnormal sites for 310 patients, and three or more abnormal sites for 296 patients. Within the lumbosacral spine 44.1% of abnormalities were equally well seen on planar and SPECT images, 24.0% better seen on SPECT, 31.4% seen only on SPECT, and 0.4% seen only on planar images. Thus there is convincing evidence that when used to examine adult patients with low back pain, SPECT detects more abnormalities than planar imaging. Furthermore, in his 1988 comparison of planar and SPECT bone scanning, Gates graded the intensity of abnormal uptake on planar images before comparing with SPECT.[35] He found that the less intense or less obvious abnormalities on the planar scans often benefit from correlation with SPECT imaging. Finally, investigators who analyzed the results of positive SPECT scans by anatomic region report that SPECT evidence for increased uptake in the articular facets, pars interarticularis, or pedicles is particularly likely to be associated with negative findings on planar studies.[35,89]

In the clinical practice of nuclear medicine, not just detection but also accurate localization of lesions favor the use of SPECT. As has been pointed out by Gates and Holder, the anatomic detail available only with SPECT bone scanning allows nuclear medicine physicians to closely correlate scintigraphic findings with available radiologic studies and thereby generate a more complete and accurate report.[35,45] This leads to a more meaningful consultation with referring clinicians, particularly when additional diagnostic studies or definitive therapy is being considered.

When interpreting SPECT bone scans of the spine and SIJ, it is well to have not just coronal, sagittal, and transaxial SPECT images but also planar images and previously performed radiographic studies available. Normal anatomy to be identified includes the lumbar vertebral bodies, pedicles, lamina, and spinous process (Figs. 4-4 and 4-5 and Box 4-6). The region of the articular facets in the lumbar spine deserves particular scrutiny in patients with low back pain, and this is conveniently seen at multiple lumbar levels on the sequential coronal images. Look carefully for left-to-right asymmetries. Vertebral bodies throughout the spine often are best imaged on the sagittal images. The transaxial images are of particular value for localizing an abnormality to a specific bony structure in the vertebrae and then correlating this finding with computed tomography (CT) or magnetic resonance imaging (MRI). SIJs usually show bilaterally symmetric uptake, although this may not be true with certain normal variants such as partial sacralization of L5.

Many nuclear medicine departments routinely film SPECT studies of the spine and SIJs; however, digital review of images often is necessary. The wide range of intensities on SPECT studies, particularly in the region of the SIJ, often can be appreciated only when using the more flexible digital display. Occasionally changes in processing, such as a sharper filter to improve resolution, may be necessary.[45] Three-dimensional displays may help to define unusual anatomy, and special oblique reconstructions have been recommended as a method of clarifying the anatomy of the lumbar spine.[77,111] Quantitation also may at times be useful.[34]

Accurate localization of increased scintigraphic uptake to a specific site within a lumbar vertebra helps to narrow the differential diagnosis. Evan-Sapir et al in a retrospective study of 233 patients (75 of whom had a history of malignancy) undergoing thoracolumbar bone SPECT found that the location of a lesion within the vertebra could be a powerful predictor of malignancy.[26] For example, all lesions appearing as increased uptake projecting beyond vertebral body surfaces were osteophytes, and all lesions appearing as increased uptake at articular facets were benign. Lesions showing increased uptake in the vertebral bodies and pedicles were usually metastases (83%). However, whenever abnormal uptake was seen in both the vertebral body and posterior elements but with an intervening normal pedicle, benign disease was the most common cause (93%).

Other patterns of abnormal uptake also have diagnostic significance. Always note whether the increased uptake is limited to vertebral body end plates or extends deep into the vertebral bodies. This can be of value when diskitis (usually increased uptake limited to adjacent end plates), osteomyelitis (usually deeper involvement into the vertebral body), tumor (usually deeper involvement into the vertebrae), or osteoporotic compression fractures (sometimes limited to one end plate) are being considered (Fig. 4-6).

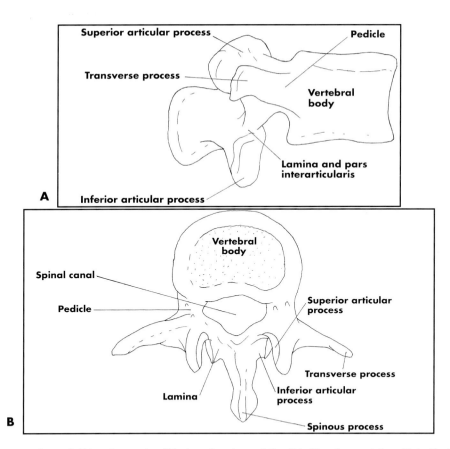

Fig. 4-4. Lateral (**A**) and superior (**B**) view drawings of the third lumbar vertebra. Note that the L3 vertebral body, pedicles, lamina, spinal canal, and spinous process can be identified on the transaxial SPECT image in Fig. 4-5.

SPONDYLOLYSIS, SPONDYLOLISTHESIS, AND STRESS FRACTURES

Spondylolysis, spondylolisthesis, and stress fractures can be detected and evaluated by bone SPECT. When examining patients with low back pain and radiographically demonstrated sites of spondylolysis or spondylolisthesis, Collier et al found SPECT to be significantly better than planar imaging with a sensitivity of 0.85 for SPECT versus 0.62 for planar imaging.[19] In a study of 18 patients Longostrevi et al found similar results with 3 of 18 patients having positive SPECT but normal planar studies.[61] Bodner reported results for 15 adolescent patients with low back pain examined with both radiographs and bone scanning.[10] Four patients had normal examinations. The remaining 11 patients had at least one positive imaging study. SPECT was positive in 11, planar bone scanning in 6, and radiography in 3 patients. The authors conclude that "SPECT was the most sensitive method of imaging and greatly enhanced our acumen for stress fractures or stress reactions of the spine." More recently, Bellah et al reviewed their 1-year experience with 162 athletic active young patients with low back pain.[7] Ninety-one of the patients had normal planar and SPECT bone scans. SPECT demonstrated lesions in the remaining 71 patients, only 32 of whom also had lesions shown on the planar images. The authors reported correlation with radiographic studies for 72 patients in this series. Interestingly there was a subgroup of 16 patients with negative radiographs, negative planar bone scans, and positive SPECT bone scans. The authors postulate that such cases represent spondylolysis with multiple microfractures. In the Bellah series therapeutic decisions to treat surgically, treat by mobilization, or return the patient to athletic activity were strongly influenced by the results of bone SPECT. In 1994 Read reported a series of 9 adolescent patients with low back pain, 5 of whom had confirmation of suspected spondylolysis demonstrated by SPECT but not planar bone scintigraphy.[85] Read emphasizes that the positive bone SPECT study has significant patient management implications. In particular, inappropriate early manipulation or too early a return to sports might convert the stress-related pars interarticular defect into a frank fracture, possibly leading to unstable spondylolisthesis.

ARTICULAR FACET OSTEOARTHRITIS

Articular facet osteoarthritis is a common cause of low back pain in adults (Fig. 4-7). In this patient population a strong correlation between increased uptake in the articular facets on SPECT images and changes of osteoarthritis as shown by CT has been demonstrated.[89] Positive SPECT findings can also be used to direct treat-

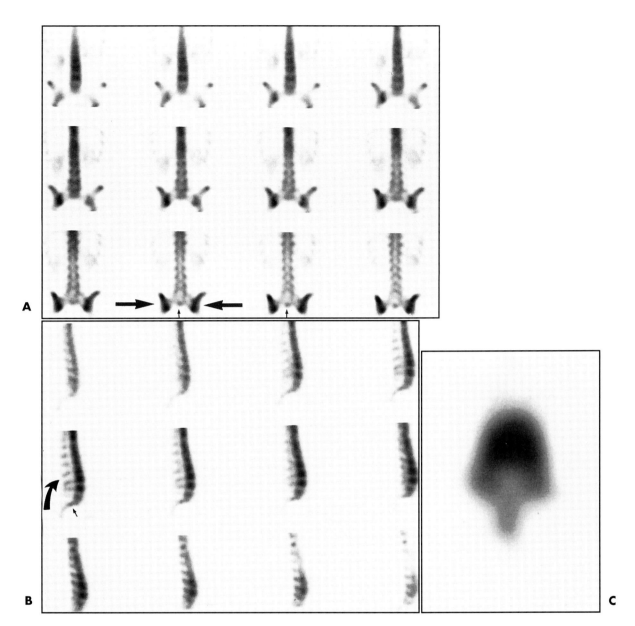

Fig. 4-5. Normal lumbosacral spine bone SPECT study of a young female adult volunteer. Twelve sequential 6-mm thick coronal (**A**) and sagittal (**B**) images show normal anatomy including sacroiliac joints (*large straight arrows*), spinous processes on midline sagittal image (*curved arrow*), and sacral promontory (*small arrows*). On the transaxial 6-mm thick SPECT image through the L3 vertebrae (**C**), much of the bony anatomy of the posterior vertebral arch can be identified.

ment. In a study that followed positive SPECT imaging with local anesthetic injection into the appropriate articular facet, Scott reported that significantly increased uptake on SPECT could be used to predict a favorable response.[94] Furthermore, in a pilot study of 10 patients, Ryan found that 60% of those with chronic back pain achieved complete relief or were markedly improved 3 months after SPECT was used to direct articular facet injection with 40 mg of methylprednisone and local anesthetic.[88] More recently Holder reported favorable results with high-resolution bone SPECT studies of 58

consecutive patients referred with a diagnosis of possible facet syndrome. The standard of reference included facet injections with a bupivacaine (Marcaine) and steroid mixture followed by review of the patient's ongoing pain journal. The 1.00 sensitivity of SPECT for the "facet syndrome" was significantly greater than the 0.71 sensitivity of planar imaging. However, the 0.71 specificity for SPECT was slightly less than the 0.76 specificity of planar imaging. Most useful in Holder's clinical practice was the high negative predictive value of 1.00 for SPECT and 0.93 for planar imaging. Holder concludes that "the high neg-

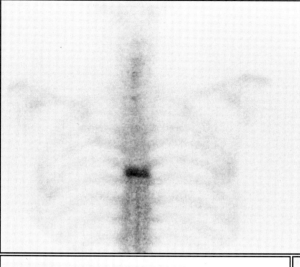

A

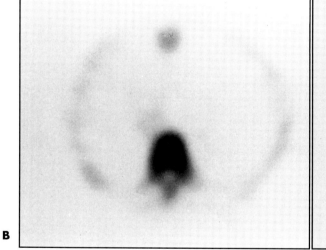

B

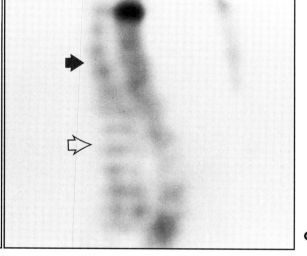

C

Fig. 4-6. Recent T6 vertebral body compression fracture. A 69-year-old female with a history of osteoporosis and recent onset of upper back pain following minor trauma. Planar image (**A**) shows a thin linear band of increased activity extending across T6 with the typical appearance of a vertebral body end plate compression fracture. Subsequent radiographs confirmed this diagnosis. The increased uptake is well localized to the vertebral body on the transaxial (**B**) and sagittal (**C**) images. Note that on the sagittal image the thoracic spine shows more intense activity (*closed arrow*) than the lumbar spine (*open arrow*). This is due to decreased soft-tissue attenuation above the diaphragm.

ative predictive value allows radionuclide bone imaging to be used to select appropriate patients to undergo the invasive facet injection procedure."[45]

INCREASED SACROILIAC JOINT UPTAKE

Increased SIJ uptake is also more frequently detected with SPECT than with planar imaging. Onsel et al reported SIJ findings on SPECT and planar images for 753 patients with chronic low back pain and no history of extraosseous malignancy.[81] They found 28 patients with unilateral and 15 patients with bilateral SIJ abnormalities for a total of 58 abnormal joints. Of these 58 joints with increased uptake, 20 were more convincingly demonstrated by SPECT (Fig. 4-8), and 5 were identified as abnormal only by SPECT. The majority of lesions were due to degenerative joint disease and previous surgery. At follow-up none of the patients were found to have malignancy or infection as the cause of increased SIJ uptake. The abnormalities in the postoperative group were thought to be due to increased impact loading on the SIJ caused by altered low back mechanics following spinal surgery. The authors conclude that for patients with a

history of lumbar spinal fusion and/or laminectomy, increased SIJ uptake usually is due to altered spinal mechanics rather than malignancy or infection. In a report of 15 patients with ankylosing spondylitis, Jacobsson et al reported SPECT to be superior to planar imaging in identifying abnormalities.[51]

CONTINUED OR RENEWED LOW BACK PAIN FOLLOWING SPINAL SURGERY

Continued or renewed low back pain following spinal surgery is a frequent indication for bone SPECT. When interpreting such studies, it is important to know the date and type of surgery including such details as iliac crest bone graft donor sites. Commonly the surgery involves interbody fusion between adjacent lumbar vertebral bodies or posterolateral fusion with bone graft applied across adjacent laminae. Metallic internal fixation devices often are used, and laminectomy or facetectomies also may be performed. By 1 year following surgery, the well-healed fusion will show no more than minimally increased activity. In this patient population, likely causes for postoperative back pain include

BOX 4-6   Bone SPECT: The Most Frequently Asked Questions

Question 1: How do I localize increased uptake in an articular facet to a specific level in the lumbar spine?
- On the coronal images the L5/S1 facets usually are just below the top of the SIJ with the L4/5 facets lying just above the top of the SIJ (Fig. 4-7).
- Use radiographs of the pelvis for anatomic correlation, making note of renal outlines, size of the 12th rib, and any other defining anatomic landmarks such as the apex of a scoliotic curve.
- Beware of the normal variant of 6 lumbar vertebral bodies or sacralization of the lowest lumbar vertebral body.

Question 2: How do I distinguish spondylolysis in the pars interarticularis from increased uptake involving a lumbar articular facet?
- The pars interarticularis usually is located at the level of the lumbar vertebral body and the articular facet at the level of the intervertebral disk space.
- Spondylolysis is a leading cause of low back pain in active adolescents and young adults, whereas articular facet disease often affects an older population.
- The oblique tomographic reconstruction as described by Nicholson may be of value.[77]

Question 3: Why is it that when viewed on the sagittal images the L4 and L5 vertebral bodies sometimes are a bit more prominent than the vertebral bodies at higher levels in the lumbar spine?
- L4 and L5 are bigger, carry a greater axial load, and more frequently are involved in early degenerative disk disease. I consider the appearance to be a normal variant and usually do not report the finding.

Question 4: Why do I so rarely see an abnormal SIJ on my SPECT studies of patients with low back pain?
- When films are properly exposed for the articular facets and vertebral bodies, the SIJs may be so dark that pathology is obscured. Lighter films or review of digital images is helpful (Fig. 4-8).

BOX 4-6, cont'd   Bone SPECT: The Most Frequently Asked Questions

Question 5: Why does S1 sometimes appear prominent on coronal images?
- The sacral promontory is a normal structure found in the same coronal images as the articular facets of the lower lumbar spine. The sacral promontory can easily be recognized as a normal finding on the sagittal views (Fig. 4-5).

Question 6: Why does the thoracic spine show increased activity relative to the lumbar spine on SPECT images?
- There is decreased attenuation above the diaphragm (Fig. 4-6).

Question 7: Why does the middle cervical spine sometimes appear to have increased activity on bone SPECT?
- There is attenuation of the upper cervical spine by the mandible and other facial structures along with more pronounced attenuation of the lower cervical spine by the shoulders and upper thorax.

Question 8: I frequently see increased activity involving the right side of several midthoracic vertebral bodies. Is this an artifact?
- Osteophytes at vertebral margins in the midthoracic spine frequently are larger on the right than on the left. When three or more levels are involved, I report the finding as being characteristic of osteoarthritis.

Question 9: Why did my first lumbosacral spine SPECT show such very poor resolution?
- Patient motion is by far the most frequently encountered problem (Fig. 4-3). If you play back the projections in a cinematic display, you can appreciate any patient motion. This should be part of routine quality control.

pseudoarthrosis within the bony fusion mass, articular facet osteoarthritis developing immediately above or below the fusion, degenerative disk disease, sacroiliitis, arachnoiditis, spinal stenosis, new or recurrent herniation of the nucleus pulposus, osteomyelitis, and myofascial pain.

PSEUDOARTHROSIS

Pseudoarthrosis—a failure of the bony fusion mass to heal solidly—is a frequent cause of continued or renewed low back pain among patients who have undergone lumbar spinal fusion.[87] Serial bone scans of a healing posterolateral lower lumbar to sacral fusion will show a progressive and uniform decrease in activity of the fusion mass beginning about 3 months following surgery and continuing on to only minimally increased activity ap-

proximately 1 year following surgery (Fig. 4-3). At a site of pseudoarthrosis, there is increased impact loading on bone with pounding of the fusion margins one on another. This continued impact loading produces a persistent, and sometimes increasingly intense, site of uptake that is better detected with SPECT than with planar imaging (Fig. 4-9). Metallic internal fixation devices limit the use of CT, and of the available radiographic techniques lateral view flexion and extension radiographs (to detect motion within the fusion) are recommended.

Slizofsky et al reported results for 26 patients with spinal fusions performed more than 6 months before scanning: 15 were symptomatic and 11 were asymptomatic at the time of imaging.[95] Focal areas of significantly increased uptake within the fusion mass were considered positive for pseudoarthrosis. For the 15 symptomatic patients, bone scintigraphy had a sensitivity of 0.78 and a specificity of 0.83, which was superior to the 0.43 sensitivity and 0.50 specificity of flexion and extension radi-

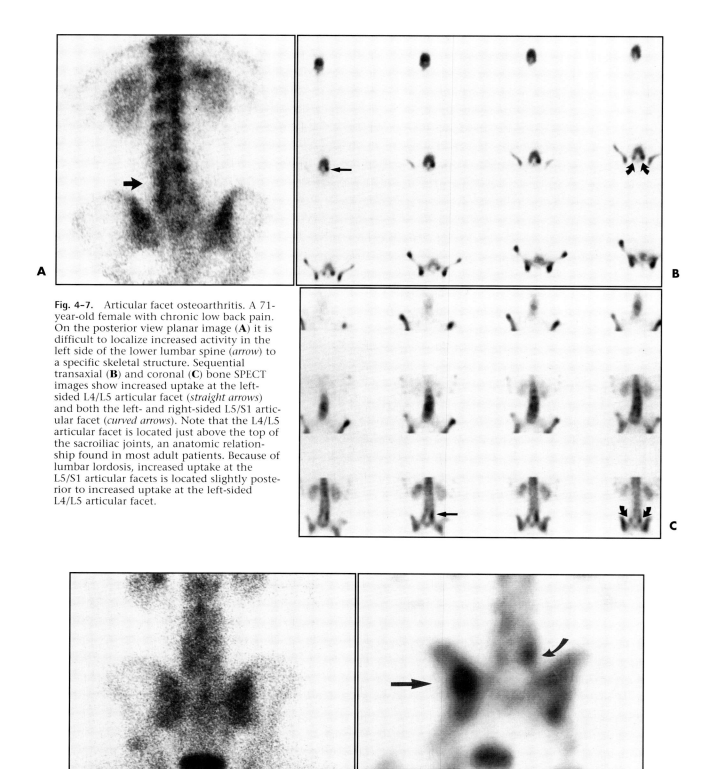

Fig. 4–7. Articular facet osteoarthritis. A 71-year-old female with chronic low back pain. On the posterior view planar image (**A**) it is difficult to localize increased activity in the left side of the lower lumbar spine (*arrow*) to a specific skeletal structure. Sequential transaxial (**B**) and coronal (**C**) bone SPECT images show increased uptake at the left-sided L4/L5 articular facet (*straight arrows*) and both the left- and right-sided L5/S1 articular facet (*curved arrows*). Note that the L4/L5 articular facet is located just above the top of the sacroiliac joints, an anatomic relationship found in most adult patients. Because of lumbar lordosis, increased uptake at the L5/S1 articular facets is located slightly posterior to increased uptake at the left-sided L4/L5 articular facet.

Fig. 4–8. Increased sacroiliac joint uptake ascribed to osteoarthritis. A 57-year-old male with chronic low back pain. Posterior planar image (**A**) shows a very subtle increase in uptake in the right sacroiliac joint. Coronal SPECT image (**B**) more clearly defines the increased uptake in the SIJ (*straight arrow*) along with demonstrating increased uptake at the left-sided L5/S1 articular facet (*curved arrow*). SIJ abnormalities are best seen when the normal portions of the joint appear in a shade of gray rather than dark black.

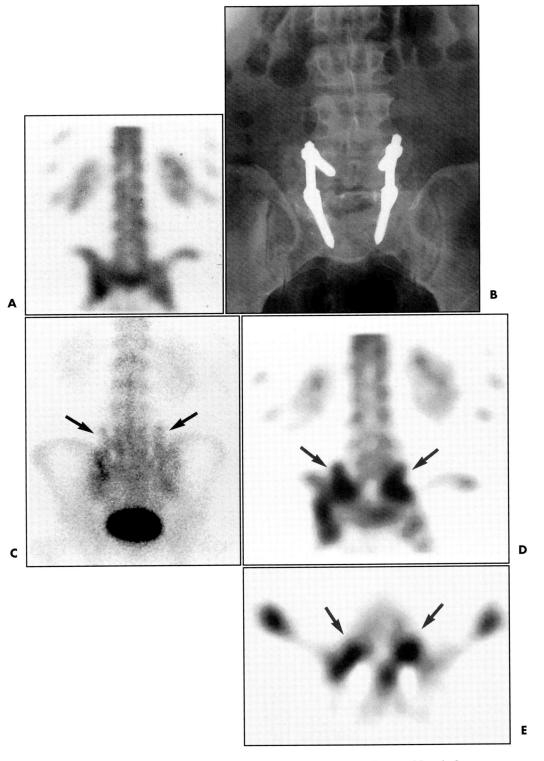

Fig. 4-9. Pseudoarthrosis with increasingly severe low back pain. A 42-year-old male 2 years after L4 to S1 spinal fusion. Coronal SPECT image (**A**) from preoperative study is normal. Postoperative radiograph two years later (**B**) shows posterolateral bony fusion mass along with metallic instrumentation. Posterior view planar image (**C**) shows slightly increased uptake in the left SIJ. Note that the bony fusion mass located to the left and right of the lower lumbar spine (*arrows*) does not show increased activity when compared with the lumbar spine. Coronal SPECT image (**D**) shows markedly increased abnormal uptake in the left and right sides of the fusion mass corresponding to sites of pseudoarthrosis demonstrated at the time of subsequent surgery (*arrows*). Apparent asymmetry in SIJ activity is due to slight rotation. Transaxial SPECT image (**E**) shows the markedly increased uptake in the left and right sides of the fusion mass (*arrows*) located anterior and slightly lateral to the photon-deficient defects created by the metallic internal fixation devices.

ographs. In the Slizofsky series, surgical findings were used as the method of proof for pseudoarthrosis. Six of the eleven asymptomatic patients had focal areas of increased activity in the bony fusion mass which were interpreted as representing painless pseudoarthrosis, a recognized orthopedic condition.[63,87] The authors felt that planar imaging was substantially enhanced by SPECT in 14 of the 26 cases. They conclude that for patients who remain symptomatic after lumbar spinal fusion, bone scintigraphy with SPECT is of significant value in detecting painful pseudoarthrosis. Lusins et al reported favorable results for SPECT bone scanning among 25 patients who continued to complain of low back pain following spinal surgery.[63] The authors note that the likelihood of a positive SPECT bone scan increases as the number of spinal segments treated with laminectomy or spinal fusion is increased. They suggest that this is due to increased potential for instability when laminectomies involve multiple spinal segments. Furthermore, increased forces of flexion/extension occurring above and below fusions extending across multiple lumbar spinal segments may be responsible.

More recently Even-Sapir et al reported results for a group of 33 patients undergoing SPECT to assess the painful late effects of lumbar spinal fusion.[27] For patients more than four years after surgery, the most common SPECT abnormality was increased uptake in the vertebral bodies and apophyseal joints at the motion-free segments adjacent to the fused segments (62.5% of patients). The authors conclude that SPECT can be used to identify both intervertebral spondylosis and apophyseal joint osteoarthritis at spinal segments adjacent to a lumbar fusion. These results suggest that SPECT is of value in assessing the painful late effects of lumbar spinal fusion.

Hathaway et al reported favorable results for bone SPECT when used to image 11 patients who had undergone spinal fusion with placement of femoral allografts.[40]

PRIMARY AND METASTATIC TUMORS OF THE SPINE

Primary and metastatic tumors of the spine have also been successfully imaged with SPECT. Wahl and Botti reported favorable results for 15 patients with suspected bone metastases undergoing lumbosacral spine bone SPECT.[109] SPECT found all lesions seen on the planar studies as well as abnormalities in an additional 5 patients. For 3 other patients SPECT added significant information to that obtained on the planar views. Anees et al, in reporting results for a large series of patients undergoing bone SPECT for low back pain, found 11 patients who had normal planar images but positive SPECT findings due to bone metastases.[4] Caluser et al, in their multimodality report for 21 patients with malignant disease, concluded that "CT scanning seems to be more sensitive than planar imaging but less than SPECT for the detection of metastatic lesions in the thoracic and lumbar spine."[15] Osteoid osteoma and other primary bone tumors of the spine in addition to such common spinal pathology as osteomyelitis, diskitis, stress fractures

and other trauma, and Paget's disease have been better imaged with SPECT than with planar technique.*

Hips

In most clinical nuclear medicine practices, osteonecrosis is the most frequently encountered indication for bone SPECT of the hips. The examination, however, can also be used for imaging arthritis, occult fractures, infection, and heterotopic ossification in or near the hip joints.

In adult populations a photon-deficient defect in the femoral head frequently is the earliest scintigraphic evidence of osteonecrosis, and bone scans often demonstrate absent or decreased femoral head activity before conventional radiography shows any morbid changes (Chapter 15). In fact, when used to image adult populations at risk for osteonecrosis, investigators have found that bone scanning may show the presence of "silent" osteonecrosis before hip pain develops. Such individuals will eventually progress through the stages of the disease, ending with collapse of the femoral head and disruption of the hip joint.[46,60] As is discussed in Chapter 5, a radiographic staging of femoral head osteonecrosis based both on conventional radiography and on MRI has been proposed.[31,59,70] Serial bone scans during the clinical course of osteonecrosis will show increased activity gradually appearing in the femoral metaphysis and in the bone adjacent to the articular surfaces of the involved hip. This progression of scintigraphic findings is probably due to ingrowth of osteoblast upward from the metaphysis as well as development of osteoarthritis within the hip joint.[22,46,66] Eventually these areas of increased activity may merge and totally obliterate the original deficient photon defect.[22,46,98] As long as the photon-deficient defect can still be imaged, the scintigraphic diagnosis of osteonecrosis can still be made with confidence. However, once the photon-deficient defect has been obliterated or obscured, it might be difficult to distinguish osteonecrosis from osteoarthritis, fracture, inflammatory arthritis, or other clinical conditions associated with increased bony repair about the hip joint.[1,62,66]

Most orthopedic procedures for femoral head osteonecrosis undertaken with the intention of preserving the hip joint must be performed in the early stages of the disease. Such joint-preserving surgeries include core decompression, bone grafting, and osteotomy.[28,31,67,100] If bone scanning is to be used in evaluating such patients for joint-preserving surgery, the task for nuclear medicine is to image at the earliest stages of osteonecrosis a photon-deficient defect within the femoral head. As is described in the following material, this task is best accomplished using SPECT. An alternative method for the sensitive and specific early diagnosis of osteonecrosis by MRI is presented in Chapter 5. In more advanced cases of femoral head osteonecrosis that have progressed to loss of articular cartilage and with secondary osteoarthritis, orthopedic treatments undertaken to relieve pain and

*References 11,73,76,101,102,105.

restore function include hemiarthroplasty and total joint replacement.

Most investigators report that SPECT has a higher sensitivity than planar imaging for detection of osteonecrosis of the femoral head[16,30,38] although one study did find similar sensitivities for the two bone scanning techniques.[99] A photon-deficient defect within the femoral head may be obscured on planar imaging by activity originating in the acetabulum or the soft tissues adjacent to the hip. Stromqvist reports that when acquiring a planar bone scan image, less than half the activity ascribed to the femoral head is derived from radioactive decay actually occurring in the femoral head.[98] SPECT by isolating the tomographic plane containing the femoral head improves image contrast and facilitates detection of osteonecrosis. Collier et al compared planar and SPECT bone scanning in 21 adult patients with the clinical diagnosis of osteonecrosis of the femoral head.[16] Using SPECT, 12 of 15 symptomatic patients and 17 of 20 involved hips (sensitivity of 0.85) were correctly identified, whereas with planar imaging only 8 of 15 patients and 11 of 20 hips (sensitivity of 0.55) were detected (Fig. 4-1). In this series there were no false-positive diagnoses on SPECT or planar scintigraphy. However, in some but not all series directly comparing bone scanning with MRI, the sensitivities and specificities for the radionuclide technique have been lower than for MRI.[2,8,41,64,99] Continued advances in MRI in addition to the introduc-

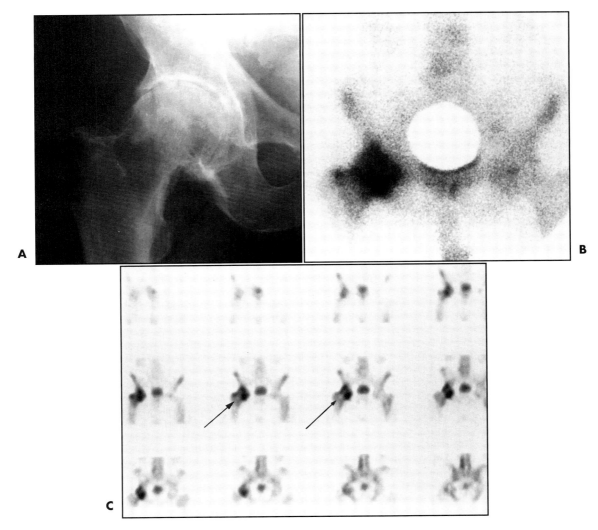

Fig. 4-10. Advanced osteoarthritis mimics appearance of osteonecrosis on bone SPECT. A 72-year-old male with right hip pain. Radiograph (**A**) shows joint space narrowing, sclerosis, and large osteophyte formation on both sides of the hip joint. Anterior view planar image (**B**) shows increased activity over the hip joint, which extends to cover the right femoral head. Sequential coronal SPECT images (**C**) cut through the activity that surrounds the femoral head. Although this to a degree mimics the appearance of osteonecrosis, note that increased activity is limited to areas involved with osteoarthritis and does not involve the femoral neck (*arrows*). Sparing of the subcapital portion of the femoral neck, which invariably shows markedly increased uptake in advanced osteonecrosis, is helpful in distinguishing on bone SPECT images between advanced osteoarthritis and osteonecrosis.

tion of high-resolution multidetector SPECT systems suggest that additional prospective studies need to be undertaken. The clinically relevant population of patients with early stage osteonecrosis for whom joint preserving surgery may be of value should be studied.

At our institution the routine examination for adults with clinical suspicion of osteonecrosis is a rapid-sequence flow study and blood pool images, high-resolution anterior and posterior planar images, and SPECT. The flow study is undertaken to exclude the possibility of an inflammatory process within the hip joint. In addition, it has been reported that increased flow in the region of the proximal femoral metaphysis and adjacent soft tissues is an occasionally encountered indirect sign of femoral head osteonecrosis. This increased flow probably represents collateral circulation from the medial circumflex artery.[16,103] When interpreting bone SPECT of the femoral head, bladder filling artifacts (see Fig. 18-9), activity associated with open or recently fused growth plates, and large marginal osteophytes (Fig. 4-10) can all make the task more difficult. When bone SPECT is either normal or nondiagnostic due to bladder filling artifacts, consideration should be given to further evaluation with MRI. For adult patients undergoing bone scintigraphy of the hips, pinhole planar views rarely provide information not available with SPECT.[38] However, as is discussed in Chapter 16, pinhole images are routinely obtained during bone scanning of the hips in children.

Bone SPECT also has been used to evaluate the viability of acetabular bone grafts. In reporting results for a series of 13 patients who had undergone acetabular bone graft replacement in order to ensure a secure fixation of an acetabulum prosthesis, Gordon et al noted that bone SPECT was superior to both planar bone scanning and radiography in assessing graft viability.[37] Similar results also were described by Transick et al.[104] Hierholzer et al reported favorable results for bone SPECT when used to evaluate pedicled pelvic bone grafts among patients treated by this surgical procedure for osteonecrosis of the femoral head.[44] In particular, these authors found bone SPECT to be superior to planar imaging for evaluation of bone graft incorporation and viability.

Knees

Bone SPECT of the knees has been used to detect and assess osteoarthritis, meniscal tears, cruciate ligament tears, osteonecrosis, osteochondritis dissecans, subchondral fractures, and tumors. The technique appears particularly well suited to assessing the extent of osteoarthritis in the three compartments of the knee and in detecting increased uptake secondary to torn menisci.

When interpreting a bone SPECT study of the knees, divide the knee into three compartments: medial, lateral, and patellofemoral. Do not interpret areas of prominent uptake in the proximal tibiofibular joint and the anterior tibial tuberosity as representing pathology. When considering abnormalities in the medial and lateral compartments, it is important to note whether both the femoral and tibial sides of the joint are involved. For example,

osteoarthritis usually involves both sides of the joint, whereas spontaneous osteonecrosis of the lateral femoral condyle usually will extend from the subchondral bony surface of the femur deep into the adjacent femoral metaphysis with little or no increased uptake on the tibial side of the lateral compartment.

To investigate the role of bone SPECT in evaluating osteoarthritis and torn menisci, Collier et al studied 27 patients with chronic knee pain.[18] Results were correlated with subsequent arthroscopic examination of the knee. For detecting increased uptakes at sites of arthroscopically proven cartilage damage and synovitis, bone SPECT showed the greatest diagnostic advantage in the patellofemoral compartment, with a sensitivity of 0.91 for bone SPECT, 0.57 for planar bone scanning, and 0.22 for conventional radiography. Collier found a sensitivity of 1.00 for bone SPECT in detecting torn menisci when examining 14 patients with chronic knee pain (Fig. 4-11). Synovitis or cartilage damage was present near the sites of torn menisci in 11 of these 14 patients, suggesting that the increased uptake might not have been in the menisci but rather was due to altered joint mechanics and secondary arthritic changes. In studying 12 patients with suspected torn menisci, Fajman also found bone SPECT to be effective in identifying increased uptake near the sites of meniscal tears.[29] Murray et al studied 33 patients with acute meniscus tears confirmed by arthroscopy and found bone SPECT to have a sensitivity of 0.88, specificity of 0.87, and a negative predictive value of 0.91.[74] These authors conclude that if a bone SPECT examination is normal, subsequent arthroscopy to detect torn menisci is not warranted. Murray et al also reported that for 10 patients with anterior cruciate ligament tears, increased uptake was seen in 5 patients at the site of avulsion of the anterior cruciate ligament from its tibial attachment. More recently Ryan et al have reported that a crescent of increased activity in the tibial plateau on transaxial bone SPECT images, often in association with increased blood pool activity, is a reliable sign of a torn meniscus.[91]

In the United States MRI is more frequently performed than bone SPECT for the investigation of torn menisci. The MRI images often provide a convincing anatomic display of meniscus tears and other frequently associated internal derangements of the knees such as tears of the anterior cruciate ligament. Five reported series show sensitivities for MRI ranging from 0.58 to 0.94, with specificities ranging from 0.37 to 1.00.[21,33,68,84,86] Arthroscopy, the standard to which MRI is compared in these five series, may be an imperfect test. However, greater use of bone SPECT as a low-cost screening procedure or as a method of confirming questionable MRI findings before arthroscopy appears warranted.

Dehdashti et al evaluated bone SPECT of the knee in 56 patients with chronic knee pain and found the technique to be superior to conventional radiography and of particular value in detecting lateral patella facet degeneration.[24] Brecht-Krauss et al, in evaluating 15 patients with osteochondritis dissecans, found that planar images detected 75% of lesions, whereas SPECT was positive in

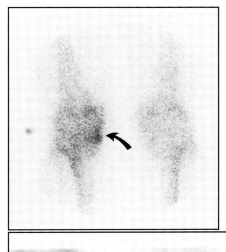

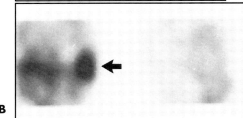

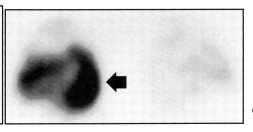

Fig. 4–11. Torn medial meniscus. A 21-year-old male who had experienced pain in the medial side of the right knee during the past 8 months. No history of trauma. Medial joint line tenderness was present, and radiographs were normal. Anterior view planar view bone scan image (**A**) shows increased uptake in the medial compartment of the painful right knee principally at the joint line (*curved arrow*). Coronal (**B**) and transaxial (**C**) SPECT images show markedly increased uptake in the medial compartment, which at the time of subsequent arthroscopy was noted to correspond to the site of a tear through the mid and posterior portion of the medial meniscus (*arrows*). *(From Collier BD, Johnson RP, Carrera GF, et al: Chronic knee pain assessed by SPECT: Comparison with other modalities. Radiology 1985; 157:795; with permission.)*

all patients with this disorder.[12] Bone SPECT of the knees also has been applied to the study of giant cell tumors,[58] osteonecrosis,[39] osteoid osteoma,[75] subchondral fractures,[65] and in children, physeal arrest.[114]

Skull and Facial Bones

In the region of the skull and facial bones, bone SPECT often has been used to detect internal derangement of the TMJ, infection of the paranasal sinuses and mastoid bones, and bone metastases. Because of the complex three-dimensional anatomy with extensive overlap of bony structures, the facial bones and base of the skull may be difficult to evaluate with planar bone scan images. For this reason, bone SPECT also has been used to assess the extent of fibrous dysplasia, histiocytosis X, and other morbid processes that frequently involve these structures. Both hyperplasia of the mandibular condyle and vascularized mandibular bone grafts have been evaluated with SPECT.

TMJ dysfunction is thought to effect as much as a quarter of the adult population.[96] Symptoms include joint pain, limited opening, locking, and an audible opening click. The TMJ is a synovial joint with superior and inferior compartments separated by a normally flexible disk. During opening of the mouth, the mandibular condyles rotate and move on this pliable disk, which "cushions" such motion. In internal derangement the disk typically is displaced anteriorly and often is deformed or perforated. Secondary osteoarthritic change, often with osteophyte formation along the anterior and superior margin of the mandibular condyle, may then develop.

Increased uptake secondary to internal derangement

of the TMJ is more clearly seen on SPECT than on planar bone scans (Fig. 4-12). The normal TMJ has activity only slightly greater than the adjacent cranium. Oesterreich et al developed a semiquantitative method for evaluating this normal scintigraphic relationship: a TMJ was considered abnormal when its uptake was more than three times that of the cranium.[80] This semiquantitative method was based on the study of 60 symptomatic patients with arthrographically confirmed TMJ internal derangement and 30 normal volunteers. A sensitivity of up to 0.89 and specificity of 0.73 was reported for this technique. Using operative findings of internal derangement as the standard for comparison, Collier et al studied the diagnostic efficacy of SPECT and planar bone scintigraphy, arthrography, and conventional radiography in 36 patients with symptomatic TMJ dysfunction undergoing preoperative testing.[17] The 0.94 sensitivity of bone SPECT was comparable to the 0.96 sensitivity of arthrography and significantly better than the 0.76 sensitivity of planar bone scanning or the 0.04 sensitivity of transcranial lateral radiographs. All patients in this series had significant symptoms. Specificity, therefore, was based on whether the symptoms were severe enough eventually to require surgical correction. Collier reported a 0.70 specificity of SPECT for internal derangement of the TMJ, suggesting that the technique measures the severity of internal joint derangement and is of value in predicting eventual need for surgical intervention. Independent reports by Katzberg, Schroeder, and Byhan also state that SPECT is superior to planar bone scintigraphy for evaluation of TMJ internal derangement.[6,53,93] Benti et al found SPECT superior to CT in 8 patients with TMJ symptoms present for less than 1 year as well as in

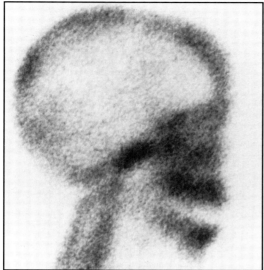

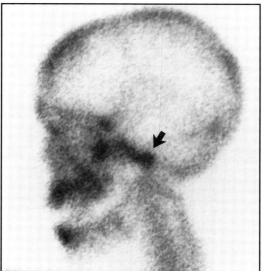

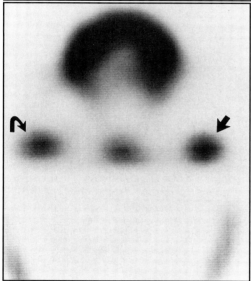

Fig. 4-12. Bilateral internal derangement of the TMJ. A 34-year-old female with joint pain and limited opening. Planar right lateral (**A**) and left lateral (**B**) views suggest increased activity in the region of the left TMJ (*arrow*). Transaxial SPECT image (**C**) obtained with a single-detector rotating gamma camera shows increased activity at both TMJs being somewhat more intense on the left (*straight arrow*) than on the right (*curved arrow*). The normal TMJ would show only slightly more intense activity than that seen in the adjacent portion of the temporal bone. *(From Collier BD: Single photon emission computed tomography: a clinical experience. In Nuclear Medicine Annual, New York, 1987, Raven Press.)*

17 patients with chronic symptoms of greater than 1 year's duration.[9] Bone SPECT also has been used to study patients in the postoperative period when symptoms either persist or recur (Fig. 4-13).

MRI frequently is used both to evaluate internal derangement of the TMJ and to study postoperative complications.[43,92] Direct visualization of the displaced TMJ disk, in addition to depiction of osteophytes, are particular strengths of MRI. Arthrography with injection of contrast material into the inferior joint space often is needed, however, to demonstrate perforation of the disk.

In a study of 21 symptomatic patients, which used arthrographic proof of disk displacement or perforation as proof of internal derangement, Krasnow et al compared MRI with planar and SPECT bone scanning.[56] MRI was slightly more sensitive: the authors report sensitivities of 0.88 for MRI, 0.76 for bone SPECT, and 0.56 for planar bone scanning. The low 0.17 specificity for bone SPECT in this series possibly was due to positive SPECT

findings in symptomatic patients with functionally abnormal joints that did not as yet display any morphologic disk abnormalities on arthrography.

SPECT of the skull and facial bones was first reported by Brown et al in 1977 and has since been extensively studied.[13,23,50] Investigators have reported using bone and occasionally gallium-67 SPECT imaging to identify sites of infection. For example, Strashun et al successfully used bone and gallium-67 SPECT studies to evaluate for malignant otitis externa.[97] Park et al used bone SPECT to evaluate 13 patients, 11 of whom were shown to have malignant otitis externa.[83] Using ROC analysis, the authors showed SPECT to have superior diagnostic efficacy when compared with planar imaging. In both the Strashun and Park series, SPECT revealed more extensive and deeper bony involvement by infection at the base of the skull. Furthermore, in a study of 12 patients with active sinusitis, Mitnick et al found that SPECT showed increased activity at 17 sites as opposed to only 7 positive

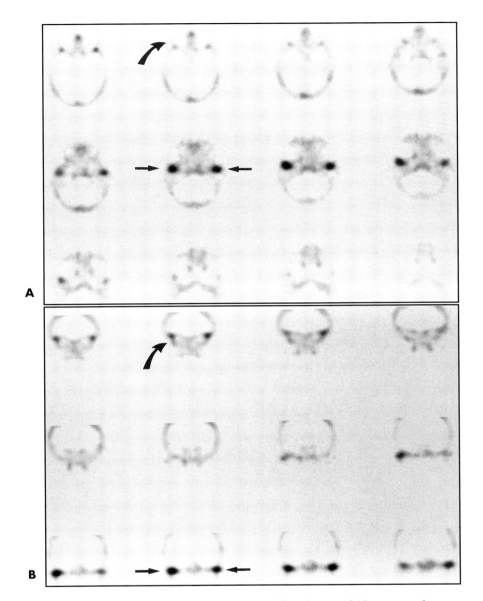

Fig. 4-13. Post-operative TMJ arthritis. A 38-year-old female treated 10 years ago for severe bilateral internal derangement of the TMJ with Silastic implants. TMJ implants subsequently revised with removal of Silastic and placement of cartilage implants. Sequential transaxial (**A**) and coronal (**B**) SPECT images obtained using a high-resolution multidetector SPECT system demonstrate markedly increased uptake at both TMJs (*straight arrows*). Other bony structures such as the lateral wall of the orbit (*curved arrows*) are well seen on these high-resolution images.

sites on planar images.[71] For tumor involvement at the base of the skull, SPECT also provides improved information about the extent and location of the disease.[54,112]

Bone SPECT of the mandible has been used to evaluate a variety of conditions including the viability of vascularized bone grafts and the metabolic activity associated with hyperplasia of the mandibular condyle. Vascularized bone grafts that receive active perfusion should be viable with uptake on bone scanning. Such grafts often are placed in the mandible of patients who have undergone radiation therapy with subsequent tumor and bone necrosis. In the early postoperative peri-

od after placement of a vascularized bone graft, patients have inflammation of the soft tissues adjacent to the mandible. In addition, a metal prothesis often is placed next to the bone graft to provide fixation and support. Early evaluation of these grafts, usually between 2 and 3 days following surgery, is desirable. Poor surgical outcomes with decreased graft perfusion secondary to hematoma, kinking of vessels, or thrombosis often can be corrected. Moskowitz and Lukash found that planar bone scanning of these grafts may be misleading as tracer may be deposited only on the surface of the graft, a phenomenon called *creeping substitution.*[72] This superfi-

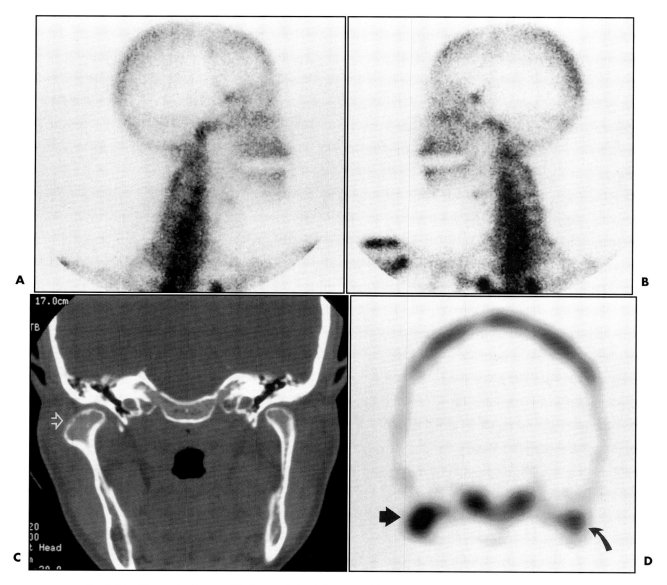

Fig. 4-14. Hyperplastic mandibular condyle. A 28-year-old female with facial deformity and bite abnormality due to hyperplasia of the right mandibular condyle. Planar right lateral (**A**) and left lateral (**B**) images fail to show abnormalities of the TMJ and mandibular condyle. Coronal CT (**C**) demonstrates the anatomy of the hyperplastic right mandibular condyle (*open arrow*). Coronal SPECT (**D**) shows markedly increased activity extending from the right TMJ deep into the hyperplastic right mandibular condyle (*straight arrow*). In addition, there is moderately intense increased uptake localized to the left TMJ (*curved arrow*), reflecting altered joint dynamics due to the bite abnormality.

cial activity may, therefore, mask an underlying photon-deficient defect due to deficient perfusion deep within the graft. Moskowitz performed bone scan imaging between 3 and 7 days after surgery on 12 patients and found that SPECT was able to remove the overlying soft-tissue activity as well as the metal prothesis, thus allowing visualization of the graft itself. For Moskowitz, SPECT successfully imaged viability throughout the entire thickness of the grafts. In a similar experience with vascularized grafts, Fig et al found SPECT to be slightly superior

to planar imaging for evaluating graft viability. The SPECT examinations were judged to be especially helpful in patients with soft-tissue swelling.[32]

Allwright et al used planar and SPECT bone scanning to evaluate 17 patients with hyperplasia of the mandibular condyle.[3] Of these 17 patients, 11 had asymmetric mandibular uptake on SPECT examinations, and in all 11 instances SPECT was thought to be superior to planar imaging in demonstrating the abnormality. The authors conclude that bone SPECT is useful in determining the site and activity of excessive growth of the mandibular condyle responsible for an asymmetry of the jaw (Fig. 4-14).

Other Clinical Applications of Bone SPECT

Given the enthusiasm and resourcefulness of nuclear medicine practitioners, it seems likely that every bone in the body has been studied at least once using SPECT. A few of these SPECT applications are particularly worthy of mention.

Wahl et al used bone SPECT to evaluate the shoulders of 21 patients.[110] Although all abnormalities were seen on both planar and SPECT images, the authors felt that the tomographic study led to better visualization of the scapular tip and coracoid process in addition to being helpful in detecting lesions in the proximal humerus.

The use of bone SPECT to image the extremities at sites other than the knees has been reported. Minoshima et al performed SPECT of the extremities on 11 pediatric patients with neuroblastoma.[69] Seven out of thirty-seven sites of metastatic disease were seen on planar images, whereas seventeen of these thirty-seven sites were detected with SPECT. Murray and Dixon used both planar and SPECT techniques to image the extremities of 5 children with osteogenic sarcoma.[73] Using cone-beam collimation for bone SPECT, Cooper et al found SPECT to be superior to planar imaging of the distal extremities.[20]

Front et al have been particularly successful with quantitation of bone SPECT data. Their initial paper validated the quantitative technique by comparing the results of SPECT examinations of the pelvis with subsequent bone biopsy specimens.[34] Later publications by the same group present the results of quantitative bone SPECT studies of the spine for normal subjects, 27 patients with hyperparathyroidism, 12 patients with thyrotoxicosis, 28 patients undergoing radiation therapy for cancer, and 16 patients with chronic renal disease.[47-49] The results indicated that quantitative bone SPECT can be used to evaluate bone metabolism. The information obtained by this quantitative procedure is a measure of bone turnover, not a measure of mineral content.

In 1984 Vanel et al reported on a large number of patients who were evaluated by various imaging techniques for pulmonary metastases from osteogenic sarcoma.[108] It previously had been shown that sites of pulmonary and other soft-tissue metastases from osteogenic sarcoma may show uptake on bone scan. There was almost a doubling of the number of pulmonary metastases detected by SPECT when compared with planar images. CT, however, was far superior to SPECT for detecting such pulmonary metastases. More recently Balingit reported the use of bone SPECT to detect renal metastases from primary osteosarcoma.[5]

Turner et al used bone SPECT to image patients treated with samarium-153-EDTMP (103-keV photon) for painful bone metastases.[107] Images showing a similar distribution of tracer were obtained when these same patients were injected with Tc-99m-MDP.

Technetium-99m-MDP SPECT also has been used to evaluate the vascularization of corallin hydroxyapatite ocular implants. For patients who have lost an eye, spheric, porous, hydroxyapatite implants are used during surgical reconstruction. Completion and attachment of this prothesis requires that the implant be revascularized by ingrowth of connective tissue. When vascularized, such implants will concentrate technetium-99m-MDP, and SPECT imaging has been used to look for complete vascularization throughout the implants. Weissman et al report that SPECT is the method of choice for detecting vascularization defects in such ocular implants.[113]

SUMMARY

In many nuclear medicine practices, bone SPECT has become a common clinical examination. Although bone SPECT of the lumbosacral spine is the most frequently requested study, nuclear medicine practitioners may be called on to perform other bone SPECT examinations including imaging of the skull and facial bones, hips, and knees. Bone SPECT, by providing otherwise unavailable diagnostic information, is a useful addition to many planar bone scan examinations. In addition, by generating new indications for radionuclide skeletal imaging, SPECT significantly increases the number of patients referred to nuclear medicine departments for bone scanning.

REFERENCES

1. Alavi A, McCloskey JR, Steinberg ME: Early detection of avascular necrosis of the femoral head by 99m-technetium disphosphonate bone scan. *Clin Orthop* 1977; 127:137.
2. Alavi A, Mitchell M, Kundel H, et al: Comparison of RN, MRI and XCT imaging in diagnosis of avascular necrosis of the femoral head. *J Nucl Med* 1986; 27:952.
3. Allwright SJ, Cooper RA, Shutter B, et al: Bone SPECT in hyperplasia of the mandibular condyle. *J Nucl Med* 1988; 29:780.
4. Anees A, Ali A, Erwin WD, et al: Evaluation of lower back pain. Improvement with SPECT imaging. *J Nucl Med* 1987; 28:654.
5. Balingit AG, Rudd S, Williams S: Clinical utility of bone SPECT scintigraphy in renal metastases from primary osteosarcoma. *Clin Nucl Med* 1994; 19:1098.
6. Bayhan H, Kinaci C, Ozguven MA, et al: Evaluation of temporomandibular joint dysfunction by Tc-99m MDP planar and SPECT bone scans. *Eur J Nucl Med* 1990; 16:527.
7. Bellah RD, Summerville DA, Treves ST, et al: Low back pain in adolescent athletes: Detection of stress injury to the pars interarticularis with SPECT. *Radiology* 1991; 180:509.
8. Beltran J, Herman LT, Burk JM, et al: Femoral head necrosis: MR imaging with clinical pathologic and radionuclide correlations. *Radiology* 1988; 166:215.
9. Benti R, Zito F, Ciancaglini R, et al: Noninvasive assessment of bone damage with CT and SPECT in temporomandibular joint (TMJ) osteoarthrosis. *Eur J Nucl Med* 1988; 14:324.

10. Bodner RJ, Heyman S, Drummond DS, Gregg JR: The use of single photon emission computed tomography (SPECT) in the diagnosis of low-back pain in young patients. *Spine* 1988; 13:1155.

11. Boyko OB, Kreipke DL, Park HM, et al: Evaluation with technetium-99m MDP and SPECT of unilateral articular pillar compression deformity in acute cervical spine trauma. *J Nucl Med* 1987; 28:751.

12. Brecht-Krauss D, Wetzel R, Weller R, et al: Bone SPECT in osteochondritis of the knee joint. *Eur J Nucl Med* 1989; 15:493.

13. Brown ML, Keyes JW, Leonard PF, et al: Facial bone scanning by emission tomography. *J Nucl Med* 1977; 18:1184.

14. Bunker SR, Handmaker H, Torre DM, et al: Pixel overflow artifacts in SPECT evaluation of the skeleton. *Radiology* 1990; 174:229.

15. Caluser CI, Macapinlac HA, Abdel-Dayem HM, et al: Role of Tc-99m MDP planar and SPECT bone scanning versus CT in evaluation of the spine in patients with malignant disease. *Radiology* 1991; 181:221.

16. Collier BD, Carrera GF, Johnson RP, et al: Detection of femoral head avascular necrosis in adults by SPECT. *J Nucl Med* 1985; 26:979.

17. Collier BD, Carrera GF, Messer EJ, et al: Internal derangement of the temporomandibular joint: Detection by single-photon emission computed tomography. *Radiology* 1983; 149:557.

18. Collier BD, Johnson RP, Carrera GF, et al: Chronic knee pain assessed by SPECT: Comparison with other modalities. *Radiology* 1985; 157:795.

19. Collier BD, Johnson RP, Carrera GF, et al: Painful spondylolysis or spondylolisthesis studied by radiography and single photon emission computed tomography. *Radiology* 1985; 154:207.

20. Cooper JA, Mahmood MM, Smith HS, McCandless BK: Tomographic imaging of the distal extremities using cone-beam collimation. *J Nucl Med* 1994; 35:914.

21. Crues JV, Mink J, Levy TL, et al: Meniscal tears of the knee: Accuracy of MR imaging. *Radiology* 1987; 164:445.

22. D'Ambrosia RD, Shoji H, Riggins RS, et al: Scintigraphy in the diagnosis of osteonecrosis. *Clin Orthop* 1978; 130:139.

23. De Roo M, Mortelmans L, Devos P: Single photon emission computerized tomography of the skull. *Nucl Med Commun* 1985; 6:649.

24. Dehdashti F, Collier BD, Johnson RP, et al: Patellar SPECT and planar imaging in orthopaedic patients with knee pain. *Radiology* 1987; 165:137.

25. Even-Sapir E, Barnes D, Iles S, Nickerson R: 180° SPECT of the spine in patients with LBP: Comparison with 360° acquisition. *J Nucl Med* 1992; 33:950.

26. Even-Sapir E, Martin RH, Barnes DC, et al: Role of SPECT in differentiating malignant from benign lesions in the lower thoracic and lumbar vertebrae. *Radiology* 1993; 187:193.

27. Even-Sapir E, Martin RH, Mitchell MJ, et al: Assessment of painful late effects of lumbar spinal fusion with SPECT. *J Nucl Med* 1994; 35:416.

28. Fairbank AC, Bhatia D, Jinnah RH, Hungerford DS: Long-term results of core decompression for ischaemic necrosis of the femoral head. *J Bone Joint Surg* 1995; 77:42.

29. Fajman WA, Diehl M, Dunaway E, et al: Tomographic and planar radionuclide imaging in patients suspected of meniscal injury: Arthroscopic correlation. *J Nucl Med* 1985; 26:77.

30. Feiglin D, Levine M, Stulberg B, et al: Comparison of planar (PBS) and SPECT scanning in the diagnosis of avascular necrosis (AVN) of the femoral head (FH). *J Nucl Med* 1986; 27:952.

31. Ficat RP: Treatment of avascular necrosis of the femoral head. In *The Hip: Proceedings of the 11th Open Scientific Meeting of the Hip Society*. CV Mosby, St Louis, 1983, p 279.

32. Fig LM, Shulkin BL, Sullivan MJ, et al: The utility of emission tomography in evaluation of mandibular bone grafts. *Arch Otolaryng Head Neck Surg* 1990; 116:191.

33. Fischer S, Fox J, Pizzo W, et al: Accuracy of diagnoses from magnetic resonance imaging of the knee. *J Bone Joint Surg* 1991; 73:2.

34. Front D, Israel O, Jerushalmi J, et al: Quantitative bone scintigraphy using SPECT. *J Nucl Med* 1989; 30:240.

35. Gates GF: SPECT imaging of the lumbosacral spine and pelvis. *Clin Nucl Med* 1988; 13:907.

36. Gillen GJ, McKillop JH, Hilditch TE, et al: Digital filtering of the bladder in SPECT bone studies of the pelvis. *J Nucl Med* 1988; 29:1587.

37. Gordon SL, Binkert BL, Rashkoff ES, et al: Assessment of bone grafts used for acetabular augmentation in total hip arthroplasty. *Clin Ortho Rel Res* 1985; 201:18.

38. Gruen GS, Mears DC, Tauxe WN, et al: Distinguishing avascular necrosis from segmental impaction of the femoral head following an acetabular fracture. *J Nucl Med* 1987; 28(suppl):664.

39. Gupta SM, Foster CR, Kayani N: Usefulness of SPECT in the early detection of avascular necrosis of the knees. *Clin Nucl Med* 1987; 12:99.

40. Hathaway R, Rao S, Stewart CA, et al: Evaluation of femoral allograft in the spine using bone SPECT. *J Nucl Med* 1991; 32:913.

41. Hawkins RA, Flynn R, Bassett LW, et al: SPECT and MRI for evaluation of aseptic necrosis of the femoral heads. *J Nucl Med* 1987; 28:564.

42. Hellman RS, Nowak D, Collier BD, et al: Evaluation of distance weighted SPECT reconstruction for skeletal scintigraphy. *Radiology* 1986; 159:473.

43. Helms CA, Kaban LB, McNeill C, et al: Temporo-mandibular joint: Morphology and signal intensity characteristics of the disk at MR imaging. *Radiology* 1989; 172:817.

44. Hierholzer J, Keske U, Cordes M, et al: Bone SPECT and 3D reconstruction in patients with hip-head-necrosis before and after implantation of a pedicled pelvic cone graft. *J Nucl Med* 1991; 32:1027.

45. Holder LE, Machin JL, Asdourian PL, et al: Planar and high-resolution SPECT bone imaging in the diagnosis of facet syndrome. *J Nucl Med* 1995; 36:37.

46. Hull A, Hattner RS, Vincente F: Prospective scintigraphic evaluation of avascular necrosis (AVN) of the femoral head in renal transplant recipients. *J Nucl Med* 1979; 20:646.

47. Israel O, Front D, Hardoff R, et al: In vivo SPECT quantitation of bone metabolism in hyperparthyroidism and thyrotoxicosis. *J Nucl Med* 1991; 32:1157.

48. Israel O, Gips S, Hardoff R, et al: Quantitative bone SPECT for prediction of bone loss in patients with chronic renal disease. *Eur J Nucl Med* 1994; 21:573.

49. Israel O, Gorenberg M, Frenkel A, et al: Local and systemic effects of radiation on bone metabolism measured by quantitative SPECT. *J Nucl Med* 1992; 33:1774.

50. Israel O, Jerushalmi J, Frenkel A, et al: Normal and abnormal single photon emission computed tomography of the skull: Comparison with planar scintigraphy. *J Nucl Med* 1988; 29:1341.

51. Jacobsson H, Larsson SA, Vesterskold L, et al: The application of single photon emission computed tomography to the diagnosis of ankylosing spondylitis of the spine. *Br J Radiol* 1984; 57:133.

52. Kanmaz B, Yu L, Uzum F, et al: SPECT vs. planar scintigraphy in patients with low back pain. *J Nucl Med* 1992; 33:868.

53. Katzberg RW, O'Mara RE, Tallents RH, et al: Radionuclide skeletal imaging and single photon emission computed tomography in suspected internal derangements of the temporomandibular joint. *J Oral Maxillofac Surg* 1984; 42:782.

54. Keogan MT, Antoun N, Wraight EP: Evaluation of the skull base by SPECT: A comparison with planar scintigraphy and computed tomography. *Clin Nucl Med* 1994; 19:1055.

55. Kouris K, Al-Ghussain NM, Higazi E, et al: Correction and evaluation of the bladder artifact in hip SPECT. *Eur J Nucl Med* 1989; 15:492.

56. Krasnow AZ, Collier BD, Kneeland JB, et al: Comparison of high-resolution MRI and SPECT bone scintigraphy for noninvasive imaging of the temporomandibular joint. *J Nucl Med* 1987; 28:1268.

57. Krasnow AZ, Collier BD, Peck DC, et al: The value of oblique angle reorientation in SPECT bone scintigraphy of the hips. *Clin Nucl Med* 1990; 15:287.

58. Krasnow AZ, Isitman AT, Collier BD, et al: Flow study and SPECT imaging for the diagnosis of giant cell tumor of bone. *Clin Nucl Med* 1988; 13:89.

59. Lang P: *Magnetic Resonance Imaging in Avascular Necrosis of the Femoral Head.* Enke, Stuttgart, 1990.

60. Lee CK, Hansen HT, Weiss AB: The "silent hip" of idiopathic ischemic necrosis of the femoral head in adults. *J Bone Joint Surg Am* 1980; 62A:795.

61. Longostrevi GP, Donelli F, Masera G: Diagnostic utility of planar bone and single photon emission tomogrpahy (SPECT) in spondylolysis and spondylolisthesis. *Eur J Nucl Med* 1988; 14:325.

62. Lull RJ, Utz JA, Jackson JH, et al: Radionuclide evaluation of joint disease. In *Nuclear Medicine Annual-1983*, Raven, New York, 1983, p 281.

63. Lusins JO, Danielski EF, Goldsmith SJ: Bone SPECT in patients with persistent back pain after lumbar spine surgery. *J Nucl Med* 1988; 30:490.

64. Markisz JA, Knowles JR, Altchek DW, et al: Segmental patterns of avascular necrosis of the femoral heads: Early detection with MR imaging. *Radiology* 1987; 162:717.

65. Marks PH, Goldenberg JA, Vezina WC, et al: Subchondral bone infractions in acute ligamentous knee injuries demonstrated on bone scintigraphy and magnetic resonance imaging. *J Nucl Med* 1992; 33:516.

66. Matin P: Bone scanning of trauma and benign conditions. In *Nuclear Medicine Annual-1982*, Raven, New York, 1982, p 81.

67. Meyers MH: The treatment of osteonecrosis of the hip with fresh osteochondral allografts and with the muscle pedicle graft technique. *Clin Orthop* 1978; 130:202.

68. Mink JH, Levy T, Crues JV: Tears of the anterior cruciate ligament and menisci of the knee: MR imaging evaluation. *Radiology* 1988; 167:769.

69. Minoshima S, Uno K, Toita T, et al: Evaluation of SPECT bone studies in the extremeties of patients with neuroblastoma. *J Nucl Med* 1989; 30:858.

70. Mitchell DG, Rao VM, Dalinka MK, et al: Femoral head avascular necrosis: Correlation with MR imaging, radiographic staging, radionuclide imaging and clinical findings. *Radiology* 1987; 162:709.

71. Mitnick RJ, Postley JE, Esser PD, et al: Comparison of planar bone scintigraphy and single photon emission computed tomography (SPECT) in evaluation of patients with paranasal sinus disease. *J Nucl Med* 1983; 24:58.

72. Moskowitz GW, Lukash F: Evaluation of bone graft viability. *Semin Nucl Med* 1988; 18:246.

73. Murray IPC, Dixon J: The role of single photon emission computed tomography in bone scintigraphy. *Skeletal Radiol* 1989; 18:493.

74. Murray IPC, Dixon J, Kohan L: SPECT for acute knee pain. *Clin Nucl Med* 1990; 15:828.

75. Murray IPC, Rossleigh MA, Van der Wall H: The use of SPECT in the diagnosis of epiphyseal osteoid osteoma. *Clin Nucl Med* 1989; 14:811.

76. Nagele-Wohrle B, Nickel O, Hahn K: SPECT bone scintigraphy of benign and malignant lesions of the spine. *Neurosurg Rev* 1989; 12:281.

77. Nicholson RL, Manglal-Lan B, Wilkins K: Reverse oblique reconstruction for SPECT of the spine. *Clin Nucl Med* 1991; 16:478.

78. Nowak DJ, Eisner RL, Fajman WA: Distance-weighted backprojection: A SPECT reconstruction technique. *Radiology* 1986; 159:531.

79. O'Connor MK, Kelly BJ: Evaluation of techniques for the elimination of "hot" bladder artifacts in SPECT of the pelvis. *J Nucl Med* 1990; 31:1872.

80. Oesterreich FU, Jend-Rossmann I, Jend HH, et al: Semiquantitative SPECT imaging for assessment of bone reactions in internal derangements of the temporomandibular joint. *J Oral Maxillofac Surg* 1987; 45:1022.

81. Onsel C, Collier BD, Kir KM, et al: Increased sacroiliac joint uptake following lumbar fusion and/or laminectomy. *Clin Nucl Med* 1992; 17:283.

82. Palmer DW, Knobel JW, Collier BD, et al: Collimator for emission tomography of the head. *Radiology* 1982; 149:231.

83. Park HM, Oppenheim BE, Philippsen L, et al: Evaluation of malignant otitis externa with 99m-MDP bone scan: Comparison between SPECT and planar imaging. *J Nucl Med* 1986; 27:978.

84. Raunest J, Oberle K, Loehnert J, et al: The clinical value of magnetic resonance imaging in the evaluation of meniscal disorders. *J Bone Joint Surg Am* 1991; 73:11.

85. Read MTF: Single photon emission computed tomography (SPECT) scanning for adolescent back pain. A sine qua non? *Br J Sports Med* 1994; 28:5657.

86. Reicher MA, Hartzman S, Duckwiller GR, et al: Meniscal injuries: Detection using MR imaging. *Radiology* 1986; 159:753.

87. Rothman RH, Booth R: Failures of spinal fusion. *Orthop Clin North Am* 1975; 6:299.

88. Ryan PJ, Divadi P, Gibson T, et al: Facet joint injection in patients with low back pain and increased facetal activity on bone scintigraphy with SPECT: A pilot study. *Nucl Med Comm* 1991; 13:401.

89. Ryan PJ, Evans PA, Gibson T, Fogelman I: Chronic low back pain: Comparison of bone SPECT with radiography and CT. *Radiology* 1992; 182:849.

90. Ryan PJ, Fogelman I, Gibson T: Bone scintigraphy with SPECT in chronic low back pain. *J Nucl Med* 1991; 33:913.

91. Ryan PJ, Taylor M, Grevitt M, et al: Bone SPECT in recent meniscal tears. An assesment of diagnostic criteria. *Eur J Nucl Med* 1993; 20:703.

92. Schellhas KP, Wilkes CH, Deeb ME, et al: Permanent Proplast temporomandibular joint implants. MR imaging of destructive complications. *AJR Am J Roentgenol* 1988; 151:731.

93. Schroeder G, Reich RH, Kleba C, et al: SPECT or planar imaging in temporomandibular joint disease? *J Nucl Med* 1986; 27:953.

94. Scott AM, Schwarzer A, Cooper R, et al: Comparison of SPECT and planar bone scintigraphy methods with zygapophyseal joint injection in the evaluation of chronic low back pain. *J Nucl Med* 1992; 3:868.

95. Slizofski WJ, Collier BD, Faltley TJ, et al: Painful pseudarthrosis following lumbar spinal fusion: Detection by combined SPECT and planar bone scintigraphy. *Skeletal Radiol* 1987; 16:136.

96. Solberg WK, Woo MW, Houston JB: Prevalence of mandibular dysfunction in young adults. *J Am Dent Assoc* 1979; 98:25.

97. Strashun AM, Nejathein M, Goldsmith SJ: Malignant external otitis: Early scintigraphic detection. *Radiology* 1984; 150:541.

98. Stromqvist B, Brismar J, Hansson LI, et al: Technetium-99m-methylenediphosphonate scintimetry after femoral neck fracture. *Clin Orthop* 1984; 182:177.

99. Stulberg BN, Levine M, Bauer TW: Multimodality approach to osteonecrosis of the femoral head. *Clin Ortho Rel Res* 1989; 240:181.

100. Sugioka Y: Transtrochanteric anterior rotational osteotomy of the femoral head in the treatment of osteonecrosis affecting the hip. *Clin Orthop* 1978; 130:191.

101. Swanson D, Blecker R, Gahbauer H, et al: Diagnosis of discitis by SPECT technetium-99m MDP scintigram: Case report. *Clin Nucl Med* 1986; 11:210.

102. Swayne LC, Dorsky S, Caruana V, et al: Septic arthritis of a lumbar facet joint: Detection with bone SPECT imaging. *J Nucl Med* 1989; 30:1408.

103. Theron J: Superselective angiography of the hip. *Radiology* 1977; 124:649.

104. Trancik CM, Stulberg BN, Wilde AH: Allograft construction of the acetabulum during revision total hip arthroplasty: Clinical, radiographic and scintigraphic assessments of the results. *J Bone Joint Surg Am* 1986; 68A:527.

105. Traughber PD, Havlinen JM: Bilateral pedicle stress fractures: SPECT and CT features. *J Comput Assist Tomogr* 1991; 15:338.

106. Tsui BMW, Gullberg GT, Edgerton ER, et al: Design and clinical utility of a fan beam collimator for SPECT imaging of the head. *J Nucl Med* 1986; 27:810.

107. Turner JH, Hoffman RF, Martindale AA, et al: Samarium-153 EDTMP therapy dosimetry and SPECT in cancer patients with disseminated skeletal metastasis. *J Nucl Med* 1988; 29:762.

108. Vanel D, Henry-Amar M, Lumbroso J, et al: Pulmonary evaluation of patients with osteosarcoma: Roles of standard radiography, tomography, CT, scintigraphy and tomoscintigraphy. *AJR Am J Roentgenol* 1984; 143:519.

109. Wahl RL, Botti J: SPECT of the thoracic and lumbar spine in patients with suspected vertebral metastases. *J Nucl Med* 1987; 28:665.

110. Wahl RL, Botti J, Ackermann R: SPECT imaging of the shoulder: Pathologic anatomy. *Radiology* 1986; 161:197.

111. Wallis JW, Miller TR: Volume rendering in three-dimensional display of SPECT images. *J Nucl Med* 1990; 31:1421.

112. Wang PW, Li CH, Chen HY: Assessment of skull base involvement in cases with nasopharyngeal carcinoma—comparison of single photon emission computed tomography with planar scintigraphy. *Eur J Nucl Med* 1990; 16:S197.

113. Weissman A, Sisson J, Nelson C, et al: Utility of Tc-99m-MDP with SPECT in coralline hydroxyapatite ocular implants. *J Nucl Med* 1993; 34:110.

114. Wioland M, Bonnerot V: Diagnosis of partial and total physeal arrest by bone single-photon emission computed tomography. *J Nucl Med* 1993; 34:1410.

A MULTI-MODALITY APPROACH TO BONE IMAGING

Guillermo F. Carrera

B. David Collier, Jr.

For many patients radionuclide bone scanning fills an important and surprisingly complex role in evaluating skeletal disorders. All diagnostic tests, including imaging examinations, serve three fundamental purposes in evaluating skeletal disease: detection, characterization, and staging. Imaging studies such as conventional radiography, computed tomography (CT), magnetic resonance imaging (MRI), and ultrasound (US) serve to display both normal and morbid anatomy and physiology in a regional or anatomic context. This is important because a fundamental part of classic clinical evaluation and many forms of treatment (e.g., surgery and radiation therapy) also rely on anatomic localization and characterization. From a multimodality imaging perspective, detection of skeletal physiology is the greatest strength of radionuclide bone scanning with limited spatial resolution and virtual absence of soft-tissue visualization relative weaknesses.

CORRELATION OF IMAGING MODALITIES AND CLINICAL INFORMATION

The value of correlating bone scanning and other imaging studies with clinical findings seems obvious. Unfortunately, however, important clinical information is all too frequently overlooked. Consider, for example, the value of an accurate history of prior wrist trauma in an athlete with focal increased uptake in the scaphoid on a bone scan, a known primary tumor in a patient with a destructive lesion seen radiographically in a long bone, or gout in an individual with focal increased uptake in a great toe on bone scan. Careful clinical correlation before beginning the imaging study allows the imaging physician to tailor an examination to the desired diagnostic goals and thereafter to intelligently interpret any positive finding in terms that will prove helpful to both patient and referring physician. The converse practice—simply detecting abnormalities and listing either the most frequent or more ominous potential causes—is rarely helpful to the referring physician. The reporting of imaging results without prior clinical correlation frequently introduces considerable confusion into the evaluation of an already complex patient.

Bone is an extraordinarily dynamic tissue. Constant turnover in response to metabolic or mechanical demands results in a steady state between new bone formation and resorption. Radionuclide bone scanning takes advantage of this constant physiologic activity. Most morbid processes involving bone result in increased turnover or new bone formation. Exquisitely sensitive detection and demonstration of focal increased bone turnover makes bone scanning extremely valuable in detecting skeletal pathology, and because bone scanning is potentially a whole-body study the entire skeleton can be evaluated at once and multiple areas of abnormality, even if asymptomatic, can be detected. Some processes such as myeloma, early stage osteonecrosis, and eosinophilic granuloma characteristically destroy bone without corresponding increased bone formation. These infrequently encountered processes may be detected as "cold" areas on bone scans. The basic principles for evaluating these lesions, however, are the same as for evaluating areas of increased uptake.[8,20,31,38]

Because there are limited responses in bone to focal pathology, and both osteodestruction and osteoproduction are manifest most usually as areas of increased bone scan uptake, correlation with other, more anatomically precise, imaging studies is extremely important. When compared with bone scanning, the most helpful difference in the way radiography, CT, MRI, or US demonstrate lesions is that these other modalities offer much greater anatomic precision. Although the spatial resolution on a clinical bone scan is no better than 7 mm, the high-resolution anatomic modalities can frequently demonstrate bone structure at the trabecular level or better. Furthermore, good discrimination between soft-tissue structures is available using the digital imaging modalities of CT and MRI. Planar and single photon emission computed tomography (SPECT) bone scanning are exquisitely sensitive modalities. Unfortunately a wide variety of benign and malignant, significant and insignificant, conditions cause findings on bone scans that can be very similar if not indistinguishable. Even the intensity of abnormal uptake and distribution of polyostotic lesions is not always a reliable guide to the correct diagnosis. The combination, however, of exquisitely sensitive detection of lesions with bone scanning and precise demonstration of pathologic anatomy with the high-resolution imaging leads to the optimal evaluation.

Many lesions first detected on high-resolution anatomic studies such as plain films or CT scans are ambiguous. Although more sensitive to anatomic variation than radioisotope scanning, these modalities are by no means perfect discriminators of focal bony abnormality. In such cases, particularly if a lesion is an incidental finding, bone scanning can serve as a second-stage diagnostic test to determinate metabolic activity. In these cases the differential diagnosis provided by anatomic imaging tests is further refined by adding the physiologic data derived from bone scanning.

As treatment for both serious and minor disease becomes increasingly complex and specific, close correlation between all available imaging modalities and clinical information becomes more important. Not all areas of markedly increased uptake in the foot of a diabetic represent infections,[30] and not all areas of increased uptake in the spine of an elderly patient with breast cancer are metastases.[28] Young athletes can avulse the insertion of hamstrings but can also develop osteogenic sarcomas at this same site. Only reasonable attention to clinical detail and careful application of all available imaging modalities, with careful correlation during interpretation, yields the most accurate diagnoses. These points can be illustrated using three commonly encountered diagnostic problems: metastatic bone disease, osteonecrosis of the femoral head, and osteomyelitis in the diabetic foot.

METASTATIC BONE DISEASE

Evaluating skeletal metastatic disease is critically important to both treating physicians and diagnostic imagers.[7,13,33,40] One of the earliest and still highly successful applications of radionuclide bone scanning is evaluation for skeletal metastases in patients with known primary neoplasms. The superior sensitivity of bone scanning when used to detect metastatic bone disease is discussed in detail in Chapter 6.

Today the search for metastatic disease usually follows one of three pathways. Some primary tumors, such as breast and prostatic cancer, typically metastasize early and often to the skeleton. An initial bone scan evaluation at the time of presentation is frequently indicated to stage the tumor. After initial evaluation, asymptomatic patients with high-risk primaries are evaluated periodically in an attempt to diagnose bone metastases as early as possible. For these individuals, examinations that allow whole-body sensitivity are critically important, and the role of radionuclide bone scanning as well as nonimaging screening tests are firmly established[15,27,36] (Fig. 5-1).

The diagnostic issues are somewhat more complex for patients who develop symptoms after the initial diagnosis and treatment of a primary malignancy. For such symptomatic patients it is important to both make a diagnosis for the specific symptoms in question and—if metastatic disease becomes a significant diagnostic possibility after initial evaluation—to screen for other asymptomatic sites of skeletal metastases.[12,23] Consider a patient several years after mastectomy for breast cancer with axillary lymph node involvement but no bone metastases detected at the initial evaluation. If such a patient now presents with hip pain, a wide differential diagnosis that includes metastasis but also more favorable diagnoses such as arthritis or mechanical pain must be considered.[24,29,34] Conventional radiographs should be the first diagnostic imaging study. If the radiographic findings are characteristic of metastatic disease, further imaging is not indicated for evaluation of the symptomatic site. Whole-body bone scanning to evaluate for possible asymptomatic sites of metastases is an important next step. If asymptomatic abnormalities are detected by bone scanning, each potential metastatic lesion will require complete anatomic evaluation with radiographs and possibly CT or MRI to differentiate malignancy from less significant benign conditions. This is particularly true in weight-bearing or other mechanically critical areas where timely radiotherapy or surgical intervention may prevent fractures and other complications (Fig. 5-2).

Finally, an occasional patient presents initially with a lesion (usually discovered radiographically) thought to represent a bone metastasis. For example, an initial radiographic examination of a patient with hand pain, perhaps thought by the family practitioner to result from arthritis or trauma, may reveal an osteodestructive lesion in one of the small bones of the hand. The radiographic differential diagnosis is wide, including many metastatic tumors as well as aggressive infection and even primary neoplasms such as fibrosarcoma or roundcell tumor. Many tumors can metastasize to the hand, but few characteristically do so.[11] For such a patient, rapid and accurate diagnosis of the symptomatic focus is essential. Such a lesion deemed likely to represent a metastasis at initial presentation must be thoroughly diagnosed to the point of histologic confirmation before embarking on costly (and frequently fruitless) search for a primary lesion. Immediate diagnosis by percutaneous needle biopsy is frequently the most efficient way to establish the neoplastic origin for such a lesion. Once the diagnosis of metastatic disease is established by biopsy or other means, both the primary site and the extent of skeletal metastatic disease must be established. In these patients the initial lesion is not well evaluated unless whole-body bone scan evaluation for multifocal skeletal disease is conducted. Whole-body bone scanning remains the best way to find other skeletal sites of metastases: high-resolution anatomic studies such as CT and MR should be applied to lesions that are bone scan–positive and radiographically normal. In all of these situations, the various imaging modalities have well-defined, closely interwoven roles.

Conventional radiography was the first imaging modality applied to diagnosing skeletal metastatic dis-

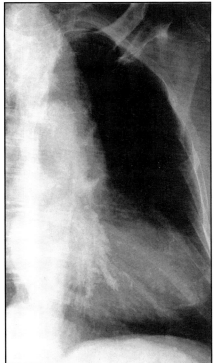

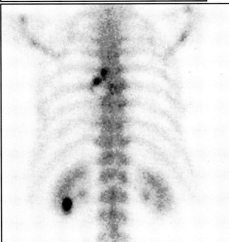

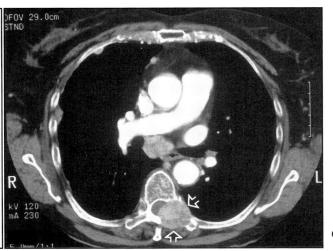

Fig. 5-1. **A,** Oblique film of the ribs and thoracolumbar junction obtained as part of an evaluation for focal midthoracic pain in a patient 3 years after the diagnosis of small cell carcinoma of the lung. This examination and complete radiographic examination of the ribs and thoracic spine are all normal. **B,** Bone scan shows two focal areas of intense abnormal increased uptake on the left side at T6 and T7. A subtle photon-deficient region is seen over the left side at T7 as well. No other abnormalities are identified on bone scan. **C,** CT scan done to evaluate bone scan abnormality reveals a highly destructive mass lesion that is responsible for the bone scan findings (*arrows*). The additional anatomic information provided by CT scanning allows diagnosis of a mass encroaching on the spinal canal as well as abutting the pleural surface of the left lung.

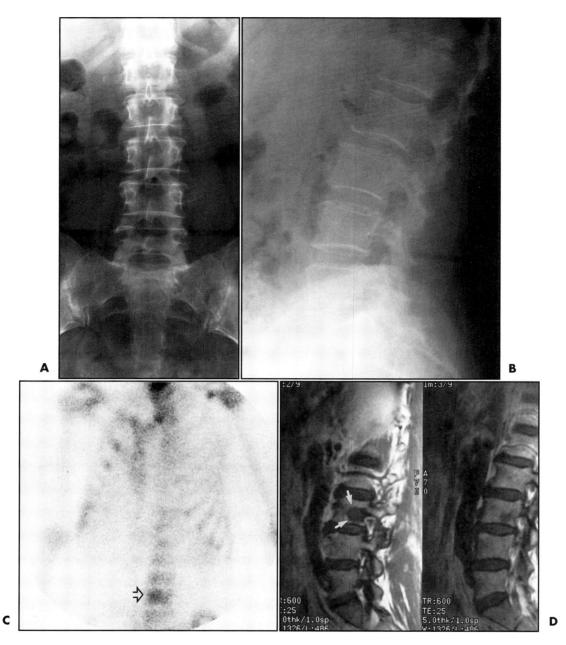

Fig. 5-2. **A** and **B,** Recent normal AP and lateral radiographs of the lumbar spine in a 65-year-old woman being evaluated for persistent midback pain 12 years after the diagnosis of breast cancer. Initial conventional radiographic evaluation and subsequent periodic examinations had revealed no evidence of metastatic bone disease. **C,** Bone scan image shows asymmetric abnormal increased uptake in the L3 vertebral body (*arrow*). Slightly oblique spot image reveals the focal area of abnormal accumulation to be anterior rather than in the posterior elements. Whole-body examination revealed no other abnormalities. **D,** Sagittal T1-weighted MR image of the lumbar spine shows a low signal lesion in the L3 vertebral body (*arrows*). This corresponds to the abnormality seen on bone scan. The signal characteristics are nonspecific.

ease, and it remains central to the diagnostic algorithm. Conventional radiographs offer numerous advantages. The equipment for conducting the examinations is widely available, and the studies are rapidly performed and inexpensive. Many abnormalities of bones and joints have characteristic radiographic appearances, so that symptoms can frequently be explained with a single, safe radiographic examination. There is widespread familiarity with the radiographic appearance of bones and joints, so the comfort level for physicians evaluating patients radiographically is high. The anatomic detail available with modern radiographic technique is excellent. Few

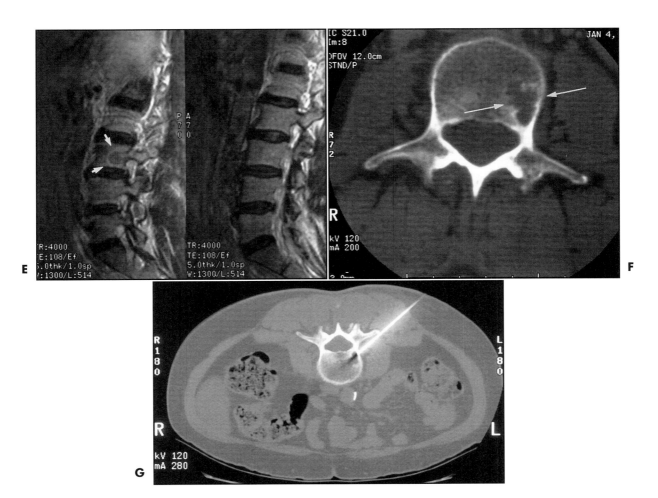

Fig. 5-2, cont'd.   E, T2-weighted sagittal MR image of the lumbar spine shows somewhat unusual findings in the L3 lesion (*arrows*). A relatively low signal intensity center surrounded by a slightly high signal intensity rim is present. Metastatic lesions demonstrate a wide variety of signal characteristics on MRI, most often low signal intensity on T1 and high signal intensity on T2. Because this abnormality was somewhat atypical, and solitary, further evaluation with CT was indicated. **F,** High-resolution computed tomogram through the L3 vertebral body reveals a destructive lesion, peripherally located, with cortical interruption as well as geographic destruction of cancellous bone (*arrows*). The appearance is typical of an aggressive lesion, in this case probably a metastasis. **G,** Because of the long interval between initial diagnosis and the development of an apparent metastasis, the presence of a solitary lesion, and the somewhat atypical MRI finding, percutaneous biopsy to confirm metastasis was performed. High-resolution CT allowed precise placement of a biopsy needle into the lesion of L3. Cytologic and histologic examination confirmed metastatic breast carcinoma.

patients who have symptoms referable to the bones or joints are evaluated without plain films, particularly since a lesion with characteristic radiographic findings is essentially fully evaluated with this single study. The main drawback to conventional radiography is that, as a diagnostic technique, it is relatively insensitive to subtle osteodestruction. Technical limitations including overlapping and often unclear anatomy, somewhat limited spatial and contrast resolution, and a relatively slow anatomic response to aggressive morbid processes. For these reasons, plain films are quite insensitive to early metastatic bone disease. Research showing that radionuclide bone scans are far more sensitive to metastases for most neoplasms than conventional radiographs is discussed in Chapter 6. The improved contrast resolution

and cross-sectional display offered by CT and MRI allow demonstration of metastatic lesions which are occult when studied with conventional radiographs. Thus, although highly specific when characteristic findings are present, a negative conventional radiographic examination should not be viewed as conclusive in evaluating symptomatic skeletal lesions.

CT has come to play a major role in the anatomic evaluation of skeletal metastases first discovered by other modalities. Modern CT is extremely rapid and shows in exquisite detail the trabecular structure of bone. In areas of complex overlying anatomy, such as the spine and pelvis, or in areas of physiologic abnormality diagnosed by radionuclide scanning that demonstrate no radiographic abnormality, CT offers a much higher degree of anatomic discrimination. Unfortunately CT cannot be used as a whole-body screening study. CT is best applied to highly detailed examinations of limited areas. Used in this fashion, CT becomes the replacement for conventional radiographic tomography and the main modality for diagnosing a radiographically occult, scintigraphically positive lesion[9] (Fig. 5-2, F).

With unsurpassed sensitivity for detecting focal soft-tissue and bone marrow abnormalities, MRI has great potential for evaluating skeletal metastases.[14] Although CT is superior for showing cortical and trabecular bony structure, in many instances the additional marrow detail depicted by MRI more than compensates for this shortcoming[37] (Fig. 5-2, D and E). Furthermore, the ability to display MRI in multiple planes and projections facilitates evaluation of such large structures as the spine or the long bones. In some instances MRI techniques which limit the signal from normal marrow fat will improve detection of metastases, and intravenously administered contrast agents also may be used for this purpose. In cases where the presence of a soft-tissue mass is a key diagnostic consideration, or if a lesion often without increased uptake on bone scan (e.g., myeloma or eosinophilic granuloma) is under evaluation, MRI becomes a primary tool for assessing extent of disease. Indeed, some authors recommend MRI as the initial imaging study for evaluating patients with multiple myeloma: the multifocal lesions in this disorder, which may be completely occult on bone scanning or conventional radiography, appear as clearly defined, high-contrast abnormalities.[26] Finally, note that the drawbacks of MRI, (including relatively high cost, relatively slow examination times, somewhat limited availability, and occasional difficulties with patient acceptance) are rapidly disappearing.

Bone scanning remains the single best screening study for patients with known or suspected metastatic disease, particularly since most lesions become positive on bone scan far earlier than on conventional radiographic examination. Whole-body evaluation is extremely important in such patients. The role of bone scan in symptomatic bone lesions is somewhat harder to define. Beyond using bone scanning to detect occult coexistent lesions, there is often great value in determining the physiologic activity of a lesion that may have specific or even diagnostic radiographic appearance. Sometimes the differential diagnosis for an abnormal skeletal radiograph includes both highly significant and active lesions and quiescent benign conditions. For example, consider a sclerotic lesion with radiographically visible chondroid matrix calcifications located in the distal femoral diaphysis. Older patients with a symptomatic joint will frequently have such a sclerotic focus with chondroid characteristics in adjacent bone. If there is no major lytic component, and if the cortex looks intact, the differential diagnosis lies between a quiescent benign chondroma, an active chondroma, and a low-grade chondrosarcoma. In such cases, bone scanning should be performed to evaluate the physiologic activity of the skeletal lesion. If the lesion is inactive on bone scan, it can be safely ignored or, at most, followed with interval radiographs. If focal

increased uptake is detected, a more aggressive course of action is followed. Although involuting benign chondromas may show increased activity on bone scan, the combination of a symptomatic focus and a physiologically active lesion with chondroid calcification requires that active chondroma or chondrosarcoma becomes the presumptive diagnosis. Biopsy then should be undertaken to evaluate for possible malignancy. Furthermore, if the bone scan shows increased activity extending beyond the margins of the radiographically visible abnormality, malignancy becomes a much more likely possibility.

Bone scans rarely are used to mark biopsy sites or plan margins for surgical resection. Biopsy using conventional radiographic or fluoroscopic guidance or CT direction is generally easy, safe, and well accepted (Fig. 5-2, G). On rare occasions when all other diagnostic studies are normal, bone scan can be used to mark an area of the skeleton for biopsy. In such cases, however, directed needle aspiration or sampling may be difficult. Open biopsy of bone scan–positive lesions, which are normal on all other imaging studies, often is necessary.

OSTEONECROSIS

Osteonecrosis of subchondral marrow, discussed in detail in Chapters 4 and 15, is a frequent comorbidity to numerous common clinical syndromes. For example, patients with chronic renal failure, marrow-packing disorders such as Gaucher's disease, chronic alcoholism, vasculitis, small-vessel occlusive syndromes such as sickle cell disease, and other conditions requiring treatment with corticosteroids are all at risk.[17,18,19] Idiopathic osteonecrosis of the femoral head or femoral condyle, although not common, is occasionally seen particularly in middle-aged or elderly women.[1,2,39] Sometimes osteonecrosis is a diagnosis of exclusion, particularly in a patient with long-standing symptoms of hip pain and disability but no predisposing factors to guide early diagnosis. In these instances the diagnosis is often radiographic and occurs late, when intervention directed at preserving the affected joint is useless. Late or end-stage diagnosis of osteonecrosis is usually radiographic.

The key to successful treatment is to establish the diagnosis of osteonecrosis before collapse of the subchondral bony plate. If the diagnosis is made during the stage of active marrow ischemia or the early reaction to infarction (e.g., edema and immediate inflammatory response), appropriate steps to protect the affected joint may be instituted. MRI is extremely effective for diagnosing marrow infarction at a very early stage.[3,5,6,16,32] Before the application of MRI to the imaging of osteonecrosis, bone scanning was recognized as the best, and indeed only, method for diagnosing early stage osteonecrosis.

Conventional radiography is of little value in early stage diagnosis of osteonecrosis of the femoral head. However, radiographs are frequently obtained to exclude other causes for the patient's hip pain (Fig. 5-3, *A*). The findings of established, late-stage osteonecrosis are radiographically characteristic.[4,22] The initial marrow edema and ischemia are radiographically invisible. Subsequent fracture due to stresses on weakened subchondral bone leads to alterations in the shape of the articular surface and the familiar radiographic "crescent sign" of osteonecrosis. As the process continues and bony response to infarction and the inflammatory response progresses, such radiographic findings as reactive sclerosis at the margins of the infarcted zone and cyst formation following liquefaction necrosis of the marrow become apparent.[35] When the constellation of findings in a symptomatic joint includes flattening of the articular surface, subchondral lucency, irregular reactive sclerosis surrounding an area of cyst formation, and finally degenerative arthritis as a secondary process, the radiographic diagnosis of osteonecrosis is obvious and accurate. Unfortunately diagnosis at the stage of advanced collapse with secondary arthritis offers little hope for protective hip therapy. Generally radiographic identification of osteonecrosis becomes part of a staging procedure, allow-

ing good diagnosis of an advanced process that frequently will require joint replacement.

Diagnosing osteonecrosis at an early stage depends on detecting either the ischemic episode or the earliest responses to it: marrow edema, acute inflammatory response, or osteoproliferative bone response before subchondral collapse. MRI is exquisitely sensitive to tissue inflammation, which is attended by changes in tissue water, microvascularity, and cellular composition. The normal adult bone marrow is largely fatty and because of this fat content is ideally suited to imaging with conventional MRI techniques. Signal changes in characteristic locations and with characteristic anatomic patterns occur very early after the ischemic episode. In clinical practice MRI has been proven highly accurate in establishing the diagnosis of femoral head osteonecrosis. Typical findings include altered signal intensity due to marrow edema surrounded by a serpiginous zone of reactive bone from both the inflammatory response and early healing reaction. When the appropriate constellation of findings is detected using MRI, conclusive early diagnosis is possible[25] (Fig. 5-3, *B* and *C*).

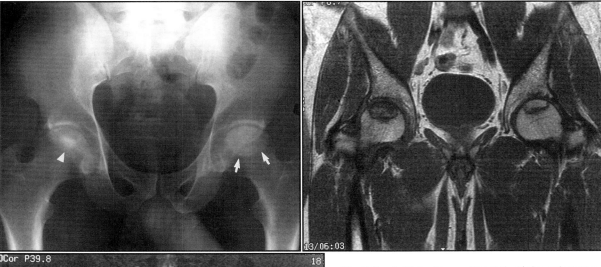

Fig. 5-3   A, Plain film radiograph of the pelvis in a patient undergoing treatment for acute leukemia, with sudden hip pain, shows a sclerotic lesion with surrounding sclerosis in the left femoral head (*arrows*). Vague sclerosis in the right femoral head (*arrowhead*) raised the possibility of bilateral disease such as osteonecrosis, but the atypical radiographic appearance (no collapse or subchondral fracture) left the diagnostic possibility of leukemic infiltration (chloroma) to be further evaluated. T1-weighted (**B**) and T2-weighted (**C**) coronal MR images show typical findings of bilateral osteonecrosis. Intermediate signal intensity abnormalities in the femoral head surrounded by a serpiginous low signal margin on T1-weighted images are classic findings in osteonecrosis. Note that the abnormalities are symmetric bilaterally and much more conclusively shown than on conventional radiographs. The T2-weighted image (**C**) demonstrates joint effusion involving the right hip (*arrows*). The MRI examination allowed definite diagnosis of osteonecrosis.

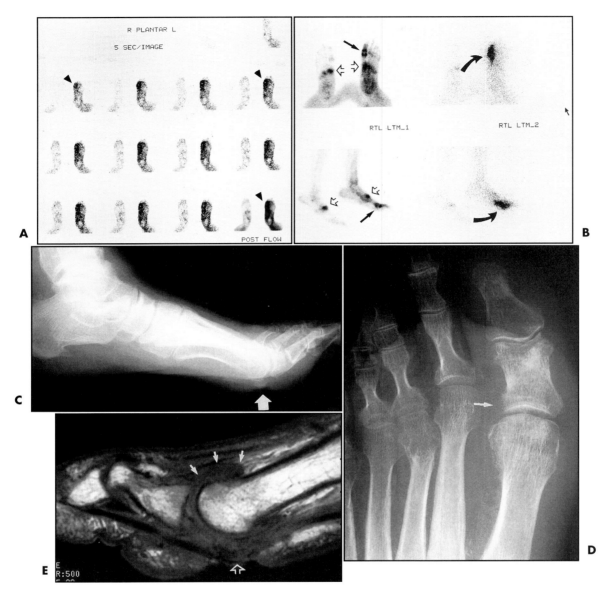

Fig. 5-4. Flow study (**A**) and simultaneously acquired bone scan and In-111 labeled white cell images (**B**) to evaluate a painful draining sinus under the first metatarsophalangeal joint of a diabetic patient. Flow study with postflow image (**A**) shows markedly increased flow along with hyperemia medially in the left forefoot (*arrowheads*). Delayed plantar and lateral view bone scan images with corresponding In-111 labeled white cell images (**B**) show increased Tc-99m-MDP uptake in the tarsometatarsal region of each foot, due to the patient's diabetic mid-foot osteoarthropathy (*open arrows*). Focal increased uptake of bone-scanning agent also is present at the base of the first proximal phalanx on the left, as well as in both sesamoids (*straight arrows*). A larger area of intense In-111 labeled white cell uptake corresponding to the left first metatarsophalangeal joint and surrounding soft tissues is present (*curved arrows*). **C**, Lateral radiograph reveals a soft-tissue defect corresponding to the ulcer (*arrow*). **D**, AP radiograph shows severe demineralization of the sesamoids, which are nearly invisible because of cortical destruction and demineralization. Close inspection reveals a focal area of cortical destruction (*arrow*) on the lateral articular corner of the first proximal phalanx. The joint width looks normal. These findings are diagnostic of osteomyelitis. **E**, Sagittal T1-weighted MR image of the first metatarsophalangeal joint shows a low signal intensity joint effusion (*solid arrows*). The ulcer on the plantar aspect of the foot, as well as the abnormal low signal intensity occupying the marrow of the medial sesamoid (*open arrow*) suggests not only soft-tissue abnormality but bone marrow involvement from osteomyelitis. The marrow in the remainder of the visualized bones is of normal, high signal intensity.

Fig. 5–4, cont'd.   Corresponding transaxial T1-weighted (**F**) and T2-weighted (**G**) transaxial MR images through the first metatarsal head show the soft-tissue defect (*open arrow*). The sesamoids show abnormally low signal intensity on T1-weighted images with correspondingly bright signal on fat-saturated T2 images (*curved arrows*). The surrounding bright soft tissue signal abnormalities demonstrate the extent of soft tissue inflammation. These findings are diagnostic of osteomyelitis involving the sesamoids as well as soft-tissue inflammation surrounding the first metatarsophalangeal joint.

Applications of planar and SPECT bone scanning to the imaging of osteonecrosis in adults are presented in Chapters 4 and 15 with pediatric applications found in Chapters 15 and 16. In the appropriate setting, bone scanning with SPECT offers good diagnostic utility for detection of osteonecrosis. The SPECT findings are generally thought, however, to be less specific, and for early disease, less sensitive than those obtained with MRI. Although MRI is becoming accepted as a superior means for diagnosing osteonecrosis, definitive proof of superiority in all clinical settings is not available. Indeed, the technical requirements for adequate MRI just like those for adequate SPECT may not be present in all cases or at all institutions. The most reasonable approach then is to view MRI and bone scanning as roughly equivalent, occasionally complementary, methods for diagnosing osteonecrosis at an early stage. Often local availability and expertise will determine the imaging method of choice.

OSTEOMYELITIS IN THE DIABETIC FOOT

Detecting osteomyelitis in the severely damaged neurotrophic foot of a diabetic patient is one of the most vexing problems facing clinicians and imaging scientists alike. Osteomyelitis is a frequent complication for diabetic patients and often occurs in ischemic extremities. It is important to separate patients with aseptic tarsal osteoarthropathy from those with osteomyelitis. Major treatment decisions, including long-term parenteral antibiotic therapy and amputation, depend on the differentiation. Strong clinical evidence of infection, when present, is very useful. Systemic evidence such as fever, leukocytosis, and other indicators, when combined with local findings of swelling, pain, and drainage favor the clinical diagnosis of infection. Unfortunately the neurotrophic foot is frequently swollen and never painful. Redness, edema, and joint instability are frequently found in aseptic neurotrophic feet. Systemic findings of infection may be present for any number of reasons in a diabetic patient, and the accurate localization of an infected site is critically important. Thus the task presented to the imager is to discriminate an infected focus in a complex anatomic area that may have extensive aseptic inflammation, osteoproliferation, deformity, and dysfunction.

Plain film radiographic findings of osteomyelitis and septic arthritis are well recognized and fully described.[21] Soft-tissue edema, periosteal reaction and new bone formation, and osteodestruction (which should be viewed as the hallmark of adult osteomyelitis) all help in defining an infected focus. Late in the course of osteomyelitis sequestrum formation may occur. Rapid destruction of articular cartilage with large joint effusions frequently are found with septic arthritis.

These radiographic findings of osteomyelitis unfortunately overlap significantly with those of neurotrophic joint disease as commonly encountered in the diabetic foot. The classic "word picture" of a neurotrophic joint as a sclerotic, disorganized structure both summarizes the salient radiographic findings and makes the problem of identifying superimposed osteomyelitis obvious. A typical neurotrophic joint is radiographically deformed, disorganized, and has abundant periosteal and juxtaarticular new bone formation. Dislocation of joints can lead to fragmentation and areas of osteodestruction. Small-vessel disease and cortical infarction causes periosteal elevation even in the aseptic bone.

Clearly the radiographic findings in the aseptic neurotrophic foot of an adult diabetic can be similar to those present in advanced osteomyelitis. It must be recognized,

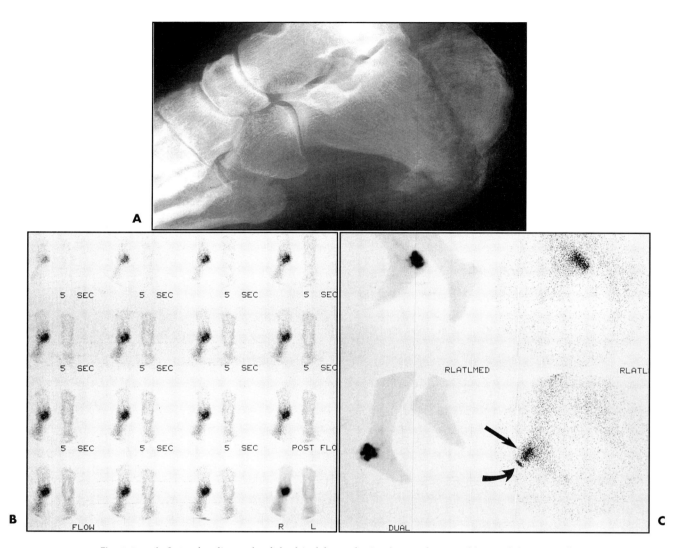

Fig. 5-5. **A,** Lateral radiograph of the hind foot, obtained to evaluate sudden inability to walk in a diabetic patient with a 3-month history of progressive heel pain. A fracture through the body of the calcaneus, displaced proximally, extending through an ill-defined lytic lesion suggesting extensive destruction of calcaneal bone is apparent. A small amount of reactive bone is present in the plantar soft tissues. This lesion was thought to represent a pathologic fracture through infected bone. The atypical appearance, however, and absence of other evidence of diabetic osteoarthropathy suggested the need for further evaluation to exclude tumor. **B,** Flow study and postflow images from a plantar view bone scan show focal increased perfusion and blood pool uptake at the right heel. **C,** Lateral view bone scan and simultaneously acquired In-111 labeled white cell images show dramatically increased uptake in the calcaneus. The In-111 labeled white cell scan shows uptake in bone at a site of osteomyelitis (*straight arrow*) with a second abnormal area plantar to the calcaneus, suggesting adjacent soft tissue infection (*curved arrow*).

however, that in both conditions radiographic change occurs late in the process. The key to radiographic diagnosis of an infected area in a neurotrophic foot is identifying a focus of osteodestruction. This is particularly supported by changes identified on sequential examinations. Regardless of whether several studies over time are available to make the diagnosis, however, the differences between a sclerotic, reactive area of neurotrophic change and an osteodestructive focus with acute periosteal elevation can for some patients be identified. Indeed, care-

ful examination of plain films may prove gratifyingly accurate in defining foci of osteomyelitis.

There is little reason to use CT in attempts to discriminate osteomyelitis from neurotrophic disease. MRI, in contrast, is being applied extensively to diagnosing osteomyelitis.[10] Subtle marrow edema, soft-tissue inflammation, and even periosteal elevation from normal cortical bone can be resolved easily if technically superior MR images are produced. For studies undertaken to diagnose osteomyelitis, the role of MRI intravenous contrast

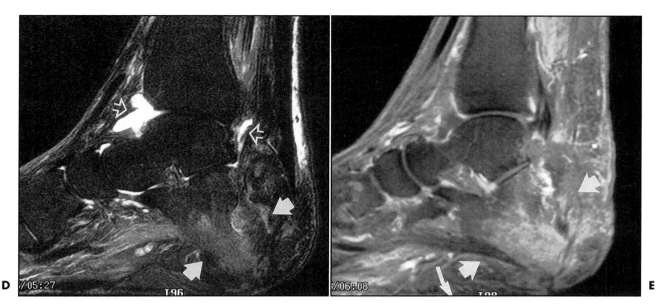

Fig. 5-5, cont'd. D, T2-weighted fat-saturated MRI shows an ankle joint effusion (*open arrows*). The marrow signal is normally dark because of fat saturation sequences. A generalized ill-defined area of increased signal intensity is present in the calcaneus and adjacent soft tissues (*solid arrows*). **E**, T1-weighted MRI sequences with fat saturation following contrast agent administration shows an ill-defined area of contrast enhancement in the calcaneus on both sides of the fracture, as well as in the adjacent soft tissues (*arrows*). These findings, together with the findings on T2-weighted sequences, indicate extensive inflammatory disease involving bone marrow as well as soft tissues. The findings are characteristic of osteomyelitis with a pathologic fracture.

agents is not yet clear. Current criteria for the diagnosis of infection in neurotrophic joints define any area of marrow edema, particularly if adjacent to a zone of soft-tissue edema or inflammation, as a focus of osteomyelitis. Using these criteria, very subtle changes can be detected and osteomyelitis diagnosed with a high degree of sensitivity. Caution is necessary, however, because any process that causes marrow inflammation or edema, including trauma or acute infarction, may lead to similar MRI findings. The possibility of a false-positive MRI diagnosis of osteomyelitis might be considered when very subtle changes of marrow edema are viewed as conclusive evidence for osteomyelitis near a neurotrophic joint (Figs. 5-4 and 5-5).

Bone scanning alone has limited usefulness in this situation. Neurotrophic joints even when aseptic typically have intensely increased uptake. If a change from a prior bone scan is identified and radiographic correlation confirms new osteodestruction, osteomyelitis can be diagnosed. Current practice, described in detail in Chapter 11, is increasingly reliant on more specific examinations for infection including In-111 or Tc-99m labeled white blood cell scanning. This combination of bone scanning and labeled white blood cell scanning offers a powerful tool for diagnosing osteomyelitis in the neurotrophic foot.

REFERENCES

1. Ahlback S, Bauer GCH, Bohne WH: Spontaneous osteonecrosis of the knee. *Arthritis Rheum* 1968; 11:705.
2. Ahuja SC, Bullough PG: Osteonecrosis of the knee. A clinicopathological study in twenty-eight patients. *J Bone Joint Surg Am* 1978; 60A:191.
3. Bassett LW, Gold RH, Reicher M, et al: Magnetic resonance imaging in the early diagnosis of ischemic necrosis of the femoral head. *Clin Orthop* 1987; 214:237.
4. Bell ALL, Edson GH, Hornick N: Characteristic bone and joint changes in compressed air workers: A survey of symptomless cases. *Radiology* 1942; 38:698.
5. Beltran J, Burk JM, Herman LJ, et al: Avascular necrosis of the femoral head: Early MRI detection and radiological correlation. *Magn Reson Imaging* 1987; 5:431.
6. Beltran J, Herman LJ, Burk JM, et al: Femoral head avascular necrosis: MR imaging and clinical-pathologic and radionuclide correlation. *Radiology* 1988; 166:215.
7. Copeland MM: Bone metastases—a study of 334 cases. *Radiology* 1931; 16:198.
8. Davis MA, Jones AG: Comparison of ^{99m}Tc-labeled phosphate and phosphonate agents for skeletal imaging. *Semin Nucl Med* 1976; 6:19.
9. DeSantos LA, Goldstein HM, Murray JA, Wallace S: Computed tomography in evaluation of musculoskeletal neoplasms. *Radiology* 1978; 128:89.
10. Erdman WA, Tamburro F, Jayson HT, et al: Osteomyelitis: Characteristics and pitfalls of diagnosis with MR imaging. *Radiology* 1991; 180:533.

11. Fam AG, Cross EG. Hypertrophic osteoarthropathy, phalangeal and synovial metastases associated with bronchogenic carcinoma. *J Rheumatol* 1979; 6:680.

12. Forbes GS, McLeod RA, Hattery RR: Radiographic manifestations of bone metastases from renal carcinoma. *AJR Am J Roentgenol* 1977; 129:61.

13. Fornasier VL, Horne JG: Metastases to the vertebral column. *Cancer* 1975; 36:590.

14. Frank JA, Ling A, Patronas NJ, et al: Detection of malignant bone tumors: MR imaging vs scintigraphy. *AJR Am J Roentgenol* 1990; 155:1043.

15. Freitas JE, Gilvydas R, Ferry JD, Gonzalez JA: The clinical utility of prostate-specific antigen and bone scintigraphy in prostate cancer follow-up. *J Nucl Med* 1991; 32:1387.

16. Gillespy T, Genant H, Helms CA: Magnetic resonance imaging of osteonecrosis. *Radiol Clin North Am* 1986; 24:193.

17. Glimcher MJ, Kenzora JE: The biology of osteonecrosis of the human femoral head and its clinical implications. I. Tissue biology. *Clin Orthop* 1979; 138:284.

18. Glimcher MJ, Kenzora JE: The biology of osteonecrosis of the human femoral head and its clinical implications. II. The pathological changes in the femoral head as an organ and in the hip joint. *Clin Orthop* 1979; 139:283.

19. Glimcher MJ, Kenzora JE: The biology of osteonecrosis of the human femoral head and its clinical implications. III. Discussion of the etiology and genesis of the pathological sequelae; comments on treatment. *Clin Orthop* 1979; 140:273.

20. Goergen TG, Alazraki NP, Halpern SE, et al: "Cold" bone lesions: A newly recognized phenomenon of bone imaging. *J Nucl Med* 1973; 15:1120.

21. Gold RH, Hawkins RA, Katz RD: Bacterial osteomyelitis: Findings on plain radiography, CT, MR and scintigraphy. *AJR Am J Roentgenol* 1991; 157:365.

22. Jaffe HL: Ischemic necrosis of bone. *Med Radiogr Photogr* 1969; 45:58.

23. Jorgens J: The radiographic characteristics of carcinoma of the prostate. *Surg Clin North Am* 1965; 45:1427.

24. Lagier R: Synovial reaction caused by adjacent malignant tumors: Anatomicopathological study of three cases. *J Rheumatol* 1977; 4:65.

25. Lang P, Jergesen HE, Moseley ME, et al: Avascular necrosis of the femoral head: High-field strength MR imaging with histologic correlation. *Radiology* 1988; 169:517.

26. Ludwig H, Fruhwald F, Tscholakoff D, et al: Magnetic resonance imaging of the spine in multiple myeloma. *Lancet* 1987; 2:364.

27. McNeil BJ: Rationale for the use of bone scans in selected metastatic and primary bone tumors. *Semin Nucl Med* 1978; 8:336.

28. McNeil BJ, Pace PD, Gray EB, et al: Preoperative and follow-up bone scans in patients with primary carcinoma of the breast. *Surg Gynecol Obstet* 1978; 147:745.

29. Meals RA, Hungerford DS, Stevens MB: Malignant disease mimicking arthritis of the hip. *JAMA* 1978; 239:1070.

30. Merkel KD, Brown ML, Dewanjee MK, Fitzgerald RH Jr: Comparison of indium-labeled leukocyte imaging with sequential technetium-gallium scanning in diagnosis of low-grade musculoskeletal sepsis: A prospective study. *J Bone Joint Surg Am* 1985; 67A:465.

31. Merrick MV: Bone scanning. *Br J Radiol* 1975; 48:327.

32. Mitchell DG, Rao VM, Dalinka MK, et al: Femoral head avascular necrosis: Correlation of MR imaging, radiographic staging, radionuclide imaging, and clinical findings. *Radiology* 1987; 162:709.

33. Mulvey RB: Peripheral bone metastasis. *AJR Am J Roentgenol* 1964; 91:155.

34. Murray GC, Persellin RH: Metastatic carcinoma presenting as non-articular arthritis: A case report and review of the literature. *Arthritis Rheum* 1980; 23:95.

35. Rosingh GE, James J: Early phases of avascular necrosis of the femoral head in rabbits. *J Bone Joint Surg Br* 1969; 51B:165.

36. Schaffer DL, Pendergrass HP: Comparison of enzyme, clinical, radiographic, and radionuclide methods of detecting bone metastases from carcinoma of the prostate. *Radiology* 1976; 121:431.

37. Sundaram M, McGuire MH: Computed tomography or magnetic resonance for evaluating the solitary tumor or tumor-like lesion of bone? *Skeletal Radiol* 1988; 17:393.

38. Teates CD, Williamson BRJ: "Hot and cold" bone lesion in acute osteomyelitis. *AJR Am J Roentgenol* 1977; 129:517.

39. Williams JL, Cliff MM, Bonakdarpour A: Spontaneous osteonecrosis of the knee. *Radiology* 1973; 107:15.

40. Young JM, Funk FJ Jr: Incidence of tumor metastasis to the lumbar spine: A comparative study of roentgenographic changes and gross lesions. *J Bone Joint Surg Am* 1953; 35A:55.

CHAPTER 6

BONE SCANNING IN METASTATIC DISEASE

Arnold F. Jacobson

Once a diagnosis of malignancy has been established, most treatment decisions are influenced by the extent of local and distant tumor involvement. At one time staging of tumors was based primarily on physical assessment and histopathology, with results of laboratory tests and occasionally exploratory surgery used to judge if distant metastases were present. However, the advances in radiologic imaging over the past several decades have provided multiple methods for noninvasive evaluation of the primary tumor and assessment for the presence of locoregional and distant metastatic disease.[161,165] The roles of different radiologic examinations have evolved with improvements in technology and accumulation of data documenting their yields for identifying the presence and extent of metastatic involvement for various malignant tumors.

Bone is a common site of involvement by metastatic disease (Table 6-1). In some tumors bone may be either an early or late site of metastatic spread, whereas in others involvement of the skeleton occurs predominantly in the late stage of widely disseminated multiorgan disease.[38,70] Diagnostic imaging to detect the presence of bone metastases is of greatest value for identification of early or limited disease, either as part of the staging of newly diagnosed malignancy or in pursuit of the etiolo-

gy of new or recurrent musculoskeletal symptoms. However, assessment of the presence and extent of bone involvement in the late stages of metastatic disease may aid in management of symptoms and identification of patients at risk for complications such as pathologic fractures or spinal cord compromise, thereby contributing to maintaining quality of life even if prognosis is not affected.[130] Imaging for detection of bone metastases can thus be useful for any cancer patient, although its greatest impact is on the management of patients with tumors known to have a predilection for early spread to bone.

Scintigraphic imaging has had a role in the evaluation of bone for metastatic disease for more than 30 years. With the evolution of bone scintigraphy radiopharmaceuticals from fluorine-18 and isotopes of strontium (Sr-85 and Sr-87m) to the technetium-99m labeled phosphate and diphosphonate compounds, improved image quality led to the increasing use of this technique as a standard element in the evaluation of cancer patients.[76,130,149] The wide acceptance of scintigraphy in the evaluation of bone metastases was due in large measure to the high sensitivity of the technique in comparison to conventional radiographs, with many studies convincingly demonstrating the superiority of bone scanning for detecting metastatic lesions.[35,37,64,72,154] Because

TABLE 6-1
Frequency of Identification of Bone Metastases at Autopsy

Malignancy	Bone Metastasis Frequency (%)
Breast	52-85
Lung	30-55
Prostate	33-85
Renal	33-40
Thyroid	28-60
Alimentary tract	3-13
Genitourinary tract	9-50

Modified from Galasko CSB, The anatomy and pathways of skeletal metastases, in Weiss L, Gilbert AH, (eds): *Bone Metastasis*, Hall Medical Publishers, Boston, 1981, p 49; with permission.

of its ability to demonstrate disease before the presence of symptoms or biochemical abnormalities on routine blood tests, bone scanning came to be frequently used during the staging of newly diagnosed cancers, as well as during later evaluations for suspected recurrence or to follow the course of known metastatic disease.

Although the utility of bone scanning in metastatic disease is well established, the appropriate role of the technique in management of the cancer patient has been the subject of frequent reevaluations.[41,67,81] A commonly expressed concern is the lack of specificity of scan findings, given the multiplicity of abnormal but benign processes affecting bone that can possibly be confused with metastatic disease. A second major issue regarding bone scanning, which also applies to other methods for early detection of metastatic disease, is whether the study results are of demonstrable value in clinical patient management. Depending upon the known metastatic disease status of the patient, detecting new or additional disease may provide no established prognostic or survival benefit, which can create an ethical dilemma for both the diagnostician and the clinician. Although an in-depth discussion of this topic goes beyond the scope of this chapter, it is important to appreciate that just because a test has a high sensitivity for detection of occult disease does not necessarily justify its routine clinical use.[18]

This chapter discusses bone scanning in metastatic disease, and the chapter is organized to emphasize basic attributes of secondary malignant involvement of bone and the general principles that affect its detection via radionuclide techniques. While pediatric studies are mentioned only briefly in this chapter, bone scanning for metastatic disease in children is covered in greater detail in Chapter 16. Extensive discussions of scan results for individual tumor types have not been presented, although a wide array of relevant references have been cited. Also, the primary focus is on the Tc-99m diphosphonate bone scan, with other radiopharmaceuticals that have been used for identification of bone metastases only briefly noted. To provide a balanced perspective on the role of scintigraphic bone imaging in cancer patients, the controversies concerning the appropriate use of scanning for different malignancies and at different stages in cancer progression are presented and critically examined. Although the extensive literature on scintigraphic bone imaging in oncology makes it virtually impossible to review all aspects of this topic in detail, the goal of this chapter is to provide a clearer understanding of the documented value of bone scanning for evaluating metastatic disease in the cancer population, serving as a counterpoint to analyses whose conclusions focused primarily on the technique's limitations.[73,111,120,135,155]

ATTRIBUTES OF METASTATIC INVOLVEMENT OF BONE

Elements of the Metastatic Cascade

Metastatic disease results from a process that begins with release of tumor cells from the site of a primary malignancy and culminates with the independent growth of lesions derived from these cells at one or more distant locations. Despite the continuing expansion of knowledge on the biology of malignant neoplasms and the factors that influence their growth and dissemination, the sequence of steps that results in the establishment of metastatic disease in different organs remains incompletely understood.[145,216,217] If the metastatic process simply involved the transport of cells from one location to another, there would be a common pattern of metastatic involvement across tumor types, reflecting primarily the vascular supply of the various tissues of the body. Instead, different tumors have well-documented tendencies to involve specific distant sites, with the liver and skeletal system being frequent end organs for the development of metastatic disease, whereas sites such as the spleen and heart rarely become involved by secondary spread of tumor.[65,217] Much of our understanding of the biology and biochemistry of the metastatic process is based on animal models of human tumors,[80,128] in vitro studies of the structure and functional behavior of tumor cells,[6,12,31,145] and results of large autopsy series of cancer patients.[70,79]

Tumor cells may potentially reach sites in the skeleton via transport through the arterial or venous circulations or lymphatic channels, or by directly invading bony structures that are contiguous with a nonosseous tumor. Differences in the frequency and distribution of skeletal involvement for various tumors is in part a reflection of the varying contribution of these routes of metastatic spread. Cancers that commonly spread to bone such as those arising in breast, prostate, lung, kidney, and thyroid have somewhat different patterns of early metastatic involvement, both to skeletal and nonskeletal locations[70,214] (Tables 6-1 and 6-2). Although, as suggested by Paget more than 100 years ago, the "seed" of a tumor cell

TABLE 6-2
Skeletal Distribution of Metastatic Lesions On Bone Scintigraphy of Patients With Breast, Prostate, and Lung Cancer

Skeletal Location	Prevalence of Metastases as Detected on Bone Scan			
	Breast: Widespread (%)*	Breast: Limited (%)†★	Prostate (%)‡	Lung (%)§
Spine (unspecified)	72-87	52-53	78	93
Cervical spine	19-67	3-8	25-51	—
Thoracic spine	47-92	12-38	63-87	93
Lumbar spine	45-78	8-18	62-85	85
Pelvis	34-66	9-20	60-87	23
Ribs	60-92	6-20	57-78	93
Skull	35-60	3-15	7-28	23
Extremities	35-54	8-12	24-41	54
Sternum	20	9-12	—	—

*References 21, 50, 55, 72, 87, 104, 155, 211.

†Limited: 1-4 bone scan lesions at first recurrence.

★References 21, 99.

‡References 50, 115, 160, 183.

§Reference 211.

requires an agreeable "soil" in the distant organ for a metastasis to develop,[151] the actual metastatic process is considerably more complex than envisioned by this simple analogy. The reason one tumor cell succeeds in becoming established at a distant site and many others fail is not specifically understood, but most research indicates that the physical and biochemical characteristics of both the tumor and the distant site are contributing factors.[58,144,145] As an aid to understanding the features of bone scintigraphy across the spectrum of skeletal metastatic disease, a brief review of the elements of anatomy and physiology that influence the metastatic cascade is instructive.

The metastatic cascade is initiated by the release of a single tumor cell, or an embolus composed of several cells, in a process mediated by various proteolytic enzymes produced by the tumor.[58,145,216] Once liberated from the primary site, the cell or embolus enters the vascular or lymphatic system, where its most likely fate is to be intercepted and destroyed by cells of the immune system. It is only the occasional cell or embolus that escapes early destruction and retains the potential to become a metastasis when it reaches a distant site. Survival of the embolus at the distant location requires that implantation occur, which typically involves adherence to receptors on the vascular endothelium or the basement membrane.[58,127,145,216,217] The tumor cells may then progress to penetrate through the vessel wall into the substance of the organ and begin to destroy the site of implantation, a process mediated by growth factors and enzymes released both by tumor cells and those of the tissue being invaded.[127,145,216] This destruction increases the poten-

tial space for tumor growth, while stimulation of angiogenesis serves to increase the vascular supply of the tumor and thereby meet its nutrient requirements.[127] Progression and growth of independent metastatic deposits may also be affected by the underlying cellular matrix, such as the components of stromal tissues and matrix molecules such as laminin.[12,31] Although growth of a metastatic lesion may initially be suppressed or at least controlled by the body's immune response, in most instances the local metastatic burden eventually overwhelms the immune system's ability to exert an inhibitory effect.[127,145]

Most bone metastases develop in the red bone marrow. Slow blood flow through the marrow sinusoids is often cited as a predisposing factor for the development of metastatic deposits, but this latter process also is dependent on compounds produced both by the tumor cells and the surrounding bony environment. A key step in producing the bone lysis required for growth of metastatic tumor is the stimulation of osteoclastic activity. Both local and systemic factors may influence the level of osteoclastic activity in metastatic lesions. Tumor cells may stimulate the activity of osteoclasts by directly releasing factors such as prostaglandins of the E series, and procathepsin D, or indirectly by their influence on production of compounds by macrophages and other cells of the immune system such as tumor necrosis factor (TNF) and interleukin-1 (IL-1).[41,144,170] Bone cells can also be stimulated to produce IL-1, TNF, and IL-6.[144] Systemic factors that have been implicated in stimulating osteoclast activity in association with development of bone metastases include parathyroid hormone–related protein, transforming growth factor alpha, and transforming growth factor beta, although their individual or combined contributions remain under investigation.[22,116,144]

Routes of Tumor Spread to Bone

Tumor emboli reaching the systemic arterial circulation would be expected to result in a distribution of bone metastases closely paralleling relative arterial blood flow. However, with the exception of primary lung neoplasms, most tumors that metastasize frequently to bone show greater involvement of the spine, particularly the thoracolumbar region, than other sites.[70,199] The observation from autopsy studies that bone metastases often occurred in the absence of metastases to the lungs also raised questions concerning the eventual fate of tumor cells and emboli entering the venous circulation, since the size of these entities would prevent their passage through the terminal arterioles of the lungs (diameter 5 to 10 μm).[70] Batson's demonstration of the importance of the vertebral venous plexus provided a major insight into how tumor emboli originating below the diaphragm could become implanted in bone without passing through the lungs.[10,11] The vertebral venous plexus is a low-pressure, valveless venous system that communicates with a variety of venous channels in the pelvis, abdomen, and chest, and retrograde flow into this system can be caused by increased intraabdominal or intrathoracic pressure, such as occurs with straining or coughing. The communication of the vertebral venous plexus with the skeletal system allows visceral tumor cells from organs such as the prostate and breast to reach virtually any location from the pelvis to the cervical spine and the skull while bypassing both cavae and the portal venous system. Although there have been challenges to Batson's conclusions, with suggestion that the lungs become a major secondary source of tumor spread to bone,[209] animal and human data from most investigators have supported the role of the vertebral venous plexus as an important determinant of the predilection of bone metastases for involvement of the axial skeleton.[70,146] The variable contributions of the arterial circulation to the spread of metastatic disease, with or without lung involvement, can be seen from the range in prevalence of metastases in different organs and bones both at autopsy[70,80,214] and in experiments in which animals received intravenous injections of suspensions of tumor cells.[146,202]

The lymphatic system is only infrequently involved in the spread of tumor to bone. Cells entering the lymphatic system are generally trapped in lymph nodes, and those that eventually reach the systemic venous circulation are indistinguishable from cells that entered the venous system directly.[127] Tumor does occasionally involve bone via direct extension from an adjacent lymph node, but this is not, strictly speaking, an example of secondary spread of tumor directly to bone.

Direct extension of tumor into bone occurs most commonly from organs that either abut or are in close proximity to a major bony structure. The lung is such an organ, and it is not uncommon for peripheral parenchymal or pleural-based tumors to invade into one or more ribs. Although these lesions are not metastatic, their presence does impact on the surgical approach to a potentially resectable primary tumor. Another form of direct tumor extension to bone involves metastatic lymph nodes, typified by sternal involvement by mediastinal lymph nodes in breast cancer patients.[121]

Factors Influencing Scintigraphic Imaging of Bone Metastases

The degree of abnormal uptake of bone-seeking radiopharmaceuticals by skeletal metastases is mediated primarily by osteoblastic activity, despite the dominant role of osteoclasts in the initial resorption phase of development of most bone metastases.[22,41,144] However, osteoclasts that have been stimulated to produce increased bony resorption also secrete factors that act on the osteoblasts involved in the remodeling process, and this interrelation between the actions of these opposing cell types accounts for the increased bone scan uptake of most lesions that appear lytic on radiographs.[63,144,170] In a few tumors, most notably prostate cancer, osteoblastic reaction is the dominant feature of skeletal lesions, and factors that stimulate osteoblastic activity are present in extracts of prostatic tissue.[78,144] Although characterization of these factors remains incomplete, urokinase-type plasminogen activator may be one of importance.[78]

The spectrum of scintigraphic findings in patients with bone metastases ranges from prostate cancer, where osteoblastic activity predominates and virtually all lesions show increased uptake,[78] to multiple myeloma, in which there is strong local osteoclast stimulation and less than 50% of lytic abnormalities seen on x-ray studies are identified scintigraphically.[130] In the middle of the spectrum are tumors with lytic lesions that produce strong osteoblastic reaction, thereby permitting their detection on the typical bone scintigraphy study. Breast and lung cancer are two common tumors whose metastases often appear lytic on radiographs but that are nevertheless usually avid for radionuclide bone agents. The lytic bone lesions of renal and thyroid carcinoma are also commonly observed on scintigraphic studies.

Metastatic lesions that may not be detected on bone scintigraphy include those which are small and still confined to the myeloid cavity and purely lytic lesions with bony destruction not associated with significant reactive changes.[63,76] In the latter situation, while there may be diminished bone uptake centrally (in proximity of the marrow cavity), this may be masked by the surrounding, as yet uninvolved bone. Purely lytic lesions may be demonstrated as photon-deficient (photopenic) abnormalities when destruction has extended into the cortical bone, but "cold" defects are generally more difficult to identify than those with increased radiotracer accumulation. It is fortunate that most of the lytic abnormalities associated with neoplasms such as renal and thyroid carcinoma, and even some of those seen with myeloma and other plasma cell disorders, appear as foci of increased uptake, indicative of the secondary osteoblastic response associated with most bone lesions that appear lytic on radiologic examination.[63]

BONE SCINTIGRAPHY WITH Tc-99m DIPHOSPHONATES

General Imaging Considerations

For more than 20 years the predominant radiopharmaceuticals for radionuclide bone imaging have been the Tc-99m labeled diphosphonates. The mechanism by which these compounds are taken up by bone and produce their characteristic imaging appearance is described in Chapters 2 and 3. Comparisons between several diphosphonate compounds in clinical use have shown modest differences in the rate of excretion and the degree of bone retention but equivalent performance for detection of metastatic lesions.[61,204] In the following discussion reference is made to a specific compound only with regard to a specific study, or if the results being presented are not generalizable to this entire category of radiopharmaceuticals.

Accurate interpretation of a bone scan for metastatic disease requires image quality sufficient to demonstrate subtle abnormalities in bone uptake (increased or decreased) and experience and skill in judging the significance of such findings. Whether acquired in the whole-body format (anterior and posterior) or as a series of overlapping spot views, it is desirable that the scan include the entire skeleton, although exclusion of the distal extremities is unlikely to result in significant underestimation of metastatic disease burden. As an initial survey of the skeletal system, the whole-body sweep has the advantage of assured image continuity, as care must be taken using the multiple spot technique to ensure that adjacent views overlap and include the entirety of bones such as the femora and humeri, particularly when gamma cameras with round crystals are used. Most modern computer systems allow display of zones of whole-body images as "spot views," but these magnified images may not be equivalent in quality to separately acquired spot images unless the original scan was acquired as a high-count study in a suitable matrix (e.g., 4 million counts in 512×1024 word mode). Whether the initial acquisition is total-body or multiple spots, additional spot images should always be acquired as needed to clarify equivocal or uncertain findings.

A variety of simple techniques can be used to improve the diagnostic yield of the planar bone scan and reduce the likelihood of important findings being missed or artifactual collections of tracer being identified as suspicious lesions. Acquisition of selected nonstandard views can be helpful for clarifying uncertain findings including oblique and lateral images of the thorax and pelvis, vertex views of the skull, upright images of the cervical and upper thoracic spine, and TOD (tail-on-detector) views of the pelvis (to better delineate the pubic bones from activity in the bladder) (Fig. 6-1). Repeat postvoid or if necessary postbladder catheterization views should be

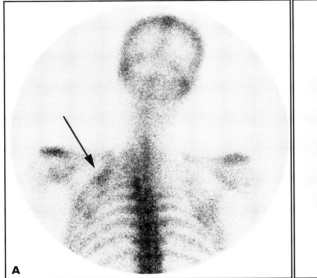 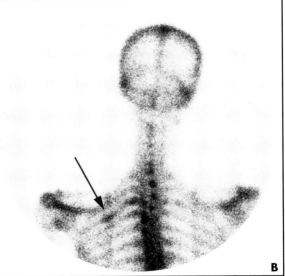

Fig. 6-1. A 60-year-old male with nasopharyngeal squamous cell carcinoma and a known pulmonary metastasis in the left lung was submitted for bone scintigraphy to evaluate increasing left arm pain. The standard supine posterior thorax and skull image (**A**) shows possible increased uptake in the left upper chest or the left medial scapula, which cannot be further delineated on this view (*arrow*). An additional upper thoracic spine view (**B**), with the camera brought closer to the head and neck by having the patient sit upright with his chin on his chest, demonstrated focal increased uptake in the left posterior third rib (*arrow*). Correlative CT image demonstrated a pulmonary mass eroding into and destroying the posterior aspect of the left third rib.

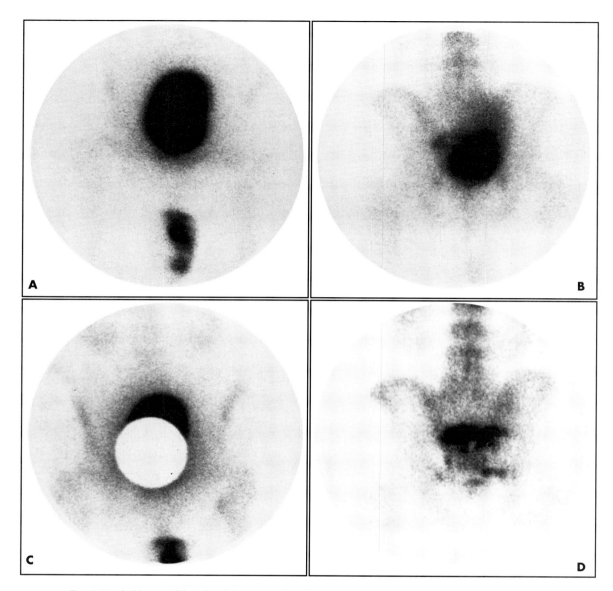

Fig. 6-2. A 56-year-old male with metastatic colon cancer was evaluated with bone scintigraphy because of severe lumbar spine and left hip pain. Anterior (**A**) and posterior (**B**) images of the pelvis demonstrate an enormous bladder residual that obscures all pelvic structures, and an additional image following placement of a bladder blocker (**C**) provides little additional information. Posterior pelvis image obtained subsequent to the patient being catheterized (**D**) shows a large area of increased uptake extending across the mid to lower sacrum into the ilia bilaterally, as well as other foci of increased uptake in the lower sacrum and pelvis. These findings corresponded to destructive lesions due to direct tumor extension from the rectosigmoid area seen on a companion CT scan.

obtained if residual bladder activity significantly interferes with visualization of pelvic structures, particularly in patients with low abdominal or pelvic tumors (see below) (Fig. 6-2). Skin or garment contamination with radioactive urine is a common finding on pelvis and proximal lower extremity images, and additional views following cleansing of the skin or removal of clothing are usually sufficient to confirm the etiology of such artifacts (Fig. 6-3).

Another adjunct to the conventional 2- to 4-hour postinjection bone scan is later delayed imaging, either on the same day (e.g., 6 to 8 hours) or the next day (24 hours). A common reason for obtaining such images is the presence of retained bladder activity obscuring pelvic structures, even after repeated voiding. Although bladder catheterization will usually resolve this problem, some patients may consider this an unacceptable option and the procedure itself may be technically difficult in others such as older men with enlarged prostates. The longer delay allows dilution and/or elimination of most activity from the bladder, with resultant improved identification of bone abnormalities, although the patient must be able

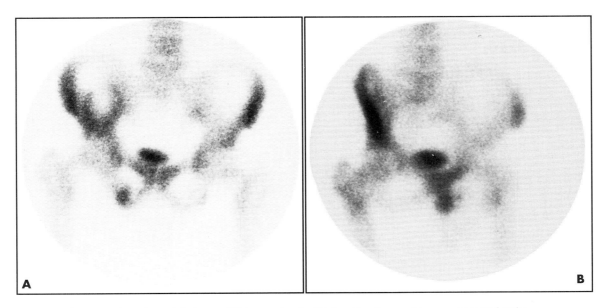

Fig. 6-3.   Anterior pelvis image (**A**) in a patient with locally advanced lung cancer and right leg pain demonstrates a large metastatic lesion in the right ilium, characterized by a central photopenic zone and a rim of increased uptake. In addition, there is an area of apparent increased activity in the region of the right ischium, but the contour of this abnormality relative to the native bone suggests it may be a nonosseous structure. A right anterior oblique pelvis view (**B**) demonstrates that this tracer activity is not in bone but rather at the tip of the penis, most likely reflecting urine contamination.

to tolerate the increased image acquisition time (up to 10 minutes) required to obtain adequate counts (Fig. 6-4). For patients with renal disease, vascular insufficiency (arterial or venous), or significant edema, delayed imaging provides additional time for soft-tissue clearance of radiotracer, thus improving the target-to-background ratio for bone detail. In circumstances where a subtle or questionable focus of increased uptake is seen on standard delayed images, later views allow an opportunity to assess for change in lesion conspicuity over time. Malignant abnormalities tend to show increasing target-to-background or target-to-nontarget ratio over time compared with benign findings, although the distributions of quantitative activity ratios (typically 24 hours vs. 3 or 4 hours) for benign and malignant lesions have considerable overlap.[89,106]

Quantitation of the skeletal uptake of bone scan agents can be used to supplement qualitative image review for assessing the extent of metastatic disease.[52,157,192,193] Methods that have been employed include measuring the total counts from specified bone regions-of-interest,[192,193] or determining the whole-body count rate using a scintillation detector placed several meters from the patient.[52,157] Increased bone uptake, indicative of disease progression, is usually positively correlated with other measures of disease severity such as radiographic findings, symptoms, and performance status, whereas decreased uptake, reflecting treatment response, may be identified even though the improvement may not be appreciated on visual examination of scan images.[52] Nevertheless, uptake quantitation has not emerged as a routine clinical procedure, mostly due to

the general success of qualitative and semiquantitative approaches to scan analysis for diagnostic and prognostic assessment of skeletal metastatic disease.[97,115,187]

Although planar imaging remains the mainstay of scintigraphic evaluation of skeletal metastases, the value of bone SPECT (single photon emission computed tomography) has become increasingly apparent in recent years.[175] Bone SPECT provides images with increased contrast and improved separation of overlapping structures, enhancing identification of known abnormalities and allowing detection of lesions that may not be seen on planar images. Although useful throughout the appendicular and proximal axial skeleton, SPECT of the spine has proven particularly valuable (Fig. 6-5). SPECT and computed tomography (CT) studies have demonstrated that 78% to 93% of vertebral metastases involve only the body or the body and pedicles.[4,28,60] In one SPECT study among 72 patients with known primary tumors, 93% (33 of 35) of abnormalities involving both the vertebral body and the pedicle proved to be metastases, whereas other patterns including focal or diffuse uptake in the vertebral body alone, abnormalities extending from the anterior aspect of the body, and those involving only the posterior elements and facet joints were usually of nonmalignant etiology (79/90, 88%).[60] With improvements in gamma cameras and nuclear medicine computers, as well as increased use of image fusion between SPECT and other cross-sectional modalities such as CT and magnetic resonance (MR), the role of bone SPECT in metastatic disease evaluation should continue to expand. Although routine use of SPECT, irrespective of findings on planar images, would likely result in improved identification of early bone metastases, it would be necessary to confirm the etiology of abnormalities identified only on SPECT to validate the increase in sensitivity. Unfortunately confirmation of the etiology of all detected lesions is frequently difficult to accomplish even in well-designed clinical trials, particularly once the diagnosis of metastatic disease has been established at one or more locations.

Interpretative Considerations

The large majority of metastatic lesions identified on bone scintigraphy appear as sites of increased uptake, and when the characteristic pattern of multiple lesions throughout the axial and proximal appendicular skeleton is present, there is little difficulty in scan interpretation (Fig. 6-6). However, the scans of many patients with bone metastases do not show this pattern, and scan interpretation thus requires appreciation of the various other ways that metastatic disease may appear. Equally important is

an understanding of the implications of the inherent low specificity of the bone scintigraphic technique, given that virtually any process that affects the local metabolic behavior of bone may result in focal increased tracer uptake.[155] Although most scan abnormalities in patients with widespread skeletal involvement are metastases, the majority of isolated new lesions in patients with malignancy but no known metastases are of nonmalignant origin.[99,155] The higher index of suspicion in patients with known malignancy can contribute to lowering the specificity of bone scanning for metastatic disease, with over-reading of scans being unavoidable if the simplistic assumption that any unexplained bone abnormality is a metastasis unless proven otherwise is employed. The data in the clinical and radiologic literature confirming this latter assumption to be faulty[98,99,155] only reinforce the need for sophistication in bone scan interpretation to avoid the many pitfalls that can result in either over-diagnosis or underdiagnosis of metastatic disease.

Both the number and location of bone scan lesions are

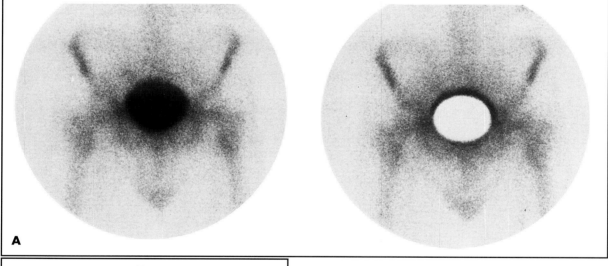

Fig. 6-4.   Anterior pelvis images (**A**) obtained at three hours post-injection demonstrate a significant bladder residual (*left*), with a repeat view with a lead blocker placed over the bladder (*right*) still compromised by scatter from the large amount of bladder activity visible around the superior aspect of the blocker. A 24-hour delayed view (**B**) obtained subsequently demonstrated increased uptake in the upper sacrum and medial left iliac wing adjacent to the left sacroiliac (SI) joint (*arrow*). Note that although there is residual bladder activity on the 24-hour view, its relative contribution to the total counts from the image is small enough that the SI joint abnormality can be identified.

correlated with the likelihood that the findings reflect metastatic disease.[94,98,99] Although it is rarely possible to confirm the etiology of every abnormality seen on a bone scintigram, even using all available noninvasive methods such as plain radiographs, CT and magnetic resonance imaging (MRI), in most clinical evaluations this does not prove necessary. In one review of bone scan results in breast cancer patients without known metastases, all patients with five or more new scan lesions had bone metastases, even though not all lesions were confirmed as malignant.[99] Among the 14 patients in this series with two to four new lesions and bone metastases, only 71% (24/34) of the scan abnormalities could be individually confirmed as malignant. If a patient is not known to have metastatic disease, definite identification of at least one lesion as a metastasis is critical, whereas in patients with known distant disease, change in disease status can generally be assessed qualitatively via comparison with results of prior studies. Although the sensitivity of competing imaging techniques is sometimes compared using expressions such as "technique A identified 18 metastatic lesions per patient versus 13 lesions per patient by technique B," such observations are of very limited clinical relevance. A more meaningful assessment of diagnostic methods focuses on their performance in equivocal cases and in patients with limited disease, in whom important treatment decisions are likely to be influenced by the presence or absence of metastatic disease.

One approach that has been used for assessing the value of bone scintigraphy in detecting early metastatic disease is the examination of scans with solitary lesions. Reviews from the 1970s reported 19% to 64% of solitary

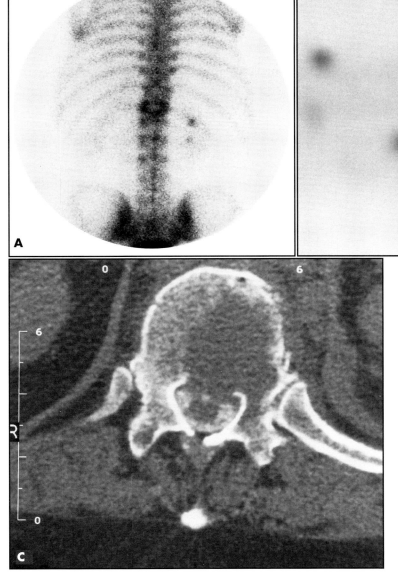

Fig. 6–5. A 40-year-old male 6 months s/p resection of a left adrenal cortical carcinoma presented with new onset of mid to low back pain, and bone scan image of the posterior spine (**A**) showed intense increased uptake in the T12 vertebra. Axial SPECT image at this level (**B**) showed this activity to involve the body and both pedicles (left greater than right). CT scan performed following completion of the bone scan demonstrates a large destructive metastatic lesion involving T12 (**C**).

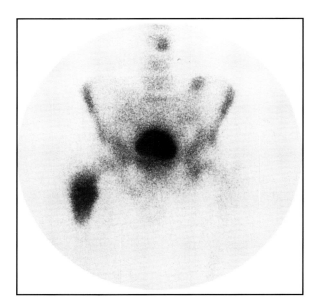

Fig. 6-6. A 55-year-old male had right hip pain out of proportion to the degenerative disease seen on plain radiographs, and bone scintigraphy demonstrated a large intense lesion in the right proximal femur extending approximately 5 cm distally from the level of the lesser trochanter. Pelvic image also demonstrates abnormalities in the left iliac crest, the left acetabulum, and the body of L3. Subsequent evaluation established the diagnosis of metastatic prostate carcinoma.

scan lesions to be malignant,[48,162,181] with one series including some patients without known tumors,[181] and these findings undoubtedly contributed to the perception that unexplained bone scan abnormalities in cancer patients were frequently metastases. Although prevalence of metastatic disease may well have been high in these small and highly selected series, these reviews were based on rectilinear scans and most involved imaging with less optimal agents such as F-18 and Tc-99m phosphate complexes, raising the possibility that some of the patients with "solitary" metastases might have had additional lesions that would have been detected with the improved image quality achievable with modern gamma cameras and radiopharmaceuticals. In more recent analyses of scans with one or two new lesions in cancer patients without known metastases, solitary lesions were confirmed as metastases in 11% of patients, whereas 24% to 35% of scans with two new abnormalities contained metastatic deposits.[94,99] Similar findings were seen in a recent review of isolated vertebral compression fractures identified on bone scintigraphy in male patients with various malignancies, with only 12% of solitary lesions (4/32) confirmed as metastases based upon clinical follow-up, imaging studies, and histology from biopsy or autopsy specimens.[96] Many patients in this series had other compression fractures of varying age on x-ray, CT, or MRI examinations, findings suggesting that the more recent fractures seen on scintigraphy were benign. Isolated rib lesions are also common and usually reflect metastases in 10% or less of cases.[94,99,201] Both recollected and unsuspected rib trauma are sufficiently common that unless a lesion has an unusual appearance (e.g.,

elongated, exceptionally intense, or associated with other discrete lesions in the same rib), the interpretation of an isolated new rib lesion as a probable metastasis is generally not justified.

As the preceding discussion concerning solitary spine and rib lesions suggests, the locations of bone scan abnormalities is strongly associated with their likely etiology. Common locations for abnormal but benign bone uptake include the articular surfaces of joints throughout the axial and appendicular skeleton, the end plates and anterior aspects of the vertebral bodies, the suture lines of the skull, and several locations in the ribs, particularly the anterior rib ends and costovertebral junctions. Abnormal uptake in the shoulders and the bones of distal extremities is also unlikely to reflect metastatic disease, regardless of the specific site involved. Nevertheless, virtually any bone in the skeleton can on occasion become a site of metastatic involvement, and the diagnostician must remain alert to detection of unsuspected or unusually intense scan findings, which may warrant further investigation (Fig. 6-7).

Knowledge of the typical distribution of benign abnormalities on bone scans is important in the identification and characterization of malignant lesions. Most bone metastases occur in the axial skeleton, with the spine being a common site of initial involvement for a number of tumors such as breast and prostate cancer[21,70,94,99] (Table 6-2). As noted earlier, the vertebral venous plexus provides a route for tumor cells that enter the venous circulation of the pelvis, abdomen, and thorax to reach the vertebral body bone marrow, particularly that of the thoracic and lumbar spine.[10,11,202] The interconnections between this system and the intercostal veins also serves as a means for tumor spread to the ribs without passing through the central venous and arterial circulations. Long bone metastases are somewhat more common in lung tumors than in those of other organs, reflecting the ready access of tumor emboli from the lungs to the pulmonary venous and systemic arterial circulations[65,118,170] (Figs. 6-8 and 6-9) (Table 6-2). The distribution of bone metastases seen on scintigraphy generally correlates with the findings of larger autopsy series in cancer patients, allowing for some underestimation in the histopathologic prevalence data due to the difficulty of performing a complete evaluation of the skeleton, particularly the spine, even in the most thorough autopsy.[70]

An issue that has been the subject of considerable debate over the years is whether patients with newly diagnosed malignancy should have a baseline bone scan, regardless of tumor stage or clinical suspicion of metastatic disease, to assure accurate interpretation of any subsequent scans. If there were no confounding medicolegal or economic issues, a baseline scan in a patient with a malignancy with known predilection for early metastasis to bone would be desirable to document preexisting bone abnormalities that could then not be confused with tumor at a later date. Baseline bone scans are rarely so abnormal as to make subsequent identification of early metastatic disease impossible; however, exceptions might include individuals with serious previous skeletal injury

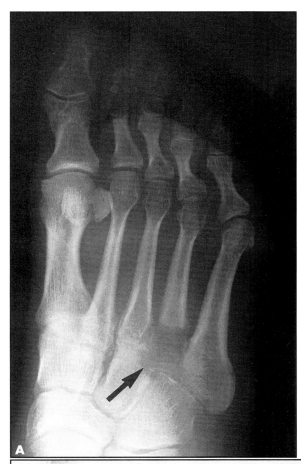

Fig. 6-7. A 61-year-old male with esophageal cancer had sudden onset of right foot pain, and a radiograph showed a lytic lesion at the base of the right fourth metatarsal (**A**, *arrow*). Bone scintigraphic anterior (**B**, *left*) and right lateral (**B**, *right*) images of the right foot demonstrated a focus of markedly increased uptake at the base of the right fourth metatarsal. Biopsy of this location demonstrated metastatic malignancy consistent with the esophageal primary. The remainder of the bone scintigraphy and other correlative imaging studies failed to demonstrate any other site of metastatic disease involving bone.

such as a major motor vehicle accident or polytrauma from a fall and those with severe inflammatory arthritides with multiple abnormal joints and skeletal deformities. However, as is discussed later for specific tumors, in most cancer patients the baseline study does not provide sufficient additional information or incremental benefit to be recommended as a routine procedure.

Lesion intensity on bone scintigraphy, although not directly an indicator of etiology, can nevertheless provide insight into the likelihood of malignancy, particularly when considered over the course of a series of scans. Lesion intensity at any one point in time is of limited value, in that acute trauma or infection can result in bone uptake as intense as any malignant deposit.

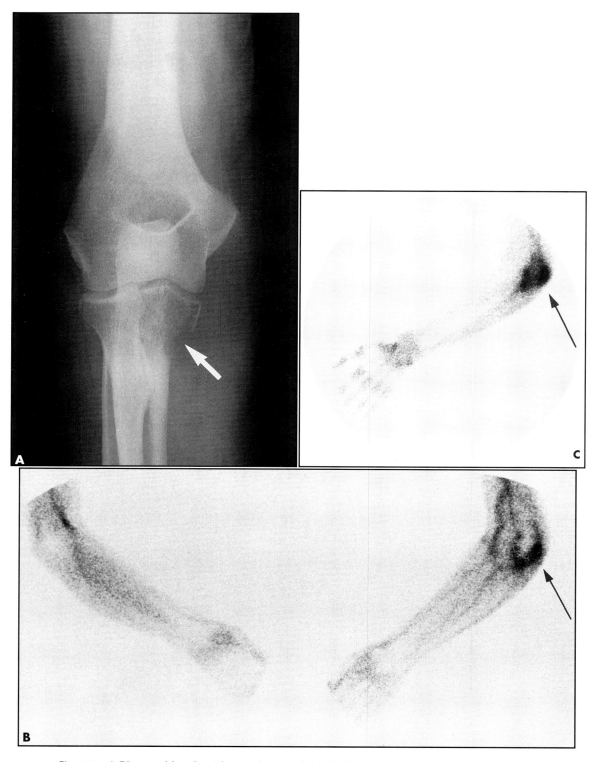

Fig. 6–8. A 70-year-old male with an enlarging right-sided pulmonary nodule, a new lytic lesion of the right ulna (**A**, *arrow*), and elevated ESR and white blood cell count was studied with a three-phase bone scan. Patient history included a fall with injury to the right elbow 2 months earlier, with negative x-rays at that time. Blood pool image (**B**) shows increased activity in the region of the right elbow, and delayed image (**C**) shows focal increased uptake in the proximal right ulna (*arrows*). These findings were considered consistent with infection or occult trauma, and the patient was initially treated with antibiotics. Subsequent biopsy of the lytic area seen on radiographs was positive for metastatic lung cancer.

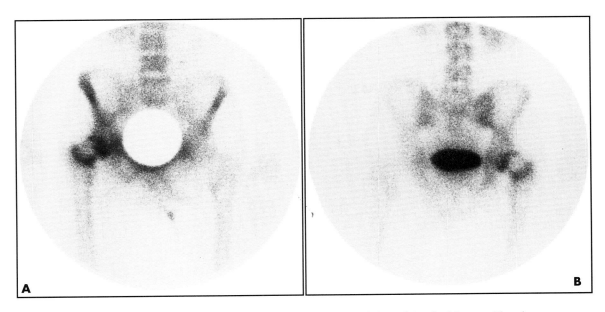

Fig. 6–9. Shown are anterior (**A**) and posterior (**B**) images of the pelvis of a 59-year-old male with a recent low-energy right femoral neck fracture and a new right upper lobe mass discovered on a routine chest radiograph. There are two curvilinear zones of increased uptake in the proximal right femur, one in the region of the base of the femoral head, the other extending from the greater to the lesser trochanter. Radiograph 2 days earlier demonstrated only an acute subcapital fracture of the right femur but no abnormal bone changes in the intertrochanteric region. At subsequent hip replacement, metastatic lung cancer was identified in the resected specimen.

However, the vast majority of benign processes that result in acutely increased bone uptake will show progressive decline in abnormal uptake over time with healing or treatment (Fig. 6-10). For example, an acute fracture typically shows maximum uptake within the first several weeks to several months of injury, with uptake gradually decreasing thereafter until in many cases the lesion can no longer be identified.[129,188] In contrast, early malignant lesions often display only mildly increased uptake, but in the absence of treatment virtually always show progressive increase in uptake over time.[94] Although some degenerative processes also result in progressive increase in uptake on serial bone scans, the typical locations of degenerative lesions usually allow them to be discriminated from metastases.

Because of the characteristic behavior of metastatic deposits on serial bone scintigraphy, patients who had equivocal scan abnormalities but no other objective findings to suggest recurrent disease were often in the past simply observed and submitted for a follow-up scan in 3 to 6 months. Increase in lesion intensity over time, with or without appearance of new abnormalities, almost always signaled the presence of metastatic disease,[94] leading to subsequent intervention with chemotherapy, hormonal therapy, or radiation therapy as appropriate. In today's medical environment, however, blood tests to assess for elevation of tumor-associated antigens (e.g., prostate specific antigen [PSA], carcinoembryonic antigen [CEA]), correlative imaging with CT and MRI to demonstrate early evidence of bone and bone marrow involvement by tumor, and bone biopsy as appropriate

have in general replaced the follow-up bone scan as a means to confirm the presence of distant metastases. Although periodic follow-up bone scans still have an accepted role in monitoring the response of metastases to therapy, serial scanning is now rarely used as a primary approach to establish the initial diagnosis of metastatic bone disease.

Although increase in the intensity of a metastatic lesion on a follow-up bone scan usually reflects disease progression, an exception is a phenomenon associated with healing known as "flare." In 6% to 23% of patients with bone metastases from breast or prostate cancer, treatment with either hormones or chemotherapy results in healing of bone lesions while the scan shows increased uptake in known lesions, often accompanied by visualization of new lesions.[40,47,100,101] Flare usually occurs during the first 3 months, occasionally up to 6 months, after initiation of treatment (Fig. 6-11) and is typically associated with increased sclerotic changes on radiographs consistent with lesion healing. One study showed that the majority of breast cancer patients who responded to a new course of therapy demonstrated flare on bone scans obtained at 3 month follow-up.[40] Awareness of the flare phenomenon will reduce the likelihood of misinterpreting this scintigraphic change as disease progression, particularly if the interval between the scan date and the date the patient began treatment is carefully noted. Continued increase in lesion number and intensity beyond 6 months after initiation of a new therapy, however, almost always reflects disease progression.[40,47]

A scan pattern that reflects an extreme level of

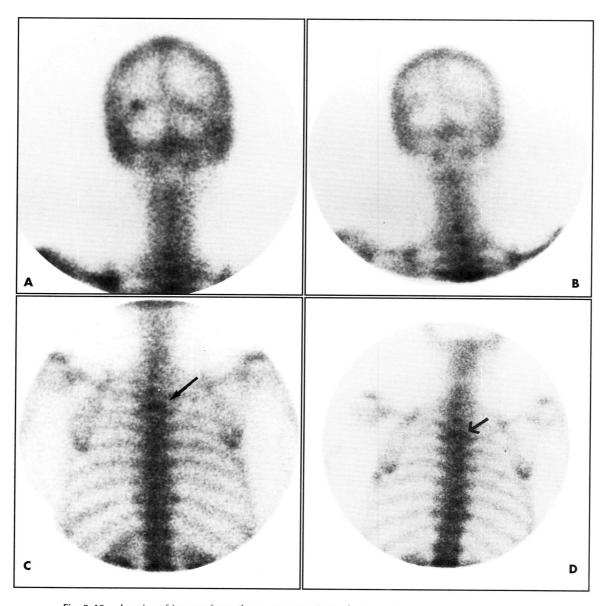

Fig. 6-10. A series of images from three cancer patients demonstrates typical changes seen in benign and malignant bone lesions on serial scintigraphy. Posterior skull images (**A** and **B**) show a focus of increased uptake along the left lambdoid suture that totally resolved in 1 year, consistent with effects of minor trauma, whereas posterior thorax views (**C** and **D**) show no change in a focus of degenerative disease at T4 (*arrow*) over 4 years.

metastatic involvement of bone is the so-called "superscan." Primarily encountered in prostate cancer patients, the superscan is characterized by markedly increased bone uptake of radiotracer, such that soft-tissue activity on 3-hour delayed images is low and renal activity is minimal to undetectable.[46,113,194] Occasionally bone uptake appears so uniform that at first observation the presence of metastatic disease may not be suspected, but the high target-to-background ratio and minimal renal activity usually serve to indicate the correct interpretation (Fig. 6-12). However, most superscans do demon-

strate a degree of focal abnormality, although the appearance may be that of heterogeneous uptake rather than the discrete "hot spots," which are usually associated with widespread bone metastases (Fig. 6-13). As discussed in Chapter 9, a superscan-type pattern may be seen in patients with nonmalignant diseases that are characterized by increased bone turnover, such as primary and secondary hyperparathyroidism and certain metabolic bone disorders.[19] However, discrimination of such patients from the population likely to present with a metastatic disease superscan is usually not difficult. Successful treat-

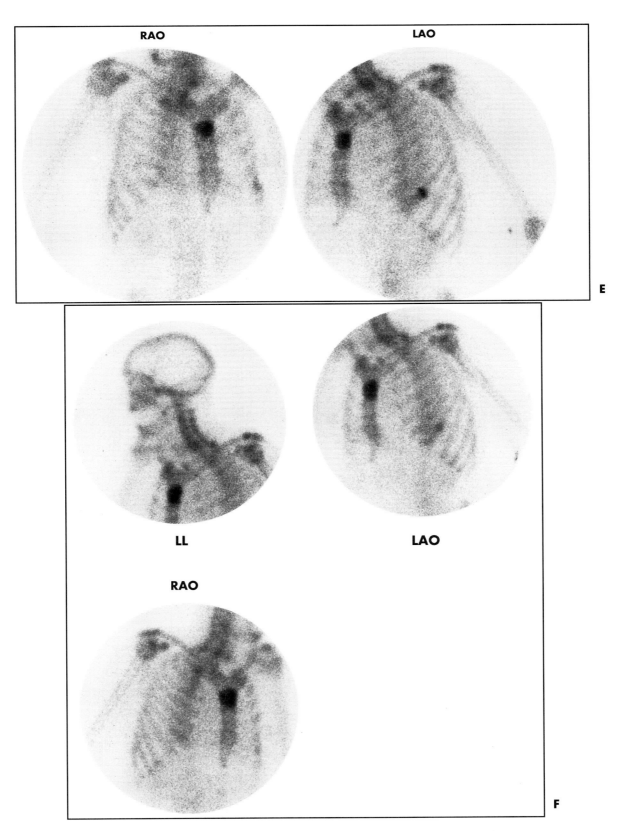

Fig. 6-10, cont'd. **E** and **F** show increasing uptake in a metastatic lesion involving the manubrium and sternum but decreasing uptake in a benign left rib fracture during the same 4 months.

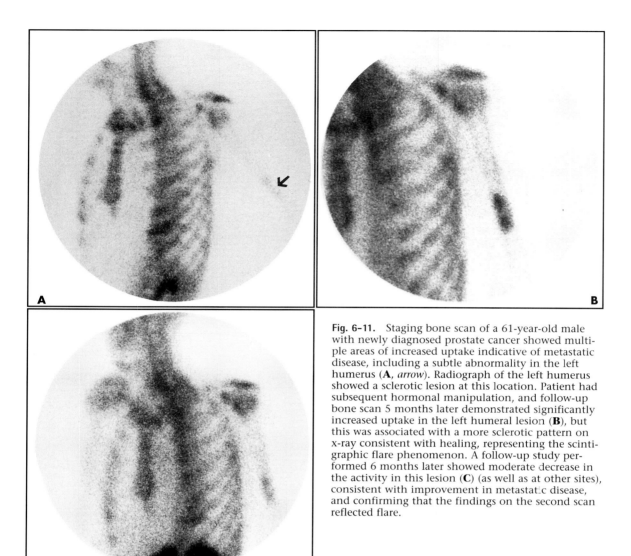

Fig. 6-11. Staging bone scan of a 61-year-old male with newly diagnosed prostate cancer showed multiple areas of increased uptake indicative of metastatic disease, including a subtle abnormality in the left humerus (**A**, *arrow*). Radiograph of the left humerus showed a sclerotic lesion at this location. Patient had subsequent hormonal manipulation, and follow-up bone scan 5 months later demonstrated significantly increased uptake in the left humeral lesion (**B**), but this was associated with a more sclerotic pattern on x-ray consistent with healing, representing the scintigraphic flare phenomenon. A follow-up study performed 6 months later showed moderate decrease in the activity in this lesion (**C**) (as well as at other sites), consistent with improvement in metastatic disease, and confirming that the findings on the second scan reflected flare.

ment which reduces the active tumor burden may cause the bone scan to revert to a more "normal" appearance, at least with regard to presence of soft tissue and renal activity, although occasionally the pattern of diffuse increased uptake is replaced by multiple focal abnormalities likely reflecting a more aggressive or resistant residual tumor population (Fig. 6-13).

Although purely photopenic metastatic lesions can be identified on scintigraphy,[63,153] considerably more bone destruction is often present in comparison to a typical blastic metastasis. Vascular compromise may contribute to occurrence of photopenic defects, possibly as a result of external compression of small vascular channels in the bone marrow by enlarging tumor deposits. Regardless of their etiology, photopenic defects can be important findings and should be sought with the same attention as foci of increased uptake (Fig. 6-14). Just as the significance of photopenic abnormalities on white blood cell scans has become better appreciated during the past 10 years,[95,132]

photopenic bone scan abnormalities are often true positive findings rather than artifacts or variants of normal, and their presence as possible malignant deposits should be evaluated as appropriate for any focal scan abnormality.

Correlation with Other Imaging Modalities

Although bone scintigraphy may provide the initial identification of a lesion, the subsequent correlative radiologic studies usually serve to confirm the diagnosis of metastatic disease. Initial correlation for scintigraphic findings is generally done with plain radiographs. A benign finding on a correlative radiograph is highly reliable in establishing lesion etiology[98]; a normal or equivocal x-ray interpretation is of much less certain value. In one series of cancer patients without known metastases, the majority of metastatic foci first seen as solitary or one or two new bone scan lesions were associated with nor-

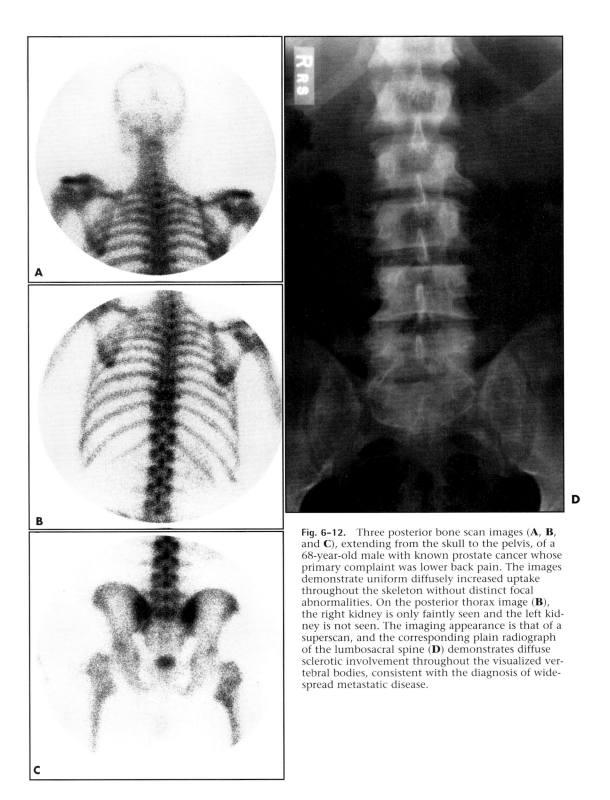

Fig. 6-12.   Three posterior bone scan images (**A**, **B**, and **C**), extending from the skull to the pelvis, of a 68-year-old male with known prostate cancer whose primary complaint was lower back pain. The images demonstrate uniform diffusely increased uptake throughout the skeleton without distinct focal abnormalities. On the posterior thorax image (**B**), the right kidney is only faintly seen and the left kidney is not seen. The imaging appearance is that of a superscan, and the corresponding plain radiograph of the lumbosacral spine (**D**) demonstrates diffuse sclerotic involvement throughout the visualized vertebral bodies, consistent with the diagnosis of widespread metastatic disease.

mal radiographs, whereas three quarters of the lesions considered suggestive of metastases radiographically turned out to be benign.[98] Radiographic correlation for rib lesions must be viewed with particular care, as early healing fractures may appear similar to metastatic deposits on radiography, emphasizing the importance of careful attention to clinical history. More commonly, isolated rib abnormalities will have no definite radiographic correlation, as documented in a study of breast cancer patients with 1 to 4 new scan abnormalities, in which 68% (40/59) of the rib lesions had negative correlative x-rays, with all but one of these lesions proving benign on

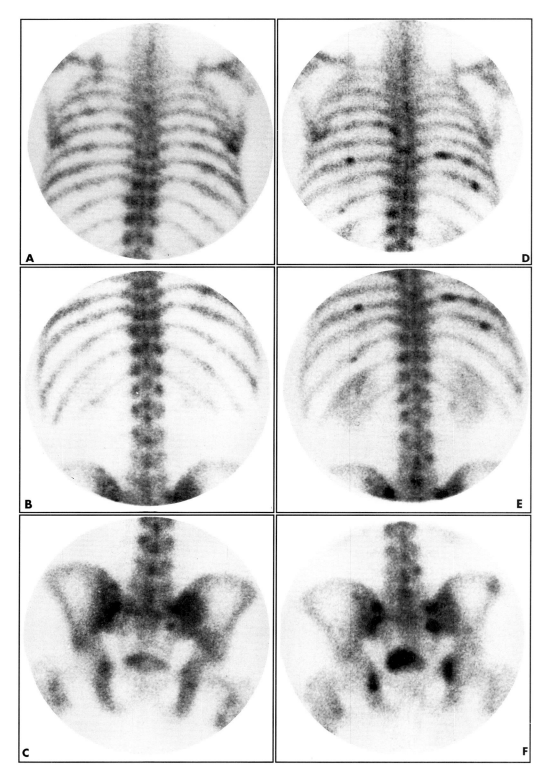

Fig. 6-13. Selected bone scan images (posterior thorax, abdomen, and pelvis [**A, B,** and **C**]) of a 66-year-old male with prostate cancer and generalized bone pain show diffuse but moderately heterogeneous increased uptake throughout the visualized skeletal structures, with minimal activity in the kidneys, consistent with a superscan. Correlative radiographs showed diffuse sclerotic changes. Comparable images (**D, E,** and **F**) from a follow-up scan obtained 9 months later, following hormonal ablation therapy, show marked improvement in the inhomogeneous bone uptake seen on the earlier study, but multiple new focal abnormalities in the pelvis, ribs and spine. More normal renal activity is evident on the second study, reflecting an overall decrease in bone uptake since the initial examination. These findings indicate a mixed response to therapy, with improvement in the superscan pattern, but appearance of possibly hormonally resistant metastatic lesions.

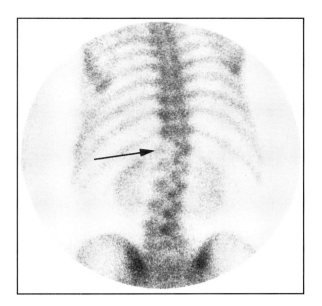

Fig. 6–14. Bone scintigraphy was obtained to evaluate a 73-year-old male with periaortic lymphadenopathy and back pain. Posterior thorax image demonstrates a photopenic defect involving the left lateral aspect of T12 (*arrow*). The patient was subsequently determined to have a poorly differentiated carcinoma of unknown primary and died several weeks after the scan. On autopsy there was destruction of the left side of T12 by tumor.

follow-up.[99] However, among the same patients, almost 60% (11/19) of scans that demonstrated metastatic disease in the thoracolumbar spine included scan-positive/x-ray negative metastases. This supports the previously noted importance of skeletal location, independent of x-ray findings, as an indicator of the likelihood that a particular lesion represents a metastasis.

The cross-sectional imaging modalities introduced in the past 20 years have proven of great utility for correlation with bone scan findings. CT is capable of demonstrating lytic and blastic abnormalities not seen on plain radiographs, particularly in the pelvis and the spine.[83,131,191] MRI is especially useful for identifying malignant involvement of bone marrow, with identification of lesions at sites other than initially detected on bone scintigraphy often serving to establish with certainty the diagnosis of metastatic disease.* Although a number of reports have described diffuse marrow abnormalities on MRI in patients with normal bone scans,[25,107,131] all such cases involved comparisons between planar scintigraphy and the tomographic MRI images. To date, a prospective comparison of bone SPECT and MRI has not been reported.

Correlation with Clinical Findings and Laboratory Results

Bone scintigraphy findings have been correlated not only with results of other imaging modalities but also

*References 51,107,131,165,185,191.

with clinical findings and laboratory data. Pain is usually the symptom that leads to initiation of an investigation for possible metastatic disease, but in fact the correlation between bone pain and bone metastases is not as strong as might be expected.[69,109] Many sites of metastatic disease are asymptomatic, especially initially, whereas many benign processes involving bone can result in significant symptoms[69] (Fig. 6-15). Patients with widespread metastases still tend to have specific local pain complaints, although patients with extensive malignant skeletal involvement do occasionally present with diffuse bony symptoms.[92] Although pain is neither sensitive nor specific for metastatic disease, it is an important indicator of various malignant and nonmalignant processes that can affect bone, and therefore is a valid reason for obtaining a bone scan.

Abnormal blood test results, such as elevation in alkaline phosphatase, calcium, prostate acid phosphatase, or erythrocyte sedimentation rate (ESR), are another common reason bone scans are obtained to evaluate patients for metastatic disease. None of these markers is specific for bone involvement by tumor, being elevated in association with many nonmalignant pathologies such as infection, hyperparathyroidism, and Paget's disease. In addition, the levels of these markers are usually not predictive of bone scan findings, and thus are of limited value in the determination of which patients will benefit from scintigraphy.[23,136,159,200] In recent years prostate acid phosphatase has given way to prostate specific antigen (PSA) for cancer screening, as is discussed below.

Organ-specific markers such as PSA are becoming increasingly important in surveillance of patients for the presence of tumor. PSA is used routinely for assessing prostate cancer patients both before and after initiation of treatment, and the development of metastatic disease is usually associated with increased PSA.[34,66,140,147] However, elevated PSA levels may also reflect only local growth of tumor, particularly in patients who have not undergone prostatectomy.[148] A recent review indicated that the pretreatment PSA was not predictive of either the likelihood of later development of bone metastases or the PSA at the time of relapse.[91] Although there is a correlation between PSA levels at initial diagnosis and the likelihood of bone metastases, once patients have undergone hormonal manipulation, either via orchiectomy or with antiandrogen or luteinizing hormone-releasing hormone (LHRH)-agonist drugs, the association between bone metastases and PSA level may be lost.[77,91] Occurrence of widespread bone metastases in patients with low or nondetectable PSA levels is presumed to reflect dedifferentiation of tumor cell populations, which no longer express the antigen found in both normal prostate tissue and well-differentiated tumor cells.[77]

Other tumor-associated markers whose elevation suggests the presence of metastases, sometimes involving bone, include CEA and thyroglobulin.[87,196] As with PSA, these markers are useful in combination with clinical assessment and as an aid in judging whether a workup for metastatic disease, which might include bone scintigraphy, is justified.

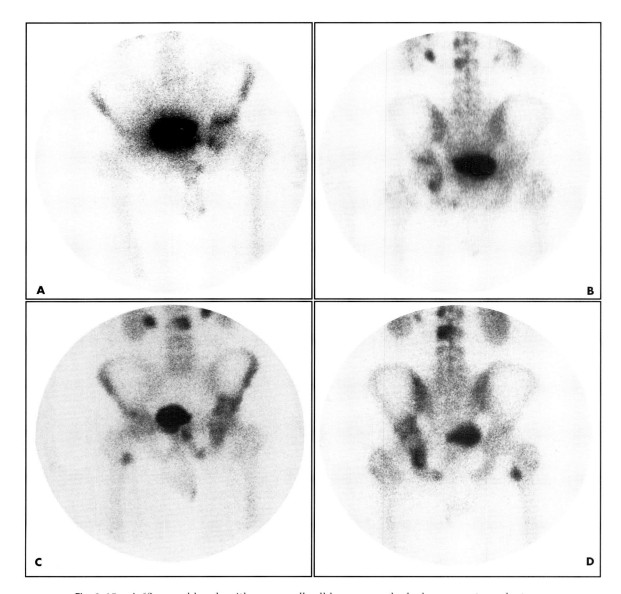

Fig. 6-15. A 63-year-old male with non–small cell lung cancer had a bone scan to evaluate complaints of proximal left thigh pain. Anterior and posterior pelvis images (**A** and **B**) demonstrate increased uptake in the left acetabulum, more prominent superiorly and inferiorly. There is also a suggestion of increased uptake in the left superior pubic ramus, although this is difficult to confirm because of the adjacent bladder activity. There is no focal abnormal uptake in the left femur in the specific area of symptoms. Pelvis images (**C** and **D**) from a follow-up bone scan performed 3 months later demonstrate increased abnormal uptake in the inferior left ilium and acetabulum, as well as more distinct abnormal uptake in the left ischium and pubic ramus, all consistent with progression of metastatic disease.

TUMOR-SPECIFIC CONSIDERATIONS

Lung

The role of bone scintigraphy in patients with lung cancer has changed as advances in other radiologic imaging techniques have resulted in improved accuracy of staging newly diagnosed malignancy. In lung malignancy, once the tissue type has been determined, patients with non–small cell (NSC) tumors are evaluated to deter-

mine whether surgical resection is possible and appropriate.[141] At one time, bone scintigraphy was commonly used as part of this staging evaluation of NSC lung cancer patients, with scans reported as positive for metastases in 34% to 49% of those studied.[57,109,137,200,208] However, since the routine availability of CT for lung cancer staging, evidence of metastatic disease is often first identified in hilar and mediastinal lymph nodes, liver, and/or adrenal glands, thereby documenting nonresectability and obviating the need for scintigraphy to

TABLE 6-3
Prevalence of Metastatic Disease on Bone Scintigraphy of Patients with Newly Diagnosed Breast Cancer Versus Clinical Stage*

Stage	Prevalence of Bone Metastases (% Range)	Aggregated Data		
		No. of Patients	No. with Metastases	Prevalence of Metastases (%)
I	0-2.5	959	8	0.8
II	0.6-12.2	1655	68	4.1
III	0-30.8	673	114	16.9

*References 3, 43, 49, 75, 110, 112, 130, 189, 210.

identify bone metastases.[141] Additionally, one study of 110 NSC lung cancer patients staged in the mid-1980s reported a true-positive bone scan yield of only 8%, at least in part reflecting preselection of patients considered to have potentially resectable tumors.[139] Bone scans are now only infrequently performed during staging of NSC lung cancer patients, usually in those with symptoms or suspicious bone findings on chest x-ray or CT.[158]

Because resectability is usually not an issue in small cell lung cancer patients, identification of metastatic disease commonly occurs as a result of studies performed to evaluate abnormal physical, laboratory, or radiologic findings. The majority of patients with small cell lung cancer already have distant metastatic involvement at the time of diagnosis;[141] thus it is not surprising that about 50% will have positive bone scans.[17,124,137] Just as for NSC patients, bone scintigraphy is used occasionally to evaluate pain complaints and document the extent of disease before initiation of chemotherapy. During follow-up, bone scanning is used for assessing symptomatic sites to determine if metastatic disease is present and if interventions such as local radiation therapy or an orthopedic procedure may be needed to prevent long-bone fracture or spinal cord compromise.

Irrespective of lung cancer cell type, scintigraphy can demonstrate the extent of metastatic bone involvement in patients with hypercalcemia and tumor-associated bone marrow suppression, which may aid in determining whether any therapy other than for symptom palliation is justified. The bone scan is also useful for documenting heterotopic pulmonary osteoarthropathy as a cause for lower extremity pain, with increased cortical bone uptake in the femora and/or tibias being the characteristic finding.[63] Scans will also occasionally demonstrate that symptoms are related to nonmalignant processes (e.g., avascular necrosis, unappreciated trauma or infection) that can be treated independent of the patient's malignant disease status.

Breast

Bone is a frequent site of metastatic disease in breast cancer and, of all malignancies, the use of bone scintig-raphy has been perhaps most extensively evaluated in this patient group. Bone scintigraphy was used in most of the large breast cancer therapy trials of the 1970s and 1980s, and the data from these trials have had a major impact on the current use of the technique in clinical practice.

Bone scintigraphy results published from the late 1960s to the mid-1970s showing positive scans for metastatic disease in up to 17% of stage I and up to 32% of stage II breast cancer patients led many investigators to recommend routine use of staging bone scans for all breast cancer patients.[36,71,81] However, by the late 1970s and early 1980s, data from trials employing improved scanning techniques and more rigorous requirements for disease confirmation began to appear, with considerably fewer early stage breast cancer patients shown to have bone metastases[26,74,130,210] (Table 6-3). These latter observations have been further validated by many subsequent studies,[3,43,49,112,189] and it is likely that the earlier overestimates of metastatic disease prevalence were due in part to categorization of unexplained scan abnormalities as metastases without independent imaging or histopathology confirmation. This conclusion is supported by later findings that many scan-positive/x-ray negative abnormalities, as well as some lesions with initial radiographic findings considered suggestive of metastatic disease, are in fact benign.[98,99]

Once it became clear that the prevalence of metastatic bone disease in clinical stage I and II breast cancer patients was much less than 10%, attention turned to whether staging bone scans were needed in these patients. Although both proponents and opponents of staging bone scans have presented reasonable arguments in favor of their respective positions,[27,33,62,142,168] the general consensus is that scans are not needed in stage I and most stage II patients, being possibly justified in some individuals with stage II disease with larger or histologically more aggressive tumors, as well as in those with symptoms or conventional radiographic studies suggestive of bone metastases.[43,55,62] Although a baseline scan may also be helpful for comparison with later examinations, as discussed earlier, the need for such a study must be individualized, with the decision based upon the clinical circumstances of an individual or a selected group of patients.

The prognosis of metastatic breast cancer patients with disease limited to bone is better than for those with other distant sites of involvement.[62,97,215] While the 1- to 2-year survival advantage of patients with bone-only relapse may be due in part to selection bias, with such patients being more closely followed, particularly in clinical trials, the subset of breast cancer patients with initial bone involvement at only one or two sites appears to have a less aggressive tumor or one that is more responsive to therapy.[97] Whether close interpretation of subtle new bone scan abnormalities to specifically identify less aggressive disease provides clinical benefit to the patient has yet to be established.[97] However, a recent randomized trial of clinical versus intensive diagnostic follow-up, the latter including biannual bone scintigraphy, demonstrated increased detection of bone metastases in the intensive study group, but no differences in 5-year overall mortality.[167]

The same cost-effectiveness and efficacy concerns that led to reduced use of staging bone scans have also influenced attitudes toward the need for routine follow-up studies. Routine follow-up scans (1–2/year) are included in the design of most protocol trials to maximize the early detection of metastatic disease.[167] However, in clinical practice, once initial staging for metastatic disease has been completed, the trend has been to limit routine follow-up procedures to those that have a demonstrable effect on patient management.[39,119,174,206] Bone scintigraphy is thus justified as a directed examination to eval-

uate new symptoms or monitor the effect of a course of therapy, and most diagnostic algorithms include follow-up bone scans for patients with symptoms, worrisome physical findings, or abnormal laboratory results or radiographs.[39,76] Because early diagnosis and treatment of limited or asymptomatic bone metastases have not been shown to improve survival, routine follow-up scans are generally not recommended in asymptomatic patients.[39,174]

Genitourinary Tract

PROSTATE

Prostate cancer is now the most common malignancy in men, with incidence increasing progressively with age. Effective treatment of prostate cancer depends upon early detection and accurate staging, and current clinical practice emphasizes regular surveillance of males over 50, beginning with digital rectal examinations and supplemented with PSA determinations based on the association between elevated PSA levels and an increased likelihood of prostate cancer.[24,171] In patients with abnormal digital rectal examinations or elevated PSA, transrectal ultrasound is often the next study performed, usually in association with six-sector or lesion-directed biopsies. Once the diagnosis of prostate cancer has been established, as bone is the most frequent site of distant metastatic involvement, a bone scan is often obtained as part of the staging workup.

Bone scan findings at the time of initial diagnosis have been examined in relation to a number of attributes

TABLE 6–4
Prevalence of Metastatic Disease on Bone Scintigraphy of Patients with Newly Diagnosed Prostate Cancer Versus Clinical Stage and Prostate Specific Antigen

Stage	No. of Patients	No. with Metastases	Prevalence of Metastases (%)	References
A1	30	0	0	34
A2	32	6	18.8	
B1	151	2	1.3	
B2	192	18	9.4	
C1	70	20	28.6	
C2	46	25	54.3	
PSA (ng/ml)	←————	Aggregated Data	————→	
<20	1297	10	0.8	34, 93, 147, 152
20-50	153	12	7.8	
50-100	88	31	35.2	
>100	93	62	66.7	

of prostate cancer. The prevalence of positive bone scans for metastases has been shown to increase with increasing clinical stage,[34,84] Gleason histologic score,[84,180] and serum levels of prostate acid phosphatase and PSA[5,34] (Table 6-4). One anomaly in the relation between clinical stage and scan findings is the higher prevalence of bone metastases in patients with stage A2 tumors than in those with either A1 or B1 tumors, presumably reflecting the more aggressive nature of these otherwise apparently localized primary tumors.

Patients with low PSA levels at the time of diagnosis of prostate cancer have a low likelihood of having bone metastases. While some authors use 10 ng/ml and others 20 ng/ml as the PSA cutoff value, the yield of bone scanning for detection of metastases in these patients is usually <1%[34,93,147] (Table 6-4). Analogous to the evolution of the workup for stage I and II breast cancer patients, a staging bone scan is generally not needed at the time of prostate cancer diagnosis for patients with PSA <10 ng/ml and may be of only marginal value when the PSA is between 10 and 20 ng/ml.[34,93,147] Baseline scans are still appropriate in patients with low PSA levels but symptoms or radiologic abnormalities that raise the suspicion of bone metastases, and for those with pre-existing skeletal conditions that might render interpretation of later scans difficult.[140]

Staging scans continue to be part of the routine workup for patients with PSA levels >20 ng/ml at the time of diagnosis of prostate cancer. In this latter group a recent study showed that 50% (3/6) of patients with PSA of 20 to 100 ng/ml and bone metastases had baseline scans with 1 to 3 suspicious abnormalities, whereas for PSA >100 ng/ml, almost all patients with metastases (8/9, 89%) had widespread skeletal involvement.[93] Thus for patients with moderately elevated PSA, there is an increased likelihood that metastatic disease may present as subtle or limited abnormalities, and appropriate radiologic follow-up should be obtained in such cases to establish lesion etiologies.

Routine follow-up bone scans are commonly obtained in prostate cancer patients enrolled in clinical trials, but for other patients, such scans are only performed for specific indications such as new bone symptoms or rising PSA levels. Once metastatic disease has developed, serial scans are often used to assess the extent of bony involvement and the effectiveness of therapy.[66,186,193,197] As prostate cancer patients with bone metastases often survive for a number of years, the bone scan provides a convenient means to monitor the severity and extent of metastatic disease and estimate prognosis, which is usually poorest in those whose scans show progressive disease despite appropriate treatment.[115,193]

The flare phenomenon may be seen in prostate cancer patients with bone metastases within the first 6 months of initiation of hormonal manipulation, whether via administered drugs or orchiectomy.[101,192] In such patients radiographic and scintigraphic follow-up are usually needed to accurately assess the eventual degree of resolution of metastatic disease and to determine if additional therapeutic interventions are needed (Fig. 6-11).

OTHER GENITOURINARY TUMORS

Bone scintigraphy has a limited role in staging and follow-up of most tumors of the genitourinary (GU) tract other than prostate cancer. In renal carcinoma, staging scans have a low positive yield (<5%) and are not recommended.[126,166] Although renal carcinoma produces lytic bone metastases, increased uptake is still frequently identified on the bone scan as a result of reactive changes and the extensive bone destruction often seen with this tumor.[78] Photopenic defects are also seen, sometimes with a border of increased uptake. The first indication of the presence of renal carcinoma is occasionally discovery of a solitary lytic lesion in a long bone such as the humerus or femur, with typically intense increased uptake on scintigraphy[92] (Fig. 6-16).

The majority of GU tract tumors are not associated with early spread to bone. The yield of bone scanning in patients with newly diagnosed bladder cancer is low,[13,125] with 4.5% prevalence of metastases among 221 patients in one large series.[54] Reviews of staging bone scan results in patients with gynecologic malignancies, including cervical, uterine, ovarian, and endometrial cancers, all showed bone metastases only in an occasional stage III or IV patient.[82,85,108,138] In one series of 160 patients with cervical cancer, only one patient had a lesion on bone scan that was subsequently confirmed to be a metastasis.[85] Similar low yields have been reported for staging studies of male patients with testicular tumors.[134]

As in any tumor population, bone scanning in patients with GU malignancy may be helpful in identifying the cause of symptoms or abnormal findings on radi-

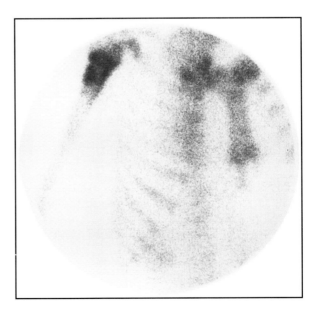

Fig. 6-16. Bone scintigraphy in a 53-year-old male with progressive right proximal shoulder pain and no history of trauma demonstrates markedly increased uptake in the proximal right humerus, with suggestion of a photopenic center surrounded by a zone of intense cortical bone uptake. Right humerus radiograph demonstrated a large erosive lytic lesion; biopsy of this site revealed renal carcinoma.

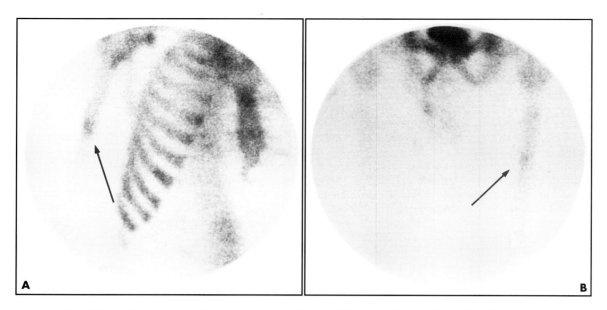

Fig. 6-17. A bone scan performed to assess a 75-year-old male with medullary thyroid carcinoma demonstrated multiple sites of increased uptake, including subtle lesions in the proximal right humerus (**A**) and proximal left femur (**B**) (*arrows*). All correlative radiographs showed no abnormalities.

ographs or blood tests. Although most metastases from GU tumors, with the exception of prostate, are lytic, several series have shown detection of more malignant lesions by scan than x-ray study.[9,154] The directed bone scan remains the most convenient method for evaluating both a local symptomatic site and the rest of the skeletal system without incurring additional radiation exposure or a significant increase in expense.

Thyroid

The most commonly used tracer for evaluation of metastatic disease from thyroid cancer is iodine-131. Metastatic surveys are usually performed 2 to 3 days following a dose of 74 to 185 MBq (2 to 5 mCi) of I-131, and are most effective following surgery and radioiodine ablation of residual thyroid tissue. The radioiodine scan, however, is useful only for papillary, follicular, and mixed tumors which produce iodine-avid metastatic lesions, and the image quality of I-131 scans is rather poor. Bone scintigraphy can sometimes provide supplementary information to radioiodine imaging, as well as offering the opportunity to identify metastases from non–iodine-avid tumors such as medullary carcinoma[102] (Fig. 6-17). In a recent study of differentiated thyroid carcinoma patients, the combination of I-131 and Tc-99m HMDP imaging studies allowed increased confidence in identification of metastatic lesions, particularly in the spine, with some metastases being identified only on the bone scan.[196] Although thyroid bone metastases are usually lytic, most lesions show increased uptake on bone scintigraphy, some with a region of increased uptake surrounding a central photopenic zone.[196]

Hematologic Malignancies

Malignancies of the hematopoietic system, such as the leukemias and lymphomas, show varying degrees of involvement of bone marrow, and as such it might be expected that metabolic changes in bone would be readily seen on scintigraphy. In fact, these malignancies often result in significantly less abnormal bone uptake than characterize metastatic lesions from visceral tumors. In patients with lymphoma, particularly Hodgkin's disease, there is frequent involvement of the appendicular skeleton,[88,133,150,173] often appearing as uniform juxta-articular increased uptake, typically in the femora and proximal tibias, suggestive of marrow expansion (Fig. 6-18). Marrow involvement with tumor may also appear in a patchy, inhomogeneous distribution, reflecting a mixture of involved and uninvolved marrow elements. Intense focal areas of increased bone uptake are relatively unusual in the lymphomas and leukemias, with more subtle areas of increased uptake being more commonly seen.[150] Distinct photopenic lesions are also seen at sites where normal marrow has been replaced by tumor as well as in zones of myelofibrosis (Fig. 6-18).

One category of hematologic malignancy that is particularly difficult to image scintigraphically is the plasma cell disorders, the most commonly encountered being multiple myeloma. The characteristic multiple lytic abnormalities of myeloma involving the bones of the axial and appendicular skeleton are often not identified on planar bone imaging with Tc-99m diphosphonates (Fig. 6-19). Less than half the lesions seen on radiographs show abnormal uptake on bone scintigraphy, including foci of increased and decreased activity.[177,195,215] Bone

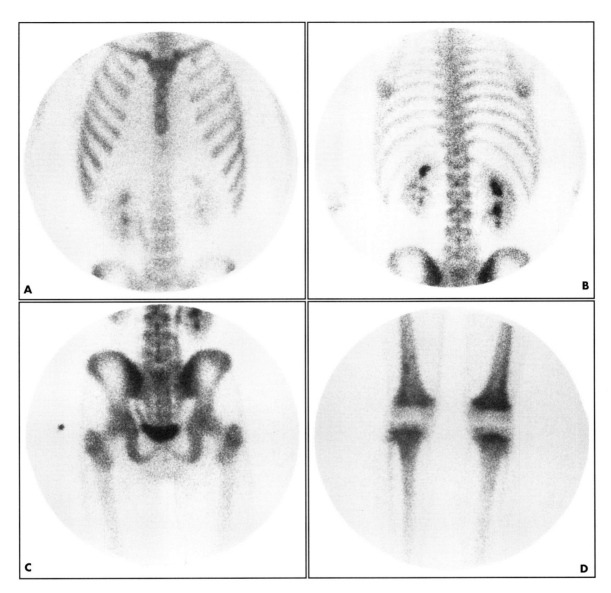

Fig. 6-18.   A 23-year-old male with non-Hodgkin's lymphoma and right hip pain was evaluated with bone scintigraphy. **A-D,** Images demonstrate relatively high skeletal target-to-background ratio, with overall increased tracer uptake in the pelvis, intertrochanteric region of the femora, the distal femora, and proximal tibias. These findings were thought most consistent with marrow expansion.

Continued.

scintigraphy may aid in assessing areas that are more difficult to visualize on radiographs such as the ribs, sternum, and the shoulder girdle, but findings in these areas rarely have significant clinical impact.[177,213] A skeletal x-ray survey is generally sufficient to evaluate patients with suspected or confirmed myeloma, and bone scintigraphy should be performed only if findings on radiography have failed to explain localizing symptoms or to examine for the presence and acuity of a pathologic fracture.

Miscellaneous

Because bone scintigraphy may be used to study any patient with a malignancy and symptoms or x-ray findings that suggest possible metastatic disease, positive scan results have been reported for most of the different tumors encountered clinically. Series examining the utility of bone scintigraphy in patients with melanoma have shown a typically low positive yield (<5%) as a staging examination in stage I and II patients,[8,169] while docu-

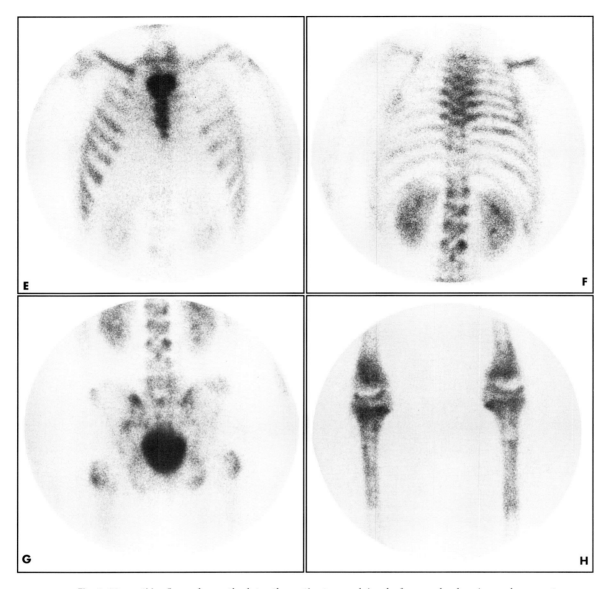

Fig. 6-18, cont'd. Several months later the patient complained of severe back pain, and a repeat bone scan (**E-H**) showed markedly inhomogeneous uptake in the skeleton, with photopenic zones in the lower thoracic spine, ribs, and pelvis, and multiple focal areas of increased uptake in the spine, pelvis, and sternum, consistent with tumor. The distal femora and proximal tibias also demonstrated marked heterogeneity consistent with tumor infiltration.

menting the value of the scan for identifying later development of metastatic disease prior to detection by radiography.[64] Several investigators have suggested that bone scans are useful for staging and follow-up of children with neuroblastoma, with more than half the patients with stage II to IV disease having positive scans for metastases prior to initiation of therapy.[53,156] Data from several groups studying patients with nasopharyngeal carcinoma have showed, as might be expected, a low yield for staging scans, but occasional utility for identifying disease in high-risk patients.[123,178,190] The literature of bone scintigraphy contains innumerable case reports that attest to the technique's value as an adjunctive diagnostic study, particularly because it provides information concerning the entire skeletal system. For this and the

various other reasons presented earlier, bone scintigraphy is usually readily justified for evaluation of oncologic patients for the presence of metastatic disease during clinical follow-up.

EFFICACY AND COST–EFFECTIVENESS OF SCINTIGRAPHIC EVALUATION FOR BONE METASTASES

Controversies

In the changing world of medicine, diagnostic and therapeutic approaches that at one time were considered the standard of care may now be subjects of controversy.

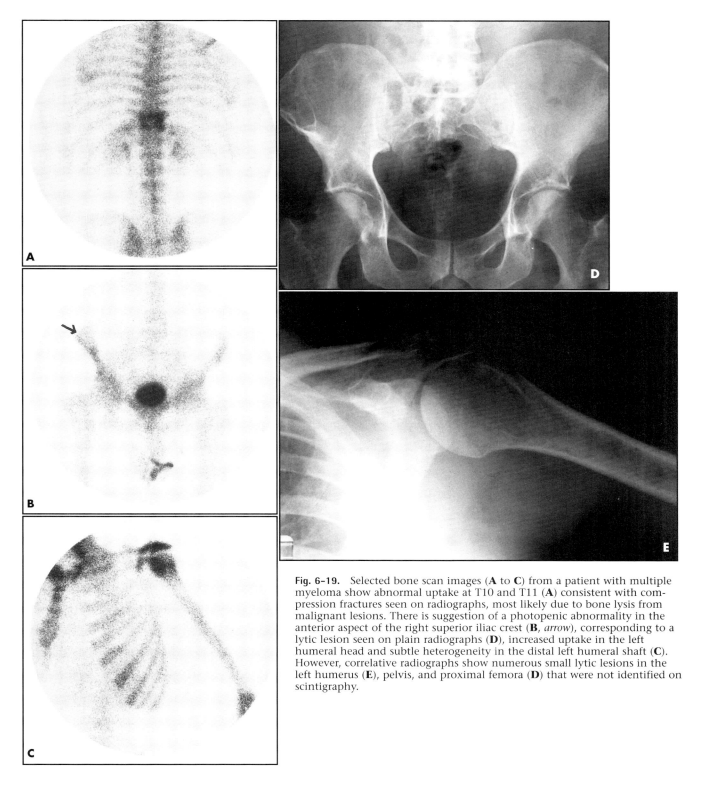

Fig. 6-19. Selected bone scan images (**A** to **C**) from a patient with multiple myeloma show abnormal uptake at T10 and T11 (**A**) consistent with compression fractures seen on radiographs, most likely due to bone lysis from malignant lesions. There is suggestion of a photopenic abnormality in the anterior aspect of the right superior iliac crest (**B**, *arrow*), corresponding to a lytic lesion seen on plain radiographs (**D**), increased uptake in the left humeral head and subtle heterogeneity in the distal left humeral shaft (**C**). However, correlative radiographs show numerous small lytic lesions in the left humerus (**E**), pelvis, and proximal femora (**D**) that were not identified on scintigraphy.

Although diagnostic imaging is a major focus in the ongoing debate over health care reform and appropriate utilization of medical resources, scintigraphic studies in general, and the bone scan in particular, have been under scrutiny for a number of years as potential targets for restriction or even elimination. Controversies concerning use of bone scintigraphy, which have been noted throughout this chapter, can be divided into four categories: the role of pretherapy staging studies; the utility and appropriateness of routine follow-up examinations; the utility of directed follow-up scans; and the value of scanning as a prognostic tool.

As noted in the discussion on specific tumor types, bone scanning has a significantly lower positive yield for metastases in low-grade compared with high-grade or stage primary malignancies. The inherent difficulty in establishing whether a staging procedure should be performed arises from the necessity of defining a population prevalence threshold below which cost-effectiveness and/or clinical management considerations render the procedure inadvisable. Although such a threshold has not been explicitly determined for bone scintigraphy, a value in the range of 5% can be reasonably inferred from the results of a number of published analyses.* In general, this value is consistent with an approach that limits staging scans to patients with clinical stage II malignancies and those with symptoms, abnormal blood tests or x-ray findings, or large or histologically more aggressive tumors.

Aside from its use in staging, the most common reason bone scintigraphy is performed in cancer patients is to determine if new or persistent bone or musculoskeletal pain is due to metastatic disease. However, as noted earlier, the correlation between bone pain and bone metastases is not particularly high. There are many causes of bone pain other than malignancy, whereas bone metastases are often asymptomatic, even occasionally in the presence of extensive disease. Bone pain in association with laboratory abnormalities is also cited as a reason for bone scintigraphy, but elevation in markers such as serum calcium, acid and alkaline phosphatase, PSA, and ESR is also nonspecific, being seen in a variety of inflammatory, infectious, and degenerative conditions. Although selection of patients based on combinations of signs and symptoms increases the positive yield of scanning somewhat, decision rules that are reliable and easily used remain elusive.

One of the more daunting tasks for the diagnostic imager is to judge whether the findings of a requested procedure are likely to have a measurable influence on either immediate care decisions or long-term patient management. The often unspoken question in cancer patients is whether earlier detection of metastatic disease will result in improvement in the effectiveness of therapies initiated thereafter. Although routine follow-up bone scans are more likely to identify metastatic disease at an earlier stage,[39,63,99,167] such identification is of little value in the absence of therapies known to influence later disease progression. Identification of asymptomatic disease can result in the appearance of benefit, such as prolonged survival, which in reality is only the result of lead-time and length-time bias.[18] If the state of available treatments is such that a late event (e.g., death) occurs at the same time as it would have in the absence of an earlier diagnosis (lead-time bias), or if diagnosis of asymptomatic disease identifies a significant number of individuals in whom that disease would not have been manifest during their lives (length-time bias), any apparent improvement in outcome for the total disease population is artifactual. Published results must be carefully examined for the often unappreciated effects of these biases, as the appearance of improved survival secondary to use of a new diagnostic test that identifies disease at an earlier

stage may be analogous to moving position markers in the middle of a playing field whose beginning (occurrence of disease) and ending locations (death) are geographically fixed.

Performance of a directed bone scan to evaluate a localizing complaint or radiographic abnormality is the most straightforward examination to justify. Identification of lesions in the long bones, which may be potential sites for fracture, or at sites in the spine, which may cause neurologic complications, is of particular clinical importance. Similarly, directed follow-up studies for examining patients with known lesions that are undergoing specific treatment (e.g., external beam or radionuclide radiation therapy) allows an objective assessment of the effectiveness of that treatment, particularly if serial studies are available to document progression or regression of one or more metastatic lesions.[16,40,45,193,197]

Bone scan findings are often used as an objective means to judge disease prognosis, and data from numerous series have confirmed that patients with extensive bone metastases have poorer survival than those with more limited disease.† Although disease progression in spite of treatment is generally an ominous sign, the scan findings in this setting probably contribute little to management decisions, given that most patients also have clinical evidence of worsening disease.[29,86,135,206] There remains a considerable need for well-designed studies to determine how best to utilize bone scanning in monitoring and follow-up of early metastatic disease, both from the perspective of treatment and quality-of-life issues that may have an effect on prognosis.

Competing Versus Complementary Imaging Modalities

As in other areas of medicine, there is competition within diagnostic radiology regarding the optimal way to image different disease processes. Most nuclear medicine procedures have been compared and/or correlated with radiographic, sonographic, CT, and MRI examinations, and the results of these comparison studies have influenced decisions concerning the clinical uses of scintigraphy.[90] For bone scans, correlation is most often obtained with plain radiographs, and the information provided by the two modalities is clearly complementary. Radiography is most helpful for confirming a benign or definitely malignant etiology for a scan abnormality.[98] Many scan lesions, particularly in the ribs and the spine, have no definite radiographic correlation,[98,99] reflecting the limits of planar anatomic imaging for identifying subtle structural changes in bone and bone metabolism. CT provides greater detail in demonstrating bone anatomy, as well as showing features of adjacent soft-tissue elements.[83,131,191] To obtain detailed information on the marrow compartment of bone where early metastatic tumor is found, MR imaging correlation for suspicious bone scan results is needed.‡ Pulse sequences such as STIR provide marrow images of high sensitivity for identifica-

---

*References 29, 34, 43, 54, 62, 63, 135.

†References 42, 97, 120, 136, 156, 197.
‡References 51, 107, 131, 165, 185, 191.

tion of tumor, and the finding of marrow involvement at sites other than those seen on the bone scan can serve to confirm the diagnosis of malignancy without the need for a biopsy. The primary limitations of MRI are that marrow signal changes are not entirely specific for malignancy,[103,184,205] the technique cannot readily provide total-body images, and a complete examination carries a relatively high cost.

Bone Scanning for Detection of Occult Malignancy

Whereas bone scanning of patients with known malignancy is a common clinical practice, scans are also not infrequently requested to evaluate obscure, often chronic musculoskeletal symptoms in patients without known malignancy. The value of bone scintigraphy for detecting the presence of occult malignancy has been

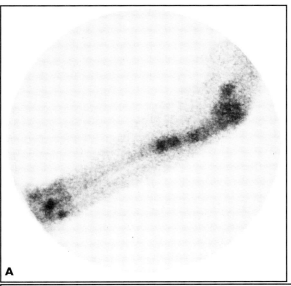

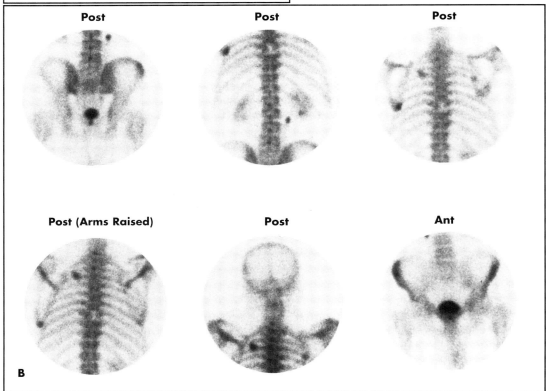

Fig. 6-20. A 77-year-old male presented with pain in his right forearm and wrist after a fall approximately 1 month earlier, and radiographs of the right elbow and wrist showed no definite abnormalities. A three-phase bone scan was obtained, and images of the hands and wrists during the initial two phases (not shown) revealed no distinct abnormality. Three-hour delayed images demonstrated multiple areas of increased activity, including the proximal half of the right radius (**A**), the right iliac wing, the left inferior scapula, and several ribs (**B**). There was also a photopenic abnormality in the eighth thoracic vertebral body. Various correlative imaging studies performed in the subsequent weeks, including CT and MRI, failed to clarify the etiology of the scintigraphic findings, which were highly suspicious for metastatic disease. A biopsy from a subsequently identified skin lesion established a diagnosis of adenocarcinoma of unknown primary.

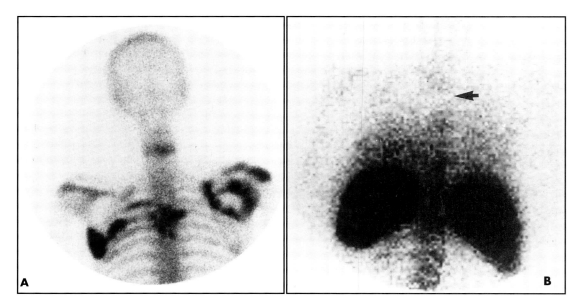

Fig. 6-21. A posterior head and upper chest bone scan image of a 62-year-old male with widely metastatic prostate cancer shows multiple areas of increased uptake, including the cervical spine and midthoracic spine, both shoulders and the left ribs (**A**). Companion image (**B**) from an indium-111 labeled white blood cell scan obtained because of concerns regarding infection shows a photopenic defect (*arrow*) in the upper thoracic spine, corresponding to the region of increased uptake on the bone image, consistent with marrow replacement by tumor.

examined in a recent review of over 400 patients without known malignancy who were scanned because of musculoskeletal complaints.[92] No positive scans suggestive of the presence of metastatic disease were found among almost 150 younger patients (<50 years of age), whereas in patients >50 years old, 10% of scans showed lesions that proved to be metastatic disease, with almost 80% of the positive scans showing multiple metastases (Fig. 6-20). These data validate the clinical impression that bone scintigraphy is an effective tool for identifying the presence of occult malignancy in older patients.[179,182]

SPECIAL APPLICATIONS

Bone Imaging with Radiopharmaceuticals Other Than Tc–99m Diphosphonates

In this chapter the primary focus has been on bone imaging using Tc-99m labeled diphosphonate compounds. Nevertheless, a variety of other tracers have been and continue to be used to examine bone for involvement by tumor. Among these are the infection and tumor imaging agent gallium-67 citrate, whose use for metastatic disease evaluation primarily involves patients with lymphomas,[68,105,143] and the cardiac perfusion agents thallium-201 and technetium-99m sestamibi. Uptake of these latter compounds is related to blood flow and/or metabolism, and their use can sometimes clarify the significance of atypical bone scan findings because of the increased uptake seen at most sites of tumor but not

in various benign lesions.[30,203] Thallium and sestamibi thus provide results analogous to those obtained with the PET (positron emission tomography) metabolic tracer F-18 FDG.[172]

Two newer classes of compounds being evaluated for tumor imaging are the monoclonal antibodies (MoAbs) and the labeled peptides. A large number of MoAbs have been developed during the past several decades, and tumor imaging antibodies directed against CEA,[15,56] tumor-associated glycoprotein-72,[44,176,212] and PSA[198] are among many that have been studied. Although MoAbs are typically less sensitive than diphosphonate bone agents, one or more of these compounds may one day be useful for clarifying the significance of equivocal bone scan findings in specific tumors. More recently there has been considerable interest in potential uses for radiolabeled peptides. The first of these agents to be approved by the Food and Drug Administration was indium-111 labeled pentreotide (OctreoScan, Mallinckrodt), which has been successful in imaging neuroendocrine tumors that contain somatostatin receptors.[117,122] For the foreseeable future, it is doubtful if this agent and other targeted receptor imaging peptides will have a significant impact on the use of bone scintigraphy.

Radionuclide Bone Marrow Imaging

Another imaging adjunct to bone scanning for metastatic disease is the radionuclide bone marrow scan. A technetium-99m labeled colloid such as microcolloid is generally used,[20,164,207] although agents such as In-111 or Tc-99m white blood cells labeled either in vitro or in vivo using antigranulocyte antibodies can also be employed.[1,14,32,59,163] Tumor is usually reflected by areas of decreased uptake on a bone marrow scan, indicating replacement of normal marrow by malignant cells* (Fig. 6-21). Bone and marrow imaging are often discordant at sites of malignancy, with increase in bone metabolic activity associated with loss of normal marrow elements and phagocytic capability. A similar dual-tracer technique has also been used for examining complicated cases of suspected osteomyelitis, with the mismatch between bone and marrow uptake indicating likely infectious pathology.[2,114]

FUTURE DIRECTIONS

Single Photon Emission Computed Tomography (SPECT)

Earlier in this chapter the role of SPECT imaging in identification of metastatic disease was briefly discussed, although the potential for expanded use of this technique was not examined in depth. As SPECT image resolution has improved, particularly with the advent of multihead cameras, it has become possible to identify smaller foci of increased uptake. The characteristic pattern of tumor involvement in the spine, with increased uptake in both the vertebral body and pedicle, is difficult to identify with planar techniques, and SPECT offers the potential for significantly improved sensitivity and specificity for evaluating this skeletal region.[60] There may come a time when SPECT is routinely performed on all patients suspected of metastatic disease, given that detection of small lesions in many skeletal locations would likely be improved over planar imaging.

Positron–Emitting Radiopharmaceuticals

There has been much interest in recent years in the use of conventional gamma cameras for imaging of positron-emitting radiopharmaceuticals, and a number of companies have already upgraded their high-energy collimators to allow performance of SPECT imaging with PET agents, most commonly F-18 FDG. The potential for performing coincidence counting using dual-head digital gamma cameras is also being actively investigated. Whether gamma camera imaging of PET tracers will have a major influence on the use of bone scans is uncertain, but the movement to increase access to agents that to date have been usable only with the relatively small number of clinical PET scanners is likely to continue.

Image Fusion

One of the more promising approaches for improving the yield of radionuclide tomographic imaging involves fusion of corresponding images from two complementary modalities. This technique has been applied to SPECT in conjunction with CT or MR, with promising preliminary results.[44] Image fusion may be able to augment the interpretation of both the radionuclide and the anatomic imaging study, and implementation of this methodology for routine clinical use is likely to increase as more imaging departments develop electronic networks for linking their computerized digital imaging systems.

SUMMARY

This chapter has presented a brief review of the pathophysiology of metastatic disease to bone and a more in-depth presentation of the major issues involved in the radionuclide imaging of this disease. The Tc-99m diphosphonate bone scan for metastatic disease evaluation has been a nuclear medicine mainstay for three decades, and although there has been some encroachment by other radionuclide and radiologic imaging techniques, the total-body data, high sensitivity, and relatively low cost of this scan remain advantages that cannot be readily matched by the competing methods. There continues to be a need to accumulate high-quality data to document that the findings on bone scintigraphy are reliable and have an effect on clinical patient management. Nevertheless, the bone scan provides valuable and often unique information and should continue to be used for its many valid indications relating to the examination of patients for the presence and extent of metastatic bone disease.

ACKNOWLEDGMENTS
The author wishes to acknowledge the important contribution to this chapter of the late William D. Kaplan, M.D., a faculty member for many years at the Harvard Joint Program in Nuclear Medicine. Dr. Kaplan taught me the clinical principles of bone scanning, introduced me to the intricacies of nuclear medicine research, and inspired me by his dedication to the highest standards in the practice of nuclear medicine.

REFERENCES
1. Aburano T, Yokoyama K, Shuke N, et al: Tc-99m HMPAO-labeled leukocytes for hematopoietic marrow imaging. *Clin Nucl Med* 1992; 17:938.
2. Achong DM, Oates E: The computer-generated bone marrow subtraction image: A valuable adjunct to combined In-111 WBC/Tc-99m in sulfur colloid scintigraphy for musculoskeletal infection. *Clin Nucl Med* 1994; 19:188.
3. Ahmed A, Glynne-Jones R, Ell PJ: Skeletal scintigraphy in carcinoma of the breast—a ten year retrospective study of 389 patients. *Nucl Med Commun* 1990; 11:421.
4. Algra PR, Heimans JJ, Valk J, et al: Do metastases in vertebrae begin in the body or the pedicles? Imaging study in 45 patients. *AJR Am J Roentgenol* 1992; 158:1275.
5. Amico S, Liehn JC, Desoize, et al: Comparison of phosphatase isoenzymes PAP and PSA with bone scan in patients with prostate carcinoma. *Clin Nucl Med* 1991; 16:643.

*References 14,20,59,163,164,207

6. Aprikian AG, Cordon-Cardo C, Fair WR, et al: Neuroendocrine differentiation in metastatic prostatic adenocarcinoma. *J Urol* 1994; 151:914.

7. Arnstein NB, Harbert JC, Byrne PJ: Efficacy of bone and liver scanning in breast cancer patients treated with adjuvant chemotherapy. *Cancer* 1984; 54:2243.

8. Au FC, Maier WP, Malmud LS, et al: Preoperative nuclear scans in patients with melanoma. *Cancer* 1984; 53:2095.

9. Babaian RJ, Johnson DE, Llamas L, Ayala AG: Metastases from transitional cell carcinoma of urinary bladder. *Urology* 1980; 16:142.

10. Batson OV: The function of the vertebral veins and their role in the spread of metastatic disease. *Ann Surg* 1940; 112:138.

11. Batson OV: The role of the vertebral veins in metastatic processes. *Ann Intern Med* 1942; 16:38.

12. Behrens J: The role of cell adhesion molecules in cancer invasion and metastasis. *Breast Cancer Res Treat* 1993; 24:175.

13. Berger GL, Sadlowski RW, Sharpe JR, Finney RP: Lack of value of routine preoperative bone and liver scans in cystectomy candidates. *J Urol* 1981; 125:637.

14. Berna L, Torres G, Carrio I, et al: Antigranulocyte antibody bone marrow scans in cancer patients with metastatic bone superscan appearance. *Clin Nucl Med* 1994; 19:121.

15. Bischof-Delaloye A, Delaloye B, Buchegger F, et al: Clinical value of immunoscintigraphy in colorectal carcinoma patients: A prospective study. *J Nucl Med* 1989; 30:1646.

16. Bitran JD, Bekerman C, Desser RK: The predictive value of serial bone scans in assessing response to chemotherapy in advanced breast cancer. *Cancer* 1980; 45:1562.

17. Bitran JD, Beckerman C, Pinsky S: Sequential scintigraphic staging of small cell carcinoma. *Cancer* 1981; 47:1971.

18. Black WC, Ling A: Is earlier diagnosis really better? The misleading effects of lead time and length biases. *AJR Am J Roentgenol* 1990; 155:625.

19. Bone Imaging: Beautiful bone scans, in Datz FL (ed): *Gamuts in Nuclear Medicine*, ed 2, Appleton & Lange, Norwalk, 1987, p 88.

20. Bourgeoi P, Malarme M, Van Franck R, et al: Bone marrow scintigraphy in prostatic carcinomas. *Nucl Med Commun* 1991; 12:35.

21. Boxer DI, Todd CEC, Coleman R, Fogelman I: Bone secondaries in breast cancer: The solitary metastasis. *J Nucl Med* 1989; 30:1318.

22. Boyce BF, Chen H: Normal bone remodeling and metastatic bone disease, in Diel IJ, Kaufmann M, Bastert G (eds): *Metastatic Bone Disease—Fundamental and Clinical Aspects*, Springer-Verlag, Berlin, 1994, p 46.

23. Brar HS, Sisley JF, Johnson RH: Value of preoperative bone and liver scans and alkaline phosphatase in the evaluation of breast cancer patients. *Am J Surg* 1993; 165:221.

24. Brawer MK, Chetner MP, Beatie J, et al: Screening for prostate carcinoma with prostate specific antigen. *J Urol* 1992; 147:841.

25. Brown B, Laorr A, Greenspan A, Stadalnik R: Negative bone scintigraphy with diffuse osteoblastic breast carcinoma metastases. *Clin Nucl Med* 1994; 19:194.

26. Burkett FE, Scanlon EF, Garces RM, Khandekar JD: The value of bone scans in the management of patients with carcinoma of the breast. *Surg Gynecol Obstet* 1979; 149:523.

27. Butzelaar RMJM, Van Dongen JA, DeGraff PW, Van Der Schoot JB: Bone scintigraphy in patients with operable breast cancer stages I and II: Final conclusion after five-year follow-up. *Eur J Cancer Clin Oncol* 1984; 20:877.

28. Caluser CI, Scott AM, Schneider J, et al: Value of lesion location and intensity of uptake in SPECT bone scintigraphy of the spine in patients with malignant tumors. *Radiology* 1992; 185P:315 (abstract).

29. Campbell RJ, Broaddus SB, Leadbetter GW: Staging of renal cell carcinoma: Cost-effectiveness of routine preoperative bone scans. *Urology* 1985; 25:326.

30. Caner B, Kitapcl M, Unlu M, et al: Technetium-99m-MIBI uptake in benign and malignant bone lesions: A comparative study with technetium-99m MDP. *J Nucl Med* 1992; 33:319.

31. Castronovo V: Laminin receptors and laminin-binding proteins during tumor invasion and metastasis. *Invasion Metastasis* 1993; 13:1.

32. Chandramouly BS, Cunningham RP, Schiano FJ: Skeletal photopenic lesions on indium-111 WBC imaging, differential diagnosis. *Clin Nucl Med* 1993; 18:439.

33. Chaudary MA, Maisey NM, Shaw PJ, et al: Sequential bone scans and chest radiographs in the postoperative management of early breast cancer. *Br J Surg* 1983; 70:517.

34. Chybowski FM, Keller JJL, Bergstralh EJ, Oesterling JE: Predicting radionuclide bone scan findings in patients with newly diagnosed, untreated prostate cancer: Prostate specific antigen is superior to all other clinical parameters. *J Urol* 1991; 145:313.

35. Citrin DL, Bessent RG, Greig WR, et al: The application of the 99mTc phosphate bone scan to the study of breast cancer. *Br J Surg* 1975; 62:201.

36. Citrin DL, Furnival CM, Bessent RG, et al: Radioactive technetium phosphate bone scanning in preoperative assessment and follow-up study of patients with primary cancer of the breast. *Surg Gynecol Obstet* 1976; 113:363.

37. Citrin DL, Tormey DC, Carbone PP: Implications of the 99mTc diphosphonate bone scan on treatment of primary breast cancer. *Cancer Treat Res* 1977; 61:1249.

38. Coleman R: Incidence and distribution of bone metastases, in Diel IJ, Kaufmann M, Bastert G (eds): *Metastatic Bone Disease—Fundamental and Clinical Aspects*, Springer-Verlag, Berlin, 1994, p 20.

39. Coleman RE, Fogelman I, Habibollahi F, et al: Selection of patients with breast cancer for routine follow-up bone scans. *Clin Oncol* 1990; 2:328.

40. Coleman RE, Mashiter G, Whitaker KB, et al: Bone scan flare predicts successful systemic therapy for bone metastases. *J Nucl Med* 1988; 29:1354.

41. Coleman RE, Rubens RD: Bone metastases and breast cancer. *Cancer Treat Rev* 1985; 12:251.

42. Coleman RE, Rubens RD: The clinical course of bone metastases from breast cancer. *Br J Cancer* 1987; 55:61.

43. Coleman RE, Rubens RD, Fogelman I: Reappraisal of the baseline bone scan in breast cancer. *J Nucl Med* 1988; 29:1045.

44. Collier BD, Abdel-Nabi H, Doerr RJ, et al: Immunoscintigraphy performed with In-111-labeled CYT-103 in the management of colorectal cancer: Comparison with CT. *Radiology* 1992; 185:179.

45. Condon BR, Buchanan R, Garvie NW, et al: Assessment of prgression of secondary bone lesions following cancer of the breast or prostate using serial radionuclide imaging. *Br J Radiol* 1981; 54:18.

46. Constable AR, Cranage RW: Recognition of the superscan in prostatic bone scintigraphy. *Br J Radiol* 1981; 54:122.

47. Coombes RC, Dady P, Parsons C, et al: Assessment of response of bone metastases to systemic treatment in patients with breast cancer. *Cancer* 1983; 52:610.

48. Corcoran RJ, Thrall JH, Kyle RW, et al: Solitary abnormalities in bone scans of patients with extraosseous malignancies. *Radiology* 1976; 121:663.

49. Cox MR, Gilliland R, Odling-Smee GW, Spence RAJ: An evaluation of radionuclide bone scanning and liver ultrasonography for staging breast cancer. *Aust N Z J Surg* 1992; 62:550.

50. Cumming J, Hacking N, Fairhurst J, et al: Distribution of bony metastases in prostatic carcinoma. *Br J Urol* 1990; 66:411.

51. Daffner RH, Lupetin AR, Dash N, et al: MRI in the detection of malignant infiltration of bone marrow. *AJR Am J Roentgenol* 1986; 146:353.

52. Dann J, Castronova FP Jr, McKusick KA, et al: Total bone uptake in management of metastatic carcinoma of the prostate. *J Urol* 1987; 137:444.

53. Daubenton JD, Fisher RM, Karabus CD, Mann MD: The relationship between prognosis and scintigraphic evidence of bone metastases in neuroblastoma. *Cancer* 1987; 59:1586.

54. Davey P, Merrick MV, Duncan W Redpath AT: Bladder cancer: The value of routine bone scintigraphy. *Clin Radiol* 1985; 36:77.

55. Derimanov SG: 'For' or 'against' bone scintigraphy of patients with breast cancer. *Nucl Med Commun* 1987; 8:79.

56. Divgi CR, McDermott K, Griffin TW, et al: Lesion-by-lesion comparison of computerized tomography and indium-111-labeled monoclonal antibody C110 radioimmunoscintigraphy in colorectal carcinoma: A multicenter trial. *J Nucl Med* 1993; 34:1656.

57. Donato AT, Ammerman EG, Sullesta O: Bone scanning in the evaluation of patients with lung cancer. *Ann Thorac Surg* 1979; 27:300.

58. Dorudi S, Hart IR: Mechanisms underlying invasion and metastasis. *Curr Opin Oncol* 1993; 5:130.

59. Duncker CM, Carrio I, Berna L, et al: Radioimmune imaging of bone marrow in patients with suspected bone metastases from primary breast cancer. *J Nucl Med* 1990; 31:1450.

60. Even-Sapir E, Martin RH, Barnes DC, et al: Role of SPECT in differentiating malignant from benign lesions in the lower thoracic and lumbar spine. *Radiology* 1993; 187:193.

61. Fogelman I, Citrin DL, McKillop JH, et al: A clinical comparison of Tc-99m HEDP and Tc-99m MDP in the detection of bone metastases: Concise communication. *J Nucl Med* 1979; 20:98.

62. Fogelman I, Coleman R: The bone scan and breast cancer, in Freeman LM, Weissman HS (eds): *Nuclear Medicine Annual*, Raven Press, New York, 1988, p 1.

63. Fogelman I, McKillop JH: The bone scan in metastatic disease, in Rubens RD, Fogelman I (eds): *Bone Metastases—Diagnosis and Treatment*, Springer-Verlag, London, 1991, p 31.

64. Fon GT, Wong WS, Gold RH, Kaiser LR: Skeletal metastases of melanoma: Radiographic, scintigraphic and clinical review. *AJR Am J Roentgenol* 1981; 137:103.

65. Frassica FJ, Sim FH: Metastatic bone disease—general perspectives, pathogenesis, pathophysiology and skeletal dysfunction. *Orthopedics* 1992; 15:599.

66. Freitas JE, Gilvydas R, Ferry JD, Gonzalez JA: The clinical utility of prostate-specific antigen and bone scintigraphy in prostate cancer follow-up. *J Nucl Med* 1991; 32:1387.

67. Front D: Bone imaging and its role in metastatic disease. *Curr Opin Radiol* 1990; 2:823.

68. Front D, Bar-Shalom R, Epelbaum, et al: Early detection of lymphoma recurrence with gallium-67 scintigraphy. *J Nucl Med* 1993; 34:2101.

69. Front D, Schneck SO, Frankel A, Robinson E: Bone metastases and bone pain in breast cancer. Are they closely associated? *JAMA* 1979; 242:1747.

70. Galasko CSB: The anatomy and pathways of skeletal metastases, in Weiss L, Gilbert AH (eds): *Bone Metastasis*, Hall Medical Publishers, Boston, 1981, p 49.

71. Galasko CSB: The significance of occult skeletal metastases, detected by skeletal scintigraphy, in patients with otherwise apparently early mammary carcinoma. *Br J Surg* 1975; 62:694.

72. Galasko CSB, Doyle FH: The detection of skeletal metastases from mammary cancer. A regional comparison between radiology and scintigraphy. *Clin Radiol* 1972; 23:295.

73. Gerber G, Chodak GW: Assessment of value of routine bone scans in patients with newly diagnosed prostate cancer. *Urology* 1991; 37:418.

74. Gerber FH, Goodreau JJ, Kirchner PT, Fouty WJ: Efficacy of preoperative and postoperative bone scanning in the management of breast carcinoma. *N Engl J Med* 1977; 297:300.

75. Glynne-Jones R, Young T, Ahmed A, et al: How far investigations for occult metastases in breast cancer aid the clinician. *Clin Oncol* 1991; 3:65.

76. Gold RH, Bassett LW: Radionuclide evaluation of skeletal metastases: Practical considerations. *Skeletal Radiol* 1986; 15:1.

77. Goldrath DE, Messing EM: Prostate specific antigen: Not detectable despite tumor progression after radical prostatectomy. *J Urol* 1989; 142:1082.

78. Goltzman D, Bolivar I, Rabbani SA: Studies on the pathogenesis of osteoblastic metastases by prostate cancer, in Karr JP (ed): *Prostate Cancer and Bone Metastasis*, Plenum Press, New York, 1992, p 165.

79. Harada M, Iida M, Yamaguchi M, Shida K: Analysis of bone metastasis of prostatic adenocarcinoma in 137 autopsy cases, in Karr JP (ed): *Prostate Cancer and Bone Metastasis*, Plenum Press, New York, 1992, p 173.

80. Harada M, Shimizu A, Nakamura Y, Nemoto R: Role of the vertebral venous system in metastatic spread of cancer cells to the bone, in Karr JP (ed): *Prostate Cancer and Bone Metastasis*, Plenum Press, New York, 1992, p 83.

81. Harbert J: Efficacy of bone and liver scanning in malignant disease, in Freeman LM, Weissman HS (eds): *Nuclear Medicine Annual*, Raven Press, New York, 1982, p 373.

82. Harbert JC, Rocha L, Smith FP, Delgado G: The efficacy of radionuclide liver and bone scans in the evaluation of gynecologic cancers. *Cancer* 1982; 49:1040.

83. Harbin WP: Metastatic disease and the nonspecific bone scan: Value of spinal computed tomography. *Radiology* 1982; 145:105.

84. Hayward SJ, McIvor J, Burdge AH, et al: Staging of prostatic carcinoma with radionuclide bone scintigraphy and lymphography. *Br J Radiol* 1987; 60:79.

85. Hirnle P, Mittmann KP, Schmidt B, Pfeiffer KH: Indications for radioisotope bone scanning in staging of cervical cancer. *Arch Gynecol Obstet* 1990; 248:21.

86. Hooper RG, Beechler CR, Johnson MC: Radioisotope scanning in the initial staging of bronchogenic carcinoma. *Am Rev Resp Dis* 1978; 118:279.

87. Hortobagyi GN, Libshitz HI, Seabold JE: Osseous metastases of breast cancer—clinical, biochemical, radiographic, and scintigraphic evaluation of response to therapy. *Cancer* 1984; 53:577.

88. Hoshi H, Nagamachi S, Jinnouchi S, et al: Bone scintigraphy as a prognostic factor in patients with adult T-cell leukemia-lymphoma. *Clin Nucl Med* 1994; 19:992.

89. Israel O, Front D, Frenkel A, Kleinhaus U: 24-hour/4-hour ratio of technetium-99m methylene diphosphonate uptake in patients with bone metastases and degenerative-bone changes. *J Nucl Med* 1985; 26:237.

90. Jacobson AF: Nuclear medicine and other radiologic imaging techniques: Competitors or collaborators. *Eur J Nucl Med* 1994; 21:1369.

91. Jacobson AF: Pre-treatment prostate specific antigen levels in newly diagnosed prostate cancer without bone metastases do not predict occurrence of metastases on follow-up bone scintigraphy. *J Nucl Med* 1994; 35:225P (abstract).

92. Jacobson AF: Yield of bone scintigraphy for identifying occult malignancy in patients with musculoskeletal pain. *J Nucl Med* 1993; 34:33P (abstract).

93. Jacobson AF, Brawer MK: Prostate specific antigen levels in patients with newly diagnosed prostate cancer: Association with occurrence and pattern of metastases on staging bone scintigraphy. *J Nucl Med* 1993; 34:218p (abstract).

94. Jacobson AF, Cronin EB, Stomper PC, Kaplan WD: Bone scans with one or two new abnormalities in cancer patients with no known metastases: Incidence and serial scintigraphic behavior of benign and malignant lesions. *Radiology* 1990; 175:229.

95. Jacobson AF, Gilles CP, Cerqueira MD: Photopenic defects in marrow-containing skeleton on indium-111 leukocyte scintigraphy: Prevalence at sites suspected of osteomyelitis and as an incidental finding. *Eur J Nucl Med* 1992; 19:858.

96. Jacobson AF, Hyman FE: Low likelihood of malignancy in isolated vertebral compression fractures on bone scans of cancer patients without known spinal metastases. *J Nucl Med* 1995; 36:26P.

97. Jacobson AF, Shapiro CL, Kaplan WD: Bone metastases in patients with breast cancer: Significance of scintigraphic patterns at presentation and follow-up. *J Nucl Med* 1993; 34:74P (abstract).

98. Jacobson AF, Stomper PC, Cronin EB, Kaplan WD: Bone scans with one or two new abnormalities in cancer patients with no known metastases: Reliability of interpretation of initial correlative radiographs. *Radiology* 1990; 174:503.

99. Jacobson AF, Stomper PC, Jochelson MS, et al: Association between number and sites of new bone scan abnormalities and presence of skeletal metastases in patients with breast cancer. *J Nucl Med* 1990; 31:387.

100. Janicek MJ, Hayes DF, Kaplan WD: Healing flare in skeletal metastases from breast cancer. *Radiology* 1994; 192:201.

101. Johns WD, Garnick MB, Kaplan WD: Leuprolide therapy for prostate cancer. An association with scintigraphic "flare" on bone scan. *Clin Nucl Med* 1990; 15:485.

102. Johnson DG, Coleman RE, McCook TA, et al: Bone and liver images in medullary carcinoma of the thyroid gland: Concise communication. *J Nucl Med* 1984; 25:419.

103. Jones RJ: The role of bone marrow imaging. *Radiology* 1992; 183:321.

104. Kamby C, Vejborg I, Daugaard S, et al: Clinical and radiologic characteristics of bone metastases in breast cancer. *Cancer* 1987; 60:2524.

105. Kaplan WD, Jochelson MS, Herman TS, et al: Gallium-67 imaging: A predictor of residual tumor viability and clinical outcome in patients with diffuse large-cell lymphoma. *J Clin Oncol* 1990; 8:1966.

106. Kashyap R, Bhatnagar A, Mondal A, Sawroop K: 24 hour/3 hour radio-uptake technique for differentiating degenerative and malignant bony lesions in bone scanning. *Aust Radiol* 1993; 37:198.

107. Kattapuram SV, Khurana JS, Scott JA, El-Khoury GY: Negative scintigraphy with positive magnetic resonance imaging in bone metastases. *Skeletal Radiol* 1990; 19:113.

108. Katz RD, Alderson PO, Rosenshein NB, et al: Utility of bone scanning in detecting occult skeletal metastases from cervical carcinoma. *Radiology* 1979; 133:469.

109. Kelly RJ, Cowan RJ, Ferree CB, et al: Efficacy of radionuclide scanning in patients with lung cancer. *JAMA* 1979; 242:2855.

110. Kennedy H, Kennedy N, Barclay M, Horobin M: Cost efficiency of bone scans in breast cancer. *Clin Oncol* 1991; 3:73.

111. Khandekar JD: Role of routine bone scans in operable breast cancer: An opposing viewpoint. *Cancer Treat Res* 1979; 63:1241.

112. Khansur T, Haick A, Patel B, et al: Evaluation of bone scan as a screening work-up in primary and local-regional recurrence of breast cancer. *Am J Clin Oncol* 1987; 10:167.

113. Kim SE, Kim DY, Lee DS, et al: Absent or faint renal uptake on bone scan—etiology and significance in metastatic bone disease. *Clin Nucl Med* 1991; 16:545.

114. King AD, Peters AM, Stuttle AWJ, Lavender JP: Imaging of bone infection with labelled white blood cells: role of contemporaneous bone marrow imaging. *Eur J Nucl Med* 1990; 17:148.

115. Knudson G, Grinis G, Lopez-Majano V, et al: Bone scan as a stratification variable in advanced prostate cancer. *Cancer* 1991; 68:316.

116. Krempien B: Morphological findings in bone metastasis, tumorosteopathy and antiosteolytic therapy, in Diel IJ, Kaufmann M, Bastert G (eds): *Metastatic Bone Disease—Fundamental and Clinical Aspects,* Springer-Verlag, Berlin, 1994, p 59.

117. Krenning EP, Kwekkeboom DJ, Bakker WH, et al: Somatostatic receptor scintigraphy with [111In-DTPA-D-Phe1]- and [123I-Tyr3]-octreotide: The Rotterdam experience with more than 1000 patients. *Eur J Nucl Med* 1993; 20:716.

118. Krishnamurthy GT, Tubis M, Hiss J, Blahd WH: Distribution pattern of metastatic bone disease—a need for total body skeletal image. *JAMA* 1977; 237:2504.

119. Kunkler IH, Merrick MV: The value of non-staging skeletal scintigraphy in breast cancer. *Clin Radiol* 1986; 37:561.

120. Kunkler IH, Merrick MV, Rodger A: Bone scintigraphy in breast cancer: A nine-year follow-up. *Clin Radiol* 1985; 36:279.

121. Kwai AH, Stomper PC, Kaplan WD: Clinical significance of isolated scintigraphic sternal lesions in patients with breast cancer. *J Nucl Med* 1988; 29:324.

122. Lamberts SW, Reubi JC, Krenning EP: Validation of somatostatin receptor scintigraphy in the localization of neuroendocrine tumors. *Acta Oncol* 1993; 32:167.

123. Leung SF, Stewart IET, Tsao SY, Metreweli C: Staging bone scintigraphy in nasopharyngeal carcinoma. *Clin Radiol* 1991; 43:314.

124. Levenson RM, Sauerbrunn FJL, Ihde DC, et al: Small cell lung cancer: Radionuclide bone scans for assessment of tumor extent and response. *AJR Am J Roentgenol* 1981; 137:31.

125. Lindner A, DeKernion JB: Cost-effective analysis of pre-cystectomy radioisotope scans. *J Urol* 1982; 128:1181.

126. Lindner A, Goldman DG, DeKernion JB: Cost effective analysis of prenephrectomy radioisotope scans in renal cell carcinoma. *Urology* 1983; 22:127.

127. Liotta LA, Stetter-Stevenson WG: Principles of molecular cell biology of cancer: Cancer metastasis, in DeVita Jr VT, Hellman S, Rosenberg SA (eds): *Cancer—Principles and Practice of Oncology*, ed 3, JB Lippincott, Philadelphia, 1989, p 98.

128. Manzotti C, Audisio RA, Pratesi G: Importance of ortho-topic implantation for human tumors as model systems: Relevance to metastasis and invasion. *Clin Exp Metastasis* 1993; 11:5.

129. Matin P: The appearance of bone scans following fractures, including immediate and long-term studies. *J Nucl Med* 1979; 20:1227.

130. McNeil BJ: Value of bone scanning in neoplastic disease. *Semin Nucl Med* 1984; 14:277.

131. Mehta RC, Wilson MA, Perlman SB: False-negative bone scan in extensive metastatic disease: CT and MR findings. *J Comput Assist Tomogr* 1989; 13:717.

132. Mello AM, Blake L, McDougall IR: "Cold" lesions on indium-111 white blood cell scintigraphy. *Semin Nucl Med* 1992; 22:292.

133. Mellor JA, Simmons AV, Barnard DL, Cartwright SC: A retrospective evaluation of mediastinal tomograms, isotope liver scans, and isotope bone scans in the staging and management of patients with lymphoma. *Cancer* 1983; 52:2227.

134. Merrick MV: Bone scintigraphy in testicular tumors. *Br J Urol* 1987; 60:167.

135. Merrick MV, Beales JSM, Garvie N, Leonard RCO: Evaluation and skeletal metastases. *Br J Radiol* 1992; 65:803.

136. Merrick MV, Ding CL, Chisholm GD, Elton RA: Prognostic significance of alkaline and acid phosphatase and skeletal scintigraphy in carcinoma of the prostate. *Br J Urol* 1985; 57:715.

137. Merrick MV, Merrick JM: Bone scintigraphy in lung cancer: A reappraisal. *Br J Radiol* 1986; 59:1185.

138. Mettler FA, Christie JH, Garcia JF, et al: Radionuclide liver and bone scanning in the evaluation of patients with endometrial caricinoma. *Radiology* 1981; 141:777.

139. Michel F, Soler M, Imhof E, Perruchoud AP: Initial staging of non-small cell lung cancer: Value of routine radioisotope bone scanning. *Thorax* 1991; 46:469.

140. Miller PD, Eardley I, Kirby RS: Prostate specific antigen and bone scan correlation in the staging and monitoring of patients with prostatic cancer. *Br J Urol* 1992; 70:295.

141. Minna JD, Pass H, Glatstern E, Ihde DC: Cancer of the lung, in DeVita Jr VT, Hellman S, Rosenberg SA (eds): *Cancer—Principles and Practice of Oncology*, ed 3, JB Lippincott, Philadelphia, 1989, p 591.

142. Monypenny IJ, Grieve RJ, Howell A, Morrison JM: The value of serial bone scanning in operable breast cancer. *Br J Surg* 1984; 71:466.

143. Mouratidis B, Gilday DL, Ash JM: Comparison of bone and 67Ga scintigraphy in the initial diagnosis of bone involvement in children with malignant lymphoma. *Nucl Med Commun* 1994; 15:144.

144. Mundy GR: Mechanisms of osteolytic bone destruction. *Bone* 1991; (suppl 1):S1.

145. Nicolson GL: Cancer progression and growth: Relationship of paracrine and autocrine growth mechanisms to organ preference of metastasis. *Exp Cell Res* 1993; 204:171.

146. Nishijima Y, Uchida K, Koiso K, Nemoto R: Clinical significance of the vertebral vein in prostate cancer metastasis, in Karr JP (ed): *Prostate Cancer and Bone Metastasis*, Plenum Press, New York, 1992, p 93.

147. Oesterling JE, Martin SK, Bergstralh EJ, Lowe FC: The use of prostate-specific antigen in staging patients with newly diagnosed prostate cancer. *JAMA* 1993; 269:57.

148. Oommen R, Geethanjali FS, Gopalakrishnan G, et al: Correlation of serum prostate specific antigen levels and bone scintigraphy in carcinoma prostate. *Br J Radiol* 1994; 67:469.

149. O'Mara RE, Weber DA: The osseous system, in Freeman LM (ed): *Freeman and Johnson's Clinical Radionuclide Imaging*, ed 3, Grune & Stratton, Orlando, 1984, p 1141.

150. Orzel JA, Sawaf NW, Richardson ML: Lymphoma of the skeleton: Scintigraphic evaluation. *AJR Am J Roentgenol* 1988; 150:1095.

151. Paget S: The distribution of secondary growths in cancer of the breast. *Lancet* 1889; 1:571.

152. Pantelides ML, Bowman SP, George JR: Levels of prostate specific antigen that predict skeletal spread in prostate cancer. *Br J Urol* 1992; 70:299.

153. Parekh JS, Teates CD: Gamut: Mixed "hot" and "cold" lesions on bone scan. *Semin Nucl Med* 1992; 22:289.

154. Parthasarthy KL, Landsberg R, Bakshi SP, et al: Detection of bone metastases in urogenital malignancies utilizing 99mTc-labeled phosphate compounds. *Urology* 1978; 11:99.

155. Perez DJ, Milan J, Ford HT, et al: Detection of breast carcinoma metastases in bone: Relative merits of x-rays and skeletal scintigraphy. *Lancet* 1983; 1:613.

156. Podrasky AE, Stark DD, Hattner RS, et al: Radionuclide bone scanning in neuroblastoma: Skeletal metastases and primary tumor localization of 99mTc-MDP. *AJR Am J Roentgenol* 1983; 141:469.

157. Prout GR, Griffin PP, Castronovo FP Jr: Quantification of changes in bone scans of patients with osseous metastases of prostatic carcinoma, in Karr JP (ed): *Prostate Cancer and Bone Metastasis*, Plenum Press, New York, 1992, p 233.

158. Quinn DL, Ostrow LB, Porter DK, et al: Staging of non-small cell bronchogenic carcinoma. Relationship of the clinical evaluation to organ scans. *Chest* 1986; 89:270.

159. Ralston S, Gardner MD, Fogelman I, Boyle IT: Hypercalcaemia and metastatic bone disease: Is there a causal link? *Lancet* 1982; ii:903.

160. Rana A, Chisholm GD, Khan M, et al: Patterns of bone metastasis and their prognostic significance in patients with carcinoma of the prostate. *Br J Urol* 1993; 72:933.

161. Rankin S: Radiology, in Rubens RD, Fogelman I (eds): *Bone Metastases—Diagnosis and Treatment*, Springer-Verlag, London, 1991, p 63.

162. Rappaport AH, Hoffer PB, Genant HK: Unifocal bone findings by scintigraphy: Clinical significance in patients with known primary cancer. *West J Med* 1978; 129:188.

163. Reske SN, Gloeckner W, Schwarz A, et al: Radio-immunoimaging for diagnosis of bone marrow involvement in breast cancer and malignant lymphoma. *Lancet* 1989; i:299.

164. Reske S, Kartsens J, Sohn M, et al: Bone marrow immunoscintigraphy compared with conventional bone scintigraphy for the detection of bone metastases. *Acta Oncol* 1993; 32:753.

165. Richards MA: Magnetic resonance imaging, in Rubens RD, Fogelman I (eds): *Bone Metastases—Diagnosis and Treatment*, Springer-Verlag, London, 1991, p 79.

166. Rosen PR, Murphy KG: Bone scintigraphy in the initial staging of patients with renal-cell carcinoma: Concise communication. *J Nucl Med* 1984; 25:289.

167. Rosselli Del Turco M, Palli D, Cariddi A, et al: Intensive diagnostic follow-up after treatment of primary breast cancer. A randomized trial (National Research Council Project on Breast Cancer follow-up). *JAMA* 1994; 271:1593.

168. Rossing N, Munck O, Nielsen P, Andersen KW: What do early bone scans tell about breast cancer patients? *Eur J Cancer Clin Oncol* 1982; 18:629.

169. Roth JA, Eilber FR, Bennett LR, Morton DL: Radionuclide photoscanning: Usefulness in preoperative evaluation of melanoma patients. *Arch Surg* 1975; 110:1211.

170. Rubens RD: Nature of metastatic bone disease, in Diel IJ, Kaufmann M, Bastert G (eds): *Metastatic Bone Disease—Fundamental and Clinical Aspects*, Springer-Verlag, Berlin, 1994, p 12.

171. Ruckle HC, Klee GC, Oesterling JE: Subject review: Prostate-specific antigen: Critical issues for the practicing physician. *Mayo Clin Proc* 1994; 69:59.

172. Sasaki M, Ichiya Y, Kuwabara Y, et al: Fluorine-18-fluorodeoxyglucose positron emission tomography in technetium-99m-hydroxymethylenediphosphate negative bone tumors. *J Nucl Med* 1993; 34:288.

173. Schechter JP, Jones SE, Woolfenden JM, et al: Bone scanning in lymphoma. *Cancer* 1976; 38:1142.

174. Schunemann H, Langecker PJ, Ellgas W, et al: Value of bone scanning in the follow-up of breast cancer patients. A study of 1000 cases. *J Cancer Res Clin Oncol* 1990; 116:486.

175. Scott AM, Larson SM: Tumor imaging and therapy, *Radiol Clin North Am* 1993; 31:859.

176. Scott AM, Macapinlac HA, Divgi CR, et al: Clinical validation of SPECT and CT/MRI image registration in radiolabeled monoclonal antibody studies of colorectal carcinoma. *J Nucl Med* 1994; 35:1976.

177. Scutellari PN, Spanedda R, Feggi LM, et al: Comparison between traditional skeletal radiography and total body bone scintigraphy in the diagnosis of multiple myeloma. *Radiol Med* 1984; 70:271.

178. Sham JST, Tong CM, Choy D, Yeung DWC: Role of bone scanning in detection of subclinical bone metastasis in nasopharyngeal carcinoma. *Clin Nucl Med* 1991; 16:27.

179. Shih LY, Chen TH, Lo WH: Skeletal metastasis from occult carcinoma. *J Surg Oncol* 1992; 51:109.

180. Shih WJ, Mitchell B, Wierzbinski B, et al: Prediction of radionuclide bone imaging findings by Gleason histologic grading of prostate carcinoma. *Clin Nucl Med* 1991; 16:763.

181. Shirazi PH, Rayudu GVS, Fordham EW: Review of solitary ¹⁸F bone scan lesions. *Radiology* 1974; 112:369.

182. Simon MA, Bartucci EJ: The search for the primary tumor in patients with skeletal metastases of unknown origin. *Cancer* 1986; 58:1088.

183. Smith PH, Bono A, da Silva FC, et al: Some limitations of the radioisotope bone scan in patients with metastatic prostate cancer. *Cancer* 1990; 66:1009.

184. Smith SR, Williams CE, Davies JM, Edwards RHT: Bone marrow disorders: Characterization with quantitative MR imaging. *Radiology* 1989; 172:805.

185. Smoker WRK, Godersky JC, Knutzon RK, et al: The role of MR imaging in evaluating metastatic spinal disease. *AJR Am J Roentgenol* 1987; 149:1241.

186. Soloway MS: The importance of prognostic factors in advanced prostate cancer. *Cancer* 1990; 66(suppl):1017.

187. Soloway MS, Hardeman SW, Hickey D, et al: Stratification of patients with metastatic prostate cancer based on extent of disease on initial bone scan. *Cancer* 1988; 61:195.

188. Spitz J, Lauer I, Tittel K, Weigand H: Scintimetric evaluation of remodeling after bone fractures in man. *J Nucl Med* 1993; 34:1403.

189. Stanchev V, Grigorov L, Ouzounov I, Mitov F: Scintigraphic diagnosis of occult bone metastases in patients with operable breast cancer. *Folia Med* 1986; 28:29.

190. Sundaram FX, Chua ET, Goh ASW, et al: Bone scintigraphy in nasopharyngeal carcinoma. *Clin Radiol* 1990; 42:166.

191. Sundaram M, McGuire MH: Computed tomography or magnetic resonance for evaluating the solitary tumor or tumor-like lesion of bone. *Skeletal Radiol* 1988; 17:393.

192. Sundkvist GMG, Ahlgren L, Lilja B, Mattson S: Dynamic quantitative bone scintigraphy in patients with prostatic carcinoma treated by orchiectomy. *Eur J Nucl Med* 1990; 16:671.

193. Sundkvist GMG, Ahlgren L, Lilja B, Mattsson S: Quantitative bone scintigraphy in prostatic carcinoma: Long-term response to treatment. *Nuklearmedizin* 1993; 32:231.

194. Sy WM, Patel D, Faunce H: Significance of absent or faint kidney sign on bone scan. *J Nucl Med* 1975; 16:454.

195. Tamir R, Glanz I, Lubin E, et al: Comparison of the sensitivity of 99mTc-methyl diphosphonate bone scan with the skeletal x-ray survey in multiple myeloma. *Acta Haematol* 1983; 69:236.

196. Tenenbaum F, Schlumberger M, Bonnin F, et al: Usefulness of technetium-99m hydroxymethylene diphosphonate scans in localizing bone metastases of differentiated thyroid carcinoma. *Eur J Nucl Med* 1993; 20:1168.

197. Terris MK, Klonecke AS, McDougall IR, Stamey TA: Utilization of bone scans in conjunction with prostate-specific antigen levels in the surveillance for recurrence of adenocarcinoma after radical prostatectomy. *J Nucl Med* 1991; 32:1713.

198. Texter JH Jr, Neal CE: Current applications of immunoscintigraphy in prostate cancer. *J Nucl Med* 1993; 34:549.

199. Tofe AJ, Francis MD, Harvey WJ: Correlation of neoplasms with incidence and localization of skeletal metastases: An analysis of 1355 diphosphonate bone scans. *J Nucl Med* 1975; 16:986.

200. Tornyos K, Garcia O, Karr B, LeBeaud R: A correlation study of bone scanning with clinical and laboratory findings in the staging of nonsmall-cell lung cancer. *Clin Nucl Med* 1991; 16:107.

201. Tumeh SS, Beadle G, Kaplan WD: Clinical significance of solitary rib lesions in patients with extraskeletal malignancy. *J Nucl Med* 1985; 26:1140.

202. Van den Brenk HAS, Burch WM, Kelly H, Orton C: Venous diversion trapping and growth of blood-borne cancer cells en route to the lungs. *Br J Cancer* 1975; 31:46.

203. Van Der Wall H, Murray PC, Huckstrep RL, Phillips RL: The role of thallium scintigraphy in excluding malignancy in bone. *Clin Nucl Med* 1993; 18:551.

204. Van Duzee BF, Schaefer JA, Ball JD, et al: Relative lesion detection ability of Tc-99m HMDP and Tc-99m MDP: Concise communication. *J Nucl Med* 1984; 25:166.

205. Vogler JB, Murphy WA: Bone marrow imaging. *Radiology* 1988; 168:679.

206. Wickerham L, Fisher B, Cronin W, et al: The efficacy of bone scanning in the follow-up of patients with operable breast cancer. *Breast Cancer Res Treat* 1984; 4:303.

207. Widding A, Stilbo I, Hansen SW, et al: Scintigraphy with nanocolloid Tc-99m in patients with small cell lung cancer, with special reference to bone marrow and hepatic metastasis. *Eur J Nucl Med* 1990; 16:717.

208. Williams SJ, Green M, Kerr IH: Detection of bone metastases in carcinoma of bronchus. *BMJ* 1977; 1:1004.

209. Willis RA: *The Spread of Tumors in the Human Body*, ed 3, Butterworth, London, 1973.

210. Wilson GS, Rich MA, Brennan MJ: Evaluation of bone scan in preoperative clinical staging of breast cancer. *Arch Surg* 1980; 115:415.

211. Wilson MA, Calhoun FW: The distribution of skeletal metastases in breast and pulmonary cancer: Concise communication. *J Nucl Med* 1981; 22:594.

212. Winzelberg GG, Grossman SJ, Rizk S, et al: Indium-111 monoclonal antibody B72.3 scintigraphy in colorectal cancer. *Cancer* 1992; 69:1656.

213. Woolfenden JM, Pitt MJ, Durie BGM, Moon TE: Comparison of bone scintigraphy and radiography in multiple myeloma. *Radiology* 1980; 134:723.

214. Wright DC, Delaney TF: Treatment of metastatic cancer, in DeVita Jr VT, Hellman S, et al (eds): *Cancer—Principles and Practice of Oncology*, ed 3, JB Lippincott, Philadelphia, 1989, p 2245.

215. Yamashita K, Ueda T, Komatsubara Y, et al: Breast cancer with bone-only metastases—visceral metastases-free rate in relation to anatomic distribution of bone metastasis. *Cancer* 1991; 68:634.

216. Yeatman TJ, Nicolson GL: Molecular basis of tumor progression: Mechanisms of organ-specific tumor metastasis. *Semin Surg Oncol* 1993; 9:256.

217. Zetter BR: The cellular basis of site-specific tumor metastasis. *N Engl J Med* 1990; 322:605.

CHAPTER 7

PRIMARY BONE TUMORS

Alan D. Waxman

Leanne L. Seeger

Charles A. Forscher

Gerald Rosen

The diagnosis, treatment, and follow-up of patients with primary tumors of bone relies heavily on information obtained from imaging techniques such as x-ray, computed tomography (CT), and magnetic resonance imaging (MRI).*

Within nuclear medicine, Tc-99m-diphosphonate and Ga-67 citrate scintigraphy have been tried with mixed results. It is known that the bone scan is nonspecific for malignancy and simply reflects levels of blood flow and available osseous receptors. Malignancy as well as bone healing may result in increased blood flow and receptors, thus resulting in a positive scan. Gallium scintigraphy is known to detect a variety of malignancies including primary bone tumors; however, uptake is often nonspecific, with gallium also reflecting uptake in tumors as well as healing, inflammation, and infection.

Recently radiopharmaceuticals as metabolic markers of tumor activity using Tl-201 and Tc-99m sesta-2-methoxyisobutyl isonitrile (MIBI) have been shown to give important information regarding tumor viability, with especially useful information obtained in the management of patients with primary tumors of bone.†

Integration of x-ray, MRI, and nuclear medicine techniques in a logical sequence will help to optimize the management of the individual patient.

THE ROLE OF PLAIN RADIOGRAPHY, COMPUTED TOMOGRAPHY, AND MAGNETIC RESONANCE IMAGING IN SARCOMA EVALUATION

Plain Radiography

Plain radiography should be the initial imaging undertaken for any patient with musculoskeletal pain or a mass. Radiography allows detection of arthritic, inflammatory, and traumatic disorders and provides the most specific noninvasive means to establish an appropriate differential diagnosis for most primary bone neoplasms.‡ Radiographic features such as lesion location, type of bone destruction, and margins should be assessed, as well as the presence and type of periosteal reaction or soft-tissue mass. These findings, when coupled with the patient's age and symptoms, usually allow differentiation

*References 5-7, 17, 20-22, 24, 28, 30, 31, 36-42, 45, 46.
†References 2, 3, 10, 11, 27, 32-35, 44, 47.

‡References 7, 28, 38, 40, 41, 45.

of benign from aggressive or malignant lesions and assist in the formation of a useful limited differential diagnosis in the majority of cases.[41] Benign bone lesions are usually relatively homogenous, show a well-defined margin, lack a periosteal reaction, and are not associated with a soft-tissue mass. Aggressive or malignant lesions generally show permeative bone destruction, ill-defined margins, aggressive periosteal reaction, and are associated with a soft-tissue mass.

Although plain radiography may be diagnostic for bone neoplasia, the appearance of a soft-tissue mass is usually nonspecific. The utility of plain radiography in the evaluation of soft-tissue masses includes documentation of exophytic bony lesions that may masquerade as a soft-tissue mass, identification of adjacent bone erosion or infiltration, identification of bone lesions with a large soft-tissue mass, and detection of mineralization within or surrounding the mass.[22]

Cross–Sectional Imaging: Magnetic Resonance Imaging and Computed Tomography

The role of cross-sectional imaging in musculoskeletal sarcoma evaluation is generally to supply information regarding tumor staging (and thus treatment planning) that is otherwise inapparent or unavailable. The goals of pretreatment cross-sectional imaging thus include determining both the bone and soft-tissue extent of the lesions, defining the relationship of tumor to major neural and vascular structures, evaluating adjacent joints for intraarticular spread, and detecting skip lesions.[5,40,45] Although different information may be derived from MRI and CT, both examinations are usually not required. The choice of which modality to use will be determined by the suspected clinical diagnosis.[40,45]

The multiplanar capability and superior soft-tissue contrast of MRI render it ideally suited for musculoskeletal tumor staging and treatment planning.[5,38,45] A major shortcoming, however, is its lack of specificity.* When dealing with bone-marrow occupying lesions, MRI may not be able to differentiate infection, trauma, benign tumors, and malignant processes. This lack of specificity is also true for soft-tissue sarcomas.[6,17,22,38,45] The majority of soft-tissue sarcomas will appear intermediate to low signal intensity on spin echo Tl-weighted images and bright on T2-weighted images. Criteria for confidently differentiating benign and malignant processes have been studied, but the magnetic resonance (MR) features are too unreliable to be clinically useful.[5,17,21,22,24] Although soft-tissue sarcomas are usually large, heterogeneous, and located below the deep fascia, they may also be small, homogeneous, and superficial.

In addition to its nonspecificity, the utility of MRI may be limited by relative contraindications such as patient tolerance (claustrophobia), patient size (too large to fit in the scanner), or metallic artifact from orthopedic hardware. Absolute contraindications include cardiac pacemakers or cerebral aneurysm clips.[31]

In some instances lesions will have signal characteristics on MRI that will allow the diagnostic possibilities to be narrowed. This occurs predominately when lesions are either high signal intensity on T1-weighted images or very low signal intensity on T2-weighted images, the opposite of the typical appearance. Bright signal on T1-weighted sequences is due to the presence of either fat or blood products.[45] Lesions that have very low signal intensity on T2-weighted imaging usually have abundant fibrous tissue, calcification, or blood. Either group may include aggressive or malignant entities, therefore biopsy is required.

MRI is often used in sarcoma evaluation; however, CT continues to play an important role and is preferred in several situations.[40,41,45] CT allows identification of fine calcifications and subtle cortical abnormalities, features that are difficult or impossible to detect with MRI. CT is useful for evaluating areas such as the ribs, where motion artifact may make MRI examinations difficult to interpret, and CT is also an appropriate alternative for imaging patients with a relative or absolute contraindication to MRI.

With CT images can be directly acquired only in the axial plane. Sagittal and coronal images can be reformatted from axial images, but this is at the expense of fine image detail. Some soft-tissue masses that are isodense to muscle or other adjacent tissue may be difficult to identify with CT, even following contrast enhancement.

Contrast Enhancement for Computed Tomography and Magnetic Resonance Imaging

The efficacy of contrast enhancement in central nervous system CT and MRI reflects the presence of blood-brain barrier. Enhancement of tissues normally protected by this barrier implies either focal or diffuse interruption and thus pathology. Since no similar structure exists in the musculoskeletal system, contrast enhancement outside the central nervous system reflects blood flow, vascular permeability, and the size of the extracellular fluid component. Contrast enhancement is therefore nonspecific.

Although exceptions do exist, contrast enhancement for musculoskeletal MRI usually aids little in establishing a differential diagnosis and provides no assistance in differentiating benign processes from malignancy. Contrast-enhanced MRI has not been shown to improve the accuracy of tumor staging or improve lesion conspicuity.[37,40,42] Contrast may, in fact, mask tumors by altering the signal characteristics of a lesion to equal those of normal surrounding tissues, especially within fatty bone marrow.[37] MRI contrast enhancement cannot accurately determine the amount of tumor necrosis following chemotherapy or radiation therapy.† In the postoperative patient, noncontrast T2-weighted sequences have been found to be the most useful means to detect tumor recurrence.[37,46]

Despite the fact that unenhanced MRI usually pro-

*References 5, 6, 17, 21, 22, 38, 39, 45

†References 7, 20, 30, 36-38, 42, 45.

vides sufficient and maximum information, there may be circumstances where additional useful information may be gained with use of contrast. The information gained must, however, outweigh the added risk and cost.

Although contrast enhancement is seldom indicated for tumor imaging with MRI, contrast enhancement is useful for CT of soft-tissue sarcomas and osseous tumors with a large soft-tissue mass.

In these instances the tumor mass may be isodense to adjacent muscle on unenhanced images.[22] Intravenous contrast is not necessary for CT evaluation of bone sarcomas where normal cortex and medullary fat contrast well against the tumor mass.[7]

Imaging After Treatment

Plain radiography, CT, and MRI also play an important role in evaluating tumor response to chemotherapy and/or radiation therapy. A favorable response is associated with a reduction in tumor bulk and tumor necrosis. Bone sarcomas are well imaged with either plain radiography or CT, where both reduced tumor bulk and increased tumor mineralization are associated with an improved prognosis.[41] CT can depict gross areas of liquefactive necrosis following therapy. However, neither CT nor MRI can provide sufficient information regarding the amount of necrosis to guide clinical decision making with respect to the need for additional chemotherapy following completion of standard courses.

The choice of imaging following surgical resection will be dictated by the presence of orthopedic hardware. If a tumor has been resected without placement of hardware, either CT or MRI may be used to evaluate for tumor recurrence. Cross-sectional studies are also useful for evaluating benign postoperative complications such as hematoma and seroma.[40] Patients with hardware following tumor resection present an imaging challenge. Plain radiography is useful for follow-up of limb-salvage surgery to assess for prosthesis failure or recurrence of mineralized tumor.[41] Extensive metallic artifact may seriously degrade image quality of both CT and MRI. These studies may nonetheless be useful, especially if the areas of clinical concern are not immediately adjacent to the prosthesis or hardware.[40]

THE ROLE OF NUCLEAR MEDICINE

Thallium-201

MECHANISM OF UPTAKE

Thallium, when administered as a chloride, behaves similarly to potassium chloride in most biologic systems.[4,8,19,23] There have been many studies demonstrating the importance of the adenosine triphosphatase (ATPase)-mediated sodium potassium pump within cell membranes, which transports the potassium ion into intact cells in high concentration relative to the extracellular space. Because of the physical and biologic similarities of thallium and potassium, thallium is concentrated in a similar manner.[9] Tumors also concentrate potassium ions and thallium in a similar manner.[29,43]

Sessler et al recently developeded a model for studying cellular uptake of thallium-201 using Ehrlich ascites tumor cells.[43] Using this model, it was demonstrated that the uptake of thallium-201 by tumor cells was inhibited by ouabain, which is known to inhibit the ATPase sodium-potassium pump. Of great interest was the finding that furosemide also inhibited thallium uptake by tumor cells. Furosemide is known to inhibit a cotransport system involving transport of potassium, sodium, as well as chloride ion into the cell. This study demonstrated an additive effect of furosemide and ouabain on the inhibition of thallium uptake. It was postulated that at least two transport systems are involved in the uptake of thallium by tumor cells. The cotransport system for thallium demonstrated a significant increase from 6-day-old Ehrlich cells to 12-day-old Ehrlich cells. In contrast, the ATPase fell as the cells became older. It was thought that the cotransport system played a dominant role in Tl-201 uptake by tumor cells. Also of interest was the discovery that following inhibition of the ATPase system, as well as the cotransport system, a minimal resting flow for ionic transport was still preserved. This flow was attributed to a calcium-dependent ion channel system.[43]

Ando[1] evaluated the biodistribution of thallium-201 in tumor-bearing animals and found that thallium was mainly accumulated by viable tumor, less well accumulated in connective tissue that contained inflammatory cells, and was barely detectable in necrotic tumor tissue. It was also determined that regardless of the length of time following administration, thallium-201 mainly exists in the free form in the fluid of the tumor. A small fraction of thallium was localized in the nuclear, mitochondrial, and microsomal fractions of these tissues. In addition, Ando demonstrated that thallium-201 was bound to protein in these fractions.[1]

THALLIUM-201 IN THE EVALUATION OF THERAPEUTIC RESPONSE

Ramanna et al demonstrated conventional bone scintigraphy to correlate poorly with chemotherapeutic effectiveness in patients undergoing chemotherapy before limb salvage.[32] This report determined that in over 80% of patients studied, the bone scan gave erroneous information in the assessment of chemotherapeutic effectiveness. The bone scan was often associated with an increasing activity following chemotherapy that was shown to be associated with healing. Therefore within 6 weeks of chemotherapy, the bone scan played no useful role because increasing activity on bone scan simply reflected healing and not necessarily aggressive tumor growth. The study also demonstrated that Ga-67 was also a relatively poor clinical correlate, with only 50% of patients successfully treated by chemotherapy demonstrating improvement on the gallium scintigraphy study.[32] Tl-201 was found to be an excellent correlate with therapeutic success with nearly 100% of patients demonstrating significant improvement on thallium scintigraphy when chemotherapy was found to be successful. Patients with greater than 95% tumor necrosis demonstrated minimal or no thallium uptake when compared with pretreatment baseline thallium scans.

Ramanna et al found that Tl-201 was able to demonstrate tumor burden as well as tumor activity and was not affected by local healing of bone. The authors recommend Tl-201 scintigraphy as the test of choice in determining effectiveness of chemotherapy before limb salvage.

In a study of 27 patients with osteosarcoma or malignant fibrous histiocytoma of bone, Rosen et al utilized serial thallium scans to assess the response of tumor to preoperative chemotherapy.[35] Patients were graded by their responses as category I (worse or no response), category II (definite response with discernible reduction but a recognizable lesion still present), or category III (previously abnormal lesion barely discernible or absent). Of the 10 patients who had category I responses, only 1 had a good histologic response. Only 5 of the patients (50%) in this group remain relapse-free survivors. There is a highly significant correlation ($p > 0.005$) of a category I response and poor histologic response to chemotherapy in the primary tumor. Nine patients were graded as having category II responses and 6 of these (67%) had good histologic responses. Eight patients had category III changes on thallium scanning, and all eight had excellent

histologic response in the primary tumor to preoperative chemotherapy.

Menendez et al demonstrated similar findings.[27] This group evaluated sequential thallium scintigraphy before and after a period of preoperative chemotherapy in 16 patients with high-grade sarcomas of the bone or soft tissue. They found that changes in thallium activity correlated extremely well with histologic findings. When no improvement in uptake on thallium scan was noted, there was a poor histologic response to chemotherapy. When there was a decrease in thallium uptake after chemotherapy, there was a good or excellent histologic response to chemotherapy (with one exception). The degree of reduced thallium uptake correlated with increasing amounts of tumor necrosis.

Figure 7-1 shows a patient with an osteogenic sarcoma prechemotherapy and postchemotherapy. Chemotherapy was done in preparation for a limb-salvage procedure of the right distal femur. The thallium study pretherapy demonstrates a large abnormality in the right distal femur, whereas the posttherapy study just before limb-salvage surgery shows complete resolution of thalli-

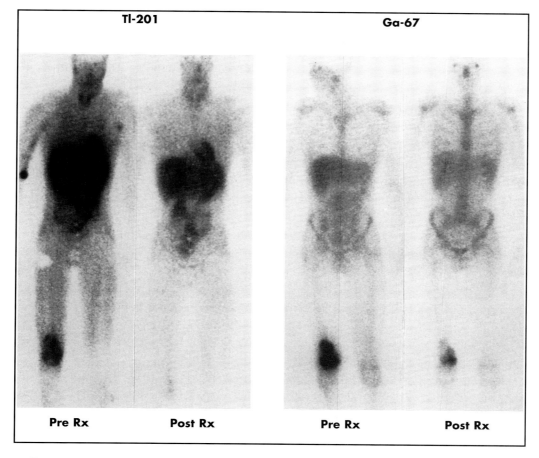

Fig. 7-1. Comparison of prechemotherapy and postchemotherapy Tl-201 Ga-67 citrate scans in a patient with an osteogenic sarcoma of the right distal femur. The posttherapy studies were performed 8 weeks after the initial chemotherapy. At limb-salvage surgery, done shortly following the posttherapy Tl-201 and Ga-67 studies, the surgical specimen demonstrated greater than 98% necrosis. The Tl-201 accurately reflected tumor viability, whereas the Ga-67 study demonstrated residual activity most probably secondary to a healing response.

um. At surgery the patient was found to have greater than 98% necrosis histologically. The gallium study, although positive on the pretherapy study, shows significant residual on the posttherapy scan. The residual gallium increase was thought to be secondary to healing, as virtually no tumor was evident in the pathologic specimen. The time interval between the pretherapy and posttherapy scan was 8 weeks.

Figure 7-2 is an example of a patient with an osteogenic sarcoma that showed no improvement posttherapy. Note the intense thallium activity on both the pretherapy and posttherapy studies, consistent with the clinical impression of no therapeutic response.

Tc-99m Methoxyisobutyl Isonitrile

MECHANISM OF UPTAKE

The exact mechanism of Tc-99m MIBI uptake by tumor cells is not yet defined. Many of the proposed mechanisms are derived from studies of myocardial tissue and tumor cells from tissue culture; therefore extrapolation to tumor cells is speculative. Currently, it is thought that in contrast to active transport involved in thallium accumulation within the myocardium, the fundamental mechanism of myocellular accumulation of Tc-99m MIBI is passive diffusion accross the sarcolemma and mitochondrial membranes in response to transmembrane potentials.[25,26] Tc-99m MIBI is a lipophilic cation that is significantly influenced by the negative charges

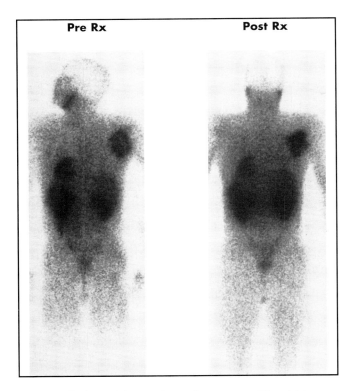

| Pre Rx | Post Rx |

Fig. 7-2. Patient with an osteogenic sarcoma of the right scapula, with persistent clinical evidence of continuing disease with no improvement. The Tl-201 scan demonstrated no significant change consistent with the patient's clinical course. Chemotherapy was modified before surgery.

on the mitochondria and increased mitochondrial density present in tumors.[18]

As in thallium accumulation within the myocardium or in tumors, adequate blood flow must be present for uptake to occur. Thus in tumors as in the myocardium, limitation of blood supply may result in a decrease of Tc-99m MIBI uptake. Extraction, however, appears to be dependent on the transmembrane potential difference developed by tumors as well as on mitochondrial density.[12-16,18,25,26]

TUMOR DETECTION AND ASSESSMENT OF THERAPY

Findings similar to those obtained with thallium have been reported for MIBI. Caner et al found MIBI to accumulate in a patient with an osteogenic sarcoma of the right proximal tibia.[10] Activity was also noted in an inguinal lymph node on the right demonstrated by biopsy to be malignant. In a separate study Caner et al demonstrated the potential of MIBI for imaging patients with primary bone tumors.[11] In this study 10 patients with malignant tumors underwent a pretherapy and posttherapy MIBI evaluation. It was demonstrated that radiotherapy or chemotherapy significantly inhibited MIBI uptake. The study showed that posttherapeutic MIBI uptake was a good reflection of the effectiveness of therapy as confirmed by histologic evaluation.

Ashok et al compared thallium-201 with MIBI in the evaluation of patients with soft-tissue as well as osteogenic sarcoma.[2,3] In 19 patients with prior or current history of osteosarcoma, Tl-201 and Tc-99m MIBI scintigraphic studies were performed on the same day. Using a semiquantitative rating system, a site-by-site comparison for thallium and MIBI was performed on each patient. Thallium-201 demonstrated a rating of 2+ or greater in 12 of 15 sites proven to be tumor. MIBI had a 2+ or greater tumor rating in all 15 sites. Response to chemotherapy was also compared in the study. In 5 patients both thallium and MIBI gave concordant information with biopsy specimens (which were evaluated for percent necrosis). The authors concluded that the sensitivity for MIBI detection of primary bone cancer is the same as that of Tl-201. However, additional abnormal sites were better detected using MIBI. Both thallium and MIBI gave excellent correlation with biopsy information in evaluating tumor response to chemotherapy before limb-salvage procedures.

Tl-201 and Tc-99m MIBI Scan Patterns in Sarcoma

Ramanna et al evaluated Tl-201 scans in 105 patients with bone and soft-tissue sarcomas.[34] All of the patients demonstrated a moderate to marked increase in Tl-201 activity. Tumors that were considered high grade demonstrated a pattern of central lucency with a peripheral zone of intense thallium uptake. This "donut" pattern was highly specific for high-grade sarcomas. Greater than 95% of the high-grade sarcomas presented with the donut sign. Low-grade sarcomas presented as solid areas of increase with no donut signs present. Ashok et al demonstrated similar findings for MIBI.[2,3] These findings

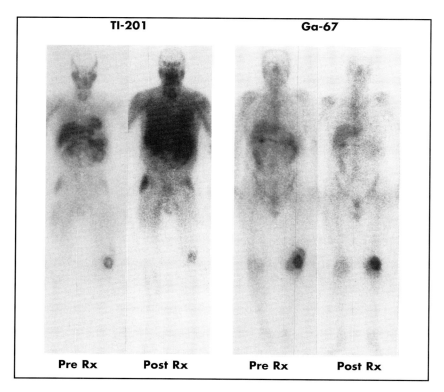

Fig. 7-3. Patient with a high-grade osteogenic sarcoma of the left distal femur. Tl-201 and Ga-67 scans were performed before and after 4 weeks of chemotherapy. Note the initial pretherapy Tl-201 scan demonstrates a "donut" lesion that loses the donut configuration but does not clear 4 weeks posttherapy. The Ga-67 scan pretherapy has a somewhat more solid appearance and shows only peripheral improvement on the posttherapy study. The patient had an incomplete response at the time the posttherapy scans were performed.

appear to parallel the natural course of sarcomas in which tumors grow extremely rapidly, with the more central areas demonstrating necrosis as the tumor outgrows its blood supply. The peripheral areas of the tumor maintain adequate vascular perfusion and pathologically demonstrate areas of active growth with little necrosis. A positive MIBI or thallium scan with a donut pattern indicates a high-grade sarcoma until proven otherwise.

Figure 7-3 shows a patient with an osteogenic sarcoma of the left distal femur. Initial biopsy demonstrated the patient to have a high-grade osteogenic sarcoma. Note the donut appearance of the high-grade tumor. Four weeks posttherapy the scan was repeated and showed a partial remission with loss of the donut pattern. The gallium scan demonstrated only a small central lucency with an intense focus in the left distal femur. Posttherapy the scan demonstrated only minimal improvement, whereas the patient's clinical symptoms improved dramatically.

Differentiation of Benign from Malignant Bone Lesions

Ramanna et al categorized skeletal lesions as benign or malignant based on Tl-201 uptake.[35] Sixteen patients with biopsy-proven benign bone lesions were included in the study. Thallium activity in the bony lesions was grad-

ed as either marked, mild, or normal. Four patients with benign abnormalities demonstrated marked increase in thallium uptake. Among the diagnoses in this group were Paget's disease of bone, fibrous dysplasia, trauma, and ossifying fibroma. Five patients demonstrated mild but definite thallium uptake. The diagnoses in this group included benign fibrous histiocytoma, benign fibrous myxoma, and three patients with Paget's disease. Seven patients with benign disease were entirely normal. The study demonstrated that thallium uptake in bone abnormalities is not specific for malignant tumor and can be seen in a variety of benign abnormalities. A negative test, however, is significant in that the probability of a malignant primary bone tumor is minimal.

Figure 7-4 is a comparison of Tc-99m methylene diphosphonate (MDP) and Tl-201 in patients with a variety of osseous abnormalities. The study on the left was performed in a patient initially diagnosed as possible osteosarcoma of the left femur on a CT scan. A biopsy that was then performed was inconclusive for the presence of osteogenic sarcoma. The bone scan with MDP was strongly positive, whereas Tl-201 was negative. A repeat CT of the area demonstrated a stress fracture. The patient was a competitive gymnast who resumed high bar competition within 1 year following the study. The final diagnosis was myositis ossificans secondary to a healing stress fracture. The study in the center is of a

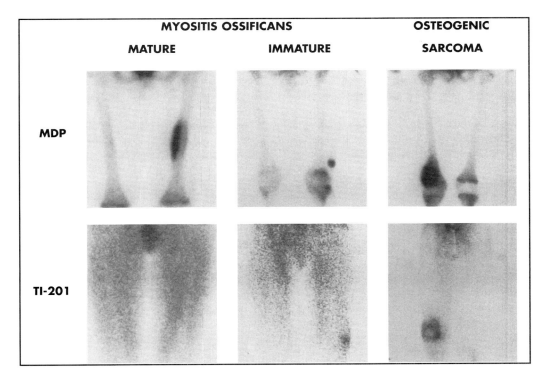

Fig. 7-4. Comparison of Tc-99m MDP bone scintigraphy with Tl-201 in three separate patients. The patient on the left was diagnosed as having mature myositis ossificans secondary to a healing stress fracture of the left femur. Note the markedly positive Tc-99m MDP study, whereas the Tl-201 study is entirely normal. The patient in the center had a biopsy-proven diagnosis of myositis ossificans. Note the markedly positive Tc-99m MDP study and the moderately positive Tl-201 scan. Tl-201 may be positive in benign disorders. However, a negative Tl-201 scan strongly suggests a benign disorder. The patient on the right demonstrates a typical pattern for osteogenic sarcoma with an intensely positive Tc-99m MDP study and a "donut" appearance of a high-grade sarcoma on Tl-201.

patient with biopsy-diagnosed myositis ossificans. The initial x-ray and CT scan suggested the possibility of an osteogenic sarcoma. Note the intense focal increase in the MDP study, whereas thallium also showed a moderately positive abnormality in the same region. The study on the right compares a bone scan done on a patient with an osteogenic sarcoma with a Tl-201 scan. Note the characteristic donut pattern consistent with a high-grade tumor confirmed by biopsy.

Caner et al evaluated Tc-99m MIBI uptake in benign and malignant lesions.[11] MIBI was positive in 36 of 42 malignant tumors (86%), whereas 11 of 31 patients (35%) with benign disease demonstrated MIBI uptake. This group concluded that malignant lesions tend to have a higher overall MIBI uptake than benign lesions but that a significant overlap between benign and malignant bone abnormalities existed.

Summary

Bone and soft-tissue sarcomas are readily detected with both MIBI and Tl-201. Significantly higher count rates are achieved using a 30-mCi dose of Tc-99m MIBI when compared with the 3-mCi dose of Tl-201. Because of the higher photon flux and more desirable imaging characteristics of Tc-99m, a higher degree of resolution is achieved. Comparative studies demonstrate sensitivity for detecting the primary sarcoma to be similar for Tl-201 and MIBI at the time of presentation. However, MIBI appears somewhat superior in detecting distant metastases, including small lymph nodes within the drainage pattern of the tumor.

Both Tl-201 and Tc-99m MIBI were found to concentrate in a variety of benign lesions. However, due to the high sensitivity of MIBI, it may be possible to establish a diagnosis of benign disease discovered on x-ray or MRI when the MIBI study is negative. Both thallium and MIBI give excellent correlative results in establishing the effectiveness of chemotherapy or radiation therapy. Significant improvement from baseline scans following tumor therapy generally indicates a good therapeutic effect. When tumor activity is minimal or undetectable on the follow-up study, necrosis of greater than 95% is usually present. Correlation with degree of improvement and survival suggests an important role for nuclear medicine techniques in managing patients with bone and soft-tissue sarcomas.

CLINICAL PERSPECTIVES OF THE ONCOLOGIST

Nuclear medicine plays an increasingly important role in the assessment of patients with bone and soft-tissue tumors. Our present approach utilizes serial scanning starting at diagnosis, during treatment to assess the effect of preoperative therapy, and during follow-up for those patients who have completed treatment.

MDP bone scans and plain skeletal radiographs remain the initial tests that should be performed for patients with suspected primary bone tumors. The bone scan is more sensitive than plain x-ray and abnormalities on bone scan can precede radiographic changes by several months. Thus an abnormal bone scan with a normal x-

ray should serve as an alert to the clinician that additional studies may be necessary, particularly if the patient's symptoms do not resolve.

Often in younger children pain may be referred (e.g., hip pain can be the complaint with a distal femoral lesion), and x-rays may be obtained of normal areas distant from the primary tumor unless a bone scan is performed at the same time. MDP scans are most likely to be positive in lesions associated with an osteoblastic or reparative process. Metastases along a bone, so-called skip lesions, are uncommonly seen by this technique, but lesions in other bones are visualized. MDP scanning is not a reliable method for evaluating the soft tissues, and although it is useful as an initial screening study, bone

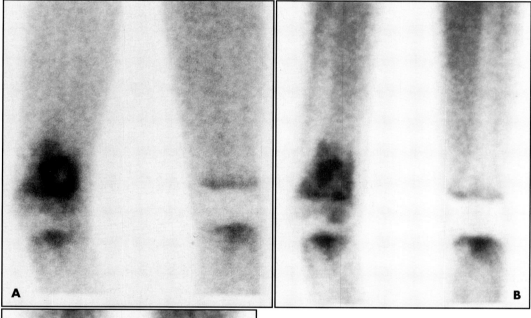

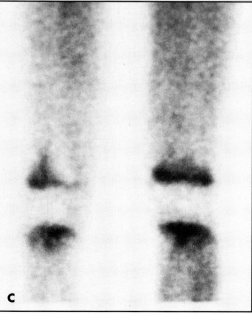

Fig. 7–5. Patient with a high-grade bone sarcoma of the right distal femur demonstrates an intense area of increased activity surrounding a central lucent area consistent with high-grade tumor (**A**). Following 4 weeks of chemotherapy, there has been moderate improvement with partial resolution of tumor as depicted by less intense Tl-201 activity and loss of the "donut" pattern (**B**). Eight weeks after chemotherapy, there has been nearly complete resolution of tumor activity before limb salvage (**C**).

scanning has major limitations. The study is nonspecific and uptake can be seen with trauma, infection, and a variety of nonmalignant conditions. MDP bone scans tend to mirror blood flow to a tumor and can be affected by the healing response (the flare phenomenon) and therefore can appear to initially worsen in the setting of a good clinical response to therapy. This makes MDP bone scanning a poor choice to monitor responses to therapy.

We also perform either thallium-201 scans or more recently Tc-99m MIBI scans at diagnosis. We have found that these scans better reflect the biologic activity of bone and soft-tissue tumors than either gallium-67 or Tc-99m MDP scans.[2,3,11,32,35] In addition, we think thallium and MIBI scans can be helpful in distinguishing benign and low-grade malignant tumors from high-grade malignancies.[34] Benign processes may be negative with thallium or MIBI, and low grade tumors can be either negative or show relatively little activity. On the other hand, high-grade malignancies will have a characteristic donut shape with more intense uptake at the periphery and less uptake in the center of a suspected lesion. This mirrors the growth pattern of high-grade sarcomas, which tend to have areas of central necrosis surrounded by areas of more rapid proliferation at the periphery. Little data exists to compare thallium with MIBI, but MIBI is labeled with Tc-99m, which has better imaging characteristics and can be used with higher doses (30 vs. 3 mCi). This should permit higher resolution using an agent with a shorter half-life.

These thallium or MIBI scans can be particularly useful in following the response to preoperative chemotherapy. Although the Tc-99m MDP bone scan is very slow to normalize during chemotherapy, either thallium or MIBI can demonstrate a marked diminution in uptake at the primary site in those patients having excellent responses to chemotherapy.[2,11,27,32,35] As the response to preoperative chemotherapy remains the most important prognostic variable for long-term disease-free survival in osteogenic sarcoma, the information gained from these scans can help to select the appropriate chemotherapy for an individual patient. The scans allow assessment of response to chemotherapy in "real-time" to permit changes in chemotherapy that appears inactive. Caution must be maintained, and it is important not to overinterpret the findings on scanning. Instead, the scan results should be evaluated in conjunction with a thorough evaluation of the patient. A scan with minimal improvement in the setting of a patient with a complete resolution of tumor-associated pain, a normalizing serum alkaline phosphatase level, and a decreasing soft-tissue mass should not prompt an immediate change of treatment. Instead, a further follow-up study has proven to be valuable as shown in Fig. 7-5. As can be seen, a MIBI scan at the completion of preoperative chemotherapy demonstrates near-complete resolution of the abnormal region.

Soft-tissue sarcomas take up thallium and MIBI at diagnosis, and uptake can decrease in response to treatment. This has been shown for a variety of histologic subtypes including synovial sarcoma, rhabdomyosarcoma, leiomyosarcoma, and malignant fibrous histiocy-toma. Improvements in scans correlate with histologic findings in patients receiving preoperative chemotherapy and radiation therapy.

Although these scans have proven valuable in evaluating extremity lesions, further efforts are necessary to refine the sensitivity in the trunk in part due to extraneous activity in the abdomen and the heart. SPECT is improving the resolution of these scans in the chest and may also be beneficial for lesions below the diaphragm.

Postoperatively scanning can help to suggest active disease in the setting where interpretation of CT scans or MRI can be difficult due to problems of anatomic distortion and the potential presence of prosthetic devices. This is an area of continuing investigation. Although lung metastases can occasionally be seen with thallium or MIBI, CT of this lung is more sensitive. However, in the postthoracotomy patient, thallium and MIBI may help differentiate active disease from postoperative changes. Thallium uptake can also be seen in nonmalignant processes such as pigmented villonodular synovitis, stress fractures, brown tumors associated with hyperparathyroidism, Paget's disease of bone, fibrous dysplasia, and ossifying fibroma. It must be remembered that uptake by these agents is not by itself diagnostic of malignancy.[33]

Thallium and MIBI scans have already demonstrated their utility in accurately predicting response to preoperative chemotherapy.[2,11,27,32,35] Further study is needed to determine whether these techniques can be correlated with survival. In addition, the relative value of thallium or MIBI scans will need to be compared with positron emission tomography (PET) in the future. Issues of cost will be important. Currently thallium and MIBI are more readily available and less expensive than PET scans. All of these tests will hopefully permit rapid, reliable, and reproducible assessment of patients with bone and soft-tissue tumors so that effective chemotherapy can be continued and exposure to ineffective chemotherapy can be limited.

REFERENCES

1. Ando A, Ando I, Katayama M, et al: Biodistribution of Tl-201 in tumor bearing animals and inflammatory lesion induced animals. *Eur J Nucl Med* 1987; 12:567.

2. Ashok G, Waxman AD, Kooba A, et al: Comparison of Tl-201 (Tl) and Tc-99m methoxyisobutyl isonitrile in the evaluation of patients with osteogenic sarcoma. *Clin Nucl Med* 1992; 9 (abstract).

3. Ashok G, Waxman AD, Kooba A, et al: Comparison of Tl-201 (Tl) and Tc-99m methoxyisobutyl isonitrile in the evaluation of patients with non-osseous sarcomas. *Clin Nucl Med* 1992; 9 (abstract).

4. Atkins HL, Budinger TF, Lebowitz E, et al: Thallium-201 for medical use, III: Human distribution and physical imaging properties. *J Nucl Med* 1977; 18:133.

5. Berquist TH: Magnetic resonance imaging of primary skeletal neoplasms, in Moser RP Jr (ed): *Imaging of bone and soft tissue tumors. Radiol Clin North Am* 1993; 31:383.

6. Berquist TH, Ehman RL, King BF, et al: Value of MR imaging in differentiating benign from malignant soft tissue masses: Study of 95 lesions. *AJR Am J Roentgenol* 1990; 155:1251.

7. Bloem JL, Kroon HM: Osseous lesions, in Moser RP Jr (ed): *Imaging of Bone and Soft Tissue Tumors. Radiol Clin North Am* 1993; 31:261.

8. Bradley-Moore PR, Lebowitz E, Greene MW, et al: Thallium-201 for medical use: II—Biological behavior. *J Nucl Med* 1975; 16:156.

9. Britten JS, Blank M: Thallium activation of the (Na+, K+) activated ATPase of rabbit kidney. *Biochem Biophys Acta* 1968; 15:160.

10. Caner B, Kitapci M, Aras T, et al: Increased accumulation of hesakis (2-methoxyisobutyl-isonitrile) technetium in osteosarcoma and its metastatic lymph nodes. *J Nucl Med* 1991; 32:1977.

11. Caner B, Kitapci M, Unlu M, et al: Technetium-99m MIBI uptake in benign and malignant bone lesions: A comparative study with technetium-99m MDP. *J Nucl Med* 1992; 33:319.

12. Carvalho PA, Chiu ML, Kronauge JF, et al: Subcellular distribution and analysis of technetium-99m MIBI in isolated perfused rat hearts. *J Nucl Med* 1992; 33:1516.

13. Chernoff DM, Strichartz GR, Piwnica-Worms D: Membrane potential determination in large unilamellar vesicles with hexakis (2-methoxyisobutyl-isonitrile) technetium (I). *Biochim Biophy Acta* 1993; 1147/2:262.

14. Chiu ML, Herman LW, Kronauge JF, Piwnica-Worms D: Comparative effects of neutral dipolar compounds and lipophilic anions on technetium 99m-hexakis (2-methoxy-isobutyl-isonitrile) accumulation in cultured chick ventricular myocytes. *Invest Radiol* 1992; 27:1052.

15. Chiu ML, Kronauge JF, Piwnica-Worms D: Effect of mitochondrial and plasma membrane potentials on accumulation of hexakis (2-methoxyisobutyl-isonitrile) technetium (I) in cultured mouse fibroblasts. *J Nucl Med* 1990; 31:1646.

16. Crane P, Laliberte R, Heminway S, et al: Effects of mitochondrial viability and metabolism on technetium-99m-sestamibi myocardial retention. *Eur J Nucl Med* 1993; 21:20.

17. Crim JR, Seeger LL, Yal L, et al: Diagnosis of soft tissue masses with MR imaging: Can benign masses be differentiated from malignant ones? *Radiology* 1992; 185:581.

18. Delmon-Moingeon LI, Piwnica-Worms D, Van den Abbeele AD, et al: Uptake of the cation hexakis (2-methoxy-isobutyl-isonitrile) technetium-99m by human carcinoma cells in vitro. *Cancer Res* 1990; 50:2198.

19. Gehring PJ, Hammond PR: The interrelationship between thallium and potassium in animals. *J Pharmacol Exp Ther* 1967; 155:187.

20. Holscher HC, Bloem JL, Nooy MA, et al: The value of MR imaging in monitoring the effect of chemotherapy on bone sarcomas. *AJR Am J Roentgenol* 1990; 154:763.

21. Kransdorf MJ: Soft-tissue tumors: An analysis of 31, 141 lesions seen in consultation over 10 years (abstract 584), in *Program and Abstracts of the 79th Scientific Assembly and National Meeting of the Radiological Society of North America*, Chicago, 1993, p. 205.

22. Kransdorf MJ, Jelinek JS, Moser RP Jr: Imaging of soft tissue tumors, in Moser RP Jr (ed): *Imaging of Bone and Soft Tissue Tumors. Radiol Clin North Am* 1993; 31:359.

23. Lebowitz E, Greene MW, Green R, et al: Thallium-201 for medical use, I. *J Nucl Med* 1975; 16:151.

24. Mankin HK, Lang T, Spanier S: The hazards of biopsy in patients with malignant primary bone and soft tissue tumors. *J Bone Joint Surg Am* 1982; 64A:1221.

25. Maublant JC, Gachon P, Moins N: Hexakis (2-methoxy-isobutyl-isonitrile) technetium-99m and thallium-201 chloride: Uptake and release in cultured myocardial cells. *J Nucl Med* 1988; 29:48.

26. Maublant JC, Moins N, Gachon P, et al: Uptake of technetium-99m teboroxime in cultured myocardial cells: Comparison with thallium-201 and technetium-99m sestamibi. *J Nucl Med* 1993; 34:255.

27. Menendez L, Fideler B, Mirra J: Thallium-201 scanning for the evaluation of osteosarcoma and soft-tissue sarcoma. *J Bone Joint Surg* 1993; 4:527.

28. Mirra JM, Picci P, Gold RH: *Bone Tumors: Clinical, Radiologic, and Pathologic Correlations*, Lea and Febiger, Philadelphia, 1989.

29. Muranake A: Accumulation of radioisotopes with tumor afinity, II: Comparison of the tumor accumulation of Ga-67 citrate and thallium-201 chloride in vitro. *Acta Med Okayama* 1981; 35:85.

30. Pan G, Raymond AK, Carrasco CH, et al: Osteosarcoma: MR imaging after preoperative chemotherapy. *Radiology* 1990; 174:517.

31. Partain CL, Jones JP, Patton JH: Physics of magnetic resonance, in Taveras JM, Ferrucci JT (eds): *Radiology: Diagnosis-Imaging-Intervention*, Vol 1, JB Lippincott, Philadelphia, 1994, Chapters 32, 33.

32. Ramanna L, Waxman AD, Binney G, et al: Thallium-201 scintigraphy in bone sarcoma: Comparison with Ga-67 and Tc-99m MDP in evaluation of chemotherapy response. *J Nucl Med* 1990; 31:567.

33. Ramanna L, Waxman AD, Rosen G: Evaluation of Tl-201 (Tl) uptake pattern in bone lesions: Differentiation of benign from malignant processes. *J Nucl Med* 1992; 33:869.

34. Ramanna L, Waxman AD, Weiss A, Rosen G: Thallium-201 (Tl-201) scan patterns in bone and soft tissue sarcoma. *J Nucl Med* 1992; 33:843.

35. Rosen G, Loren G, Brien E, et al: Serial thallium-201 scintigraphy in osteosarcoma: Correlation with tumor necrosis after preoperative chemotherapy. *Clin Orthop* 1993; 293:302.

36. Sanchez RB, Quinn SF, Walling A, et al: Musculoskeletal neoplasms after intraarterial chemotherapy: Correlation of MR images with pathologic specimens. *Radiology* 1990; 174:273.

37. Seeger LL: Contrast agents in musculoskeletal MR imaging: Uses and abuses, in syllabus: *Categorical Course of Body Magnetic Imaging*, American College of Radiology Annual Meeting, 1993.

38. Seeger LL: MR imaging of musculoskeletal tumors, in *Categorical Course Syllabus: Spine and Body MRI*. American Roentgen Ray Society Annual Meeting, 1991.

39. Seeger LL, Dungan DH, Eckardt JJ, et al: Nonspecific findings on MRI: The importance of correlative studies and clinical information. *Clin Orthop* 1991; 270:306.

40. Seeger LL, Eckardt JJ, Bassett LW: Cross-sectional imaging in the evaluation of osteogenic sarcoma: MRI and CT. *Semin Roentgenol* 1989; 24:174.

41. Seeger LL, Gold RH, Chandnani VP: Diagnostic imaging of osteosarcoma. *Clin Ortho* 1991; 270:254.

42. Seeger LL, Widoff BE, Bassett LW, et al: Preoperative evaluation of osteosarcoma: Value of gadopentetate dimelumine-enhanced MR imaging. *AJR Am J Roentgenol* 1991; 157:347.

43. Sessler MK, Geek P, Maul FD, et al: New aspects of cellular Tl-201 uptake T+Na+-2CI-cotransport in the central mechanism of ion uptake. *Nucl Med* 1986; 25:24.

44. Stoller DW, Waxman AD, Rosen G, et al: Comparison of thallium-201, gallium-67, technetium 99m MDP and magnetic resonance imaging of musculoskeletal sarcoma. *Clin Nucl Med* 1986; 12(suppl):P15 (abstract).

45. Sundaram M, McLeod RA: MR imaging of tumor and tumorlike lesions of bone and soft tissue. *AJR Am J Roentgenol* 1990; 155:817.

46. Vanel D, Shapeero LG, BeBaere T, et al: MR imaging in the follow-up of malignant and aggressive soft-tissue tumors: Results of 511 examinations. *Radiology* 1994; 190:263.

47. Waxman AD: Thallium-201 in nuclear oncology, in Freeman LM (ed): *Nuclear Medicine Annual*, Raven Press, New York, 1991, p 193.

RADIONUCLIDE IMAGING OF BONE MARROW

Brian C. Lentle

Daniel F. Worsley

David B. Coupland

The red bone marrow is an organ of immense importance to the normal functioning of the body. However, this importance is sometimes lost to sight. Bone marrow is clearly a discrete organ in functional terms, but its diseases are sometimes wrongly attributed to bone since secondary effects on the skeleton are more readily perceived clinically and revealed by radiography. Magnetic resonance imaging (MRI), with its lack of signal from bone, has more recently reemphasised the importance of bone marrow as a site of disease.[48]

ANATOMY AND PHYSIOLOGY

In young children the red or proliferative bone marrow occupies the entire marrow space of the skeleton. This extent slowly decreases until by adulthood red marrow is present only in the central skeleton. This distribution includes all of the vertebrae and ribs, the bony pelvis, pectoral girdle, the sternum, and base of skull. In addition, but somewhat variably, it extends into the very proximal ends of the humeri and femora.[68]

Crucial to an understanding of imaging the red marrow is the realization that under conditions of stress (e.g., primary and secondary anoxia, anemia) or disease (tumor invasion) the adult pattern of marrow distribution may revert in some degree to that present in children. This phenomenon is known as bone marrow extension, or, more properly, reexpansion. Ultimately mesenchymal cells may differentiate into red marrow in parts of the body where marrow is not usually found, if marrow disease is sufficiently severe and protracted. The result is known as *extramedullary hematopoiesis* (EH).

In normal adults the balance of the bone marrow space not occupied by proliferating cells is occupied by fat (yellow marrow), which is of little consequence in disease. However, when the red marrow is atrophic, as in aplastic anemia, this central marrow may also be replaced by fat to an abnormal degree, this being reflective of the underlying dysfunction.

The red or proliferative marrow is the site of formation of erythrocytes, platelets, and granulocytes, and it has a role in the maturation of lymphocytes. This process is continuous, although subject to homeostatic regulation.

Red marrow is vascular with large sinusoids. These sinusoids contains cells belonging to the reticuloendothelial (RE) system. Fortunately diseases of the hematopoietic marrow usually equally affect the RE cells. It should be borne in mind, however, that this congruence is usual but not invariable.

PATHOPHYSIOLOGY

Red bone marrow is subject to a great number of diseases. These may be classified as primarily arising with the proliferative marrow cells such as aplasia, toxic hypoplasia, or dysplasia, or resulting from the rich blood supply to the marrow or its compromise such as blood-borne infection, metastases, or infarction. Thus diseases such as osteomyelitis, which are implicitly considered to be diseases of bone, probably most often begin as blood-borne infections of the marrow space.

Indeed Ito et al have shown that so-called bone metastases are, in an animal model, revealed more sensitively by radionuclide (RN) imaging of bone marrow rather than by bone imaging itself.[26] This suggests that "bone" metastases are in fact most often marrow metastases. Until recently the lack of a technique as simple and readily available as radiophosphate imaging of bone by which to interrogate the marrow has been a contributory factor in preventing this lesson being translated into everyday clinical practice.

RADIONUCLIDE IMAGING OF BONE MARROW

Radiopharmaceuticals

It is possible to image the red cell precursor population of the marrow using a salt of iron-59. Certainly counting marrow and red cell activity after injecting Fe-59 citrate is the basis of the conceptually important, if rarely used, technique called ferrokinetics, chiefly used to explore the possibility of ineffective hematopoiesis.[49] However, the long physical half-life (45.1 days) and energetic gamma-radiation (1.099 MeV, 59% abundance; 1.292 MeV, 45% abundance) of Fe-59, with the resultant high radiation dose and poor detection efficiency, imply that this method is now rarely used to image the marrow in everyday clinical practice. Similarly, the positron-emitting RN Fe-52 can be used to image red marrow, particularly with detectors appropriate to the 511-keV gamma-rays. There is, however, a poor match between the physical half life of this RN (8.28 hours) and the rate of metabolism of iron, so that again this RN has very limited day-to-day use.[18] It has been used to image EH.[8]

Until recently the techniques available to image bone marrow have largely depended on imaging of the RE marrow components. Initially radioactive gold (Au-198) was used in this context. With the development of Mo-99/Tc-99m generators, a number of Tc-99m labeled particles have been used in this context including Tc-99m labeled sulfur colloid, antimony colloid, and albumin microspheres. The relative distribution of colloid into the RE cells of liver, spleen, and bone marrow is inflenced by particle size with the fractional distribution into marrow being greater for smaller particles such as those of antimony colloid and albumin microspheres.[31,38] Thus these radiopharmaceuticals may be used to advantage in limiting scatter from organs other than bone marrow. This scatter may limit image quality. A further minor disadvantage that results from the use of colloids of smaller particle size is that their rate of clearance from blood is slower.[18]

Indium-111 chloride has also been used to image bone marrow. Indium belongs to group III of the periodic table, but like iron is readily bound by the serum protein transferrin. Thus there was initial optimism that In-111 marrow images might reflect the distribution of hematopoietic tissue. However, only about 4% of an injected dose of indium appears in red cells, a much smaller fraction than of ferrous salts. The plasma clearance of indium cations is much slower than those of iron, and it has become apparent that the indium space differs from the transferrin space.[18] A substantial fraction of indium chloride is now known to form a colloid after intravenous injection, and its biodistribution appears to reflect in large part the location of RE cells.[15,40] However, the biodistributions of In-111 chloride and Tc-99m colloid are not always identical.[27]

Investigators have attempted to address some of the uncertainties relating to the use of In-111 by incubating it with transferrin in vitro before injection.[4] This strategy does not seem to overcome the limitations on the use of this RN previously discussed and implicit in animal studies comparing the kinetics and metabolism of iron with indium.[6]

As previously indicated, there is usually a parallel distribution of red cell precursors and RE cells in the marrow space (congruence). It should nevertheless be borne in mind in making diagnostic inferences from marrow images that a few exceptions to this rule have been noted, in particular in patients with leukemia[18,63] as well as following radiotherapy.[36]

Newer techniques employ labeled monoclonal antibodies. The antibodies cross-react with a surface marker on granulocytes. They portray the marrow space elegantly[52] as do granulocytes labeled with In-111 oxine and its analogs, or Tc-99m hexamethylene amine oxime (HMPAO).[5,7]

Vallabhajosula et al have also shown that Tc-99m labeled low-density lipoproteins (LDLs) imaged 4 hours after injection are found chiefly in the liver and spleen with limited uptake in either central or peripheral marrow. On the other hand five patients with myeloproliferative disease (two with polycythemia rubra vera [PRV], two with myeloid metaplasia following PRV, and one with agnogenic myeloid metaplasia) had marked splenic uptake of this tracer and evidence of peripheral marrow reexpansion. The uptake of Tc-99m LDLs paralleled that of sulfur colloid. The results are of interest in revealing sites of catabolism of LDLs but do not seem to offer any striking advantage as a method of marrow imaging, particularly with the long interval necessary between injection and imaging.[62]

Gallium-67 citrate is a special case. Gallium, like indium, belongs in group III of the periodic table. It was initially used at low specific activities to image bone. Gallium binds to transferrin like indium. At high specific activities, with the transferrin binding sites not saturated, it came to be used for detecting cancers and inflammatory disease. While scintigraphy with Ga-67 citrate 24 to 72 hours after injection incidentally reveals "bone" localization, that is probably a complex mixture of uptake in red marrow and in bone mineral.[18,42]

Fortunately from the perspective of making diagnostic inferences from marrow scans, the findings and their implications are similar irrespective of the radiopharmaceutical used, if allowance is made for any other characteristics of the particular radiopharmaceutical.

In the same context it is important to realize that liver and spleen uptake of radiocolloids and In-111 chloride does not necessarily reflect hematopoiesis in these organs.

Techniques

Brief reflection will suggest that radionuclide marrow imaging requires forethought. The injection of an appropriate tracer and image acquisition to some given count-density will very likely produce some demonstration of the marrow space. Should the space be depleted, as in aplastic anemia or diffuse tumor infiltration, imaging times may be unduly long and make great demands on a patient. Therefore it is necessary for an adequate assessment of bone marrow to image for a preset time to assess marrow activity, and if activity is adequate to a preset count-density to assess marrow integrity. The former images in particular need to be calibrated by an understanding of the normal findings in a given laboratory under standardized conditions relating to the type and activity of radiopharmaceutical injected (by body weight) and the imaging parameters used.

The Tc-99m labeled radiocolloids are apt to obscure the low dorsal and upper lumbar spine by virtue of their intense uptake in liver and spleen and resulting scatter. In examining the low thoracic and upper lumbar spine in particular, it is often advantageous to use single photon emission computed tomography (SPECT). Otherwise some shielding of these organs will often improve image quality (e.g., Fig. 8-4), but it is in this context that the use of a colloid particle of smaller size will also help. It may be that immunoscintigraphy of the marrow will be particularly effective in this context.[50,52]

Nonimaging Methods of Examining the Bone Marrow

Although not within the scope of this review, any complete understanding of RN studies of bone marrow must include studies of iron kinetics, iron uptake, and use by the marrow.[49] The methods for and limitations of cohort or pulsed labeling of formed blood elements for investigative analyses of cell survival and localization complete such a perspective.[49]

Summary

It is possible to image the red marrow space directly as previously discussed. Nevertheless, in day-to-day clinical nuclear medicine practice, intimations of marrow space disorders are most often derived from an awareness of how these disorders influence conventional bone scintigraphy (Figs. 8-1 and 8-2).

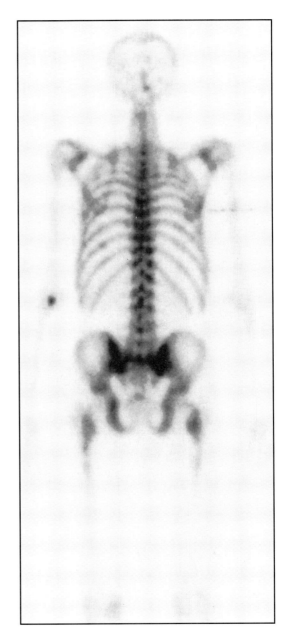

Fig. 8-1. Delayed static posterior whole-body Tc-99m phosphate bone scan image demonstrates diffuse increased uptake throughout the axial skeleton ("superscan"), proximal femora, and base of skull secondary to diffuse metastatic spread of prostatic cancer through the distribution of red marrow.

INCIDENTAL IMAGING OF THE MARROW SPACE

Note has already been made that disorders of "bone" may often in reality be disorders of marrow.[26] Certainly this realization immediately makes more comprehensible the distribution of osteomyelitis in children and adults, and that of metastates of solid tumors in bone.[50,56] The Tc-99m radiophosphate bone scan, however, may reflect the fact that tumor is replacing red marrow in other more subtle ways. The so-called bone "superscan," when due to diffuse malignant cell invasion of the marrow, reveals increased uptake of tracer mirroring the distribution of red marrow. Indeed it may also indicate increased bone turnover associated with marrow reexpansion into the long bones in adults (Figs. 8-1 and 8-2).[54]

Fatty replacement of the red marrow may be seen, like other collections of fat cells, on later images of the lung made with radioxenon (Xe-127 or Xe-133) (Fig. 8-3).[21] This phenomenon reflects the differential solubility of xenon, which is greater in fat than water.

Focal tumor replacement of bone marrow by metas-

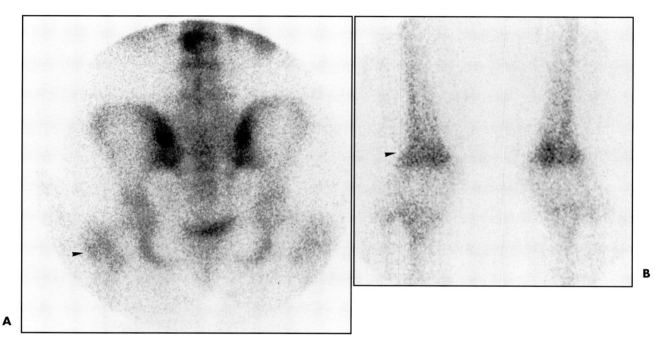

Fig. 8-2. Delayed static anterior images of the knees and posterior image of the pelvis from a Tc-99m phosphate bone scan demonstrate increased accumulation of activity within the proximal (**A**) and distal (**B**) femoral metaphyses bilaterally (*arrowheads*) secondary to bone marrow expansion in a patient with polycythemia rubra vera.

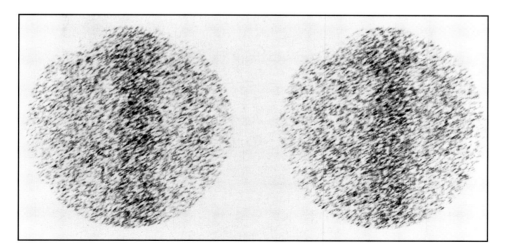

Fig. 8-3. Serial images of the posterior thorax obtained following the inhalation and washout of xenon-133 gas demonstrates retention of radioxenon within fatty marrow in the thoracic spine.

tases may be seen incidentally on colloid images of the liver or spleen and are worth briefly searching for, in an appropriate clinical setting, by increasing the intensity on planar or appropriate tomographic images (Fig. 8-4).[33,34,58]

Last, marrow hyperemia may be recognized as an incidental finding in imaging with those Tc-99m chelates which, in particular, do not localize in bone but which have a relatively long residence time in blood—for example, Tc-99m diethylene triamine pentacetic acid (DTPA) (Fig. 8-5).[30] Diffuse marrow hyperemia results from a variety of causes including tumor invasion of the marrow, myelofibrosis, and possibly from chemotherapeutic marrow toxicity. Abdel-Dayem et al have also described increased localization of Tl-201 thallous chloride, again presumably reflecting hyperemia, in a patient with severe leukopenia that was successfully treated with granulocyte colony-stimulating factor (G-CSF).[1]

FINDINGS IN DISEASE

The patterns of marrow replacement, which are continuously interrelated rather than discrete, are illustrated in Fig. 8-6.

Focal Marrow Replacement

Bone marrow is normally present uniformly through the space it occupies. However, focal or multifocal replacement of the marrow occurs from lesions occurring both in bone and bone marrow. In the former category are diseases such as Paget's disease with its expanded matrix,[35,53] hemangiomas of bone, and in vertebrae, compression fractures as well as adjacent to both intervertebral disk disease,[14] particularly when there is associated discogenic sclerosis, and diskitis.[67] Focal marrow defects in the ribs have also been noted at the sites of healed fractures.[13] Although marrow replacement may occur in Paget's disease of bone, the marrow scan may also reveal either normal or increased uptake of the radiopharmaceutical. This has been suggested as a possible method of distinguishing between Paget's disease and metastases when the radiographic findings are ambiguous.[53]

Metastatic disease is by far the most common cause of focal marrow defects in older adults (Fig. 8-4). Clearly in resolving this differential diagnosis, radiography will play a very similar role to that which it has in conventional skeletal scintigraphy, in excluding false-positive diagnoses of metastatic disease.[33,34]

Following the observations of Ito et al[26] a number of

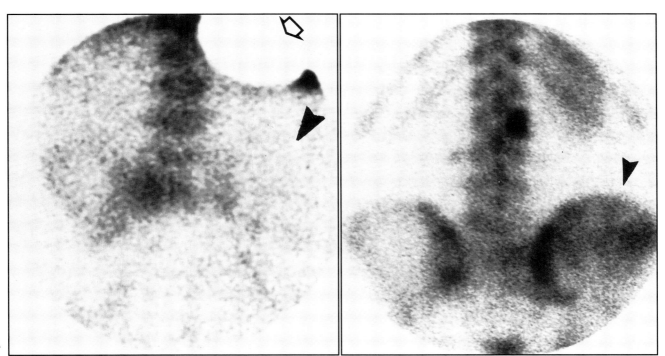

A   B

Fig. 8-4. A, Delayed static posterior images of the pelvis obtained during a Tc-99m sulfur colloid liver-spleen scan demonstrates decreased accumulation of activity within the right ilium (*arrowhead*) secondary to bone metastases. Lead shielding (*open arrow*) has been used to reduce scatter from activity in the liver and spleen. **B,** Posterior image of the lumbar spine and pelvis from a Tc-99m phosphate bone scan in the same patient within days confirms the presence of bone metastases within the right ileum and second lumbar vertebra. *(Reprinted by permission of the Society of Nuclear Medicine, from Lentle BC, et al: Detecting bone marrow metastases at the time of examining the liver with radiocolloid.* J Nucl Med *1987, 28:184-187.)*

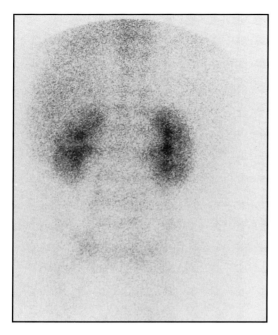

Fig. 8–5. Posterior frame from a Tc-99m DTPA renal scan demonstrates diffuse hyperemia of the red marrow within the lower thoracic spine, lumbar spine, and pelvis following recent chemotherapy. *(Courtesy of Dr. Helen Nadel.)*

investigators have examined the relative sensitivities of bone and marrow scintigraphy in diagnosing metastatic disease of the skeleton. Using the improved diagnostic agents recently made available, Reske et al have used marrow immunoscintigraphy in breast cancer and Hodgkin's disease, finding the technique more sensitive than bone scintigraphy.[52] Reporting in a second communication, Reske et al described 15 patients with breast cancer, all of whom had marrow defects, and 17 with lymphoma, 10 of whom had marrow defects. These investigators were only able to conclude that they detected more lesions using bone marrow compared with bone imaging.[51] Duncker used a similar technique in 32 patients with breast cancer and reported a sensitivity of bone marrow scintigraphy of 0.72 and of bone scintigraphy of 0.53, the former technique again revealing more sites of disease.[16] However, Bourgeois et al, also using marrow immunoscintigraphy, examined 101 patients with breast cancer and found the examination abnormal in 38 of 41 with skeletal metastases, whereas 3 of the 32 patients with normal examinations had other evidence of skeletal involvement by cancer.[9] In a second report concerning 73 patients with prostate cancer, examined by the same method, the sensitivity of marrow scintigraphy was 0.83 and of bone scintigraphy was 0.86 at one of the thresholds used and was lower than bone scintigraphy at all thresholds.[10] Nearly all of these data were obtained with some form of tissue examination as validation.

These results are inconsistent. They certainly do not confirm the findings of Ito et al in an animal model.[26] Any slight advantage to bone marrow scintigraphy is at present outweighed by the convenience of conventional bone scintigraphy, which has the added advantage of being a "hot-spot" technique. The conspicuousness of hot-spots is greater than cold for a given signal-to-noise ratio.

A number of investigators have examined the role of radiocolloid scintigraphy in diagnosing metastases. Widding et al found focal marrow replacement in patients with prostatic cancer to be a more sensitive reflection of metastatic disease than reexpansion,[65] which can be nonspecific. Bourgeois et al examined 52 patients with small cell lung cancer, using biopsy for validation, and found marrow scintigraphy to be of a sensitivity equal to or greater than bone scintigraphy depending on the diagnostic threshold used,[11] whereas Langer et al could not confirm these observations in patients with breast cancer.[32] Siddiqui et al have shown in children that even with radiocolloids it is sometimes possible to demonstrate metastatic disease that is not otherwise apparent on other imaging examinations.[59] These data suggest a selective rather than ubiquitous role for marrow scintigraphy.

Effectively treated metastases in the marrow space may still leave focal defects on a marrow scan,[59] although it is more usual for marrow recovery to occur.

An important cause of focal marrow defects is marrow infarctions. These may be multiple, particularly in the hemoglobinopathies such as sickle cell disease. In this condition the marrow may have a complex pattern compounded of bone and bone marrow infarcts and marrow reexpansion. Because patients with sickle cell disease are prone to the further complication of osteomyelitis, they may need intensive investigation with bone, marrow, and either labeled white cell or Ga-67 scintigraphy to explain their presenting symptoms.[2,15,28,37]

Diffuse Marrow Involution or Replacement

The scintigraphic appearance of diffuse marrow disease is simply that of a global reduction in marrow activity. However, the recognition that this is taking place, particularly in the early stages, may be challenging, as previously described in techniques.

Diffusely reduced marrow activity occurs from a great number of diseases primarily affecting the marrow or skeleton including the myeloproliferative diseases, myelofibrosis, mastocytosis, and aplastic anemia.* In addition, it may result from skeletal disorders such as osteopetrosis.[17,46]

Most often, however, it results from the diffuse spread of metastases from solid tumors through the marrow, a finding most commonly seen in carcinomas of the breast and prostate. However, the finding is not confined to these cancers as it is less frequently seen, for example, in metastatic small cell lung carcinoma.

Despite the striking appearance of marrow scintigraphy in the diseases causing diffuse marrow replacement, its role in this context proves to be selective rather than

*References 4, 15, 18, 25, 47, 55, 64.

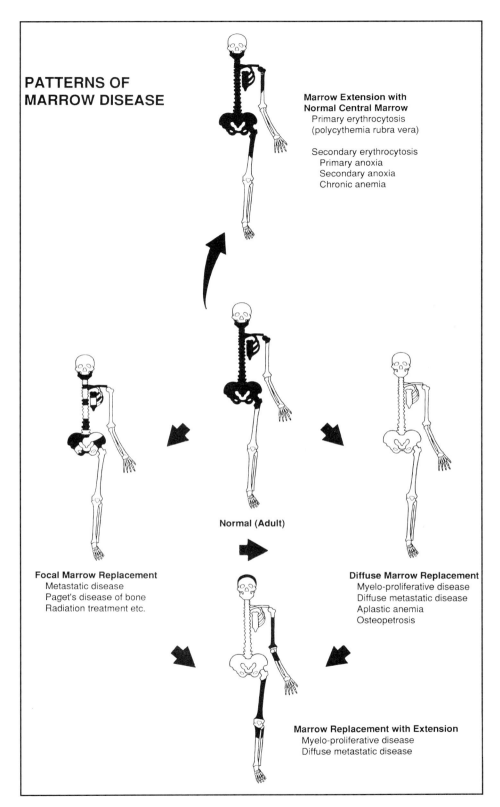

PATTERNS OF MARROW DISEASE

Marrow Extension with Normal Central Marrow
Primary erythrocytosis (polycythemia rubra vera)

Secondary erythrocytosis
Primary anoxia
Secondary anoxia
Chronic anemia

Normal (Adult)

Focal Marrow Replacement
Metastatic disease
Paget's disease of bone
Radiation treatment etc.

Diffuse Marrow Replacement
Myelo-proliferative disease
Diffuse metastatic disease
Aplastic anemia
Osteopetrosis

Marrow Replacement with Extension
Myelo-proliferative disease
Diffuse metastatic disease

Fig. 8-6. Stylized diagram of patterns of marrow replacement found in various disease states. These patterns are not discrete, but a given patient may have one finding change to another as a disease progresses or regresses.

invariable. Marrow scintigraphy may explain the occasional conflicts between clinical and laboratory data and will provide a good measure of marrow reserve free of the sampling errors associated with biopsies.[15,18]

Marrow Extension

Normal marrow may reexpand given some demand for increased hematopoiesis as in primary or secondary hypoxia and chronic anemias such as those due to blood loss, hemolysis, or the hemoglobinopathies. The result is usually the appearance of red marrow along the shafts of some or all long bones.

The same marrow extension occurs in patients with primary erythrocytosis (PRV) (Fig. 8-2).

A recent report also suggests that marrow expansion may result from treatment with colony-stimulating factor used to treat leukopenia.[39]

In addition marrow extension or reexpansion may result when the normal marrow space is replaced by tumor. This compensatory response is, however, selective, and it often does not provide a remedy for primary

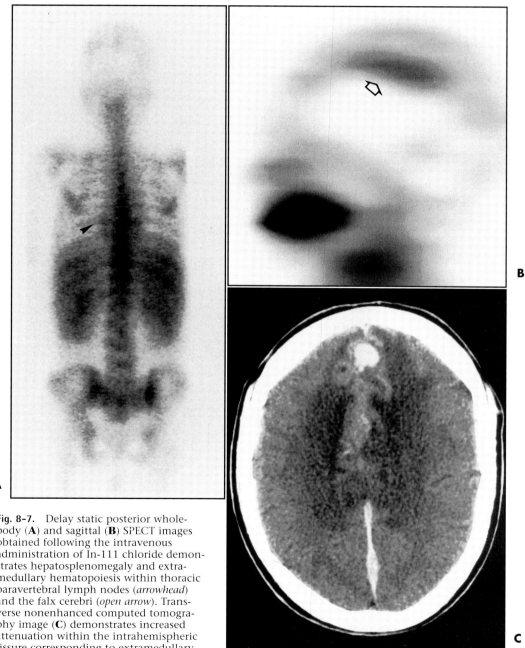

Fig. 8-7. Delay static posterior whole-body (**A**) and sagittal (**B**) SPECT images obtained following the intravenous administration of In-111 chloride demonstrates hepatosplenomegaly and extramedullary hematopoiesis within thoracic paravertebral lymph nodes (*arrowhead*) and the falx cerebri (*open arrow*). Transverse nonenhanced computed tomography image (**C**) demonstrates increased attenuation within the intrahemispheric fissure corresponding to extramedullary hematopoiesis at the falx cerebri.

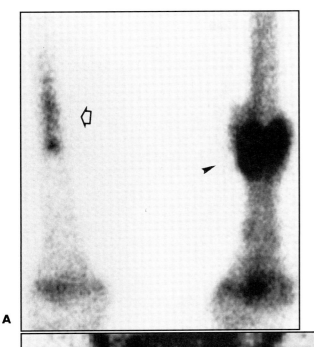

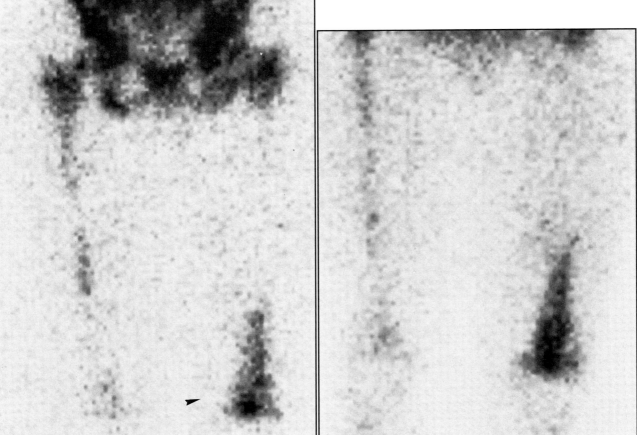

Fig. 8–8. Delayed static anterior images from a bone scan (**A**) demonstrates markedly increased activity within the mid-diaphysis of the left femur related to a previous fracture (*arrowhead*) and mild diffuse increased uptake within the proximal diaphysis of the right femur (*open arrow*). An anterior image obtained following the administration of indium-111 labeled white blood cells (**B**) demonstrates increased activity within the proximal two-thirds of the right femur and distal one-third of the left femur (*arrowhead*). Images of the femora obtained following the intravenous administration of Tc-99m sulfur colloid (**C**) demonstrate a similar pattern of activity compared with the labeled white blood cell images. Radiolabeled white cell imaging and radiocolloid marrow imaging can be helpful in distinguishing sites of infection from sites of expanded or displaced marrow. The congruent pattern of the two images (**B** and **C**) confirmed the presence of expanded marrow within the right femur and displaced marrow secondary to the insertion of an intramedullary rod within the distal left femur.

marrow diseases such as aplastic anemia or myelofibrosis. The scintigraphic appearance is the same as reexpansion of normal marrow except that the central marrow space will be depleted either uniformly or by multiple focal lesions.[19]

Although marrow reexpansion may be diagnosed directly from marrow scintigraphy, it is most commonly inferred from secondary changes noted on bone scintigraphy (Figs. 8-1 and 8-2).

Extramedullary Hematopoiesis

Marrow failure from whatever cause may, if it is sufficiently severe and prolonged, result in extramedullary hematopoiesis (EH). It chiefly affects RE organs such as liver, spleen, and lymph nodes. A paravertebral mass is a common manifestation (Fig. 8-7, A).[12,15,18] Less frequently it involves the kidneys, skin, heart, pleura, and mesentery. Rarely even the central nervous system may be involved with sites of EH along the falx cerebri (Figs. 8-7, B and C).[61]

It should be noted that a false-negative finding has been reported concerning the use of RE cell imaging to diagnose EH. Therefore this method cannot be used with certainty to exclude this diagnosis.[24]

The diagnosis of EH is an important application of marrow scintigraphy, using the radiopharmaceutical most appropriate to the site and the laboratory in question, because it provides tissue-specific evidence that may negate the need for biopsy or exploratory surgery.

Marrow Damage

The most common iatrogenic causes of marrow damage are irradiation and drug toxicity. Generalized bone marrow hypoplasia may also result from chronic exposure to benzene. Local irradiation of the marrow causes a focal defect if the dose is above a threshold and it has also been reported, chiefly in animal experiments, that there is some dissociation of the effect on RE cells and red cell precursors.[6,41]

Marrow irradiation in the short term has also been reported to result in an increase in radiolabeled granulocyte localization in the irradiated volume, presumably as a result of a local increase in capillary permeability.[45]

Bone Marrow Imaging in the Context of Fractures

Bone marrow scintigraphy has been explored in particular for its potential value in recognizing avascular necrosis of the femoral head complicating femoral neck fractures. It is true that marrow obliteration will result from avascular necrosis, and Tawn and Watt found colloid marrow scintigraphy to be more sensitive than bone scintigraphy in this context.[60] They were, however, not able to infer specificity. Since there are differences from patient to patient in the presence, amount, and distribution of bone marrow in the femoral head,[66] the negative predictive value of this method may be too poor to per-

mit reliance on its use in practice as suggested by the findings of Langer et al [3] (see Chapter 15).

As noted, already healed rib fractures and potentially fractures at other sites may result in focal marrow defects.[13]

Bone Marrow Imaging and Hip Replacements

In distinguishing a loose from an infected hip prosthesis, bone and labeled granulocyte scintigraphy are often used. Marrow present in heterotopic bone in proximity to the joint may result in a false-positive granulocyte scan. Thus a limited radiocolloid marrow examination used for comparison may increase the specificity of the combined examinations.[29,44] Marrow "displacement" from the femoral head to the shaft may also occur in the presence of hip prostheses, so that localized marrow examinations may again prevent false-positive scans made with radiolabeled granulocytes (Fig. 8-8, A and B)[57] (see Chapter 11).

COMPARATIVE IMAGING

Before the advent of MRI, this section might have been brief or nonexistent. However, MRI has proved to be an elegant way of examining bone marrow noninvasively.[48] It has three disadvantages when compared with RN marrow examinations. It is globally less readily available, more expensive, and less amenable to whole-body imaging than RN methods. Clearly it provides better resolution as well as information about structures adjacent to bone and marrow. However, one elegant combined use of RN methods and MRI combines the sensitivity and whole-body scope of Tc-99m phosphate imaging with the specificity of MRI by using the latter tool to explore solitary or ambiguous findings seen on the RN bone scan.[22,48]

PRESENT CLINICAL UTILITY OF RADIONUCLIDE MARROW IMAGING

Given the limitations of the techniques now available for RN marrow imaging, it is not and is unlikely to become a high-volume procedure. However, as a specific tool, particularly where MRI is not available, it is of considerable use in characterizing masses as due to EH; occasionally in complementing Tc-99m phosphate imaging in increasing specificity in diagnosing metastatic disease[43]; and rarely in documenting the extent and amount of bone marrow involvement in the myeloproliferative diseases. In particular it may have value in documenting marrow reserves and before irradiation the location of such reserves.[23] As previously noted it has a limited but particular place in examinations of hip prostheses when infection of these is suspected.[29,44,57] A further application is in relation to patients with a hemoglobinopathy such as sickle cell disease in resolving the differential diagnosis of acute bone pain.[15,37,59] A little used application might be to plan sites for marrow biopsies because these are known to be subject to substantial sampling errors.[15,20]

To a large extent marrow scintigraphy has probably suffered from the lack of a radiopharmaceutical that can be used readily and conveniently and that will result in good image quality. It is possible that the newer immunoscintigraphic agents will redress this lack.[50]

ACKNOWLEDGMENTS

We wish to acknowledge the help of the Biomedical Illustration Department of the University of British Columbia and of Ms. Virginia Zepeda.

REFERENCES

1. Abdel-Dayem HM, Sanchez J, al-Mohannadi, Kempf J: Diffuse thallium-201-chloride uptake in hypermetabolic bone marrow following treatment with granulocyte stimulating factor. *J Nucl Med* 1992; 33:2014.
2. Alavi A, Heyman S: Bone marrow imaging, in Gottschalk A, Hoffer PB, Potchen EJ (eds): *Diagnostic Nuclear Medicine.* Baltimore, 1988, Williams & Wilkins, p 707.
3. Alberts KA, Dahlborn M, Ringertz H, Soderborg B: Comparison of skeletal and bone marrow radionuclide scintimetry of femoral neck fracture. *Acta Orthop Scand* 1984; 55:612.
4. Arrago JP, Rain JD, Vigneron N, et al: Diagnostic value of bone marrow imaging with 111-indium-transferrin and 99m-technetium-colloids in myelofibrosis. *Am J Hematol* 1985; 18:275.
5. Axelsson B, Kalin B, Von Krusenstierna S, Jacobsson H: Comparison of In-111 granulocytes and Tc-99m albumin colloid for bone marrow scintigraphy by the use of quantitative SPECT imaging. *Clin Nucl Med* 1990; 15:473.
6. Beamish MR, Brown EB: The metabolism of transferrin bound In-111 and Fe-59 in the rat. *Blood* 1974; 43:703.
7. Bennett JD, Dubeau RA, Driedger AA: Polymorphonuclear leukocytes labeled with technetium-99m HMPAO: A potential bone marrow imaging agent. *Clin Nucl Med* 1988; 13:44.
8. Borgies P, Ferrant A, Leners N, et al: Diagnosis of heterotopic bone marrow in the mediastinum using ^{52}Fe and positron emission tomography. *Eur J Nucl Med* 1989; 15:761.
9. Bourgeois P, Gassavelis C, Malarme M, et al: Bone marrow scintigraphy in breast cancer. *Nucl Med Commun* 1989; 10:389.
10. Bourgeois P, Malarme M, Van Franck R, et al: Bone marrow scintigraphy in prostatic carcinomas. *Nucl Med Commun* 1991; 12:35.
11. Bourgeois P, Thimpont J, Feremans W, Malarme M: Bone marrow scintigraphy in lung carcinomas using nanosized colloids: When is it useful and how useful is it? *Nucl Med Commun* 1992; 13:421.
12. Bronn LJ, Paquelet JR, Tetalman MR: Intrathoracic extramedullary hematopoiesis: Appearance on ^{99m}Tc sulfur colloid marrow scan. *AJR Am J Roentgenol* 1980; 134:1254.
13. Chafetz N, Slivka J, Taylor A, et al: Decreased Tc-99m sulfur colloid activity in healed rib fractures. *Radiology* 1978; 126:735.
14. Cooper M, Miles KA, Wraight EP, Dixon AK: Degenerative disc disease in the lumbar spine: Another cause for focally reduced activity on marrow scintigraphy. *Skeletal Radiol* 1992; 21:247.
15. Datz FL, Taylor A Jr: The clinical use of radionuclide bone marrow imaging. *Semin Nucl Med* 1985; 15:239.
16. Duncker CM: Radioimmune imaging of bone marrow in patients with suspected bone metastases from primary breast cancer. *J Nucl Med* 1990; 31:1450.
17. Elster AD, Theros EG, Key LL, Stanton C: Autosomal recessive osteopetrosis: Bone marrow imaging. *Radiology* 1992; 182:507.
18. Fordham EW, Ali A: Radionuclide imaging of bone marrow. *Semin Hematol* 1981; 18:222.
19. Fordham EW, Ali A, Turner DA, Charters JR: *Atlas of Whole Body Radionuclide Imaging,* vol 1, Philadelphia, 1982, Harper and Row, p 749.
20. Gilbert EH, Earle JD: 111-Indium bone marrow scintigraphy as an aid in selecting marrow biopsy sites for the evaluation of marrow elements in patients with lymphoma. *Cancer* 1976; 38:1560.
21. Gordon L, Spicer KM, Yon JW Jr: Bone marrow uptake of xenon-133. *Clin Nucl Med* 1985; 10:891.
22. Gosfield E, Alavi A, Kneeland B: Comparison of radionuclide bone scans and magnetic resonance imaging in detecting spinal metastases. *J Nucl Med* 1993; 34:2191.
23. Haddock G, Gray HW, McKillop JH, et al: ^{99m}Tc-nanocolloid bone marrow scintigraphy in prostatic cancer. *Br J Urol* 1989; 63:497.
24. Harnsberger HR, Datz FL, Knochel JQ, Taylor AT: Failure to detect extramedullary hematopoiesis during bone-marrow imaging with indium-111 or technetium-99m sulfur colloid. *J Nucl Med* 1982; 23:589.
25. Horn NL, Bennett LR, Marciano: Evaluation of aplastic anemia with indium chloride In-111 scanning. *Arch Intern Med* 1980; 140:1299.
26. Ito Y, Okuyama S, Suzuki M, et al: Bone marrow scintigraphy in the early diagnosis of experimental metastatic bone carcinoma. *Cancer* 1973; 31:1222.
27. Itoh H, Kanamori M, Takahashi N: Dissociation between In-111 chloride and Tc-99m colloid bone marrow scintigraphy in refractory anemia with excess blasts. *Clin Nucl Med* 1990; 15:124.
28. Kahn CE Jr, Ryan JW, Hatfield MK, Martin WB: Combined bone marrow and gallium imaging: Differentiation of osteomyelitis and infarction in sickle hemoglobinopathy. *Clin Nucl Med* 1988; 13:443.
29. King AD, Peters AM, Stuttle AW, Lavender JP: Imaging of bone infection with labelled white blood cells: Role of contemporaneous bone marrow imaging. *Eur J Nucl Med* 1990; 17:148.
30. Klein HA, Bolden RO, Simone FJ: Vertebral hyperemia associated with bone marrow insult and recovery. *Clin Nucl Med* 1984; 9:307.
31. Kloiber R, Damtew B, Rosenthall L: A crossover study comparing the effect of particle size on the distribution of radiocolloid in patients. *Clin Nucl Med* 1981; 6:204.
32. Langer SW, Kamby C, Thomsen HS, et al: The value of bone marrow scintigraphy in patients with recurrent breast cancer. *Ugeskr Laeger* 1993; 155:778.
33. Lentle BC, Camuzzini G, Styles C, Penney H: Focal marrow replacement observed with colloid liver imaging. *Clin Nucl Med* 1982; 7:409.

34. Lentle BC, Kotchon T, Catz Z, Penney HF: Detecting bone marrow metastases at the time of examining the liver with radiocolloid. *J Nucl Med* 1987; 28:184.

35. Lentle BC, Russell AS, Heslip PG, Percy JS: The scintigraphic findings in Paget's disease of bone. *Clin Radiol* 1976; 27:129.

36. Lentle BC, Styles CB: Iatrogenic alterations in the biodistribution of radiotracers as a result of radiation therapy, surgery and other invasive medical procedures, in Hladik WB, Saha GB, Study KT (eds): *Essentials of Nuclear Medicine Science*, Baltimore, 1987, Williams & Wilkins, p 220.

37. Lutzker LG, Alavi A: Bone and marrow imaging in sickle cell disease: Diagnosis of infarction. *Semin Nucl Med* 1976; 6:83.

38. Martindale AA, Papadimitriou JM, Turner JH: Technetium-99m antimony colloid for bone-marrow imaging. *J Nucl Med* 1980; 21:1035.

39. McAfee JG, Carrasquillo JA, Camera L, et al: Changes in skeletal images induced by granulocyte-macrophage colony-stimulating factor (GM-CSF) in patients with locally advanced and metastatic breast cancer. *J Nucl Med* 1994; 35:89P (abstract).

40. McAfee JG, Subramanian G, Aburano T, et al: A new formulation of Tc-99m minimicroaggregated albumin for marrow imaging: Comparison with other colloids, In-111 and Fe-59. *J Nucl Med* 1982; 23:21.

41. Nelp WB, Gohil MN, Larson SM: Long-term effects of local irradiation of the marrow on erythron and RE cell function. *Blood* 1970; 36:617.

42. Ohnishi T, Jinnouchi S, Hoshi H, et al: The evaluation of the bone marrow accumulation of Ga-67 citrate [Japanese]. *Kaku Igaku* 1989; 26:1371.

43. Otsuka N, Fukunaga M, Sone T, et al: The usefulness of bone-marrow scintigraphy in the detection of bone metastasis from prostatic cancer. *Eur J Nucl Med* 1985; 11:319.

44. Palestro CJ, Kim CK, Swyer AJ, et al: Total-hip arthroplasty: Periprosthetic indium-111-labelled leukocyte activity and complementary technetium-99m-sulfur colloid imaging in suspected infection. *J Nucl Med* 1990; 31:1950.

45. Palestro CJ, Kim CK, Vega A, et al: Acute effects of radiation therapy on indium-111-labeled leukocyte uptake in bone marrow. *J Nucl Med* 1989; 30:1889.

46. Park H, Lambertus J: Skeletal and reticuloendothelial imaging in osteopetrosis: Case report. *J Nucl Med* 1977; 18:1091.

47. Perry MC, Holmes RA: The radioindium bone-marrow image in acute (malignant) myelofibrosis. *J Nucl Med* 1980; 21:139.

48. Porter BA, Shields AF, Olson DO: Magnetic resonance imaging of bone marrow disorders. *Radiol Clin North Am* 1986; 24:269.

49. Price DC, McIntyre PA. The hemopoietic system, in Harbert J, da Rocha AFG (eds): *Textbook of Nuclear Medicine*, Philadelphia, 1984, Lea & Febiger, p 535.

50. Reske SN: Recent advances in bone marrow scanning: Review article. *Eur J Nucl Med* 1991; 18:203.

51. Reske SN, Karstens JH, Glockner WM, et al: Detection of bone marrow involvement in breast cancer and malignant lymphoma using immunoscintigraphy of the hematopoietic bone marrow. *Fortschr Rontgenstr Nuklearmed* 1990; 152:60.

52. Reske SN, Karstens JH, Gloeckner W, et al: Radioimmunoimaging for diagnosis of bone marrow involvement in breast cancer and malignant lymphoma. *Lancet* 1989; 1:299.

53. Rudberg U, Ahlbäck S-O, Uden R: Bone marrow scintigraphy in Paget's disease of bone. *Acta Radiol Diagn* 1990; 31:141.

54. Rudberg U, Udem R, Ahlbäck S-O: Colloid scintigraphy showing red bone marrow extension in patients with prostatic carcinoma. *Acta Radiol* 1992; 33:97.

55. Sayle BA, Helmer RE, Birdsong BA, et al: Bone-marrow imaging with indium-111 chloride in aplastic anemia and myelofibrosis: Concise communication. *J Nucl Med* 1982; 23:121.

56. Scher HI, Yagoda A: Bone metastases: Pathogenesis, treatment and rationale for the use of resorption inhibitors. *Am J Med* 1987; 82(suppl 2A):6.

57. Seabold JE, Nepola JV, Marsh JL, et al: Post-operative bone marrow alterations: Potential pitfalls in the diagnosis of osteomyelitis with In-111-labeled leukocyte scintigraphy. *Radiology* 1991; 180:741.

58. Shih W-J, Domstad PA, DeLand FH, Purcell M: Incidental vertebral lesions identified during technetium-99m sulfur colloid liver-spleen imaging. *Clin Nucl Med* 1986; 11:585.

59. Siddiqui AA, Oseas RS, Wellman HN, et al: Evaluation of bone-marrow scanning with technetium-99m sulfur colloid in pediatric oncology. *J Nucl Med* 1979; 20:379.

60. Tawn DJ, Watt I: Bone marrow scintigraphy in the diagnosis of post-traumatic avascular necrosis of bone. *Br J Radiol* 1989; 62:790.

61. Urman M, O'Sullivan R, Nugent RA, Lentle BC: Intracranial extramedullary hematopoiesis: CT and bone marrow scan findings. *Clin Nucl Med* 1991; 16:431.

62. Vallabhajosula S, Gilbert HS: Low density lipoprotein (LDL) distribution shown by ^{99m}technetium-LDL imaging. *Ann Intern Med* 1989; 110:208.

63. Van Dyke D, Shkurkin C, Price D: Differences in distribution of erythropoietic and reticuloendothelial marrow in hematological disease. *Blood* 1967; 30:364.

64. Widding A, Smolorz J, Franke M, et al: Bone marrow investigation with technetium-99m microcolloid and magnetic resonance imaging in patients with malignant myelolymphoproliferative diseases. *Eur J Nucl Med* 1989; 15:230.

65. Widding A, Stilbo I, Hansen SW, et al: Scintigraphy with nanocolloid Tc-99m in patients with small cell lung cancer, with special reference to bone marrow and hepatic metastases. *Eur J Nucl Med* 1990; 16:717.

66. Williams AG, Mettler FA, Christie JH: Sulfur colloid distribution in normal hips. *Clin Nucl Med* 1983; 8:490.

67. Wiseman J, McHenry C: Focal marrow replacement in intervertebral disc space infection: Demonstrated by Tc-99m sulfur colloid imaging. *Clin Nucl Med* 1984; 9:291.

68. Woodard HQ, Holodny E: A summary of the data of Mechanik on the distribution of human bone marrow. *Phys Med Biol* 1960; 5:57.

CHAPTER 9

METABOLIC BONE DISEASE

Leonard Rosenthall

Metabolic bone disease leads to generalized involvement of the skeleton, which in the early stages of evolution may render normal-appearing bone images with any of the radiophosphate complexes. As the disease progresses, there is increased accretion, most noticeably in the periarticular bones, vertebral column, calvarium, mandible, rib ends, sternum, and long bones. Quantitative radiophosphate uptake measurements will disclose the increases before they are visually appreciated. Various methods have been proposed such as femoral-condyle-to-adjacent-soft-tissue ratio, lumbar-spine-to-adjacent-soft-tissue ratio,[74] and lumbar-spine-to-kidney ratio.[36] These approaches have been partially successful, but they are relatively crude and may not reflect the complete picture, because the accelerated bone remodeling is not necessarily uniform throughout the skeleton. Total-body measurements of the 24-hour retention of radiophosphate, as obtained with the shadow-shield monitor, is more accurate in rendering an index of average skeletal bone remodeling, and uses about 1/300th of the diagnostic imaging dose of radiophosphate.[23] Since this device is not generally available, other methods have been tried with equipment commonly present in service laboratories.

A compromise can be achieved by performing the total-body counts with a simple thyroid uptake detector and a 15- to 20-mCi radiophosphate imaging dose.[72] In a crossover study comparing this method and the shadow-shield monitor, a coefficient of correlation of 0.99 was obtained.[47] A gamma camera equipped with a fishtail collimator has also been adapted for total-body 24-hour retention studies, and a crossover comparison with the shadow-shield monitor yielded a coefficient of correlation of 0.98.[54] Total-body retention of radiophosphate can also be estimated by assaying the 24-hour urine collection and comparing it against a standard to determine the percentage of administered dose excreted.[89] It is less reliable than taking postinjection counts because a complete urine collection is obligatory, and this is not always achieved with elderly and confused patients. Normal renal function is necessary for these studies to be valid. In renal osteodystrophy the 24-hour retention can be estimated by taking the immediate postinjection counts at a fixed time (e.g., 5 hours) before renal dialysis and at 24 hours to obtain the ratio. The same time relationship to dialysis must be maintained in follow-up studies for the comparisons to be valid.

It has been shown that no more than 30% of the 24-hour total-body retention resides in the soft tissues of normal patients, and the absolute amount remains constant whether the retention is normal or abnormal. Thus in patients with increased bone metabolism, the elevated total-body uptake is almost entirely due to the skeletal contribution.[82]

MECHANISM OF ^{99m}Tc–PHOSPHATE UPTAKE IN BONE

It is accepted that the rate of concentration in bone is a function of blood flow and extraction efficiency, and that an increase can be achieved by increasing one or both components. Still under debate is the precise site of deposition of the radiophosphate complexes. The thesis that the circulating ^{99m}Tc labeled phosphate is adsorbed selectively onto the mineral phase of forming bone was based on in vivo autoradiographs that ostensibly showed localization of ^{99m}Tc to mineralized tissue and not to unmineralized osteoid in the osteosarcoma and fracture healing animal models.[33,63] Similar conclusions about ^{99m}Tc-phosphate were derived from microautoradiography of excised human osteoarthritic femoral heads and the analysis of the deposition in the epiphyseal growth plates of rats.[9,10] It was further stated that the adsorption occurred preferentially onto amorphous calcium phosphate before it matured into the hydroxyapatite crystal, because in vitro incubation experiments demonstrated a greater affinity for the former.[28] Despite these revelations it must be recognized that microautoradiographic techniques cannot distinguish with certainty between the spatially superimposed organic matrix and inorganic phases and the relative uptakes within each.

In vitro incubation studies on demineralized and ashed bone clearly demonstrated that phosphate complexed with ^{99m}Tc behaved differently from phosphate in which a constituent of the molecule, either P or C, was replaced with ^{32}P or ^{14}C, respectively. ^{47}Ca, ^{32}PPi, and ^{14}C-HEDP demonstrated a higher uptake in bone that had the organic matrix removed by ashing than in bone demineralized by hydrochloric acid. These anticipated results were contrary to the observation of greater uptake of ^{99m}Tc-pertechnetate, ^{99m}Tc-HEDP, and ^{99m}Tc-PPi in matrix rather than mineral. In vivo experiments wherein rachitic and uremic rats were analyzed for the percent dose uptake of ^{99m}Tc-PPi, ^{32}PPi, and ^{45}Ca (or ^{47}Ca) in various segments of the femur demonstrated no difference in the radiocalcium or ^{32}PPi uptake between diseased and normal control femurs. However, the ^{99m}Tc-PPi concentration was higher in the rachitic and uremic rats than normals.[50,73] These findings indicated that there was a nonmineral supplemental site for binding, in addition to hydroxyapatite as propounded by others.

Recently it was shown by chemical separation of mineral and matrix in a rat bone repair model that with the intravenous delivery of a double labeled phosphate, ^{99m}TcMD-^{32}P, there was preferential binding of ^{99m}Tc to the organic matrix and MD-^{32}P to the mineral phase. In contrast, the injection of ^{99m}Tc, as a pertechnetate, did not demonstrate bone uptake significantly above back-

ground. The deduction from these observations was that ^{99m}Tc-MDP is taken up by bone initially, but ^{99m}Tc is released at the site by hydrolysis and then concentrates in newly formed matrix, whereas the MDP moiety remains attached to the mineral phase.[76,80] Therefore it would seem that the accretion of ^{99m}Tc seen on bone images is primarily a reflection of osteoid formation (i.e., osteoblastic activity) and not the calcification process. This thesis does not preclude the existence of bone mineral adsorption of the intact molecule of ^{99m}Tc-MDP, or other ^{99m}Tc complexed phosphates—as such, it is simply not the major source of the radioactivity seen on the bone images. In metastatic and dystrophic calcification, mineral adsorption of the intact ^{99m}Tc-MDP is the most likely mechanism.

PRIMARY HYPERPARATHYROIDISM

Primary hyperparathyroidism is associated with an increased secretion of parathyroid hormone that causes hypophosphatemia and hypercalcemia and possible sequelae consisting of nephrolithiasis, peptic ulcer, mental changes, pseudogout, and less frequently excessive bone resorption. In over 80% of the cases this is due to a single benign adenoma. Multigland adenomata and hyperplasia, either symmetric or asymmetric, account for the remainder of the benign lesions. A distinction between adenoma and hyperplasia can be difficult histologically. The frequency of carcinoma is reported to occur in 1% to 3% of the cases. It has been calculated that the incidence of hyperparathyroidism is about 27 in 100,000 persons per year.[55] Most patients are asymptomatic, and their disclosure stems from the increased use of multiphasic screening of blood and the serendipitous finding of an elevated serum calcium level. As a result of this diagnosis early in the evolution of the disease, visible radiographic and radiophosphate changes are usually not present. In fact, the frequency of the advanced radiographic stigmata of osteitis fibrosa cystica—namely, subperiosteal bone resorption of the radial aspect of the fingers, generalized demineralization, erosion of the outer cortical bone surfaces, and locally destructive lesions by cysts or brown tumors is low (Fig. 9-1). This is also true of the number of patients presenting with symptoms of osteitis fibrosa cystica: between 1930 and 1949, 53%; 1949 and 1960, 21%; 1965 and 1973, 9%;[35] 1980 and 1983, 0%.[69] All patients with hyperparathyroidism have increased bone turnover on histomorphometry, but not all depict bone mineral loss.[61] Bone densitometry measurements early in the disease may show normal mineral content in the largely trabecular lumbar vertebrae, but reduced mineral content in the compact cortical bone of the appendicular skeleton.[4,93]

A comparison between visually graded ^{99m}Tc-HEDP images for metabolic features and radiography showed that the former detected 7 of the 14 patients (50%) with primary hyperparathyroidism, whereas the latter disclosed 3 (21%) of them.[24] In another crossover study

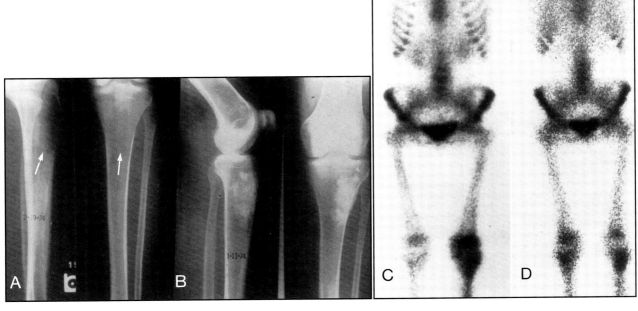

Fig. 9-1. Involution of a brown tumor following parathyroidectomy in a patient with primary hyperparathyroidism. **A**, Radiograph of the left tibia before parathyroidectomy. There is demineralization of the bone with a cyst in the proximal portion (*arrows*). **B**, At 7 months after surgery the brown tumor appears as a sclerotic mass. **C**, ^{99m}Tc-MDP scans show diffuse increased uptake in the tibia before surgery. **D**, There was bone remodeling 7 months after surgery, but it was limited to the site of the tumor, corresponding to the lesion on the radiograph. Note the partial regression of the radionuclide beading at the costochondral junctions.

measurements of the 5-hour bone to soft-tissue ratios were abnormal in 4 of 20 hyperparathyroid patients (20%), but radiography demonstrated subperiosteal bone resorption in 7 of the 20 patients (35%). Overall the 5-hour bone-to-soft-tissue ratios were not significantly different from the control group.[91] A similar lack of significance was found for a 4-hour bone-to-soft-tissue ratio by another group of investigators, but 24-hour total-body retentions in these same patients demonstrated an increase relative to the control group.[23] Thus the most sensitive radionuclide method is the 24-hour total-body retention measurement, which can be achieved with a simple probe detector in the absence of a dedicated total-body monitor.

Following parathyroidectomy the observed increased uptake of radiophosphate does not subside immediately but may remain elevated up to a year or more.[22,91] The mechanism by which the elevated uptake is sustained after surgical removal of the hyperactive gland is not clear.

Metastatic calcification of the lungs can occur in advanced hyperparathyroidism, and it may be detected with radiophosphate imaging (Fig. 9-2). All reports have been anecdotal, and there are no data on the frequency of occurrence of histologic lung calcification or on the sensitivity of the radiophosphate scan to detect its presence. Following excision of the offending gland, the lungs appear to return to normal before the bones (Fig. 9-3).[15,38] This lung response to parathyroidectomy differs from that of end-stage renal osteodystrophy where the metastatic lung calcifications may be refractory to washout.

OSTEOMALACIA

Osteomalacia is a disorder of adults in which there is defective mineralization of newly formed organic matrix. Before the closure of the epiphyseal growth plates, this defect is called rickets. A common etiologic factor is a lack of vitamin D caused by insufficient dietary intake, reduced intestinal absorption following partial gastrectomy and intestinal bypass surgery, intestinal loss in the various forms of malabsorption syndrome, and decreased endogenous production of vitamin D in skin due to insufficient exposure to ultraviolet light. Other causes are vitamin D resistance in chronic renal failure, renal tubular disorders, liver disease, excessive metabolism of vitamin D by anticonvulsant therapy, aluminum toxicity in renal dialysis, and anorexia nervosa. A rare form of tumor-associated hypophosphatemia, also called tumorous phosphaturic osteomalacia or oncogenic osteomalacia, has been reported in association with tumors of mesenchymal origin. These include hemangiomas of bone, sclerosing hemangioma of soft tissue, giant cell reparative granuloma, malignant giant cell tumor, pleomorphic sarcoma, nonossifying fibroma of bone, ossifying mesenchymal tumor, hemangiopericytoma, and neurofibromatosis.[16,64] Complete removal of the lesions is often fol-

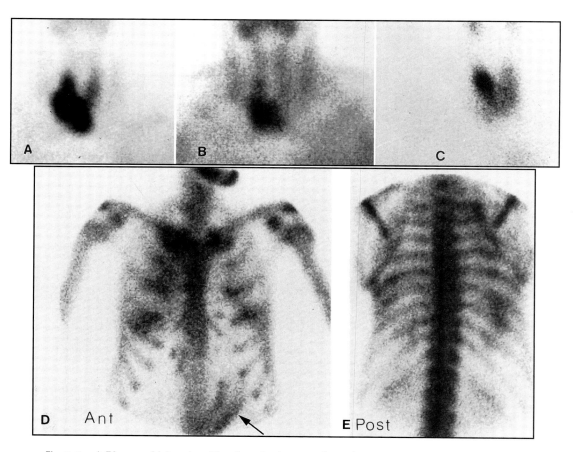

Fig. 9-2. A 78-year-old female with a functioning parathyroid carcinoma. The 5-minute (**A**) and 2-hour (**B**) ^{99m}Tc-sestamibi scans depict a mass on the right crossing the midline. **C,** Comparative pertechnetate thyroid scan. **D** and **E,** Anterior and posterior ^{99m}Tc-MDP images exhibit diffuse increased skeletal uptake. There are also a patchy lung and a uniform gastric (*arrow*) deposition, these reflecting metastatic calcification.

lowed by a remission of the osteomalacia, whereas the osteomalacia persists with partial removal. It is speculated that these tumors secrete a peptide having a parathyroid hormone (PTH)–like action on the renal transport of phosphate with resultant hyper-phosphaturia, or a humeral substance that suppresses the renal production of 1,25-hydroxycholecalciferol.

Vitamin D is made available to the body by ultraviolet photogenesis in the skin and by intestinal absorption. It is first hydroxylated in the liver to 25-hydroxycholecalciferol [25-OHD$_3$], which in turn is converted in the kidney to 1,25-dihydroxycholecalciferol [1,25-(OH)$_2$D$_3$] and 24,25-dihydroxycholecalciferol [24,25-(OH)$_2$D$_3$]. The lack of vitamin D results in decreased plasma calcium and a subsequent stimulation of PTH elaboration to sustain a normal calcium level. This in turn causes enhanced renal excretion of phosphate and hypophosphatemia. Below a critical level of extracellular fluid phosphate concentration, normal mineralization of bone cannot proceed. Phosphate depletion is probably the cause of osteomalacia in some of the renal disorders, but it does not account for all of them.

Radiographic signs of osteomalacia include loss of bone density due to the presence of nonmineralized osteoid, loss of longitudinal and transverse trabeculae with blurring of those remaining, thinning of the cortices, and pseudofractures. The pseudofractures, also called Looser's zones or milkman's fractures, are often apparent early in the disease and are usually symmetric. They occur perpendicular to the bone surface and are most frequently seen in the scapula, medial aspect of the femoral neck, pubic rami, ulna (proximal third), radius (distal third), ribs, clavicle, metacarpals, metatarsals, and phalanges. It has been suggested that these pseudofractures are caused by pulsating vessels eroding the softened cortex, which later become filled with uncalcified osteoid.[83]

The bone scan appearance of osteomalacia is that of generalized increased radiophosphate accretion, most visible at the periarticular zones, vertebral column, calvarium, mandible, costochondral junctions, and sternum. In a comparative study with conventional radiography, one report stated that of the 15 patients with the disease all were diagnosed by bone scan, whereas only 9 (60%) by radiography. Additionally, more pseudofractures were seen on the bone scan as areas of focally increased uptake than were appreciated by radiography.[24] Another study related that all 11 elderly patients,

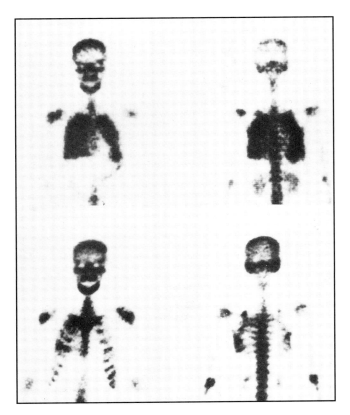

Fig. 9-3. Response to parathyroidectomy in a patient with primary hyperparathyroidism and metastatic lung calcification. *Upper panel*: Anterior and posterior views. Presurgical ^{99m}Tc-MDP scans depict an intense uniform deposition in both lungs due to metastatic calcification. *Lower panel*: At 3 months after surgery, there is a marked reduction in the radiophosphate lung uptake, but the skeletal activity has not diminished appreciably. *(Courtesy of K. Itoh, M.D., and M. Furudate, M.D., Hokkaido University, Sapporo, Japan.)*

who were between 70 and 95 years of age, with proved osteomalacia had positive ^{99m}Tc-MDP bone scans manifesting generalized increased uptake, minimal visualization of the kidneys, and focal concentrations at the costochondral junctions, pseudofractures, and true fractures. Treatment with calcium and vitamin D reversed these changes in the 5 patients who had follow-up studies.[68] The better sensitivity of radiophosphate imaging over conventional radiography has been confirmed by others who have also cautioned that the pseudofractures should not be misconstrued as metastatic disease when they occur proximal to the knees and elbows.[27,51,81]

RENAL OSTEODYSTROPHY

Renal osteodystrophy is a term encompassing the changes in bone metabolism as a result of prolonged chronic renal disease. The tubular forms of the disease—such as vitamin D–resistant rickets, renal tubular acidosis, and Fanconi's syndrome—induce osteomalacia and only rarely is there an associated secondary hyper-

parathyroidism. Acquired diseases of glomerular origin (e.g., chronic glomerular nephritis and chronic pyelonephritis) present a mixed histologic picture of osteomalacia and hyperparathyroidism (osteitis fibrosa cystica). The mechanisms involved in the development of renal osteodystrophy are complex, and there are numerous interactive factors. With progressive nephron loss the hydroxylation capacity of the kidney is reduced and with it a failure of the conversion of vitamin D to its active form, $1,25-(OH)_2D_3$. This deficiency leads to impaired calcium absorption from the gut, hyperphosphatemia, a reciprocal reduction in plasma calcium, and increased PTH elaboration in response to the hypocalcemia. The PTH increases phosphate excretion by reducing tubular reabsorption, but as renal impairment proceeds, the amount of phosphate filtered by the glomerulus decreases and PTH becomes less effective in controlling the hyperphosphatemia. In an attempt to sustain a normal calcium plasma level, there is further increased PTH secretion, far exceeding concentrations found in patients with primary parathyroid adenomas. The bone reacts to the high PTH levels with enhanced osteoclasis and mobilization of calcium. Histologic stigmata can vary from osteomalacia to severe osteitis fibrosa cystica, featuring a marked increase in the number of osteoclasts and osteoblasts, and fibrosis of the marrow. Calcification of overly abundant osteoid may lead to sclerosis by radiography. This sclerosis is not restricted in location, but in the axial skeleton sclerosis of the upper and lower vertebral end plates imparts a "rugger jersey" portrayal in the radiograph.

Osteomalacia associated with renal dialysis is largely a product of aluminum toxicity. The aluminum is derived from the dialysis bath and phosphate binding agents. There is a reduction of the function and number of osteoblasts, and mineralization is blocked by the aluminum deposited at the calcification front. Patients with this low-turnover, or adynamic, bone disease suffer from bone pain and are at increased risk for fracture. There are recent reports indicating that this adynamic bone disease can occur in the absence of excess aluminum deposition, and that it may be related to the increasing age of the patients receiving dialysis and who are diabetic.[52]

Bone Imaging

Bone uptake of radiophosphate varies with the underlying histology (Fig. 9-4). In osteomalacia secondary to aluminum toxicity, the concentration can be visibly reduced to less than normal, because of the paucity of osteoblasts and newly formed osteoid. Osteitis fibrosa cystica, the other end of the spectrum, features abundant osteoblastic activity and, therefore manifests supranormal uptakes of the test agent. Between the two extremes the radiophosphate uptake is usually normal or increased.* The increased uptake, as is commonly found in most metabolic disorders, is diffuse but most prominent in the calvarium, mandible, sternum, periarticular

*References 5, 40, 43, 56, 57, 88.

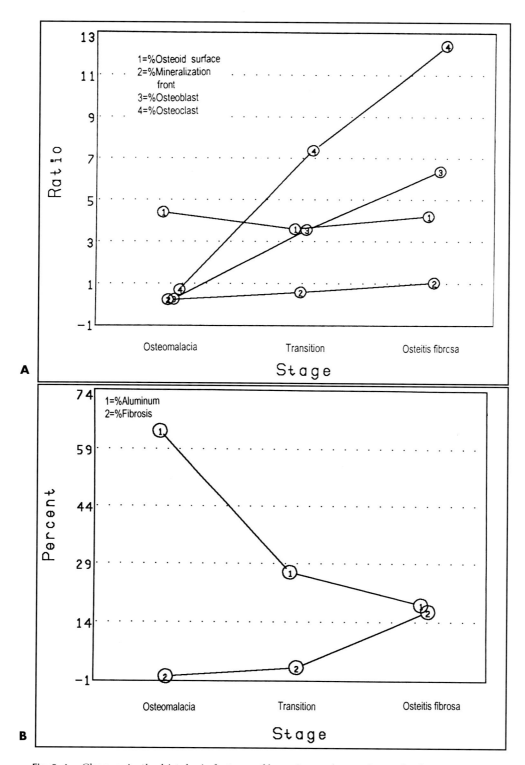

Fig. 9–4. Changes in the histologic features of bone in renal osteodystrophy from osteomalacia to osteitis fibrosis cystica. **A**, Ratios of mineralization, osteoid surface, osteoblasts and osteoclasts relative to normal. **B**, Mean percentage of aluminum and fibrosis present in each category. *(Data from Kinnaert P, Van Hooff I, Schoutens A, et al: Differential diagnosis between secondary hyperarathyroidism and aluminum intoxication in uremic patients: Usefulness of 99mTc-pyrophosphate bone scintigraphy,* World J Surg *1989; 13:219; Merz WA, Schenk RK: Quantitative structural analysis of human cancellous bone,* Acta Anat *1970; 75:54; Merz WA, Schenk RK: A quantitative histological study on bone formation in human cancellous bone,* Acta Anat *1970; 76:1; Brodier P, Zingraff J, Gueris J, et al: The effect of 1-alpha (OH)D_3 and 1-alpha 25(OH)_2D_3 on the bone in patients with renal osteodystrophy,* Am J Med *1978; 64:101.)*

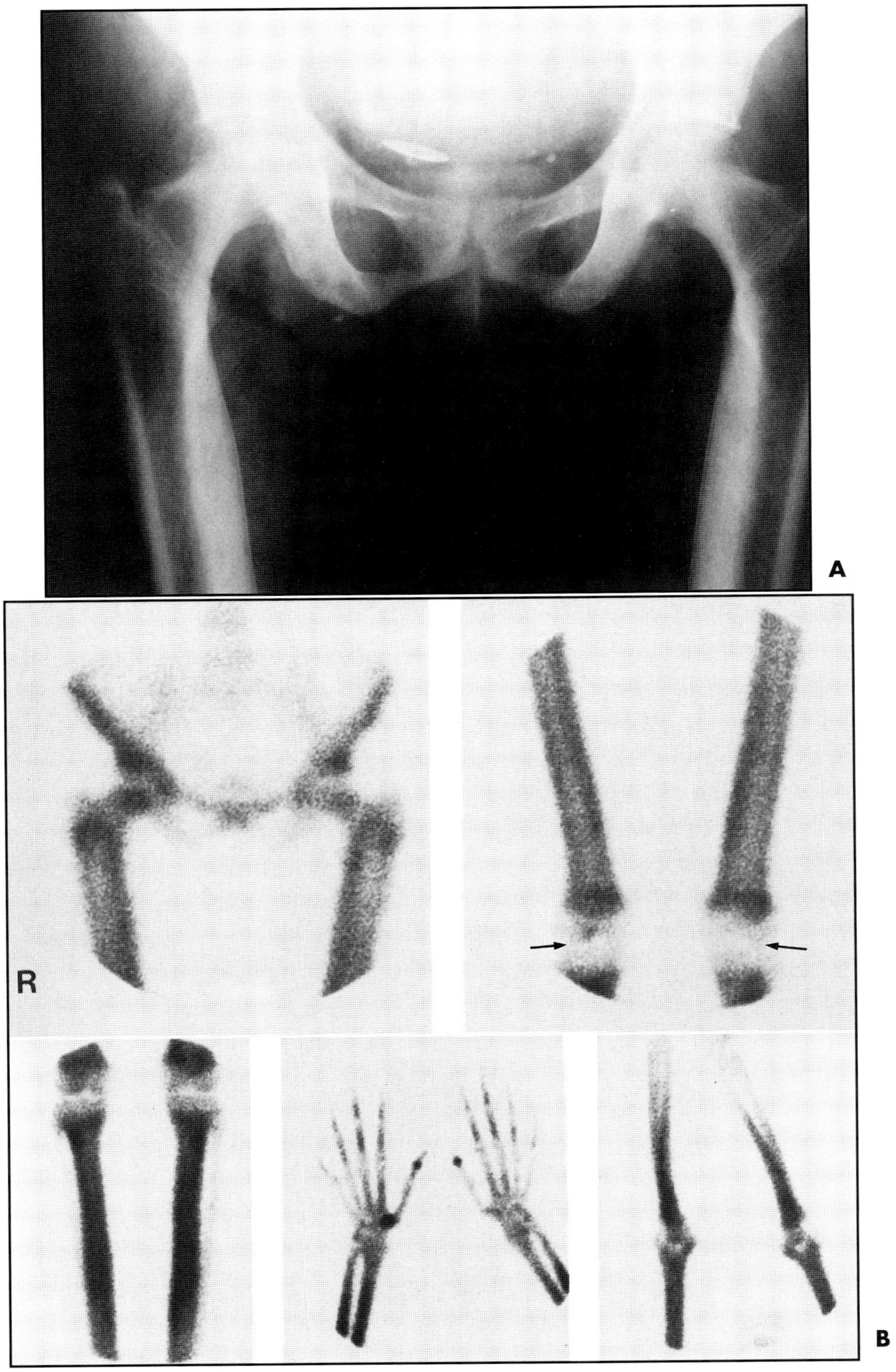

Fig. 9-5. Subperiosteal bone formation in renal osteodystrophy and the postparathyroidectomy changes. **A,** Radiograph of the femurs before total parathyroidectomy demonstrates marked thickening of the medial cortex of the shafts. Other long bones showed a similar subperiosteal reaction. **B,** Contemporary ^{99m}Tc-MDP bone scans depict the subperiosteal concentration in the long bones, involving the diaphyses and sparing the bare areas of the periarticular regions; most apparent at the knees (*arrows*).

Continued.

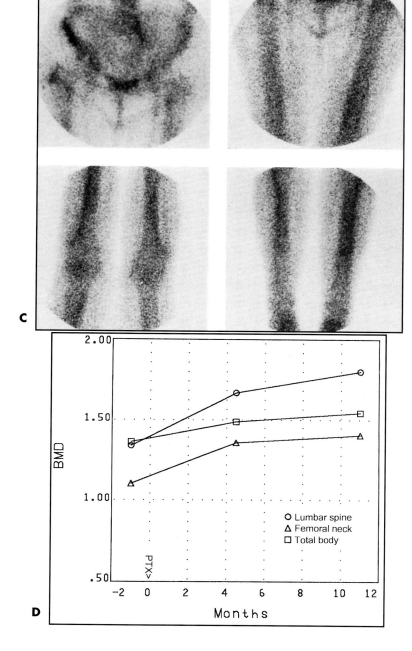

Fig. 9-5, cont'd.   C, One year after total parathyroidectomy (PTX), there is a large decrease in the ^{99m}Tc-MDP uptake in bone to levels that are probably below normal, when judged by the relatively high soft-tissue background. **D**, During the same time interval, the bone mineral density (BMD) increased in the lumbar spine, femoral neck, and total body by 34%, 28%, and 14%, respectively.

regions, rib ends, and vertebral column, but not all of these features may be present at the same time. With quantitative imaging increased uptake in the long bones can be demonstrated even when they appear normal visually.[17] Uncommonly, there may be a periosteal neostosis, or subperiosteal new bone formation, of the long bones, which manifests increased radiophosphate deposition in the diaphysis while sparing the bare area of the joint (Fig. 9-5).[75] Changes in renal osteodystrophy are diffuse and symmetric, which is in contradistinction to advanced primary hyperparathyroidism with cystic lesions and brown tumors wherein uptakes are often asymmetric. The increased accretion of radiophosphate should not be equated with increased mineral content, as many are osteopenic by bone densitometry. Mineral content is mostly the result of net osteoblastic and osteoclastic activity.

Twenty-four-hour total-body retentions are very high as might be expected when there is little or no renal excretion of radiophosphate. Bone-to-soft-tissue ratios are also abnormally high in most of these patients, but they are not sensitive to small changes in bone uptake because the prevailing high soft-tissue activity tends to buffer the ratio numerically.[23,50] It has been shown that the sensitivity of the ratios and quality of the images can be markedly improved by initiating hemodialysis after

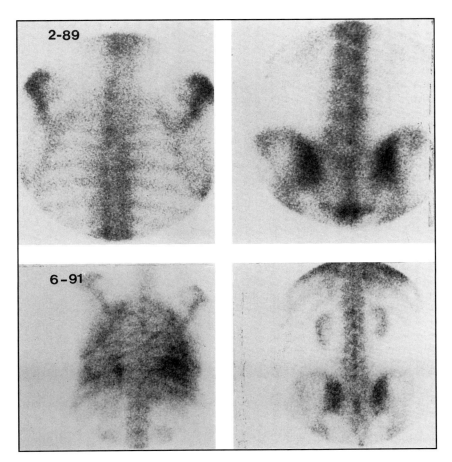

Fig. 9-6. Metastatic lung and kidney calcification in a patient with renal osteodystrophy. *Upper panel:* ^{99m}Tc-MDP scans in February 1989 were normal and the kidneys were not visible. *Lower panel:* In June 1991 there was deposition in the lungs and kidneys, indicative of calcification therein.

administration of radiophosphate to maintain normal blood levels of the tracer.[18]

Comparisons of radiophosphate and conventional radiography attest to the greater sensitivity of the former. In one study all 24 patients (100%) had ^{99m}Tc-HEDP images suggestive of a metabolic bone disorder, whereas only 14 (58%) had radiographic abnormalities.[24] Another report of 30 patients with histologically proved renal osteodystrophy related an 83% sensitivity using ^{99m}Tc-HEDP compared with 46% for radiography.[18]

The frequency of pulmonary calcification in adult patients with long-standing uremia is 60% to 70% at autopsy,[13,46] and about 25% in children.[60] Despite this high incidence visibly increased radiophosphate deposition in the lungs is uncommon, and it occurs only when the degree of calcification is severe (Fig. 9-6).[19,65,84] This is attributed to the fact that uremic pulmonary calcifications are not of the apatite structure, but rather an amorphous or microcrystalline compound high in magnesium and pyrophosphate content.[2,14,48] The molar ratio of the components Ca/Mg/P is reported to be 4.9:1:4.6.[70] In vitro the amorphous compound absorbs 24% of the ^{99m}Tc-phosphate from the medium compared with 98%

for the apatite crystal.[12] This reduced affinity of the amorphous material probably accounts for the infrequent disclosure of pulmonary calcification in chronically uremic patients. The nonvisceral calcification (i.e., of the eyes, arteries, periarticular sites, and skin) in uremia is of the apatite structure (Ca/Mg/P ratio of 30:1:18), and it is not unusual to see radiophosphate accretion by imaging in the cutaneous and periarticular regions (Fig. 9-7).

In renal osteodystrophy gastric calcification occurs in about 50% of adults and in 13% of children at autopsy.[13,46,60] Anecdotal reports on the visualization of this process with radiophosphate imaging have appeared.[31,86,87,90] The precise chemical composition of the gastric calcification has not been elucidated, but the disparate frequency of autopsy occurrence and detection by radiophosphate imaging suggests that it might be akin to the amorphous calcium/magnesium/phosphate compound.

Renal calcification is another common feature at autopsy, varying from 50% to 90% in adults and about 25% in the pediatric group.[13,46,60] Residual renal function in these dialyzed patients may weakly concentrate the radiophosphate and thereby render a false impression of metastatic calcification. The distinction may be resolved by radiographic computed tomography, which is usually sensitive to the presence of soft-tissue mineral. A more confident radionuclide diagnosis is derived from longitudinal studies in which previously unvisualized kidneys become visible with the bone tracer (Fig. 9-6).

Deposition of the amorphous Ca/Mg/P compound is seen in the myocardium and small myocardial arteries at autopsy in about 55% and 15% of adults and children, respectively.[13,18,75] In contrast, literature reports of detection of these deposits by radiophosphate imaging are few and anecdotal.[3,8,39,42,77]

Calciphylaxis is a syndrome of uncertain pathogenesis that features ischemic necrosis of the skin, subcutaneous fat and muscles, and vascular calcification in patients with severe secondary hyperparathyroidism or after successful renal transplantation.[30] There is usually a favorable response to parathyroidectomy. Radiophosphates concentrate avidly in the necrotic areas, and it can be used to monitor the regression after surgical extirpation of the glands (Fig. 9-8).

Following complete parathyroidectomy for symptomatic secondary hyperparathyroidism, the high uptake of radiophosphate in bone gradually subsides, but it may take as long as a year to achieve normal levels. Some seem to reach subnormal accretions judging by the relative bone-to-background activity, which is understandable since the PTH stimulus has been removed. In contrast to the quiescent scan appearance, bone densitometry indicates that the mineral levels are either sustained or exhibit a remarkable increase (Fig. 9-5). The explanation for the latter is not clear unless it simply reflects calcification of the large amount of osteoid present in this disorder.[41]

Amyloidosis

Secondary amyloidosis complicates many chronic diseases including chronic renal insufficiency. The amyloid in renal osteodystrophy consists of beta$_2$-microglobulin, which differs from other types of amyloid. Deposition occurs in bone, tenosynovium, vertebral disk, articular cartilage, capsule, ligament, and muscle. The frequency and extent of amyloidosis seems to vary with the duration of hemodialysis. Amyloid cysts are seen in the phalanges and carpals, most commonly the scaphoid, lunate, and capitate but have also been reported in the humoral head, patella, and hip region.[62] Individual cysts were observed to grow with time while the patients were being

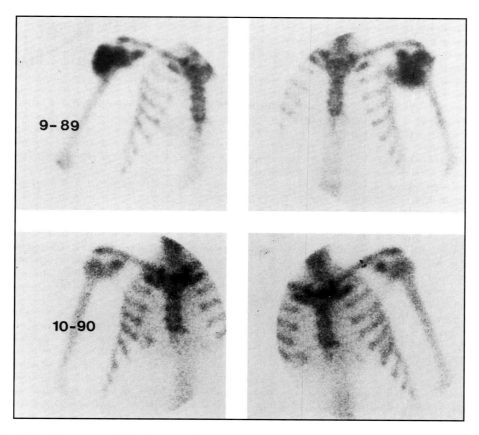

Fig. 9-7. Tumorous calcification at both shoulders in patient with renal osteodystrophy who was sustained on hemodialysis and treated with total parathyroidectomy. *Upper panel*: The ^{99m}Tc-MDP scans depict large clumps of radioactivity adjacent to both glenohumeral joints. *Lower panel*: There was complete resolution 8 months after total parathyroidectomy.

hemodialyzed.[29] Soft-tissue masses of amyloid may cause bone erosion and joint destruction. These various insults make their detection by radiophosphate imaging feasible.[32,78] Nevertheless, the enhanced accretion of radiophosphate is nonspecific and of limited value as the findings could be secondary to periarticular calcification and erosion, and not amyloid.

A more specific disclosure of amyloid lesions can be achieved with ^{123}I–serum amyloid P[11,34] and ^{131}I beta$_2$-microglobulin.[20,21] With these radiopharmaceuticals amyloid deposits were detected in both asymptomatic and symptomatic sites at the shoulders, vertebral column, knees, and carpal bones.

OSTEOPOROSIS

In involutional osteoporosis (i.e., due to aging) there is an overall depletion of bone mass with thinning of the cortex and trabeculae and a reduction in the number of trabeculae. It is an invariable accompaniment of age.

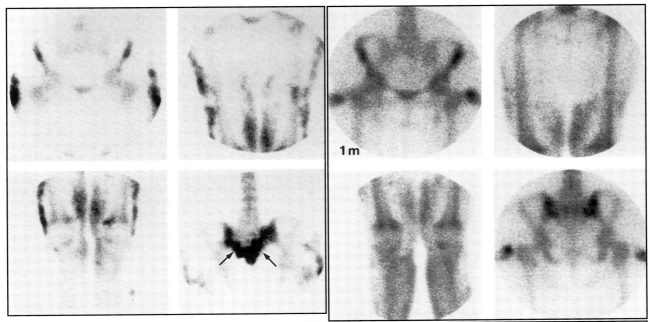

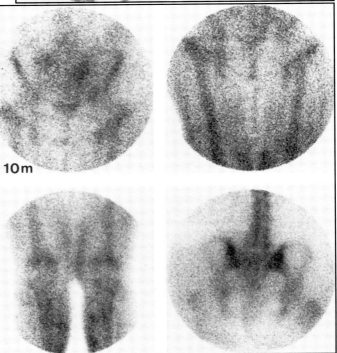

Fig. 9-8. Calciphylaxis in a patient with renal osteodystrophy who was treated by total parathyroidectomy. **A**, ^{99m}Tc-MDP images before surgery demonstrate intense soft-tissue deposition from the buttocks peripherally. The degree of uptake exceeded that of the bones. Note the very high deposit posterior to the sacrum (*arrows*). **B**, At 1 month postparathyroidectomy the extent and intensity of ^{99m}Tc-MDP accretion shows considerable regression. **C**, At 10 months after surgery there is further decrease in the soft-tissue concentration. The bone uptake relative to background has also decreased owing to absence of the PTH stimulus.

Bone loss is more pronounced in females, with a relative rapid decrease beginning soon after menopause and lasting until about the age of 60 years, when the rate of loss slows down, but persists. There can be a 40% to 50% depletion of bone tissue between the fifth and ninth decades of life. In addition to age, osteoporosis may occur in patients receiving steroid therapy, in association with various endocrinopathies such as thyrotoxicosis and Cushing's syndrome, in prolonged immobilization or weightlessness.

Various conflicting reports on radiophosphate kinetics have appeared. One extensive study evaluated the quality of the images made with ^{99m}Tc-pyrophosphate as a function of age. It showed a linear relationship between the proportion of poor-quality scans obtained at 3 hours and the age of the patient.[92] A similar deterioration was found using ^{99m}Tc-diphosphonate and sacrum-to-soft-tissue ratios.[6] This is contrary to three reports on the correlation of the 24-hour total-body retention of radiophosphate and patient age. All three demonstrated a fall in male and female retentions between 20 and 35 years, after which the males showed a linear rise. Female retention was parallel until the menopause years at which point it rose above the male values and remained higher.[53,54,85] Another communication compared the 24-hour total-body retention of ^{99m}Tc-imidodiphosphate in premenopausal and postmenopausal women. The former had a mean retention of 49% compared with 57% for the latter.[49] This increasing 24-hour total-body retention reflects an increasing rate of bone formation in the presence of a net progressive bone loss. The accelerated bone remodeling could be missed by the 3- or 5-hour bone-to-soft-tissue ratios because of higher background activity caused by a progressively normal loss of renal function in the elderly. The reduced rate of radiophosphate clearance from the background will affect the early measurements more than 24-hour retention wherein the background has more time to clear. Further confirmation of increased bone remodeling stems from the biochemical parameters, which showed that serum alkaline phosphatase and osteocalcin levels and hydroxyproline excretion increased as a function of age.[85]

Aside from these general observations, the occasional patient will present with extremely low radiophosphate uptake in the skeleton. If an iatrogenic cause can be excluded, it may represent a case of end-stage osteoporosis that is characterized by a marked deficiency or absence of osteoblasts.[49]

The geriatric population, with decreased bone mineral and quality, is at high risk for fragility or low-trauma fractures. These fractures are readily revealed with radiophosphate imaging, but the findings are not specific and may be difficult to distinguish from metastatic cancer. They are especially vexatious to decision making in a patient with a known primary malignancy.

Osteoporosis may develop secondary to hyperthyroidism. If the disease is of short duration, bone loss is minimal, partly because thyroxine is less potent than PTH. In chronic hyperthyroidism, especially in post-menopausal women, the bone loss may accelerate and become clinically significant. The ineffective reactive compensatory osteoblastic activity can result in a visibly high radiophosphate deposition. The portrayal is that of diffuse increased uptake with usual metabolic features.[45] Using ^{99m}Tc-MDP a mean 24-hour total-body retention of 40.6% (normal 30%) was obtained in group of toxic patients.[79]

Corticosteroid excess is known to induce osteoporosis by virtue of suppression of osteoblastic activity and the absorption of calcium from the gut. One report related a mean 24-hour total-body retention of 17.3% for ^{99m}Tc-MDP in patients on long-term treatment, which was considerably lower than the mean normal of 30%.[79] In contrast, another communication described a small increase after 30 days of steroid treatment.[7] There is no clear explanation for these divergent results.

OSTEOPETROSIS

Osteopetrosis is a familial disorder that is usually non–sex linked and inherited by autosomal dominant or recessive transmission. It is caused by a failure of the osteoclasts to resorb the cartilage and bone matrix as part of the remodeling process. Bone is deposited on the unresorbed, calcified cartilage, and this accumulation of bone appears on the radiograph as sclerosis along with impaired modeling at the metaphyses.

Malignant osteopetrosis is a manifestation of the recessive form: it is characterized in infancy by anemia, recurrent infections, fractures, failure to thrive, and progression to early death.[58] The radiographic findings consist of marked universal and symmetric sclerosis of the skeleton, with loss of distinction between cortex and medulla. These bones are fragile despite the imposing sclerosis and are susceptible to low-trauma fracture. Bone images with radiophosphate depict an intense uptake throughout the skeleton in malignant osteopetrosis (Fig. 9-9).[1,66] Marrow imaging with radiocolloid features a paucity of deposition in the marrow and a large liver and spleen due to the displaced hematopoiesis.

The benign form of osteopetrosis, the dominant type, is more common and it is compatible with survival. It is often not revealed until adulthood, when the patient is radiographed for other reasons. If the pathologic process is intermittent, an inset of dense bone may be framed within the confines of a larger sclerotic perimeter resulting in a "bone-within-bone" appearance (Fig. 9-10).[71] Other forms of osteoporosis have been described.[37]

PSEUDOHYPOPARATHYROIDISM

Pseudohypoparathyroidism is a rare hereditary disorder characterized by signs and symptoms of hypoparathyroidism and skeletal developmental defects; most

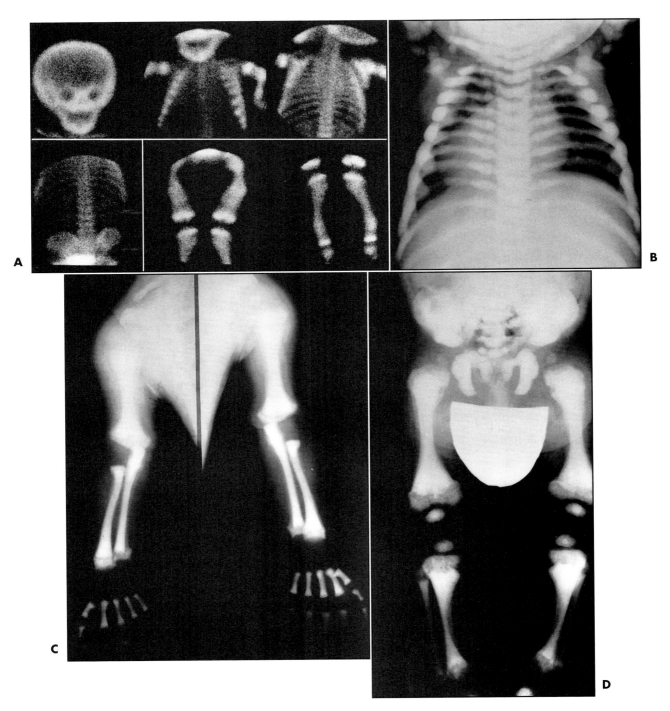

Fig. 9–9.   Malignant osteopetrosis. **A**, Radiophosphate scan demonstrates diffuse increased uptake in the skeleton. **B** to **D**, Radiographs of the thorax and upper and lower extremities showing the osteosclerosis. They were taken about 1 year before the radiophosphate study, during which time the infant had suffered bilateral femoral fractures.

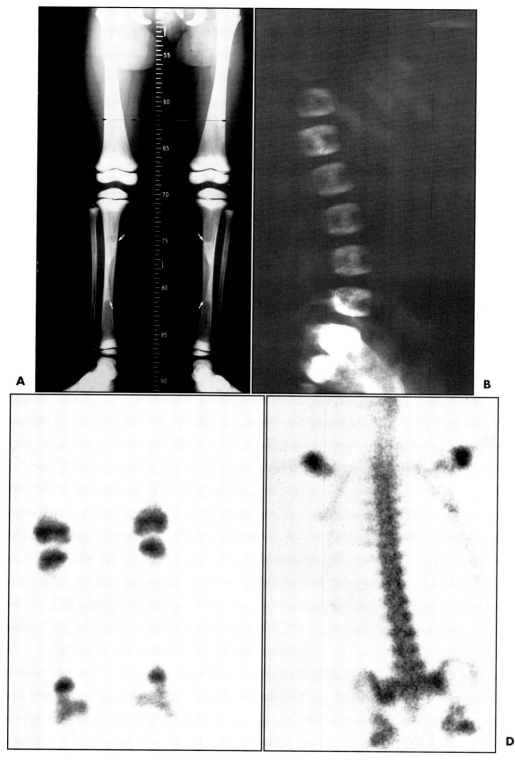

Fig. 9-10. A 3.5-year-old female with benign osteopetrosis. Selected radiographs and 99mTc-MDP bone images. **A,** Radiographs of the lower extremities show a lack of metaphyseal modeling of the distal femurs, and sclerosis of the epiphyses and metaphyses of the tibiae, femurs, and proximal fibulae. There is also a segment of sclerosis in both midtibial diaphyses having the configuration of a fetal tibia (*between arrows*), signaling a previous episode of osteopetrosis, and presenting as "bone-within-bone." **B,** Lateral spine depicts vertebral body end plate sclerosis and the "bone-within-bone" sign. **C,** 99mTc-MDP images of the lower extremities. There is intense concentration in the epiphyses and metaphyses, virtually obscuring the normal high uptakes in the growth plates. There is no apparent increased uptake in the fetal sclerosis in the midshafts of the tibiae, indicating either normal or less than normal bone remodeling. **D,** Posterior scan of the vertebral column and pelvis. Generalized enhanced uptake is registered in the spine and humeral heads; partially confirmed by a lack of kidney visualization. *(From Rosenthall L: Benign osteopetrosis. Clin Nucl Med 1990; 15:412; with permission.)*

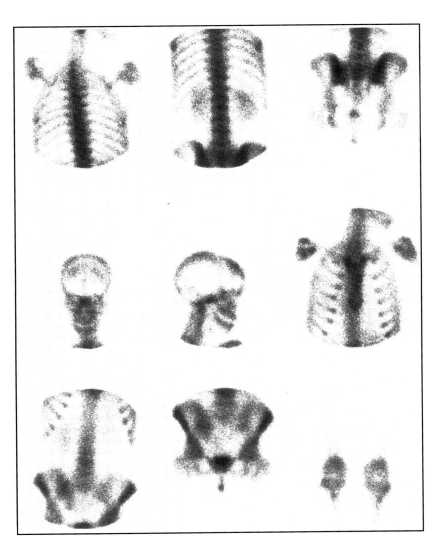

Fig. 9-11. A 27-year-old female with biochemical pseudohypoparathyroidism. She had bilateral cataracts but no developmental or anatomic aberrations. Blood chemistries revealed decreased levels of calcium, increased phosphorus, increased magnesium and normal alkaline phosphatase. Renal function was normal, except for hypophosphaturia. PTH levels were three times normal. There was no increase in urinary excretion of cyclic AMP in response to an infusion of PTH, which confirmed the biochemical pseuohypoparathyroidism. Normal calcemia was obtained with oral calcium supplements and vitamin D_3. The ^{99}Tc-MDP images depict the usual metabolic features. Bone-to-soft-tissue ratio at the lumbar spine was 9; twice normal.

notably, short stature and short metacarpals and metatarsals. There is deficient end-organ response to the endogenous PTH, which results in parathyroid hyperplasia and increased PTH blood levels. Patients with pseudohypoparathyoidism generally fail to respond to high doses of PTH, with an increase in urinary phosphate excretion and nephrogenous cyclic adenosine monophosphate (AMP). It has not been determined whether bone and kidney are refractory to PTH or just the kidney. Osteitis fibrosa has been seen by radiography and proven by biopsy in some reports. Radiophosphate images are nonspecific, and they may show increased periarticular uptake in the hands, feet, or the skeleton diffusely.[44] Biochemical forms of the disease can exist without anatomic stigmata (Fig. 9-11). Pseudo-pseudohypoparathyroidism is a condition in which the anatomic abnormalities exist without the biochemical aberrations.

No radiophosphate bone scans in this rare condition have been reported.

ACROMEGALY

Hypersecretion of growth hormone by the acidophils of the anterior pituitary lobe of the pituitary causes acromegaly. Growth hormone induces subperiosteal appositional bone development, which by radiography appears to involve predominantly the skull and small bones of the hands and feet. The radiophosphate images are more sensitive to the disorder and in the active phase may portray all the features of metabolic disease—namely, augmented axial skeleton and long-bone uptake, prominent calvarium and mandible, increased costochondral junction uptake, prominent sternum, and faint kidney visualization. A good correlation between the number of these features in a given individual and the corresponding human growth hormone radioimmunoassay levels has been found.[25] In another study a quantitative comparison of various regions in the skull and hands between 7 active acromegalics, 3 inactive acromegalics, and 12 controls showed significant differences between acromegaly and controls. No difference was found between the active and inactive patients with acromegaly.[67]

HYPERVITAMINOSIS A

The clinical appearances of vitamin A overdose are skin desquamation, lip fissuring, bone pain and overlying tender soft-tissue lumps, irritability, alopecia, hepatosplenomegaly, and pseudotumor cerebri. Cortical hyperostosis of the diaphysis of long bones and the metatarsals are seen with radiography. Radiophosphate images are more sensitive in that they may antedate the radiographic stigmata. A case report of a 3-year-old boy on megadoses of vitamin A for a year related an increased subperiosteal deposition of radiophosphate in the ulnas, femurs, tibiae and fibulae, and along the sutures of the calvaria. The changes regressed completely within 4 months of vitamin A withdrawal.[59]

HYPERVITAMINOSIS D

Hypervitaminosis D results from excessive intake of vitamin D. Osteosclerosis may develop in the growing child if the condition is left untreated, and in the adult calcific deposits can be found. Bone sclerosis can also develop in idiopathic hypercalcemia in the infant, a condition speculated to be secondary to hypersensitivity to vitamin D. These pathologic features suggest a potential for high radiophosphate bone and soft-tissue uptakes. There is very little information in the literature on the radionuclide aspects of these disorders. Three cases of hypervitaminosis D were reported wherein there was a generalized increased skeletal concentration and faint kidney visualization. All three had a history of remote renal disease, and although the PTH serum levels were normal, histologic sections suggested hyperparathyroidism.[26]

REFERENCES

1. Adams BK: Scintigraphy in a patient with complicated osteopetrosis. *Clin Nucl Med* 1989; 14:323.
2. Alfrey AC, Solomons CC: Bone pyrophosphate in uremia and its association with extraosseous calcification. *J Clin Invest* 1979; 57:700.
3. Atkins HL, Oster ZH: Myocardial uptake of a bone tracer associated with hypercalcemia. *Clin Nucl Med* 1984; 9:613.
4. Bilezikian JP, Silverberg SJ, Shane E, et al: Characterization and evaluation of asymptomatic primary hyperparathyroidism. *J Bone Miner Res* 1991; 6(suppl 2):S85.
5. Brodier P, Zingraff J, Gueris J, et al: The effect of 1-alpha (OH)D$_3$ and 1-alpha 25(OH)$_2$D$_3$ on the bone in patients with renal osteodystrophy. *Am J Med* 1978; 64:101.
6. Buell V, Kleinhaus E, Zorn-Bopp E, et al: A comparison of bone imaging with Tc-99m DPD and Tc-99m MDP. *J Nucl* 1982; 23:214.
7. Caniggia A, Nute R, Lore F, et al: Pathophysiology of the adverse effects of glucoactive corticosteroids on calcium metabolism in man. *J Steroid Biochem* 1981; 15:153.
8. Choy D, Murray IPC: Metatstatic visceral calcification identified by bone scanning. *Skeletal Radiol* 1980; 5:151.
9. Christensen SB, Arnoldi CC: Distribution of Tc99m phosphate in osteoarthritic femoral heads. *J Bone Joint Surg* 1980; 62A:90.
10. Christensen SB, Krogsgaard OW: Localization of Tc99m-methylene diphosphonate in epiphyseal growth plates of rats. *J Nucl Med* 1981; 27:237.
11. Cohen AS, Skinner M: New frontiers in the study of amyloidosis. *N Engl J Med* 1990; 8:542.
12. Conger JD, Alfrey AC: In comment: Letter to the editor. *Ann Intern Med* 1976; 84:224.
13. Conger JD, Hammond WS, Alfrey AC, et al: Pulmonary calcifications in chronic dialysis patients. Clinical and pathological studies. *Ann Intern Med* 1975; 83:330.
14. Contiguglia SR, Alfrey AC, Miller NL, et al: Nature of soft tissue calcification in uremia. *Kidney Int* 1973; 4:229.
15. Cooper RA, Riley JW, Middleton WR, et al: Transient metastatic calcification in primary hyperparathyroidism. *Aust N Z J Med* 1978; 8:285.
16. Daniels RA, Weisenfeld I: Tumorous phosphaturic osteomalacia. *Am J Med* 1979; 67:155.
17. de Graaf P, Pauwels EKT, Vos PH, et al: Observations on computerized quantitative bone scintigraphy in renal osteodystrophy. *Eur J Nucl Med* 1984; 9:419.
18. de Graaf P, Schicht IM, Pauwels EKJ, et al: Bone scintigraphy in renal osteodystrophy. *J Nucl Med* 1979; 19:1289.
19. de Graaf P, Schicht IM, Pauwels EKJ, et al: Bone scintigraphy in uremic pulmonary calcification. *J Nucl Med* 1979; 20:201.
20. Floege J, Burchert W, Brandis A, et al: Imaging of dialysis-related amyloid (AB-amyloid) deposits with ^{131}I-beta$_2$-microglobulin. *Kidney Int* 1990; 38:1169.
21. Floege J, Nonnast-Daniel B, Gielow P, et al: Specific imaging of dialysis-related amyloid deposits using ^{131}I-beta$_2$-microglobulin. *Nephron* 1989; 51:444.
22. Fogelman I, Bessant RG, Beastall GB: Estimation of skeletal involvement in primary hyperparathyroidism. *Ann Intern Med* 1980; 92:65.
23. Fogelman I, Bessent RG, Turner JG, et al: The use of whole body retention of Tc-99m diphosphonate in the diagnosis of metabolic bone disease. *J Nucl Med* 1978; 19:270.
24. Fogelman I, Carr D: A comparison of bone scanning and radiology in the evaluation of patients with metabolic bone disease. *Clin Radiol* 1980; 31:321.
25. Fogelman I, Hay ID, Citron DL, et al: Semi-quantitative analysis of the bone scan in acromegaly: Correlation with growth hormone values. *Br J Radiol* 1980; 53:874.
26. Fogelman I, McKillop JH, Cowden EA, et al: Bone scan findings in hypervitaminosis D. *J Nucl Med* 1977; 18:1205.
27. Fogelman I, McKillop JH, Greig WR, et al: Pseudo-fractures of the ribs detected by bone scanning. *J Nucl Med* 1977; 18:1236.

28. Francis MD, Ferguson DL, Tofe AL, et al: Comparative evaluation of the three diphosphonates: In vitro adsorption (C-14 labeled) and in vivo osteogenic uptake (Tc99m complexed). *J Nucl Med* 1980; 27:1185.

29. Gielen JL, van Holsbeeck J, Hauglustaine D, et al: Growing bone cysts in long-term hemodialysis. *Skeletal Radiol* 1990; 19:43.

30. Gipstein RM, Coburn JW, Adams JA, et al: Calciphylaxis in man: A syndrome of tissue necrosis and vascular calcification in 11 patients with chronic renal failure. *Arch Intern Med* 1976; 136:1273.

31. Goldstein R, Ryo UY, Pinsky SM: Metastatic calcifications of the stomach imaged on the bone scan. *Clin Nucl Med* 1984; 9:591.

32. Grateau G, Zingraff J, Fauchet M, et al: Radionuclide exploration of dialysis amyloidosis: Preliminary experience. *Am J Kidney Dis* 1988; 11:231.

33. Greiff J: Autoradiographic studies of fracture healing using Tc99m-Sn-polyphosphate. *Injury* 1977; 9:271.

34. Hawkins PN, Myers MJ, Lavender JP, Pepys MB: Diagnostic radionuclide imaging of amyloid: Biological targeting by circulating human serum amyloid P component. *Lancet* 1988; 1:1413.

35. Helstrom J, Ivemark BI: Primary hyperparathyroidism: Clinical and structural changes in 138 cases. *Acta Chir Scand* 1961; 294:1.

36. Holmes RA: Quantification of skeletal Tc-99m labeled phosphates to detect metabolic bone disease. *J Nucl Med* 1978; 19:330.

37. Horton WA, Schmike RN, Iyama T: Osteopetrosis: Further heterogeneity. *J Pediatr* 1980; 97:580.

38. Itoh K, Furudate M: Diffuse lung uptake on bone imaging in primary hyperparathyroidism before and after excision of a parathyroid adenoma. *Clin Nucl Med* 1979; 4:382.

39. Janowitz WR, Serafini AN: Intense myocardial uptake of 99mTc-diphosphonate in a uremic patient with secondary hyperparathyroidism and pericarditis. *J Nucl Med* 1976; 17:896.

40. Karsenty G, Vineron N, Jorgetti V, et al: Value of 99mTc-methylene diphosphonate bone scan in renal osteodystrophy. *Kidney Int* 1986; 29:1058.

41. Kaye M, Rosenthall L, Hill RO, Tabah RT: Long-term outcome following total parathyroidectomy in patients with end-stage renal disease. *Clin Nephrol* 1993; 39:192.

42. Kida T, Hujita Y, Sasaki M, Inoue J: Myocardial and vascular uptake of a bone tracer associated with secondary hyperparathyroidism. *Eur J Nucl Med* 1986; 12:151.

43. Kinnaert P, Van Hooff I, Schoutens A, et al: Differential diagnosis between secondary hyperparathyroidism and aluminium intoxication in uremic patients: Usefulness of 99mTc-pyrophosphate bone scintigraphy. *World J Surg* 1989; 13:219.

44. Krishnamurthy GT, Brickman AS, Blahd WH: Technetium-99m-Sn-pyrophosphate pharmacokinetic and bone image changes in parathyroid disease. *J Nucl Med* 1977; 18:236.

45. Kukar N, Sy WM: Selected endocrine disorders, in Sy WM (ed): *Gamma Images in Benign and Metabolic Bone Diseases*, Vol 2, Boca Raton, Fla, CRC Press, p 1.

46. Kuzela DC, Huffer WE, Conger JD, et al: Soft tissue calcification in chronic dialysis patients. *Am J Pathol* 1977; 86:403.

47. Lang P, Bull U: Measurement of 24 hour whole body retention of Tc99m diphosphonate by a simple thyroid probe. *Nucl Med Commun* 1984; 5:627.

48. LeGros RZ, Contiguglia SR, Alfrey C: Pathological calcifications associated with uremia: Two types of calcium phosphate deposits. *Cacif Tissue Res* 1973; 13:173.

49. Levine SB, Haines JE, Larson SM, Andrews TM: Reduced skeletal localization of 99m-Tc-diphosphonate in two cases of severe osteoporosis. *Clin Nucl Med* 1977; 2:318.

50. Lien JWK, Wiegmann T, Rosenthall L, et al: Abnormal Tc99m-Sn-pyrophosphate bone uptake in chronic renal failure. *Clin Nephrol* 1976; 6:509.

51. MacFarlane JD, Lutkin JE, Burwood RJ: The demonstration by scintigraphy of fractures in osteomalacia. *Br J Radiol* 1977; 50:369.

52. Malluche HH, Monier-Faugere MN: Risk of adynamic bone disease in dialysed patients. *Kidney Int* 1992; 38(suppl):S62.

53. Martin P, Schoutens A, Manicourt D, et al: Whole body retention of ^{99m}Tc pyrophosphate at 24 hours: Physiological basis of the method for assessing the metabolism of bone in disease. *Calcif Tissue Int* 1983; 35:37.

54. Martin W, Fogelman I, Bessant RG: Measurement of 24 hour whole-body retention of Tc99m HEDP by a gamma camera. *J Nucl Med* 1981; 22:542.

55. Melton LJ: Epidemiology of primary hyperparathyroidism. *J Bone Miner Res* 1991; 6(suppl 6):S25.

56. Merz WA, Schenk RK: A quantitative histological study on bone formation in human cancellous bone. *Acta Anat (Basel)* 1970; 76:1.

57. Merz WA, Schenk RK: Quantitative structural analysis of human cancellous bone. *Acta Anat (Basel)* 1970; 75:54.

58. Milgran KJ, Jasty WM: Osteopetrosis: A morphological study of twenty-one cases. *J Bone Joint Surg Am* 1982; 64A:912.

59. Miller JH, Hayon II: Bone scintigraphy in hypervitaminosis A. *AJR Am J Roentgenol* 1985; 144:767.

60. Milliner DS, Zeissmeister AR, Lieberman E, Landing B: Soft tissue calcifications in pediatric patients with end-stage renal disease. *Kidney Int* 1990; 38:931.

61. Mitlack BH, Daly M, Potts JT, et al: Asymptomatic primary hyperparathyroidism. *J Bone Miner Res* 1991; 6(suppl 2):S103.

62. Murphey MD, Sartoris DJ, Quale JL, et al: Musculoskeletal manifestations of chronic renal insufficiency. *Radiographics* 1993; 13:357.

63. Nakshima H, Ochi M, Yasui N, et al: Uptake and localization of Tc99m-MDP in mouse osteosarcoma. *Eur J Nucl Med* 1982; 7:531.

64. Nuovo MA, Dorfman HD, Sun CC, Chalew SA: Tumor-induced osteomalacia and rickets. *Am J Surg Pathol* 1989; 13:588.

65. Olgaard K, Heerfordt J, Madsen S: Scintigraphic skeletal change in uremic patients on regular dialysis. *Nephron* 1976; 17:325.

66. Park H-M, Lambertus J: Skeletal and reticuloendothelial imaging in osteopetrosis. *J Nucl Med* 1977; 18:1091.

67. Peretiano JD, Grigoire D, Popescu F, Zaharescu J: Bone scintigraphy in acromegaly. *Endocrinologie* 1990; 28:199.

68. Rai GS, Webster SGP, Wraight EP: Isotopic scanning of the bone in the diagnosis of osteomalacia. *J Am Geriat Soc* 1981; 29:45.

69. Rao DS: Primary hyperparathyroidism: Changing patterns in presentation and treatment decisions in the eighties. *Henry Ford Hosp Med J* 1981; 33:194.

70. Resnick D: Abnormalities of bone and soft tissue following renal transplantation. *Semin Roentgenol* 1978; 13:329.

71. Rosenthall L: Benign osteopetrosis. *Clin Nucl Med* 1990; 15:412.

72. Rosenthall L, Arzoumanian A: Total body retention measurements of Tc99m-MDP using a simple detector. *Clin Nucl Med* 1983; 8:210.

73. Rosenthall L, Kaye M: Observations on the mechanism of Tc99m labeled phosphate complex uptake in metabolic bone disease. *Semin Nucl Med* 1976; 6:59.

74. Rosenthall L, Kaye M: Technetium-99m pyrophosphate kinetics and imaging in metabolic bone disease. *J Nucl Med* 1975; 16:33.

75. Rosenthall L, Rush C: Radiophosphate disclosure of subperiosteal new bone formation in renal osteodystrophy. *J Nucl Med* 1986; 27:1572.

76. Schwartz Z, Shani J, Soskoline A, et al: Uptake and biodistribution of Tc-99m-MD (P-32) during rat tibial bone repair. *J Nucl Med* 1993; 34:104.

77. Seid K, Lin D, Flowers WM: Intense myocardial uptake of Tc-99m-MDP in a case of hypercalcemia. *Clin Nucl Med* 1981; 6:565.

78. Sethi D, Naunton Morgan TC, Brown EA, et al: Technetium-99m-labelled methylene diphosphonate uptake in scans in patients with dialysis arthropathy. *Nephron* 1990; 54:202.

79. Seto H, Futasuya R, Kamei T, et al: Measurement of 24 hour whole body retention of Tc-99m MDP with a thyroid probe: Quantitative assessment of metabolic and metastatic bone disease. *Proceedings of the 3rd World Congress in Nuclear Medicine and Biology,* Paris, France, Sept. 1982.

80. Shani J, Amir D, Soskoline A, et al: Correlations between uptake of technetium, calcium, phosphate and mineralization in rat tibial bone repair. *J Nucl Med* 1990; 31:2011.

81. Singh BN, Kesala A, Mehta SP: Osteomalacia on bone scan simulating skeletal metastases. *Clin Nucl Med* 1977; 2:181.

82. Smith ML, Martin W, Fogelman I, Bessent RG: Relative distribution of diphosphonate between bone and soft tissue at 4 and 24 hours: Concise communication. *J Nucl Med* 1983; 24:208.

83. Steinbach HL, Kolb FO, Gilfillan R: A mechanism of production of pseudofractures in osteomalacia (milkman's syndrome). *Radiology* 1954; 62:388.

84. Sy WM, Mittal AK: Bone scan in chronic dialysis patients with evidence of secondary hyperparathyroidism and renal osteodystrophy. *Br J Radiol* 1975; 48:878.

85. Thomsen K, Johansen J, Nilas L, Christiansen C: Whole body retention of ^{99m}Tc-diphosphonate: Relation to biochemical indices of bone turnover and to total body calcium. *Eur J Nucl Med* 1987; 13:32.

86. Valentzas C, Meindok H, Oreopoulos DG, et al: Detection and pathogenesis of visceral calcification in dialysis patients and patients with malignant disease. *Can Med Assoc J* 1978; 118:45.

87. Van Diemen-Steenvoorde, Donckerwolcke RA, Der Haas G: Generalized soft tissue calcification in children and adolescents with end-stage renal failure. *Eur J Pediatr* 1986; 145:293.

88. Vanherweghem J-L, Schoutens A, Bergmann P, et al: Usefulness of Tc99m-pyrophosphate bone scintigraphy in aluminum disease. *Trace Elements Med* 1984; 1:80.

89. Vattimo A, Cantalupi D, Righi G, et al: Whole body retention of Tc99m-MDP in Paget's disease. *J Nucl Med Allied Sci* 1981; 25:5.

90. Venkatesh N, Polycyn RE, Norback DH: Metastatic calcification: The role of bone scanning. *Radiology* 1978; 129:755.

91. Weigmann T, Rosenthall L, Kaye M: Technetium-99m-pyrophosphate bone scan in hyperparathyroidism. *J Nucl Med* 1977; 18:231.

92. Wilson MA: The effect of age on the quality of bone scans using technetium-99m pyrophosphate. *Radiology* 1981; 139:703.

93. Wishart J, Horowitz M, Need A, Nordin BEC: Relationship between forearm and vertebral mineral density in postmenopausal women with primary hyperparathyroidism. *Arch Intern Med* 1990; 150:1329.

IN THIS CHAPTER

CHAPTER 10

BONE SCANNING IN PAGET'S DISEASE

Ignac Fogelman

Paul J. Ryan

Paget's disease of bone (osteitis deformans) is a common disorder particularly in England and Northern European countries and areas populated by their descendants. A prevalence rate of 5% has been estimated for the United Kingdom.[3,17] In the great majority of affected individuals, the disease is asymptomatic and may only be discovered incidentally following the detection of an elevated level of serum alkaline phosphatase or as an incidental finding on x-rays or radionuclide bone scans. In the past it was regarded as an untreatable disorder and to a degree neglected. However, in recent years, with the advent of powerful antiresorption agents, effective therapies are now available, and the condition is recognized as being treatable.

ETIOLOGY

The etiology of Paget's disease remains the subject of controversy and active research, but a familial aggregation of the disorder has been recognized for some years,[13,41] and marked geographic variation in its prevalence has also been recognized with the condition strikingly uncommon in Asia and Africa.[41] More recently it has been discovered that viral nuclear capsids are present in a nuclei of osteoclasts, although they are also found in other conditions such as osteopetrosis and pyknodysostosis.[44] These viral nuclear capsids most probably belong to the paramyxo-virus groups (e.g., measles or respiratory syncytial virus).[28] Canine distemper virus has also been suggested as a cause of Paget's disease, with nucleic acids from this virus detected in the bone cells of pagetic patients.[14] This is supported by some data suggesting that there is a relationship between dog ownership and disease incidence.[16] A viral cause is supported by evidence showing the probability of a bone being infected correlates with the amount of trabecular bone present; the distribution of the disease is similar to that of hematogenous osteomyelitis.[15] The disease does not appear to progress from bone to bone during the patient's lifetime, and it progresses only in preinvaded bones, in keeping with an initial invasion by a virus with a long incubation period.[27]

RADIOLOGIC APPEARANCES

Paget's disease is usually polyostotic but can be monostotic in 20% of cases.[11] The disease is characterized in its initial phase by excess resorption of bone with a lytic front apparent on x-ray films. This is followed by an intense osteoblastic reaction with the deposition of woven bone.[1] Skeletal architecture becomes disorganized and on x-ray there is a mixed pattern of lytic and sclerotic disease. Subsequently the imbalance of bone remodeling in favor of formation leads to cortical thickening with bone expansion. This phase is identified as sclerotic on x-ray films. With aging a secondary mixed phase can occur, with lytic and sclerotic disease replacing the sclerotic stage.[23]

CLINICAL FEATURES

The most common symptom is pain, the usual presenting complaint. The cause is not well understood but may relate to stretching of the periosteum or local edema. Pagetic bone is also extremely vascular and this may be contributory. Coexistent arthritis is frequently present in weight-bearing areas and should always be considered as a possible alternative explanation for pain, particularly when there is a poor response to treatment. Pagetic bone is mechanically weak, and there is an increased susceptibility to fracture. Stress fractures may also occur and should be considered as a cause for pain.[5] Enlarging bones may cause nerve root entrapment, and rarely pain may be due to sarcomatous change. Paget's disease of the skull may be associated with deafness, the mechanism of which is unclear but is not solely attributable to auditory nerve entrapment.[19] Another serious complication of skull disease is basilar invagination with consequent severe neurologic disturbance. Paget's disease of the skull can sometimes produce headaches, although other causes of headache are more common. In the spine the patient may rarely present with progressive paraparesis, often responding well to medical therapy. Osteosarcomas occur in approximately 1% of patients, and giant cell tumors have also been described. High-output congestive cardiac failure, commonly described as a complication, is extremely rare.

TREATMENT

Calcitonin has been used successfully for some years but has largely been superseded by the bisphosphonates. This is because of poorer efficacy, resistance, and common side effects of nausea, vomiting, and flushing. Bisphosphonates can produce dramatic relief from bone pain and normalization of biochemistry.[5] Disodium etidronate has been available for some years. However, continuous high-dose usage can produce inhibition of mineralization and may result in osteomalacia; it should therefore only be given for continuous periods of up to 6 months. Particular caution should be exercised in patients with extensive lytic disease, especially in a weight-bearing bone. The second-generation bisphosphonate, pamidronate, is 10 times more powerful than

etidronate in inhibiting osteoclastic activity and has not been associated with significant mineralization defects. Although only recently licensed for use in Paget's disease in the United Kingdom, it is being used in many centers and produces striking responses in most patients.[33] Other bisphosphonates are also being investigated, with promising responses described with tiludronate,[32] alendronate,[30] and clodronate.[18] Mithramycin is now rarely used due to its toxicity. Gallium nitrate has appeared promising in recent studies, but data are limited at present.[4]

BONE SCAN APPEARANCES

The bone scan is essentially a functional display of skeletal metabolism, and technetium-labeled diphosphonate uptake in bone is dependent upon osteoblastic activity and to a lesser extent skeletal vascularity.[12] Paget's disease induces a marked increase in skeletal metabolism and blood flow, and there is high uptake of bone-seeking radiopharmaceuticals. Tracer uptake is directly related to the degree of activity of the disease process.[39] The bone scan appearances in Paget's disease are usually characteristic, with the predominant feature being striking increased uptake distributed throughout most or all of the affected bone[38] (Figs. 10-1 and 10-2). The only common exception to this is osteoporosis circumscripta (lytic disease involving the skull), in which tracer uptake may be intense only in the margins of the lesion.[31] Paget's disease, in contrast to other skeletal pathology, tends to preserve or even enhance the normal anatomy of bone. The appearance of individual lesions may be quite dramatic, and pagetic bone appears to be picked out as the borders between normal and abnormal are clearly delineated (Fig. 10-3). In affected vertebrae the transverse spinous processes frequently are involved, which may be an important factor with regard to the differential diagnosis.[31] The vertebral appearance of Paget's disease has been described as a "Mickey Mouse" sign, with uptake having an inverted triangular pattern.[9] Other case reports have described the "black beard" sign of monostotic disease of the mandible and "short pants" sign of spine, pelvis, and upper femora disease.[22,26] Expansion and distortion of involved bones can often be recognized (Fig. 10-4). In the appendicular skeleton lesions are bound by the articular surface and progress into the shaft. The advancing lesion may be seen to have a sharp V-shaped edge that corresponds to the lytic flame-shaped resorption front seen on radiographs. Rare reports have been produced showing Paget's disease confined to the diaphyseal region of the tibia or even the anterior tibial tubercle.[29,37]

The typical findings for Paget's disease are easily recognizable, and when polyostotic disease is present there is seldom any doubt as to the diagnosis. Indeed it is usually possible to differentiate between Paget's disease and metastatic disease when they coexist.[8] However, both are common conditions and inevitably some diagnostic dif-

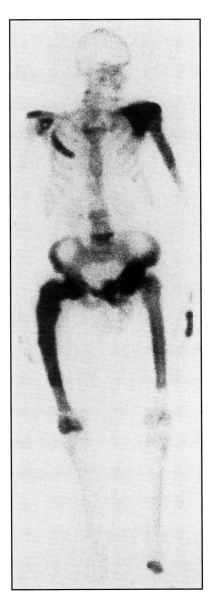

Fig. 10-1. Polyostotic Paget's disease affecting the femora, left hemipelvis, L4, scapulae, left humerus, and right third rib.

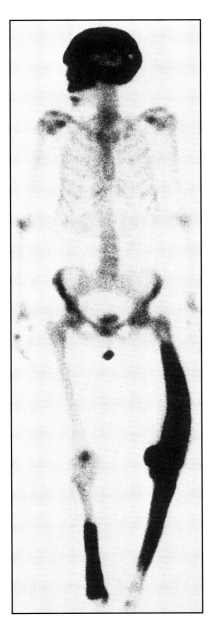

Fig. 10-2. Polyostotic Paget's disease affecting the skull, tibiae, and left femur.

ficulty can arise, particularly when the scan appearances are somewhat atypical. Furthermore, metastases do occur in pagetic bone, but in view of its high vascularity this situation occurs perhaps less often than one would expect. A frequent situation that arises is that when a patient with a known primary tumor has a bone scan performed to screen for skeletal metastases, Paget's disease is found incidentally. It must be accepted that a bone scan is nonspecific, and when any uncertainty exists, individual sites of involvement must be carefully evaluated and radiographs obtained. Rarely, when the bone scan appearances are atypical, a computed tomography (CT) scan or biopsy is required. In general, lesions involving the spine are most problematic, particularly when verte-

bral collapse and degenerative change are present. A single lesion on the bone scan can commonly be identified as pagetic but may on occasion be difficult to evaluate. With increasing experience of bone scanning in Paget's disease, unusual and atypical manifestations may occur. Following successful treatment, uptake may be seen in previously unaffected bone and at the border of former lytic lesions, suggesting that some osteoclasts from the lytic front remain viable, and with reactivation of disease resorb adjacent normal bone, which is less well protected by bisphosphonate.[22]

Single photon emission computed tomography (SPECT) bone scintigraphy has not at present found a definite role in Paget's disease, but it has been reported as

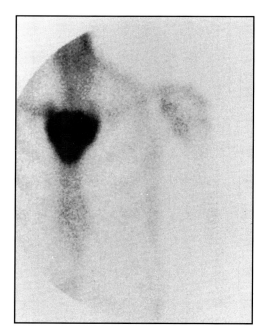

Fig. 10-3. Paget's disease affecting the manubrium of the sternum.

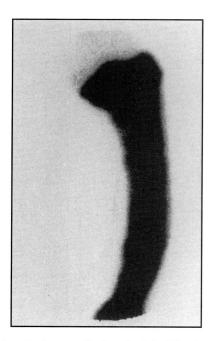

Fig. 10-4. Paget's disease affecting the left tibia, showing expansion and deformity.

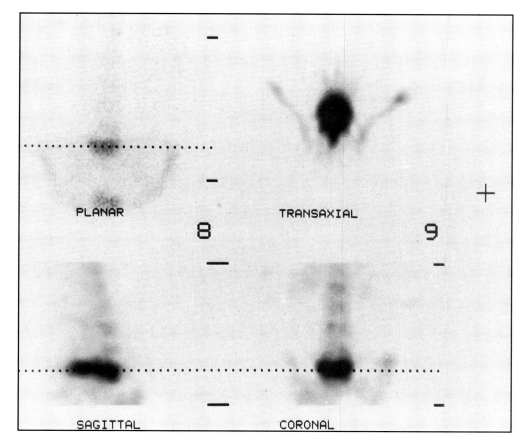

Fig. 10-5. Paget's disease affecting L4, showing increased activity on SPECT throughout the vertebra.

being useful for evaluation of cranial Paget's disease,[7] and in our experience can help distinguish Paget's disease from other pathology in the spine[35] (Fig. 10-5). Following therapy for Paget's disease, particularly with more powerful bisphosphonates, the uniform uptake on the bone scan may change to a more focal distribution, which may be particularly apparent as reactivation occurs (Fig. 10-6, *A* and *B*). Confusion with metastases could occur if this is not recognized as reflecting response to treatment.[36] On occasion, the bone scan can detect coexistent unsuspected pathology, especially in the kidneys (Fig. 10-7, *A* and *B*).

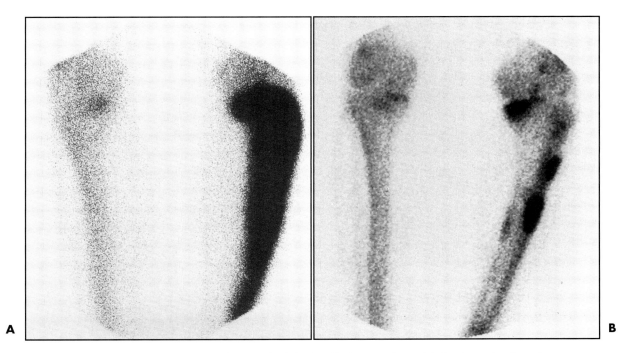

Fig. 10-6. **A**, Paget's disease affecting the left tibia. **B**, Same patient with focal reactivation of disease following pamidronate therapy.

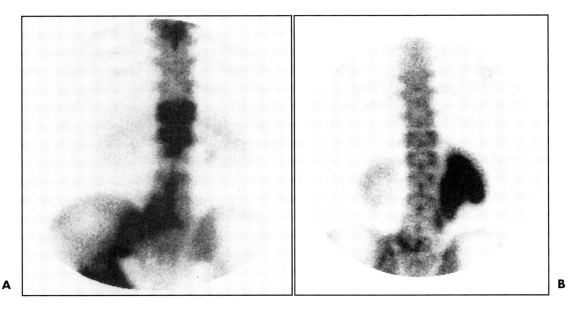

Fig. 10-7. **A**, Paget's disease affecting the spine and left hemipelvis. **B**, Same patient following pamidronate therapy who has now developed a right pelvi-ureteric junction obstruction. Note the dramatic improvement in pagetic lesions.

It is generally believed that Paget's disease does not progress from bone to bone during a patient's lifetime. However, the course of progression of Paget's disease is very slow, rarely diagnosed in its preclinical stage, and seldom followed sequentially over the course of many years. Thus the natural history in an individual case is usually a matter of conjecture.

COMPARISON OF BONE SCANNING AND RADIOGRAPHY

Bone scanning is more sensitive than radiography in detecting sites of Paget's disease throughout the skeleton. Fogelman and Carr[11] studied 23 patients with symptomatic disease and compared radiographic skeletal surveys and bone scans. Of 127 sites of pagetic involvement, 120 (95%) were detected by bone scanning and only 94 (74%) by x-ray. Other series have confirmed these findings. The bone scan also has the obvious advantage of ease of visualization of the whole skeleton.

A more recent study by Vellenga et al[49] evaluated the x-rays of abnormal sites on bone scan of patients with Paget's disease and found that 16% did not show any radiographic abnormality. Most of these sites probably represent early Paget's disease. Meunier et al[27] also reported a series of 170 cases of untreated Paget's disease and found the bone scan to be more sensitive than routine x-rays, but there was a difference of only 8%. The variance in these studies may reflect a variation in the skill of the radiograph observers.

A small number of lesions detected radiographically are not visible on bone scan but are probably largely due to burnt-out disease. Vellenga et al[49] in his series reported 9 such lesions: 2 osteolytic, 2 sclerotic, and 5 mixed. Meunier et al[27] reported bone scan-negative, radiographic-positive lesions in 2.7% of their cases, but these were either in sclerotic disease or cases of osteoporosis circumscripta.

The bone scan is generally of value in detecting a fracture[24] (Fig 10-8, A and B). In the case of stress fractures, the bone scan may be positive at a time when radiographs are negative.[25] The scan appearance will show focal increased tracer uptake superimposed on generalized increased uptake. However, with pagetic bone, activity due to Paget's disease may mask that due to fractures or pseudo-fractures, and they therefore may not always be possible to detect (Fig. 10-9, A and B). A similar problem may exist with the detection of osteosarcoma. However, an expansion of lesions outside the normal anatomic borders or the presence of a photon-deficient lesion should particularly raise this possibility. Furthermore, the majority of cases of osteosarcoma are associated with reduced tracer uptake, although normal or increased uptake can occur.[21,42] The combination of gallium and bone scans can be helpful; Yeh et al[52] found increased gallium uptake at the site of the sarcoma to be always greater than the relative diphosphonate uptake. Overall, the bone scan should not be viewed as reliable in the detection of fracture or sarcomatous change, and x-ray films should always be obtained, and a CT scan and/or biopsy may be required.

The distribution of lesions on the bone scan differs little from that found on radiography. The most common sites are the pelvis, spine, femur, tibia, and skull—but the

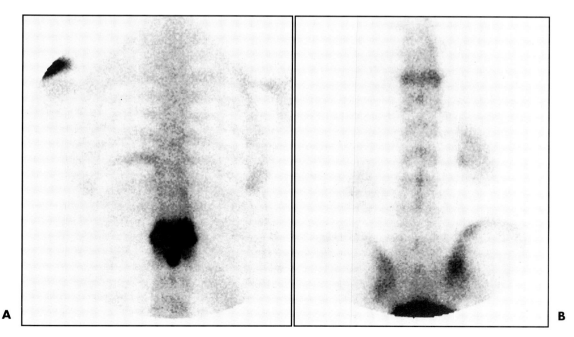

Fig. 10-8. **A**, Paget's disease affecting T11. **B**, Same patient following pamidronate therapy who later developed pain due to vertebral collapse as seen on this scan.

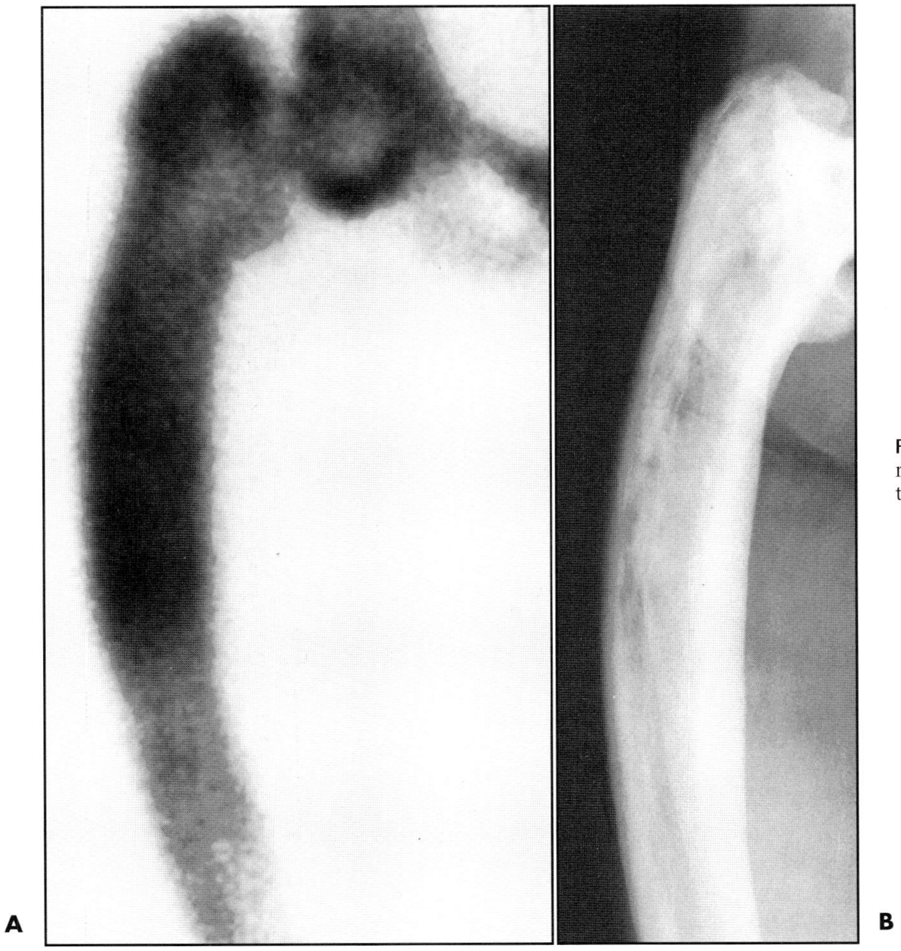

Fig. 10-9. **A**, Paget's disease affecting the right femur. **B**, X-ray reveals several stress fractures that are not apparent on the bone scan.

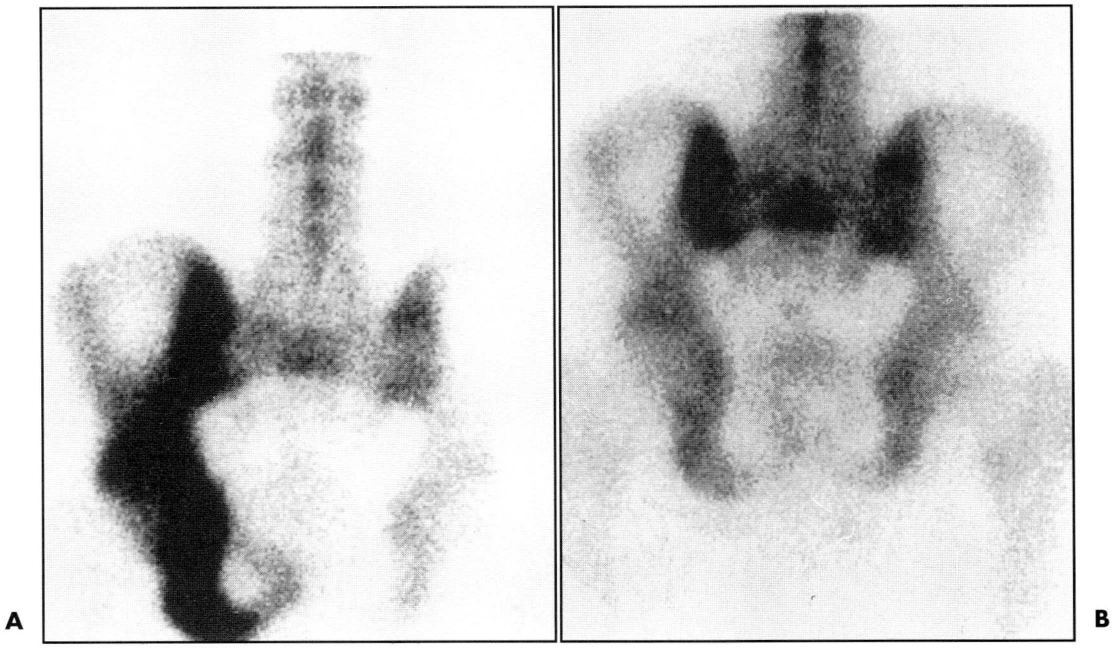

Fig. 10-10. **A**, Paget's disease affecting the left hemipelvis. **B**, Same patient after pamidronate therapy.

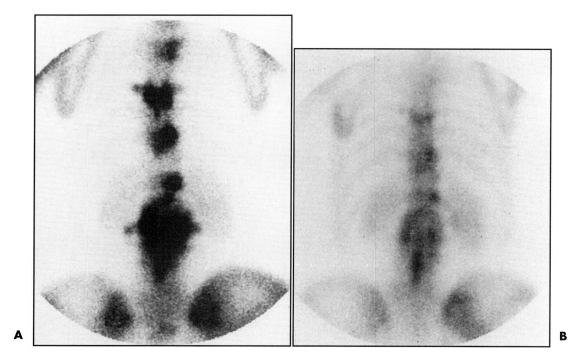

Fig. 10-11. **A**, Paget's disease affecting multiple vertebrae. **B**, Same patient 6 months after pamidronate therapy.

disease can affect virtually any bone in the body. Twenty percent of cases are monostotic, but it is of interest that when a patient is suspected of having monostotic disease on radiography, the bone scan will often identify further sites of involvement. Although the amount of tracer uptake at an involved site is probably determined by the phase of the disease activity, the clinical relevance of this is not well understood. However, symptoms may correlate with the degree of severity of individual lesions; with increase in bone scan and radiographic abnormality the frequency of symptoms rises fourfold.[50] It has also been suggested that metabolically active lesions are more likely to cause symptoms and severe structural deformation than those with low activity. There is little doubt in clinical practice that symptomatic lesions usually appear markedly abnormal on bone scan. However, only a minority of lesions are symptomatic, and there is not a clear relationship between tracer avidity and symptoms.[27] It is of note that the most frequently symptomatic bones are those that are weight-bearing. Overall factors that may be relevant with regard to development of symptoms are skeletal vascularity, the weight-bearing role of a bone, and whether there is deformity of bone with stretching of the periosteum.

EVALUATION OF TREATMENT

In Paget's disease the bone scan will demonstrate alteration in disease activity following either calcitonin[20] or bisphosphonate therapy.[45] This corresponds in a general way to biochemical findings, although the scan changes

occur slower and may lag behind by several months.[51] Early in the course of treatment, changes in serum alkaline phosphatase and urinary hydroxyproline levels are better diagnostic indicators. Bourdreau et al[6] found that the scan evaluation of response to therapy can be improved by obtaining radionuclide blood flow studies, and these are generally in good agreement with alkaline phosphatase results. However, although blood flow studies appear equally as sensitive as alkaline phosphatase, they are limited in that the technique is largely restricted to the appendicular skeleton and the extent of disease that can be included in the gamma camera field of view.

A visual display of bone scan activity can be used to assess the disease activity from 3 to 6 months following the initiation of therapy. A semiquantitative visual technique can also be used, reducing the need for subjective evaluation and increasing sensitivity for alteration in disease activity. Vellenga et al[48] compared a 6-point qualitative score with computer quantitation and concluded that visual assessment correlated well with quantitative results. However, in many lesions response was detected only by quantitation alone. Nevertheless, dramatic scan improvements can occur following successful therapy (Fig. 10-7), invariably with bisphosphonates but conversely often there is limited improvement or even no detectable change (Figs. 10-10 to 10-12). Furthermore, not all pagetic lesions in an individual will respond equally well. Ryan et al[34] described the effect of 30-mg infusions of pamidronate given once weekly for 6 weeks in 25 patients with Paget's disease. Of 136 pagetic lesions, 10% completely resolved, 65% improved, and 24% remained unchanged. There were no significant differences noted in the scan responses at different sites,

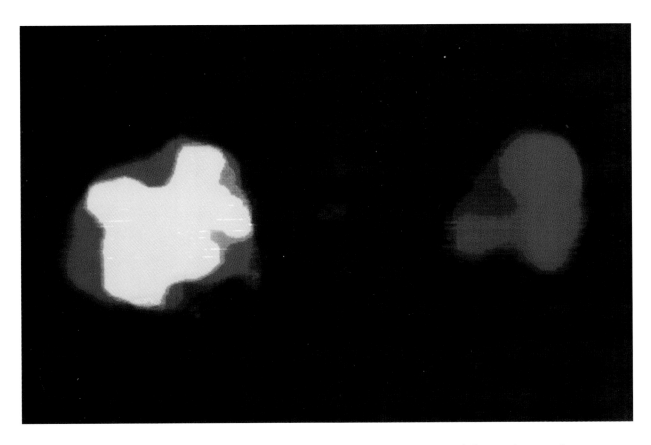

Plate 1. A 66-year-old female had an open reduction and internal fixation following fracture of the distal right femur. This became infected and the hardware was removed, the wound debrided, and the patient given a course of antibiotics. The patient did poorly and continued to spike a fever. This plate shows a representative transverse SPECT image. The red color represents pixels with Tc-99m MDP counts. The green represents pixels with In-111 labeled leukocyte counts (i.e., cellulitis). The yellow represents areas with both In-111 labeled leukocyte and Tc-99m MDP counts (i.e., osteomyelitis). See discussion in Chapter 11 of Figure 11-8, *G* (Plate 1 reproduced in black-and-white), for further information.

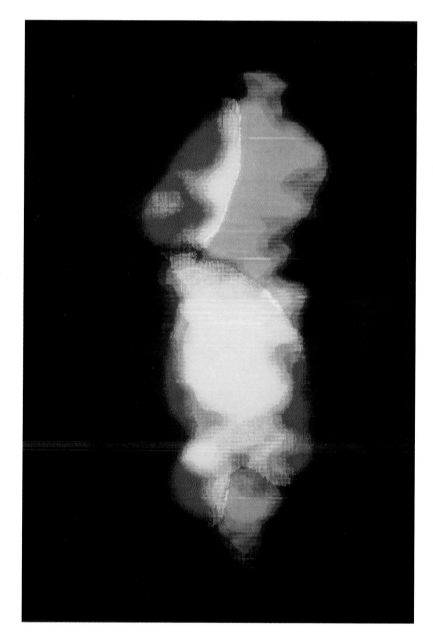

Plate 2. A 66-year-old female had an open reduction and internal fixation following fracture of the distal right femur. This became infected and the hardware was removed, the wound debrided, and the patient given a course of antibiotics. The patient did poorly and continued to spike a fever. This plate shows a representative coronal SPECT image. The red color represents pixels with Tc-99m MDP counts. The green represents pixels with In-111 labeled leukocyte counts (i.e., cellulitis). The yellow represents areas with both In-111 labeled leukocyte and Tc-99m MDP counts (i.e., osteomyelitis). See discussion in Chapter 11 of Figure 11-8, *H* (Plate 2 reproduced in black-and-white), for further information.

Fig. 10-12. **A**, Paget's disease affecting the left tibia. **B**, Same patient 6 months after pamidronate therapy.

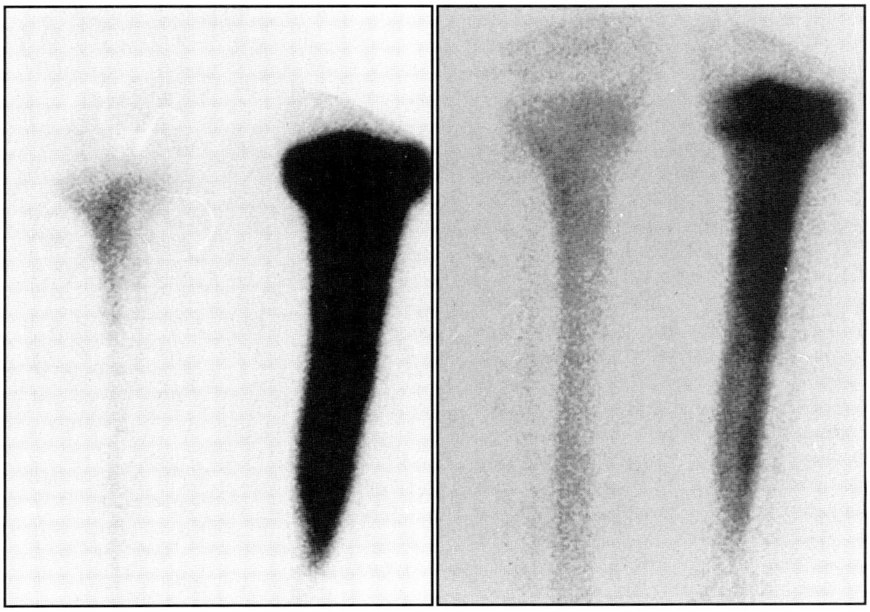

although less active lesions were more likely to resolve completely. Moreover there was no significant correlation between bone scan changes and alkaline phosphatase levels. However, bone scan activity both before and after treatment and the percentage change in bone scan visual score were significantly associated with the requirement for further therapy. Patients with grade 1 lesions (increased activity just detectable) after treatment did not require further pamidronate therapy for at least 2 to 3 years. Patients may show normalization of biochemistry but still have activity on bone scan. Possibly such patients would benefit from further treatment to normalize bone scan activity, which presumably reflects ongoing altered bone metabolism and may be a better marker of long-term response than biochemical measurements. However, in some cases it may not be possible to normalize diphosphonate uptake, particularly if a bone is grossly thickened and sclerotic when the absolute amount of bone may be considerably greater than normal. The bone scan does appear to be a sensitive means of anticipating relapse during clinical remission and can identify this before changes in biochemistry. However, the predictive value of a stable bone scan is poor, and there seems little justification in obtaining serial bone scans simply to anticipate relapse.

A more global assessment of skeletal metabolism can be obtained by 24-hour whole-body retention of technetium diphosphonate.[43,47] This can also be used to monitor therapies. The use of a bisphosphonate for therapy does not appear to interfere with the interpretation of the bone scan and does not invalidate this technique. The 24-hour whole-body retention of diphosphonate correlates well with changes in serum biochemistry.[43] A more recent approach to predicting the dose of pamidronate required for patient treatment has been

described by Evans et al[10] and in more detail by Stone et al[46] from the same group. They described the technique of bisphosphonate space measurement, which is a quantitative measurement of skeletal uptake of technetium HMDP. Some bisphosphonates are extracted by the kidney as well as taken up by bone and soft tissue, and therefore quantitative skeletal uptake needs to be corrected for renal excretion, which can be assessed using 51 chromium EDTA (ethylene diamine tetra acetic acid) as it is handled by the kidney in the same way as technetium HMDP. The ratio of the two tracers in the plasma following combined injection can be used as an index for uptake of bisphosphonate into bone; this has been called the *bisphosphonate space*. The bisphosphonate space has been shown to correlate with serum alkaline phosphatase and fasting urine creatinine/hydroxyproline ratio. The same group has shown that the ratio between the log dose pamidronate to pre-treatment bisphosphonate space measurement accurately predicts the dose of pamidronate that should be administered to produce suppression of alkaline phosphatase and urinary hydroxyproline excretion. This is a promising approach but is probably too complex to find use in routine clinical practice.

CLINICAL USE OF BONE SCANNING

The bone scan is the most sensitive technique for the detection of Paget's disease. It seems reasonable to suggest that the bone scan should be the imaging technique of choice, with radiography used to provide supplementary information when required. The bone scan is the ideal screening test in suspected Paget's disease and in patients with unexplained bone pain, bone deformity, or an elevated serum alkaline phosphatase level. The bone scan allows an accurate assessment of the extent of the disease and is simple and straightforward to perform. It can be used to monitor progression of disease and give an indication as to the requirement for further therapy, even when biochemical parameters have been normalized. The bone scan is also useful for the evaluation of new symptoms that may be related to other pathology.

REFERENCES

1. Alexandre C, et al: Effects of EHDP (5mg/kg/day dose) on quantitative bone histology in Paget's disease of the bone. *Metab Bone Dis Rel Res* 1981; 23:309.
2. Anderson DC, et al: Relapse of osteoporosis circumscripta as a lytic ring after treatment of Paget's disease with intravenous 3-amino-1 hydroxypropylidene bisphosphonate. *Br J Radiol* 1988; 61:996.
3. Barker DJ, et al. Paget's disease of bone in 14 British towns. *Br Med J* 1977; 1:1181.
4. Blockman R, et al: Treatment of Paget's disease of bone with low dose subcutaneous gallium nitrate. *J Bone Min Res* 1989; 4(suppl 1):167.
5. Bone HG, Kleerekoper M: Clinical review: Paget's disease of bone. *J Clin Endocrinial Metab* 1992; 75:1179.
6. Bourdreau RJ, Lisbona R, Hadjipavlou A: Observation on serial radionuclide blood flow studies in Paget's disease: Concise communications. *J Nucl Med* 1983; 24:880.
7. Brixen K, et al: SPECT bone scintigraphy in assessment of cranial Paget's disease. *Acta Radiol* 1990; 6:549.
8. Citrin DL, McKillop JH (eds): Paget's disease, in *Atlas of Technetium Bone Scans*. WB Saunders, Philadelphia, 1978, p 126.
9. Estrada WN, Kim CK, Alari A: Paget's disease in a patient with breast cancer. *J Nucl Med* 1993; 34:1214.
10. Evans A, et al: The diphosphonate space: A useful quantitative index of disease activity in patients undergoing hexamethylene diphosphonate (HMDP) bone imaging for Paget's disease. *Eur J Nucl Med* 1991; 18:757.
11. Fogelman I, Carr D: A comparison of bone scanning and radiology in the assessment of patients with symptomatic Paget's disease. *Eur J Nucl Med* 1980; 5:417.
12. Fogelman I: Bone scanning in Paget's disease, in Freeman LM (ed): *Nuclear Medicine Annual*, Raven Press, New York, 1991, p 99.
13. Galbraith HJ: Familial Paget's disease of bone. *Br Med J* 1954; 2:29.
14. Gordon MT, Anderson DC, Sharpe PT: Canine distemper virus localised in bone cells of patients with Paget's disease. *Bone* 1991; 12:195.
15. Harnick HIJ, et al: Relation between signs and symptoms in Paget's disease of bone. *Q J Med* 1980; 58:133.
16. Holdaway IM, et al: Previous pet ownership and Paget's disease. *Bone Miner* 1990; 8:53.
17. Kanis JA: *Pathophysiology and Treatment of Paget's Disease of Bone*, Carolina Academic Press, Durham, NC, 1991.
18. Kanis JA: Treatment of Paget's disease—an overview. *Semin Arthritis Rheum* 1994; 23:254.
19. Khetarpal U, Schuknecht HF: In search of pathologic correlation for hearing loss and vertigo in Paget's disease. *Ann Otol Rhinol Laryngol* 1990; 99(suppl 145).
20. Lavender JP, et al: A comparison of radiography and radioisotope scanning in the detection of Paget's disease and in the assessment of response to human calcitonin. *Br J Radiol* 1977; 50:243.
21. McKillop JH, et al: Bone scan appearances of a Paget's osteosarcoma: Failure to concentrate HEDP. *J Nucl Med* 1977; 18:1039.
22. Mailander JC: "The black beard" sign of monostotic Paget's disease of the mandible. *Clin Nucl Med* 1986; 11:325.
23. Maldague B, Malghem J: Dynamic radiologic patterns of Paget's disease of bone. *Clin Orthop* 1987; 217:126.
24. Marty R, et al: Bone trauma and related benign disease: Assessment by bone scanning. *Semin Nucl Med* 1976; 6:107.
25. Matin P: Bone scintigraphy in the diagnosis and management of traumatic injury. *Semin Nucl Med* 1983; 13:104.
26. Matthews J, Karimeoblini MK, Spencer RP: "Short pants" finding on bone images in Paget's disease with paralysis. *Clin Nucl Med* 1986; 11:221.
27. Meunier PJ, Salson C, Mathieu L: Skeletal distribution and biochemical parameters of Paget's disease. *Clin Orthop* 1987; 217:37.
28. Mills BG, et al: Evidence for both respiratory syncytial virus and measles virus antigens in the osteoclasts of patients with Paget's disease of bone. *Clin Orthop* 1984; 183:303.
29. Moser RP Jr, Vinh TN, Ros PR, et al: Paget's disease of the anterior tibial tubercle. *Radiology* 1987; 164:211.
30. O'Doherty DP, et al: Effects of five daily 1h infusion of alendronate in Paget's disease of bone. *J Bone Min Res* 1992; 7:81.
31. Rauseh JM, et al: Bone scanning in osteolytic Paget's disease: Case report. *J Nucl Med* 1977; 18:699.
32. Reginster JY, et al: Paget's disease of bone treated with a 5 day course of oral tiludronate. *Ann Rheum Dis* 1993; 52:54.
33. Ryan PJ, et al: Treatment of Paget's disease by weekly infusion of 3-aminohydroxypropylidene 1-1 bisphosphonate (APD). *Br J Rheumatol* 1992; 31:97.
34. Ryan PJ, Gibson T, Fogelman I: Bone scintigraphy following pamidronate therapy for Paget's disease of bone. *J Nucl Med* 1992; 33:1589.
35. Ryan PJ, Fogelman I: The role of nuclear medicine in orthopaedics. *Nuc Med Commun* 1994; 15:341.
36. Ryan PJ, Fogelman I: Paget's disease—five years follow up after pamidronate therapy. *Br J Rheumatol* 1994; 33:98.
37. Schubert F, Siddle KJ, Harper JS: Diaphyseal Paget's disease: An unusual finding in the tibia. *Clin Radiol* 1984; 35:71.
38. Serafini AN: Paget's disease of bone. *Semin Nucl Med* 1976; 6:47.
39. Shirazi PH, Ryan WG, Fordham EW: Bone scanning in evaluation of Paget's disease of bone. *Crit Res Clin Radiol Nucl Med* 1974; 5:523.
40. Siris ES, Canfield RE: Paget's disease of bone, in Becker KL (ed): *Principles and Practice of Endocrinology and Metabolism*, JB Lippincott, Philadelphia, 1990, p 504.
41. Siris ES, et al: Familial aggregation of Paget's disease of bone. *J Bone Miner Res* 1991; 6:495.
42. Smith J, Bodet JF, Yeh SDJ: Bone sarcoma in Paget's disease: A study of 85 patients. *Radiology* 1984; 152:585.

43. Smith ML, et al: Correlation of skeletal uptake of [99mTc] diphosphonate and alkaline phosphatase before and after oral diphosphonate therapy in Paget's disease. *Metab Bone Dis Rel Res* 1984; 5:167.

44. Smith R: Paget's disease of bone: Advance and controversy. *Br Med J* 1992; 305:379.

45. Stein I, et al: Evaluation of sodium etidronate in the treatment of Paget's disease before and after calcitonin treatment. *Clin Orthop* 1977; 122:347.

46. Stone MD, et al: Bisphosphonate space measurements in Paget's disease of bone treated with APD. *J Bone Min Res* 1992; 7:295.

47. Vattimo A, et al: Whole body retention of [99mTc] MPD in Paget's disease. *J Nucl Med Allied Sci* 1981; 25:5.

48. Vellenga CJLR, et al: Bone scintigraphy in Paget's disease treated with combined calcitation and diphosphonate (EHAP). *Metab Bone Dis Rel Res* 1982; 4:103.

49. Vellenga CJLR, et al: Evaluation of scintigraphic and roentgenologic studies in Paget's disease of bone studies by scintigraphy. *Radiology* 1984; 153:799.

50. Vellenga CJLR, Bijvoet OLM, Pauwels EKJ: Bone scintigraphy and radiology in Paget's disease of bone: A review. *Am J Physiol Imaging* 1988; 3:154.

51. Waxman AD, et al: Evaluation of [99mTc]-diphosphonate kinetics and bone scan in patients with Paget's disease before and after calcitonin treatement. *Radiology* 1977; 125:761.

52. Yeh SDJ, Rosen G, Benua RS: Gallium scan in Paget's sarcoma. *Clin Nucl Med* 1982; 7:546.

CHAPTER 11

THE ROLE OF NUCLEAR MEDICINE IN OSTEOMYELITIS

Donald S. Schauwecker

Multiple radiographic and scintigraphic procedures have been proposed to diagnose osteomyelitis. Some work well in certain clinical situations but are almost totally useless in others. This chapter emphasizes scintigraphic diagnosis of osteomyelitis in adult patients. Pediatric bone scanning is discussed in Chapter 16; the complementary use of radiographic and scintigraphic techniques for the complex diagnosis of the diabetic foot is discussed in Chapter 5.

Plain radiography should be the first study in every patient with suspected osteomyelitis. Most of the time the plain radiograph will not be pathognomonic because at least 10 to 14 days are required for the classic bone changes to develop.[17] Even if the plain radiograph cannot make the definitive diagnosis, it is still useful in deciding which further studies are required. Incidentally, if antibiotic therapy is begun early enough to arrest the bone mineral loss, the definitive plain radiographic findings may never develop.[27]

THREE-PHASE BONE SCAN

The three-phase bone scan is the routine nuclear medicine procedure for the diagnosis of osteomyelitis. The first phase, the nuclear angiogram or flow phase, consists of serial 2- to 5-second images of the area of suspected osteomyelitis that are obtained during injection of the radiopharmaceutical. The second phase, the blood pool image, is obtained within 5 minutes after injection. In areas of inflammation, capillaries dilate, causing increased blood flow and blood pooling. The third phase, the bone image, is obtained about 3 hours later, when urinary excretion has decreased the amount of the radionuclide in the soft tissues. Classically, with cellulitis, diffuse increased uptake occurs in the first two phases, but uptake is normal or diffusely increased in the third phase (Fig. 11-1). Diffuse increased uptake, if present on the third phase, is probably due to regional hyperemia caused by the cellulitis[55] (Fig. 11-l). Osteomyelitis causes focally increased uptake in all three phases (Fig. 11-2).

In adults with normal radiographs (i.e., no lesions that cause increased bone remodeling, except questionable radiographic changes consistent with osteomyelitis) the three-phase bone scan has a sensitivity and specificity of about 95%.[13,21,25,27,28] In addition, the three-phase bone scan can accurately diagnose osteomyelitis within 3 days of the development of symptoms, which is much earlier than can be seen with the plain radiograph.[21] Because of its high accuracy and relatively low cost, the three-phase bone scan is a very effective method to image osteo-

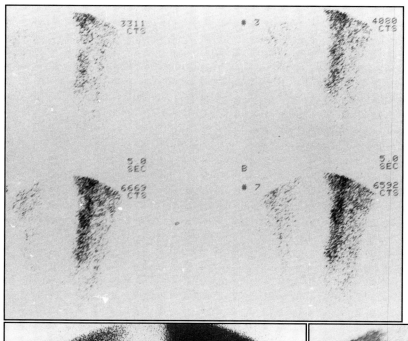

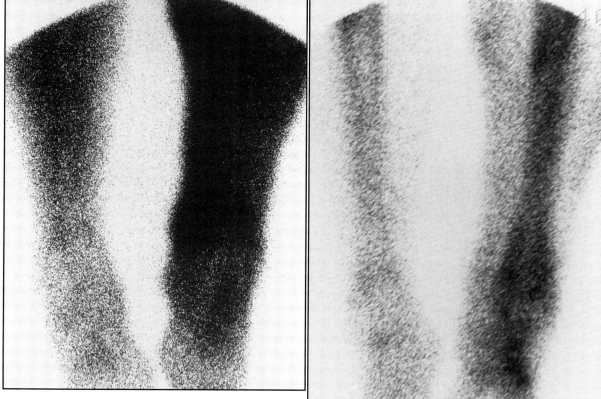

Fig. 11–1. A 78-year-old female presented with chronic venous stasis ulcer and cellulitis overlying the left medial malleolus. On the anterior view there is increased blood flow (**A**) and blood pool activity (**B**) throughout the distal left leg. There is no area of focal increased activity in the bone images (**C**); however, there is diffuse increased activity throughout the entire tibia. This extended pattern is caused by the increased radiopharmaceutical delivered to all of the bones in the left leg.[55]

myelitis in the routine clinical practice. The three-phase bone scan can also diagnose septic arthritis and septic arthritis with extension into the adjacent bone.

There are two general situations in which the three-phase bone scan has difficulty. The first is shortly after the development of osteomyelitis in young children where the sensitivity is reduced by falsely normal or cold

defects seen on the three-phase bone scan 22% to 68% of the time.[1,4,52] This is discussed more fully in Chapter 16.

The second situation in which the three-phase bone scan breaks down is where there is some process that causes increased bone remodeling (e.g., a healing fracture, neuropathic osteoarthropathy). In this situation the underlying process causing the bone remodeling can

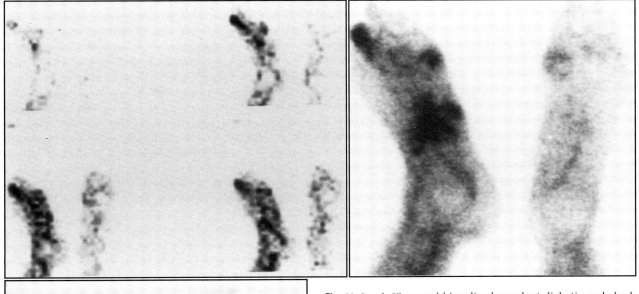

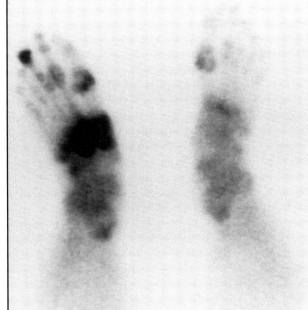

Fig. 11-2. A 60-year-old insulin-dependent diabetic male had right foot ulcer and normal radiographs of the foot. There is intense focal increased activity in the right fourth toe on the flow (**A**), blood pool (**B**), and bone images (**C**) on the plantar view. This is classic for osteomyelitis.

cause increased uptake on all phases of the three-phase bone scan that can be indistinguishable from osteomyelitis.* Fortunately most causes of increased bone remodeling can be detected on the plain radiograph. Gallium-67 and In-111 labeled leukocytes have been used to try to diagnose osteomyelitis superimposed on a disease process that causes increased bone remodeling.

GALLIUM-67

The chief advantage of Ga-67 is that it is commercially available and requires no preparation. Results in the evaluation of suspected osteomyelitis are variable, with a

*References 22, 26, 31, 38, 46, 51.

sensitivity of about 80% and a specificity of about 70%.[25,30,50,51]

Gallium-67 citrate localizes in areas of osteomyelitis by granulocyte or bacterial uptake and by binding to lactoferrin at the site of infection.[20] However, gallium citrate was originally proposed as a bone-scanning agent[8] and shows increased uptake in areas of increased bone remodeling, such as bones with neuropathic changes[14,18] or pseudoarthrosis.[16]

To overcome this problem, some authors have proposed comparing the Ga-67 citrate uptake in the lesion with the uptake on a bone scan; disparate distribution of uptake or increased intensity would constitute osteomyelitis.[40,61] If these findings are present, the specificity is very high; however, these findings are only present in about 25% of the cases of osteomyelitis.[46] In complicating cases Ga-67 citrate can be sensitive or specific,

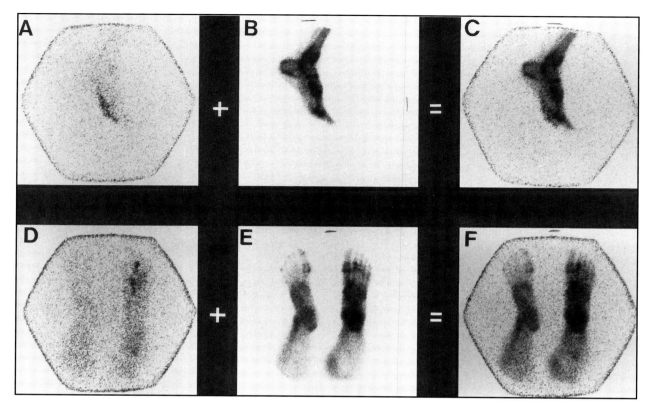

Fig. 11-3. A 58-year-old insulin-dependent diabetic female had an infected ulcer on the ball of the foot. **A** and **D**, The left medial and plantar 4-hour In-111 labeled leukocyte images, respectively. **B** and **E**, The simultaneous left medial and plantar Tc-99m MDP bone images, respectively. **C** and **F**, The superimposition of (**A**) on (**B**) and (**D**) on (**E**), respectively. On the plantar view the In-111 labeled leukocyte activity overlies the bone, but on the lateral view the In-111 labeled leukocyte activity lies in the soft tissue inferior to the bone. This is cellulitis without evidence of osteomyelitis in the soft tissue of the plantar surface of the foot.

but it is difficult to obtain high sensitivity and high specificity simultaneously.[46] When Ga-67 citrate and In-111 labeled leukocytes have been directly compared in the same patient, the labeled leukocytes are usually significantly better for the diagnosis of osteomyelitis.[30,46,48] Currently Ga-67 citrate is rarely used for the diagnosis of osteomyelitis when In-111 labeled leukocytes are available. A few authors believe Ga-67 may be more sensitive for chronic osteomyelitis than In-111 labeled leukocytes, but this is in dispute.[49]

INDIUM-111 LABELED LEUKOCYTES

The separation and labeling of the leukocytes with In-111 is a long, labor-intensive process that originally limited its availability to a few large hospitals. When In-111 oxine became commercially available, many smaller institutions could also perform In-111 labeled leukocyte studies. Currently approximately 40 to 50 ml of blood can be withdrawn from the patient, sent to the local commercial radiopharmacy for preparation, and In-111 labeled leukocytes reinjected 2 to 3 hours later. Large,

high-volume institutions may continue to prepare their own In-111 labeled leukocytes, generally by the method of Thakur or with some slight modification.[53,54]

Leukocytes normally migrate to an area of infection. If they are separated and labeled in a gentle manner, they will maintain their function. The key to good results with In-111 labeled leukocytes is the gentle, careful handling of the cells during the separation and labeling process which will preserve normal cellular function. Well-prepared cells have a sensitivity of about 90% and a specificity of about 85% for the evaluation of suspected osteomyelitis superimposed on a process that causes increased bone remodeling.[26,29,44,48,63] Note that these results were obtained for suspected complicating osteomyelitis in cases difficult to evaluate by other methods. In noncomplicating osteomyelitis (i.e., normal radiograph), the three-phase bone scan is more accurate and less expensive.

If the plain radiograph reveals a fracture, prosthesis, neuropathic osteopathy, or other problem that causes increased bone remodeling, an In-111 labeled leukocyte scan is performed. If the suspected site of osteomyelitis is in the marrow-containing skeleton, the In-111 labeled leukocyte scan is combined with a bone marrow scan. If

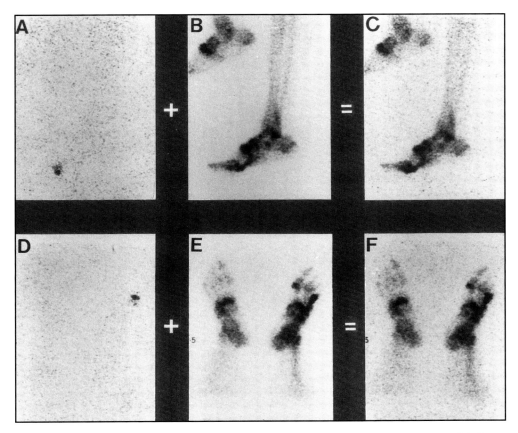

Fig. 11-4. A 47-year-old diabetic had prior osteomyelitis and resection through the midshaft of the left fifth metatarsal. Currently the patient has cellulitis and ulcer in the lateral aspect of the distal left foot. **A** and **D**, The left lateral and plantar 24-hour In-111 labeled leukocyte images, respectively. **B** and **E**, The simultaneous left lateral and plantar Tc-99m MDP bone images, respectively. **C** and **F**, The superimposition of (**A**) on (**B**) and (**D**) on (**E**), respectively. On both views the focal intense In-111 labeled leukocyte and Tc-99m MDP activity superimpose. This is osteomyelitis in the head of the left fourth metatarsal.

the suspected osteomyelitis is not in the marrow-containing skeleton and the plain radiograph reveals an abnormality that causes increased bone remodeling, the In-111 labeled leukocyte scan can be combined with the three-phase bone scan. The sensitivity and specificity of the In-111 labeled leukocyte scan are both approximately 90% in the peripheral skeleton. Since there are no landmarks on the In-111 labeled leukocyte scan, the problem is to differentiate soft-tissue infection from bone infection. By combining the three-phase bone scan with the In-111 labeled leukocyte scan, cellulitis (Fig. 11-3) can be differentiated from osteomyelitis (Fig. 11-4) in almost 90% of the cases.[45]

The combined three-phase bone/In-111 labeled leukocyte scan is performed on a camera that simultaneously captures and separates the 140-keV Tc-99m peak, and the 173- and 247-keV In-111 peaks. The In-111 labeled leukocyte image is acquired for 50-K counts or 15 minutes, whichever comes first, at both 4 and 24 hours after injection of the In-111 labeled leukocytes. For simplicity we use a 10% window at the 140-keV Tc-99m peak and a 20% window at the 247-keV In-111 peak for both the 4-

and 24-hour images. Some authors use the 247-keV peak only at 4 hours and use a 20% window at 247-keV plus a 10% window on the 173-keV peak at 24 hours. They feel intense Tc-99m localization may interfere with the 173-keV In-111 peak at 4 hours.[10] However, by 24 hours the Tc-99m has mostly decayed, thus decreasing the interference, while the additional counts from the 173-keV In-111 peak add significantly to the count-poor In-111 labeled leukocyte image. One needs to evaluate possible spectral overlap on each of the camera systems used for imaging because there appears to be some variations among different equipment.

Using the combined three-phase bone/In-111 labeled leukocyte scan, the In-111 labeled leukocytes produce the sensitivity and specificity, and the Tc-99m bone image provides the anatomic landmarks. The bone images and In-111 labeled leukocyte images are photographed on separate sheets of film. By carefully overlaying the films, one can determine if the activity is inside or outside of the bone. If the In-111 labeled leukocyte activity overlies the bone in both orthogonal projections, it is osteomyelitis (Fig. 11-4). If the In-111 labeled leukocyte activity is outside of the bone on either of the orthogonal projections, the diagnosis is cellulitis (Fig. 11-3). Oblique views or single photon emission computed tomography (SPECT) may be obtained if the orthogonal views are not diagnostic.

COMBINED BONE MARROW/In-111 LABELED LEUKOCYTE STUDY

Acute osteomyelitis can be readily diagnosed anywhere in the body, whereas chronic osteomyelitis with its lower influx of labeled leukocytes is detected accurately in the peripheral skeleton only.[44] The In-111 labeled leukocytes accumulate in active bone marrow, which reduces the sensitivity for detection of chronic osteomyelitis in the central skeleton.[44]

One way to improve specificity in the central skeleton is to perform a Tc-99m bone marrow/In-111 labeled leukocyte study.[23,34,37] The Tc-99m sulfur or antimony colloid will clearly delineate the extent of the bone marrow. Any incongruity of the bone marrow and In-111 labeled leukocyte images would be considered significant. Recently this study has been found to increase both the sensitivity and specificity for complicating osteomyelitis in the central skeleton.[36] Thus the Tc-99m bone marrow scan and In-111 labeled leukocyte study are the procedures of choice for diagnosing complicating osteomyelitis in the marrow-containing skeleton.

One of the more common applications for the combined bone marrow/In-111 labeled leukocyte study is the diagnosis of osteomyelitis of the spine because In-111 labeled leukocytes alone have poor sensitivity.[43,62] When performing In-111 labeled leukocyte scans of the spine, one occasionally encounters a "cold" defect, which can be confusing (Fig. 11-5). The "cold" defect occurs in 10% to 40% of such studies for suspected osteomyelitis in the central skeleton.[7,9,32,44,62] Although the cold defect could represent osteomyelitis, it also is seen in metastases, fractures, Paget's disease, surgical defects, and after irradiation.[7,9,32,44,62] The cold defect is consistent with, but not diagnostic of, osteomyelitis. Palestro et al[35] have performed serial studies in patients with vertebral osteomyelitis and found a progression from hot to cold as the lesions became more chronic. Perhaps the most interesting situation is when the uptake in the area of infection matches the uptake of the normal bone marrow of the spine (Fig. 11-6). Yet even in this situation, the addition of the Tc-99m bone marrow scan allows one to determine if infection is present.

Another major use of the combined bone marrow/In-111 labeled leukocyte study is the evaluation of suspected infected prosthesis. When a prosthesis is in place, it can displace and/or activate the surrounding bone marrow. An In-111 labeled leukocyte study alone could be confusing, yet it can be readily evaluated if combined with the bone marrow scan (Fig. 11-7).

The procedure for the sulfur colloid/In-111 labeled leukocyte study is analogous to that of the In-111 labeled

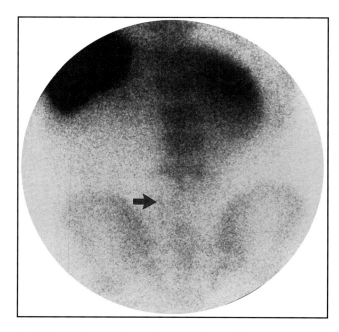

Fig. 11-5. A 67-year-old male complained of low back pain. A 24-hour In-111 labeled leukocyte study revealed a "cold defect" (*arrow*). Since In-111 labeled leukocytes normally localize in the bone marrow, liver, and spleen, this is abnormal. This study would be read as "consistent with but not diagnostic of" osteomyelitis. If a bone marrow study was also performed and was incongruent, this would be diagnostic of osteomyelitis (Fig. 11-6). Subsequently this was proven to be metastatic prostate cancer.

leukocyte/bone scan, except 10 mCi of Tc-99m sulfur colloid is used. The intense localization of the sulfur colloid in the liver and spleen renders evaluation of suspected osteomyelitis in the lower thoracic spine virtually uninterpretable by this approach, except with the possible use of SPECT. Otherwise, there is virtually never any interference from 140-keV Tc-99m counts in the 10% 173-keV In-111 window.

SPECT

The most common use of SPECT for the evaluation of suspected osteomyelitis is in the spine. Vertebral osteomyelitis will be localized within one vertebral body, thus the disk space should be preserved. In diskitis the zone of decreased activity representing the disk space is lost, and the lower margin of the upper vertebral body and the upper margin of the lower vertebral body have intense uptake.

Less commonly there are occasions when the planar images of the combined three-phase bone/In-111 labeled leukocyte study or bone marrow/In-111 labeled leukocyte study cannot differentiate cellulitis from osteomyelitis. In these situations it may be necessary to evaluate the combined study using SPECT. An example would be a case of extensive cellulitis that essentially surrounds the bone (Fig. 11-8). Any planar view will show the In-

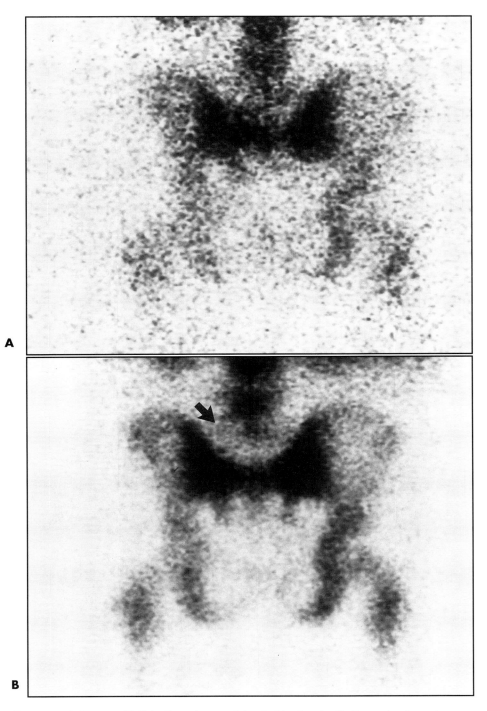

Fig. 11-6. A 47-year-old diabetic male complained of back pain. Radiographs showed questionable end plate irregularity at L5 S1. The clinicians doubted osteomyelitis but requested a combined bone marrow/In-111 labeled leukocyte scan. The In-111 labeled leukocyte 4-hour image of the lumbar spine (**A**) would probably be read as normal if interpreted alone. However, the Tc-99m sulfur colloid bone marrow image taken simultaneously (**B**) shows a cold defect (*arrow*). Thus the interpretation was osteomyelitis, which was confirmed by MRI. The patient did well after antibiotic therapy.

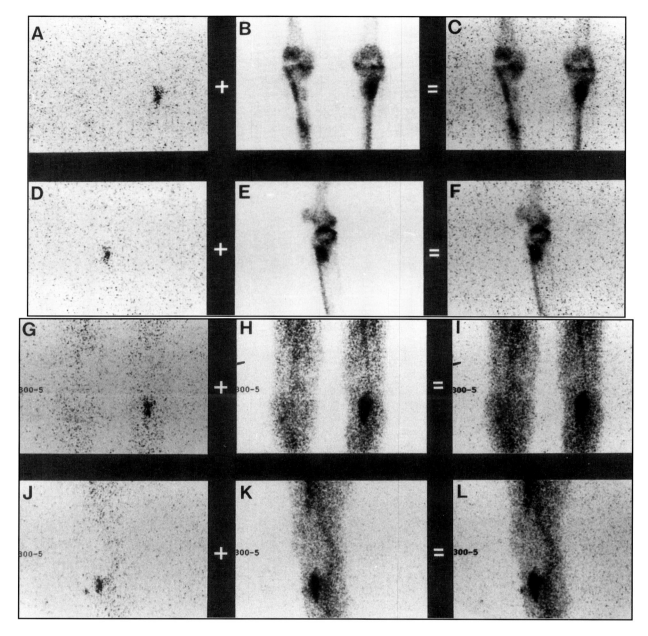

Fig. 11–7. A 28-year-old male had an open reduction and internal fixation of the proximal left tibia after being struck by a car 10 years before the study. The rod was removed and serial radiographs revealed continued remodeling of the proximal tibia. **A** and **D**, The anterior and left lateral 24-hour In-111 labeled leukocyte images, respectively. **B** and **E**, The anterior and left lateral simultaneous Tc-99m MDP bone images, respectively. **C** and **F**, The superimposition of (**A**) on (**B**) and (**D**) on (**E**), respectively. On both views the In-111 labeled leukocyte activity superimposes on an area of increased bone activity in the proximal left tibia, consistent with osteomyelitis. This was an area of bone remodeling on the radiograph where the rod had been removed from the bone. Four years earlier identical results had been obtained and were read as osteomyelitis. However, at 48 hours an injection of Tc-99m sulfur colloid was given and a bone marrow/In-111 labeled leukocyte study was obtained. **G** and **J**, The anterior and left lateral 48-hour In-111 labeled leukocyte images, respectively. **H** and **K**, The anterior and left lateral sulfur colloid images, respectively, obtained simultaneously with (**G**) and (**J**). (**I**) and (**L**) are (**G**) superimposed on (**H**) and (**J**) superimposed on (**K**), respectively. There is intense sulfur colloid bone marrow localization corresponding to the In-111 labeled leukocyte activity. Thus this represents displaced or activated bone marrow and not osteomyelitis.

111 activity superimposed on the bone activity. Yet the infection may simply be surrounding the bone, and the bone may not be involved. Notice how SPECT easily solved the problem in this case (Fig. 11-8).

A second example where there are so many superimposed structures that it is hard to determine the exact location of the In-111 labeled leukocyte activity (Fig. 11-9). Since the In-111 labeled leukocyte study is identical to the activity seen on the bone marrow scan, there is no infection.

To perform a simultaneous bone or bone marrow/In-111 labeled leukocyte SPECT study requires a sophisticated camera and computer system that can simultaneously acquire, separate, and store both the Tc-99m counts and the In-111 counts. Figs. 11-8 and 11-9 were obtained with 360-degree rotation, 64 frames at 30 seconds a frame. A 64×64 matrix was individually used for the 10% window 140-keV Tc-99m counts and for the 20% window 247-keV In-111 counts. The Tc-99m images were reconstructed with a 0.5 Butterworth filter, order 6. The In-111

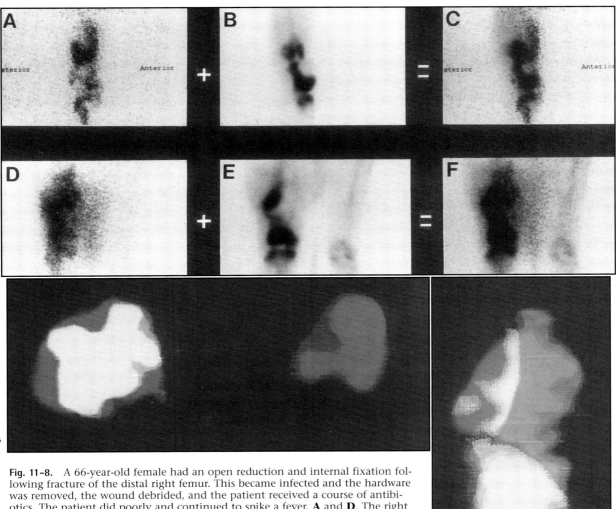

Fig. 11-8. A 66-year-old female had an open reduction and internal fixation following fracture of the distal right femur. This became infected and the hardware was removed, the wound debrided, and the patient received a course of antibiotics. The patient did poorly and continued to spike a fever. **A** and **D**, The right lateral and anterior In-111 labeled leukocyte images, respectively. **B** and **E**, The right lateral and anterior bone images, respectively, obtained simultaneously with (**A**) and (**D**), respectively. (**C**) is (**A**) superimposed on (**B**) and (**F**) is (**D**) superimposed on (**E**). Unfortunately the cellulitis is massive and seems to surround the bone, thus it is impossible to tell if osteomyelitis is present, even using orthogonal views. **G**, A representative transverse SPECT image. See Plate 1 for color reproduction. **H**, A representative coronal SPECT image. See Plate 2 for color reproduction.

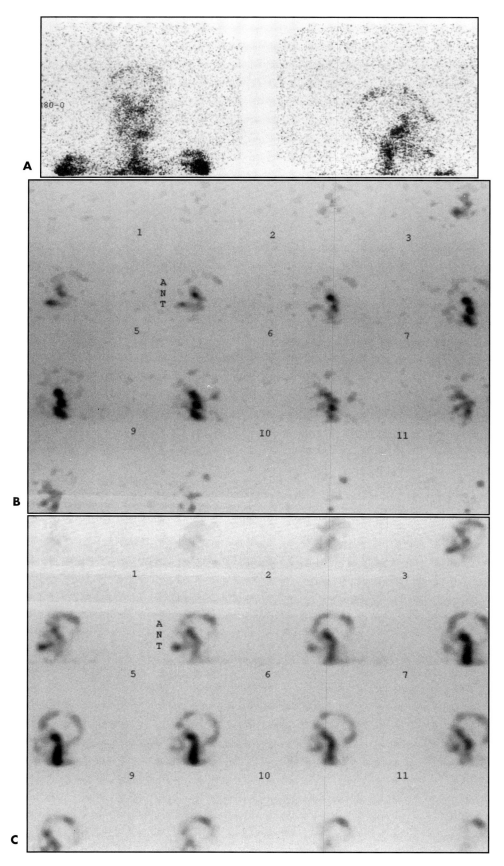

Fig. 11-9. A 29-year-old female had a right orbital blow-out fracture and reconstructive surgery using a section of a rib. The patient presented with nasal swelling, migraine headaches, and sinusitis. The anterior and right lateral 24-hour In-111 labeled leukocyte images (**A**) are hard to interpret due to overlaying bone marrow–containing structures. **B**, Sagittal 48-hour In-111 labeled leukocyte SPECT slices. **C**, The corresponding sagittal Tc-99m sulfur colloid slices obtained simultaneously. In all of the slices the In-111 labeled leukocyte uptake corresponds to uptake in the bone marrow. Thus no infection was present.

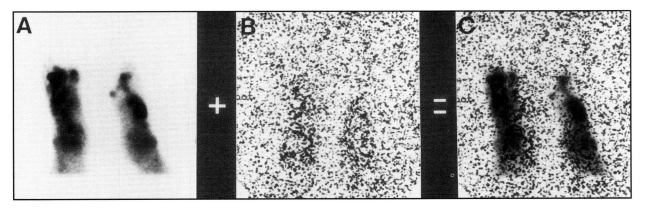

Fig. 11-10.   A 65-year-old diabetic male had a chronic right foot ulcer. **A,** The 4-hour plantar bone image of the three-phase bone scan, which was hot on all three phases. **B,** The In-111 labeled leukocyte 24-hour image. (**C**) is (**A**) superimposed on (**B**). By comparing the faint uptake in the right fourth toe with the background, it was decided that the uptake was too faint to read as positive. Subsequently this proved to be osteomyelitis. By reading the faint uptake in the right fourth toe, the sensitivity of the study could be increased. However, this would be more than offset by the decrease in specificity.

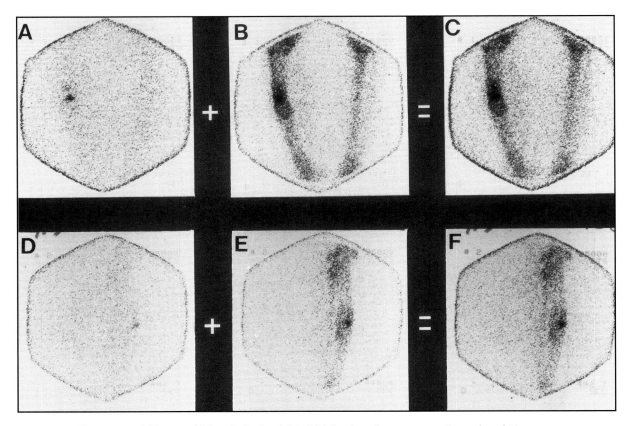

Fig. 11-11.   A 50-year-old female had a right tibial fracture 7 years ago and now has drainage from the scar. **A** and **D,** The anterior and right lateral 24-hour In-111 labeled leukocyte images, respectively. **B** and **E,** The simultaneous anterior and right lateral Tc-99m MDP bone images, respectively. **C** and **F,** The superimpositions of (**A**) on (**B**) and (**D**) on (**E**), respectively. This is another case of chronic osteomyelitis. The In-111 labeled leukocyte accumulation seen in (**A**) is about the lowest compared with the normal soft-tissue background that would be called abnormally increased uptake.

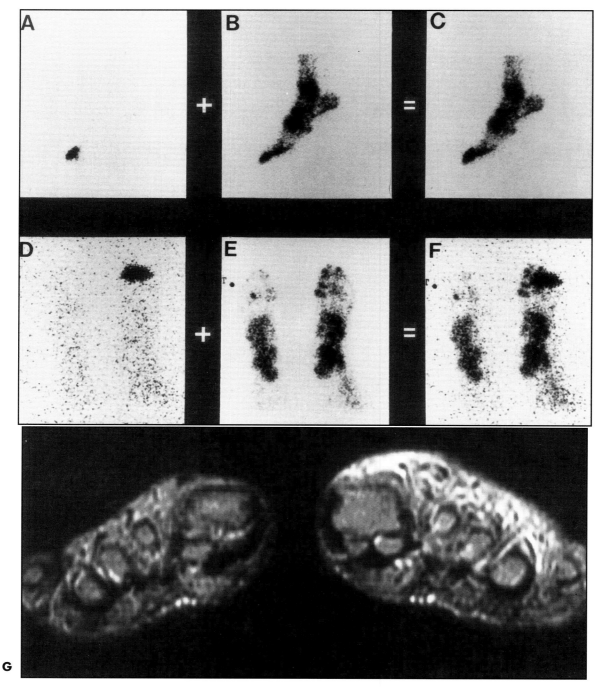

Fig. 11-12. A 50-year-old human immunodeficiency virus (HIV) positive male diabetic had extensive left foot ulcers between the left first, second, and third toes. **A** and **D**, The left lateral and plantar 24-hour In-111 labeled leukocyte images of the feet, respectively. **B** and **E**, The simultaneous left lateral and plantar Tc-99m MDP bone images, respectively. **C** and **F**, The superimposition of (**A**) on (**B**) and (**D**) on (**E**), respectively. In both projections the In-111 labeled leukocyte activity superimposes on the Tc-99m MDP activity. However, there is no increased Tc-99m MDP activity in the region of the increased In-111 labeled leukocyte activity. Therefore this study was read as extensive cellulitis surrounding the bones but no osteo-myelitis. This was confirmed by MRI (**G**).

labeled leukocyte images were reconstructed with a 0.35 Butterworth filter, order 6.

CLINICAL EXPERIENCE

A significant variable between different nuclear medicine laboratories is "What constitutes a positive In-111 labeled leukocyte scan?" Some have maintained that any accumulation of In-111 labeled leukocytes represents a positive study. With the present digital cameras, one can always see some counts in the area of interest. If these were called positive, it would result in high sensitivity but specificity would suffer. The uptake in the lesion can be compared with background activity in normal tissues (Figs. 11-10 and 11-11) or normal bone marrow in the central skeleton. There should be definite, not question-

able, increased uptake for the lesion to be called positive. Some diagnoses may be missed (e.g., Fig. 11-10), but there is a constant trade-off between sensitivity and specificity, and this approach seems to lead to the most accurate results.

Using the combined three-phase bone/In-111 labeled leukocyte study or the Tc-99m bone marrow/In-111 labeled leukocyte study can result in an error caused by In-111 counts falling into the Tc-99m window or the 140-keV Tc-99m counts overlapping the 173-keV In-111 window.[10] There are never enough counts from Tc-99m sulfur colloid to interfere with the In-111 labeled leukocyte image; however, if the region of interest overlies the liver or spleen, no meaningful information can be obtained without SPECT. Intense areas of Tc-99m uptake on the bone scan, such as a healing fracture, may cause an unacceptably large number of counts to fall within the 173-keV In-111 window on the 4-hour images. As a

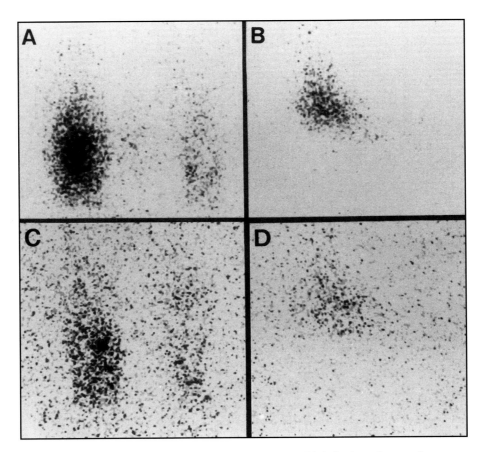

Fig. 11-13. Over 7 months, the radiograph of this 34-year-old diabetic male went from near normal to almost complete destruction of the right metatarsal bones. This was interpreted as rapidly progressive neuropathic osteoarthropathy; however, infection was possible. A combined bone/In-111 labeled leukocyte study was performed. The bone images (not shown) showed increased activity in the right metatarsal region corresponding to the activity seen on the In-111 labeled leukocyte study. **A** and **C**, The 4- and 24-hour plantar In-111 labeled leukocyte images, respectively. **B** and **D**, The 4- and 24-hour right lateral In-111 labeled leukocyte images, respectively. When the 24-hour images are compared with the corresonding 4-hour images, there appears to be an interval decrease in the diffuse activity as compared with the blood pool. This was rapidly progressive neuropathic osteoarthropathy. *(From Schauwecker DS: Differentiation of infected from non-infected rapidly progressive neuropathic osteoarthopathy.* J Nucl Med *1995; 36:1427; with permission.)*

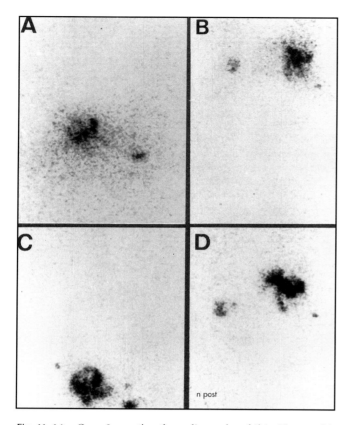

Fig. 11–14. Over 6 months, the radiographs of this 67-year-old diabetic female went from moderate degenerative changes to almost complete destruction of the right metatarsal bones. She had cellulitis and foot ulcers that did not respond to antibiotic therapy. Thus the possibility of osteomyelitis was considered. A combined bone/In-111 labeled leukocyte study was performed. The bone images (not shown) showed increased activity in the right metatarsal region corresponding to the activity seen on the In-111 labeled leukocyte study. **A** and **C**, The 4- and 24-hour plantar In-111 labeled leukocyte images, respectively. **B** and **D**, The 4- and 24-hour posterior of the left foot and lateral of the right foot In-111 labeled leukocyte images, respectively. When (**C**) is compared with (**A**) and (**D**) is compared with (**B**), there has been an interval increase in the areas of focal activity compared with the blood pool. At amputation, the neuropathic right metatarsal joints were infected. Incidental note is made of cellulitis of the left heel. *(From Schauwecker DS: Differentiation of infected from non-infected rapidly progressive neuropathic osteoarthopathy.* J Nucl Med *1995; 36:1427; with permission.)*

result, during the early imaging, only the 247-keV In-111 window should be used. For the delayed images the difference in half-lives virtually eliminates this problem, so a narrow window can be used for the In-111 173-keV peak. The reverse problem can occur when scatter from intense In-111 activity appears in the 140-keV Tc-99m window on the delayed images. This is readily recognized as an artifact because it is unlikely that the Tc-99m activity in a bone scan will markedly increase between the 4- and 24-hour studies.

The bone scan portion can be helpful for more than just anatomic landmarks. The problem with the three-phase bone scan in cases of complicating osteomyelitis is

that it is sensitive but not specific. Its sensitivity is actually higher than that of the In-111 labeled leukocyte study. Although it should occur rarely, occasionally there will be a case where the In-111 labeled leukocyte activity appears to project within the bone, but the bone scan does not show increased uptake (Fig. 11-12). In this situation one is generally dealing with soft-tissue infection adjacent to and perhaps surrounding the bone, but not osteomyelitis. An exception may be if the bone has lost its blood supply.

In an effort to save time and/or cost, some obtain only one set of In-111 labeled leukocyte images. This is a mistake. Both the early and delayed images are useful and should be obtained in virtually all cases for the following reasons. First, the In-111 labeled leukocytes continue to migrate into the area of infection for a longer period than 4 hours. It is possible to see some infections, particularly chronic infections, on the delayed images that may be missed on the earlier images. Second, since the In-111 labeled leukocyte activity increases in size between the early and delayed images, the early image is often better for localizing the activity to the bone or soft tissue. Third, comparison of activity in 4- and 24-hour In-111 labeled leukocyte images may allow one to correctly suspect an artifact. If the intensity of the lesion does not increase from early to delayed images, it is likely that one is dealing with an artifact or something other than infection (Fig. 11-13). Another aid in differentiating infection from artifact is that infections often have nonuniform uptake (Fig. 11-14), while noninfectious cases of inflammation may give more diffuse uniform activity (Fig. 11-13).

RECENTLY DEVELOPED RADIO-PHARMACEUTICALS

Technetium-99m hexamethyl propylene amine oxime (HMPAO) labeled leukocytes have two distinct advantages over In-111 labeled leukocytes. First, approximately 40 times as much radioactivity is injected, which produces prettier images, particularly with SPECT. Second, Tc-99m HMPAO is easily produced from a kit and is always available. Indium-111 may not be readily available in some hospitals. The chief advantage of using leukocytes labeled with In-111 is the ability to perform simultaneous Tc-99m imaging of bone or bone marrow, which can better localize the infection to bone or soft tissue. This advantage is lost using Tc-99m HMPAO labeled leukocytes alone (Fig. 11-15). By designing a foot holder to allow both radiographs and nuclear scans to be performed without moving the patient, it is possible to partially overcome this problem in limited clinical settings[19] (Fig. 11-16).

Currently only a relatively small number of studies have been performed using Tc-99m HMPAO labeled leukocytes for the evaluation of suspected osteomyelitis; however, the results are similar to those obtained using In-111 labeled leukocytes.[39,43,58,59] The largest comparison study to date by Uzum et al showed similar specifici-

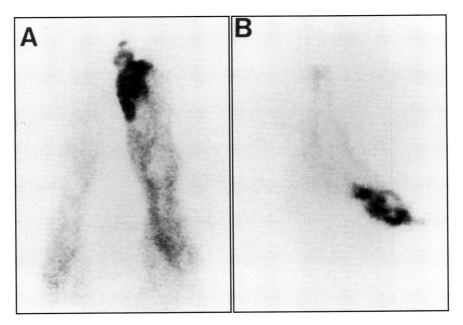

Fig. 11–15. A 57-year-old male who had an amputation of the left second metatarsal and toe presented with cellulitis and suspected osteomyelitis. A combined bone/In-111 labeled leukocyte study was ordered; however, no In-111 was commercially available. (**A**) is the plantar and (**B**) is the left medial 4-hour Tc-99m HMPAO labeled leukocyte image. Because of the extent of the cellulitis, it was impossible to determine if osteomyelitis was present. When cellulitis is extensive, it might not be possible to make the differentiation without SPECT (Figs. 11-8 and 11-12).

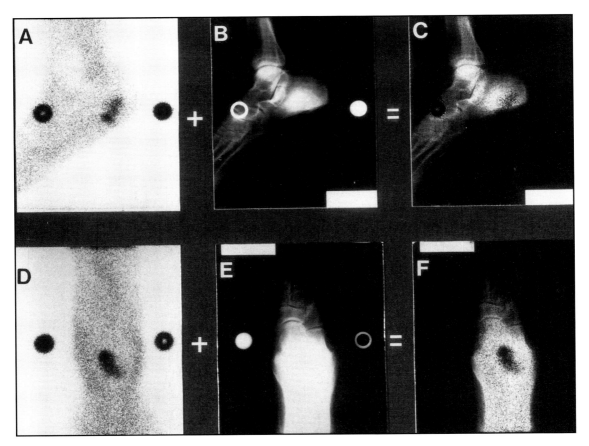

Fig. 11–16. A 40-year-old diabetic male had a long-standing ulcer of the left heel. **A** and **D**, The Tc-99m HMPAO labeled leukocyte left lateral and plantar views, respectively. A special foot-holding device allowed the nuclear images to be taken, then a radiograph cassette was inserted above the camera surface without moving the patient's foot.[19] **B** and **E**, The radiographs obtained immediately after completing the nuclear study. **C** and **F**, The superimposition of (**A**) on (**B**) and (**D**) on (**E**), respectively. The Tc-99m labeled leukocytes localized both inside and outside of the bone. The diagnosis was cellulitis and osteomyelitis, which was proven at surgery. *(Case courtesy of Dr. Robert Burt[19].)*

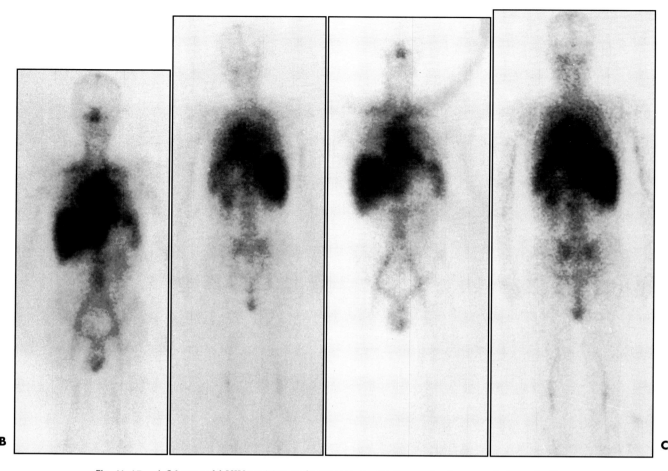

A, B

C, D

Fig. 11-17. A 26-year-old HIV-positive male presented with fever of unknown etiology. **A,** The anterior and (**B**) the posterior whole-body images obtained 6 hours after injection of the In-111 labeled human polyclonal IgG. **C,** The anterior and (**D**) the posterior whole-body images obtained 21 hours after injection. This is a normal study, and no site of infection was found. Notice the large amount of activity in the blood pool on both the early and delayed images. Although this biodistribution is quite typical for monoclonal antibodies, it is markedly different from labeled leukocytes where the activity is in the liver, spleen, and bone marrow by the time of the delayed images.

ty of In-111 and Tc-99m HMPAO labeled leukocytes. The sensitivity of Tc-99m HMPAO labeled leukocytes was 67% and In-111 labeled leukocytes was 85% for the evaluation of suspected osteomyelitis.[57] They preferred the clarity of the Tc-99m HMPAO labeled leukocyte images but found the simultaneous In-111 labeled leukocyte/bone scan combination more helpful in localizing the infection to bone or soft tissue.[57] In general, leukocytes labeled with Tc-99m HMPAO and leukocytes labeled with In-111 would be expected to have similar causes for false-positive and false-negative results because both procedures use leukocytes to carry the radionuclide to the site of infection.

Although leukocytes labeled with In-111 or Tc-99m HMPAO provide good sensitivity and specificity, both require extensive separation and labeling. This procedure takes about 2 hours and requires considerable skill to ensure that the cells are not damaged. New agents available as kits are being developed that will alleviate this difficulty.

Preliminary results from European studies[24,43,47] that used either Tc-99m or iodine-123 labeled antigranulocyte antibodies appear favorable. The agent is available as a kit in Europe, and phase III clinical trials are currently being conducted in the United States. Antigranulocyte antibodies are produced from mouse antibodies, and rare, generally mild, adverse reactions have been reported. Further work is required to establish the role of antigranulocyte antibodies in the diagnosis of osteomyelitis.

Recently In-111 labeled human polyclonal immunoglobulin G (IgG) against inflammation has been developed.[12,42] Preliminary results show a high sensitivity of over 95%, with a specificity of about 85%.[5,6,33,41] Because this agent is a human antibody, it should not produce any human antimouse antibody (HAMA) reaction that is seen rarely with antigranulocyte antibody. The biodistribution of In-111 labeled human polyclonal IgG is considerably different from that of labeled leukocytes (Fig. 11-17). Thus approximately four times the activity can be administered, which may result in prettier images. When

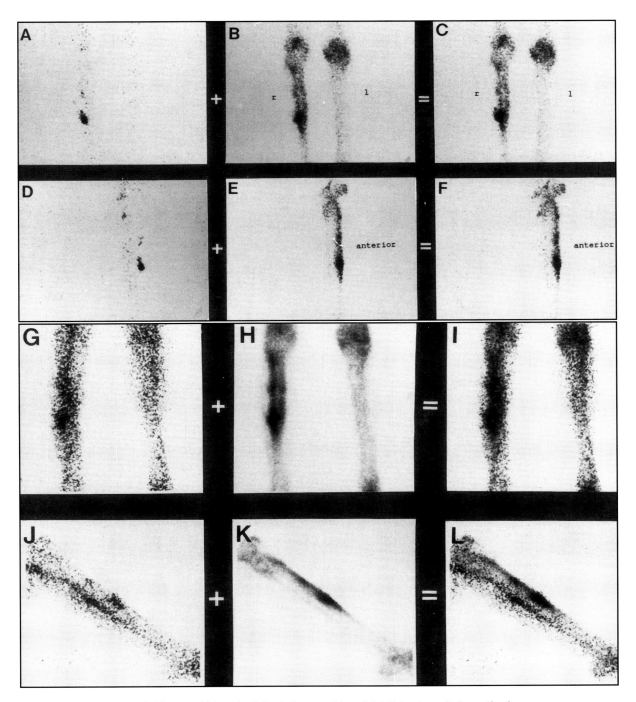

Fig. 11–18. A 48-year-old female diabetic fractured her right tibia at age 8. Recently she bumped the same area of her right leg and developed ulcers and drainage. **A** and **D**, The anterior and right lateral 24-hour In-111 labeled leukocyte images, respectively. **B** and **E**, The anterior and right lateral Tc-99m MDP bone scan images obtained simultaneously. **C** and **F**, The superimposition of (**A**) on (**B**) and (**D**) on (**E**), respectively. **G** and **J**, The anterior and right lateral 24-hour In-111 labeled IgG images, respectively. **H** and **K**, The Tc-99m MDP bone scan images obtained simultaneously with (**G**) and (**J**). **I** and **L**, The superimposition of (**G**) on (**H**) and (**J**) on (**K**), respectively. Notice that both studies show osteomyelitis in the anterior tibial cortex. Due to the higher background activity of the In-111 labeled IgG, the MDP study was not necessary for the interpretation of the IgG study.

In-111 labeled IgG is directly compared with In-111 labeled leukocytes in the same patients, they generally give similar results (Fig. 11-18). Phase III trials have been completed in the United States. Indium-111 labeled IgG is currently available in Europe.

The main problems with labeled antibodies are slow blood clearance and relatively low lesion-to-background ratios. Very recently bacterial chemotactic peptides composed of three amino acid residues have been proposed that give higher lesion-to-background ratios and faster blood clearance. Recent work suggests that the chemotactic peptides labeled with Tc-99m actually have higher lesion-to-background ratios than labeled leukocytes.[2] Work with these agents is very preliminary and mainly restricted to animal studies; however, this may be a very important commercial product in the future. Fischman et al wrote an excellent review on this subject.[11]

CONCLUSION

In conclusion, how does one approach the patient with suspected osteomyelitis? The first study is always the plain radiograph. If it is diagnostic, the evaluation is complete. If not, it can determine which studies should follow.

Current scintigraphic diagnosis of osteomyelitis in various clinical situations can be summarized as follows: (1) If the suspected osteomyelitis is in a location that is normal on the radiograph, the three-phase bone scan is highly sensitive and specific. In routine clinical practice this situation should be the most common. (2) Suspected complicating osteomyelitis in the non–marrow-containing skeleton can be evaluated by using the combined three-phase bone scan/In-111 labeled leukocyte study. (3) Suspected complicating osteomyelitis in the bone marrow–containing skeleton (e.g., spine, hips, and knees) can be evaluated by using the combined bone marrow/In-111 labeled leukocyte study.

Computed tomography (CT) gives excellent images of the bone cortex and is still used to determine the cortical extent of bone infection. In addition, it is used to guide the biopsy in vertebral osteomyelitis or other procedures when fluoroscopy would be suboptimal. However, in most situations CT has been replaced by magnetic resonance (MR) imaging.

MR imaging has the best resolution of soft-tissue versus bone infection of any imaging technique. Sensitivity is quite high at about 95%, and specificity is about 85% to 90%.[56,60,64,65] However, any disease process that replaces bone marrow and causes increased tissue water (e.g., healing fractures or tumors) may resemble osteomyelitis.[3,56] In addition, artifacts caused by joint implants may degrade the images sufficiently to make diagnosis of infected joint arthroplasty impossible.[3] For osteomyelitis with a normal radiograph, MR imaging gives results similar to the three-phase bone scan but is considerably more expensive. At our institution MR imaging is rarely used to diagnose osteomyelitis; however, its excellent resolution is often used to determine the extent of infection. This use of MR imaging is similar to that proposed by Gold.[15]

By carefully choosing the study or combination of studies, the correct diagnosis can usually be made. In the future new radiopharmaceuticals with simple preparation will become available that should make the job easier.

ACKNOWLEDGMENTS

I wish to express my appreciation to Kathy Carlson and Katie Natalie for their help in the preparation of this manuscript. The studies at Indiana University and a portion of their salaries were supported in part by National Institutes of Health grant RO1 AR 36460.

REFERENCES

1. Ash JM, Gilday DL: The futility of bone scanning in neonatal osteomyelitis: Concise communication. *J Nucl Med* 1980; 21:417.
2. Babich JW, Graham W, Barrow SA, et al: Technetium-99m-labeled chemotactic peptides for infection imaging: Comparison with In-111-labeled leukocytes in infected rabbits. *J Nucl Med* 1993; 34:2176.
3. Beltran J, Wenzel W: Experimental infections of the musculoskeletal system: Evaluation with MR imaging and Tc-99m MDP and Ga-67 scintigraphy. *Radiology* 1988; 167:167.
4. Berkowitz ID, Wenzel W: "Normal" technetium bone scans in patients with acute osteomyelitis. *Am J Dis Child* 1980; 134:828.
5. Buscombe JR, Lui D, Ensing G, et al: 99mTc-human immunoglobulin (HIG): First results of a new agent for the localization of infection and inflammation. *Eur J Nucl Med* 1990; 16:649.
6. Datz FL, Anderson CE, Ahluwalia R, et al: The efficacy of indium-111 polyclonal IgG for the detection of infection and inflammation. *J Nucl Med* 1994; 35:74.
7. Datz FL, Thorne DA, Taylor A: Cold bone defects on the In-111 labeled leukocyte scans. *J Nucl Med* 1986; 27:977 (abstract).
8. Edwards CL, Hayes R, Ahumada J, et al: Gallium-68 citrate: A clinically useful skeletal scanning agent. *J Nucl Med* 1966; 7:363.
9. Eisenberg B, Powe JE, Alavi A: Cold defects in In-111 labeled leukocyte imaging of osteomyelitis in the axial skeleton. *Clin Nucl Med* 1991; 16:103.
10. Fernandez-Ulloa M, Hughes JA, Krugh KB, et al: Bone imaging in infections: Artifacts from spectral overlap between a Tc-99m tracer and In-111 leukocytes. *J Nucl Med* 1983; 24:589.
11. Fischman AJ, Babich JW, Strauss HW: A ticket to ride: Peptide radiopharmaceuticals. *J Nucl Med* 1993; 34:2253.
12. Fischman AJ, Rubin RH, Khaw BA, et al: Detection of acute inflammation with In-111 labeled nonspecific polyclonal IgG. *Semin Nucl Med* 1988; 18:335.
13. Gilday DL, Paul DJ, Paterson J: Diagnosis of osteomyelitis in children by combined blood pool and bone imaging. *Radiology* 1975; 117:331.
14. Glynn TP: Marked gallium accumulation in neurogenic arthropathy. *J Nucl Med* 1981; 22:1016.
15. Gold R: Diagnosis of osteomyelitis. *Pediatr Rev* 1991; 12:292.

16. Hadjipavlou A, Lisbona R, Rosenthall L: Difficulty of diagnosing infected hypertrophic pseudoarthrosis by radionuclide imaging. *Clin Nucl Med* 1983; 8:45.

17. Handmaker H, Leonards R: The bone scan in inflammatory osseous disease. *Semin Nucl Med* 1976; 6:95.

18. Hetherington VJ: Technetium and combined gallium and technetium scans in the neurotrophic foot. *J Am Podiatr Med Assoc* 1982; 72:458.

19. Hindi MY, Burt RW, Siddiqui AR, et al: A novel radionuclide to radiograph overlay technique for precise localization of osteomyelitis and its differentiation from cellulitis using Tc-leukocytes. *Clin Nucl Med* 1992; 17:523 (abstract).

20. Hoffer P: Gallium: Mechanisms. *J Nucl Med* 1980; 21:282.

21. Howie DW, Savage JP, Wilson TG, et al: The technetium phosphate bone scan in the diagnosis of osteomyelitis in childhood. *J Bone Joint Surg Am* 1983; 65-A:431.

22. Keenan AM, Tindel NL, Alavi A: Diagnosis of pedal osteomyelitis in diabetic patients using current scintigraphic techniques. *Arch Intern Med* 1989; 149:2262.

23. King AD, Peters AM, Stuttle AWJ, et al: Imaging of bone infection with labeled white cells: Role of contemporaneous bone marrow imaging. *Eur J Nucl Med* 1990; 17:148.

24. Lind P, Langsteger W, Koltringer P, et al: Immunoscintigraphy of inflammatory processes with a technetium-99m-labeled monoclonal antigranulocyte antibody (MAb BW 250/183). *J Nucl Med* 1990; 31:417.

25. Lisbona R, Rosenthall L: Observations on the sequential use of 99mTc-phosphate complex and 67-Ga imaging in osteomyelitis, cellulitis, and septic arthritis. *Radiology* 1977; 123:123.

26. Magnuson JE, Brown ML, Hauser MF, et al: In-111-labeled leukocyte scintigraphy in suspected orthopedic prosthesis infection: Comparison with other imaging modalities. *Radiology* 1988; 168:235.

27. Majd M, Frankel RS: Radionuclide imaging in skeletal inflammatory and ischemic disease in children. *AJR Am J Roentgenol* 1976; 126:832.

28. Maurer AH, Chen DCP, Camargo EE, et al: Utility of three-phase skeletal scintigraphy in suspected osteomyelitis: Concise communication. *J Nucl Med* 1981; 22:941.

29. McCarthy K, Velchik MG, Alavi A, et al: Indium-111-labeled white blood cells in the detection of osteomyelitis complicated by a pre-existing condition. *J Nucl Med* 1988; 29:1015.

30. Merkel KD, Brown ML, Fitzgerald RH Jr: Sequential technetium-99m HMDP-gallium-67 citrate imaging for the evaluation of infection in the painful prosthesis. *J Nucl Med* 1986; 27:1413.

31. Modic MT, Pflanze W, Feiglin DHI, et al: Magnetic resonance imaging of musculoskeletal infections. *Radiol Clin North Am* 1986; 24:247.

32. Mok YP, Carney WH, Fernandez-Ulloa M: Skeletal photopenic lesions in In-111 WBC imaging. *J Nucl Med* 1984; 25:1322.

33. Oyen WJG, Claessens RAMJ, van Horn JR, et al: Scintigraphic detection of bone and joint infections with indium-111-labeled nonspecific polyclonal human immunoglobulin G. *J Nucl Med* 1990; 31:403.

34. Palestro CJ, Kim C, Swyer AJ, et al: Total hip arthroplasty: Periprosthetic indium-111-labeled leukocyte activity and complementary technetium-99m-sulfur colloid imaging in suspected infection. *J Nucl Med* 1990; 31:1950.

35. Palestro CJ, Kim C, Swyer AJ, et al: Radionuclide diagnosis of vertebral osteomyelitis: indium-111-leukocyte and technetium-99m-methylene diphosphonate bone scintigraphy. *J Nucl Med* 1991; 32:1861.

36. Palestro CJ, Roumanas P, Kim CK, et al: Improved accuracy for diagnosing osteomyelitis using combined In-111 leukocyte and Tc-99m sulfur colloid imaging. *J Nucl Med* 1991; 32:962 (abstract).

37. Palestro CJ, Swyer AJ, Kim CK, et al: Infected knee prosthesis: Diagnosis with In-111 leukocyte, Tc-99m sulfur colloid, and Tc-99m imaging. *Radiology* 1991; 179:645.

38. Park HM, Wheat LJ, Siddiqui AR, et al: Scintigraphic evaluation of diabetic osteomyelitis: Concise communication. *J Nucl Med* 1982; 23:569.

39. Roddie ME, Peters AM, Danpure HJ, et al: Inflammation: Imaging with Tc-99m HMPAO-labeled leukocytes. *Radiology* 1988; 166:767.

40. Rosenthall L, Kloiber R, Damtew B, et al: Sequential use of radiophosphate and radiogallium imaging in the differential diagnosis of bone, joint and soft tissue infection: Quantitative analysis. *Diagn Imaging* 1982; 51:249.

41. Rubin RH, Fischman AJ, Callahan RJ, et al: Indium-111 labeled nonspecific immunoglobulin scanning in the detection of focal infection. *N Engl J Med* 1989; 321:935.

42. Rubin RH, Young LS, Hansen WP, et al: Specific and non-specific imaging of localized Fisher immunotype *Pseudomonas aeruginosa* infection with radiolabeled monoclonal antibody. *J Nucl Med* 1988; 29:651.

43. Ruther W, Hotze A, Moller F, et al: Diagnosis of bone and joint infection by leukocyte scintigraphy: A comparative study with 99mTc-HMPAO-labeled leukocytes, 99mTc-labeled antigranulocyte antibodies and 99mTc-labeled nanocolloid. *Arch Orthop Trauma Surg* 1990; 110:26.

44. Schauwecker DS: Osteomyelitis: Diagnosis with In-111 labeled leukocytes. *Radiology* 1989; 171:141.

45. Schauwecker DS, Park HM, Burt RW, et al: Combined bone scintigraphy and indium-111 leukocyte scans in neuropathic foot disease. *J Nucl Med* 1988; 29:1651.

46. Schauwecker DS, Park HM, Mock BH, et al: Evaluation of complicating osteomyelitis with Tc-99m MDP, In-111 granulocytes, and Ga-67 citrate. *J Nucl Med* 1984; 25:849.

47. Seybold K, Locher JT, Coosemans C, et al: Immunoscintigraphic localization of inflammatory lesions: Clinical experience. *Eur J Nucl Med* 1988; 3:587.

48. Seabold JE, Nepola JV, Conrad GR, et al: Detection of osteomyelitis at fracture nonunion sites: Comparison of two scintigraphic methods. *AJR Am J Roentgenol* 1989; 152:1021.

49. Sfakianakis GN, Al-Sheikh W, Heal A, et al: Comparison of scintigraphy with In-111 leukocytes and Ga-67 in the diagnosis of occult sepsis. *J Nucl Med* 1982; 23:618.

50. Shafer RB, Marlette JM, Browne GA, et al: The role of Tc-99m phosphate complexes and gallium-67 in the diagnosis and management of maxillofacial disease: Concise communication. *J Nucl Med* 1981; 22:8.

51. Sugarman B: Pressure sores and underlying bone infection. *Arch Intern Med* 1987; 147:553.

52. Sullivan DC, Rosenfield NS, Ogden J, et al. Problems in the scintigraphic detection of osteomyelitis in children. *Radiology* 1980; 135:731.

53. Thakur ML, Lavender JP, Arnot RN, et al: Indium-111-labeled autologous leukocytes in man. *J Nucl Med* 1977; 18:1014.

54. Thakur ML, Segal AW, Louis L, et al: Indium-111-labeled cellular blood components: Mechanism of labeling and intracellular location in human neutrophils. *J Nucl Med* 1977; 18:1022.

55. Thrall JH, Geslien GE, Corcoron RJ, et al: Abnormal radionuclide deposition patterns adjacent to focal skeletal lesions. *Radiology* 1975; 115:659.

56. Unger E, Moldofsky P, Gatenby R, et al: Diagnosis of osteomyelitis by MR imaging. *AJR Am J Roentgenol* 1988; 150:605.

57. Uzum F, Akansel G, Ozker K, et al: In-111 WBC vs Tc-99m WBC imaging for the detection of osteomyelitis. *J Nucl Med* 1994; 35:88P (abstract).

58. Verlooy H, Mortelmans L, Verbruggen A, et al: Tc-99m HMPAO labeled leukocyte scanning for detection of infection in orthopedic surgery. *Prog Clin Biol Res* 1990; 355:181.

59. Vorne M, Lantto T, Paakkinen S, et al: Clinical comparison of Tc-99m-HMPAO labeled leukocytes and Tc-99m-nanocolloid in the detection of inflammation. *Acta Radiol* 1989; 30:633.

60. Wang A, Weinstein D, Greenfield L, et al: MRI and diabetic foot infections. *Magn Reson Imaging* 1990; 8:805.

61. Wellman HN, Siddiqui A, Mail JT, et al: Choice of radiotracer in the study of bone or joint infection in children. *Ann Radiol (Paris)* 1983; 26:411.

62. Whalen JL, Brown M, McLeod R, et al: Limitations of indium leukocyte imaging for the diagnosis of spine infections. *Spine* 1991; 16:193.

63. Wukich DK, Abreu SH, Callaghan JJ, et al: Diagnosis of infection by preoperative scintigraphy with indium-labeled white blood cells. *J Bone Joint Surg Am* 1987; 69-A:1353.

64. Yuh WTC, Corson JD, Baraniewski HM, et al: Osteomyelitis of the foot in diabetic patients: Evaluation with plain film, 99mTc-MDP bone scintigraphy, and MR imaging. *AJR Am J Roentgenol* 1989; 152:795.

65. Zynamon A, Jung T, Hodler J, et al: Osteitis-imaging with magnetic resonance tomography. *Helv Chir Acta* 1989; 56:561.

CHAPTER 12

ARTHRITIS AND ALLIED DISORDERS

Leonard Rosenthall

RADIOPHARMACEUTICALS

The joint disorders can be divided into two general categories for purposes of radionuclide scanning: primary synovial and primary bone. They may blend in that a primary synovial disease could cause bone erosion, and a primary bone lesion may be associated with synovitis. The inflammatory joint diseases consist of rheumatoid arthritis, Reiter's syndrome, psoriasis, gout, ankylosing spondylitis, systemic lupus erythematosus, infection, and other less common disorders. Osteoarthritis is the most frequently occurring noninflammatory bone disorder, but other entities in the primary bone group include osteonecrosis, reflex sympathetic dystrophy, neuroarthropathy, trauma, mechanical abnormalities, infection, and others.

Initial radionuclide applications to assess joint disease consisted of an intracavitary administration of the test agent and a measurement of its rate of disappearance by means of an external counting probe. Agents used for that purpose were ^{131}I-albumin, ^{131}I-globulin, Na[131]I, [24]Na, and ^{133}Xe in saline solution.[1,14,18,31,74] The rate of disappearance of these agents was found to increase as the intensity of the inflammation increased. Steroids and other antiinflammatory drugs reduced the clearance rates from the synovial cavity. This method had merit as a quantitative research tool, but it was time consuming, limited to large joints for technical reasons, and not amenable to screening a large number of patients with diffuse joint symptoms. The method has been abandoned for routine clinical use and reserved for specific animal research indications, measurement of the effectiveness of new antiinflammatory drugs, and assessment of the status of postsynovectomy joints. The advent of intravenously injected ^{131}I-albumin, which portrayed the expanded blood pool of the inflamed synovium, facilitated the study of all the joints with a single administration.[100]

A variety of radioactive test agents for intravenous use have been introduced over the years. They can be categorized into three groups of compartment markers:

(1) Vascular Compartment
[131]I-albumin
[131]I-iodopamide[56]
[99m]TcO$_4$ (pertechnetate)[28]
[99m]Tc-albumin[10]

^{113m}In[54]
^{99m}Tc-DTPA[57]
^{99m}Tc-erythrocytes[78]
(2) Bone Compartment
^{85}Sr[35]
^{87m}Sr
^{18}F[38]
^{99m}Tc-phosphate complexes[17]
(3) Inflammatory Site Compartment
^{67}Ga citrate[93]
^{111}In-leukocytes and ^{99m}Tc-leukocytes[2,95]
^{99m}Tc-liposomes[91]
^{99m}Tc-albumin nanocolloid[90]
^{111}In-chloride[82]
^{99m}Tc–polyclonal human immunoglobulin G[7]
Monoclonal antibody to granulocytes[40]
^{99m}Tc-CD4 specific antibody[40]
^{111}In-anti-E-selection
^{111}In-somatostatin

There is increased blood flow, enlargement of the vascular pool, and interstitial edema in synovitis, whether aseptic or septic. Vascular compartment markers reflect these features by increased transit of the ^{99m}Tc labeled agents on first-pass intravenous radionuclide angiography and by enhanced concentration relative to surrounding normal tissue in the equilibrium blood pool phase immediately thereafter. Anastomotic blood vessels between the synovium and juxtaarticular bone extend the hyperemia of the synovitis to the dependent bone. This results in increased accretion of bone-seeking agents, such as the ^{99m}Tc-phosphate complexes, at the site of synovitis. When there is subchondral bone destruction, the local increased uptake represents the normal bone response to the insult.

The mechanism of indium and gallium uptake, inflammatory site markers, is still not clearly established. It is suggested that the injected ^{111}In, or ^{67}Ga, binds to intravascular transferrin and is then carried to the transferrin receptors that are abundant in the inflamed synovium. Alternatively, they can bind directly to the transferrin located in the synovium.[13] Radioactive leukocytes, whether labeled in vitro with ^{111}In or ^{99m}Tc, or in vivo with monoclonal antibodies to granulocytes, accumulate at sites of leukocyte migration. They are excellent for identifying septic synovitis, but leukocytes are also present in relatively small and variable numbers in rheumatoid arthritis. A distinction between the two entities may be difficult on occasion. It is speculated that liposomes and perhaps nanocolloids are phagocytosed by the macrophages present in the synovial tissue. Because the number of macrophages increases with the degree of inflammation, the radioactive uptake varies with the intensity of the inflammatory process.[91] There is still no consensus regarding the events by which radiolabeled immunoglobulin G (IgG) accumulates at the inflammatory sites. Exudation of plasma proteins through the abnormally permeable capillary wall and specific trapping of the Fc part of IgG by Fc receptors located on the inflammatory cells (i.e., neutrophils, lymphocytes, and macrophages) has been proposed as a mechanism of

uptake.[80] In rheumatoid arthritis the localization of IgG at sites of synovial inflammation might also be due to binding of the Fc part to rheumatoid factor, which is produced by the B lymphocytes that are present. The anti-CD4 monoclonal antibodies recognize the CD4 molecule expressed on the T helper cells, and, with lower density, on macrophages. Both of these cellular elements are abundant in the inflammatory infiltrates of rheumatoid arthritis.

SYNOVITIS

Synovial inflammation induces changes in the terminal arterioles, capillaries, and venules with resultant hyperemia, increase in the number and size of the vessels, and vascular permeability. In rheumatoid arthritis and related disorders, there is also an accumulation of polymorphonuclear leukocytes in the acute phase, located primarily in the joint fluid. Infiltration of lymphocytes, macrophages, and plasma cells becomes evident in the chronic phase, but these elements are found in the interstitium, whereas the polymorphonuclear leukocytes are still confined for the most part to the joint effusion. These cellular infiltrations are probably the basis for the low-grade migration of the radiolabeled leukocytes to the site.

The normal synovium is not visualized by the various blood compartment markers used in practice, because the concentration does not exceed that of the adjacent soft tissue. When synovial inflammation intervenes, the selective accumulation at the site of test agents, like radiopertechnetate and ^{99m}Tc-albumin, exceeds background and are resolvable by scanning. These agents are primarily confined to the blood vessels and interstitium of the membrane, as very little activity is recovered in aspirated joint fluids.[28]

In a rabbit model of arthritis induced by the intraarticular injection of ovalbumin into sensitized animals, radiopertechnetate and radiophosphate were found in bone and soft tissue. The maximum uptake of radiophosphate was in bone, whereas radiopertechnetate was predominantly in the synovium.[75] Using the rabbit model of zymosan-induced arthritis, the highest concentration of ^{67}Ga-citrate occurred in the inflamed synovium, but there was also increased accretion in the fat pad, patella, meniscus, and adjacent tendons.[93] No ^{67}Ga was found in the juxtaarticular bone. A correlation between ^{67}Ga knee-to-femur count rate ratios and leukocyte content in the aspirated fluid of patients who have active rheumatoid arthritis indicated that the ratios vary with the degree of synovial inflammation.[58]

Blood compartment and inflammatory site markers are preferable to the radiophosphates whose uptake in bone is secondary to synovial hyperemia. Periarticular bone uptake may be due to other causes, such as transient osteoporosis and reflex sympathetic dystrophy (i.e., it is not specific). Few false-positive results occur with blood compartment markers, and these are caused mainly by overlying cellulitis and edema. Osteoarthritic joints usually are normal, unless complicated by synovitis. Despite the theoretical advantages of blood compartment markers, they are disadvantaged by low target-to-background ratios for peripheral joints relative to those obtained with radiophosphates. This is caused by a shift of some of the radiopertechnetate and labeled albumin from the intravascular space to the extravascular space of the background during the time that it takes to complete the imaging survey. ^{99m}Tc-erythrocytes have been used to avoid this undesirable space shift, but its efficacy relative to radiophosphate is not yet established (Fig. 12-1). Hips, sacroiliac joints, and shoulders are surrounded by a greater soft-tissue mass than the peripheral joints, and this further reduces the effectiveness of the blood compartment markers at these sites.

[67]Ga-citrate has been used extensively in synovitis, and although its accretion is more closely associated with the cellular component of the inflammatory process, it does have several drawbacks (Fig. 12-2). There is at least a 24-hour delay before imaging, which entails two patient visits, and the count rate is low for the conventional diagnostic doses given. Since the time to obtain total-body joint scans is inordinately prolonged because of these low count rates, ^{67}Ga imaging is usually reserved for the study of specific joints and perhaps for monitoring treatment when indicated. The efficacies of ^{111}In-chloride, ^{99m}Tc or ^{111}In labeled IgG, ^{99m}Tc-CD4 monoclonal antibody and labeled liposomes are yet to be fully determined. These test agents are recent introductions and clinical experience is limited. Monoclonal antibodies to granulocytes have been used experimentally in septic joint models, but there is some potential in its application to aseptic synovitis as well.

Many comparative crossover studies have been reported. In 16 patients who had synovitis due to rheumatoid arthritis, psoriasis and Reiter's syndrome (Fig. 12-3), radiopertechnetate disclosed fewer abnormal joints than clinical assessment in 12 patients, but all clinically affected joints were seen with ^{99m}Tc-polyphosphate. ^{99m}Tc-polyphosphate showed more joint involvement than clinical examination in 15 of the 16 patients, but this occurred in only 2 patients with radiopertechnetate.[17] A comparison of the efficacy of radionuclide and radiographic and clinical assessment was made in another group of patients with synovitis.[26] This study demonstrated 11% more abnormal joints by ^{99m}Tc-polyphosphate imaging than clinical impression, and 72% more abnormalities than by radiography in 191 abnormal joints. A closer analysis of the data showed that the radionuclide study performed less well than clinical judgment in large joints such as the shoulders, elbows, and knees, but the reverse was obtained in the peripheral joints—namely, the wrists, hands, ankles, and feet. There was no difficulty when large joints were asymmetrically inflamed; however, symmetrically small but equal increases in accretion were difficult to discern from the normally higher and variable concentrations that exist at these articulations. It is in these areas that blood compartment markers such as radiopertechnetate, ^{99m}Tc-albumin, or ^{99m}Tc-erythrocytes, may be useful as an adjunctive procedure, because the synovium will not be

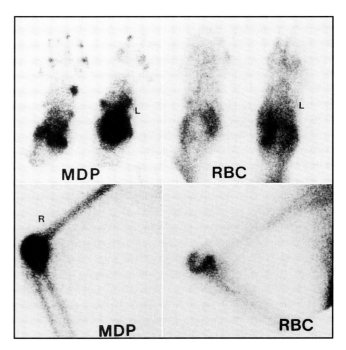

Fig. 12-1. Rheumatoid arthritis. Comparison of ^{99m}Tc-MDP and ^{99m}Tc–red blood cells in a 55-year-old female. *Upper panel:* Intense accretion of radiophosphate in both ankles and relatively less in the left tarsus and several metatarsophalangeal joints and toes. Abnormal labeled red cell activity is confined primarily to the ankles and left tarsus. The other joints that are also abnormal by ^{99m}Tc-MDP do not exhibit appreciable synovitis by labeled red cells. This suggests that there is bone remodeling, perhaps due to erosive disease or osteoarthritis, but no synovitis. *Lower panel:* Avid periarticular concentration of ^{99m}Tc-MDP at the right elbow. There is a corresponding intense labeled red cell accumulation in the distribution of the synovium indicative of synovitis. (*From Rosenthall L: The bone scan in arthritis, in Fogelman I:* Bone Scanning in Clinical Practice, *Springer-Verlag, Berlin, 1987; with permission.*)

seen unless it is inflamed. The use of inflammatory site markers (e.g., ^{67}Ga, ^{99m}Tc-IgG) would be an alternative for the larger joints. Other authors have attested to the high sensitivity of radiophosphate imaging, particularly of the peripheral joints.[4,99]

In juvenile rheumatoid arthritis, there is a fairly high false-negative frequency owing to the interference of the avid uptake of radiophosphate by the growth plates.[39,94] Unlike adults, this is particularly troublesome in the small peripheral joints, where limited resolution frustrates the discrimination of periarticular uptake of synovitis from that of the growth plates. When there is asymmetry, or some of the joints are not involved and can therefore function as reference points, the differentiation may be less difficult. An exception is the knee, because increased accretion in the patella, resulting from its vascular anastomosis with the synovial network, can be seen in the lateral projection free of growth plate activity. ^{67}Ga-citrate, or any other inflammatory site marker, may be more successful when radiophosphate fails, but its efficacy has not been fully explored for juvenile rheumatoid arthritis. The synovitis of rheumatic

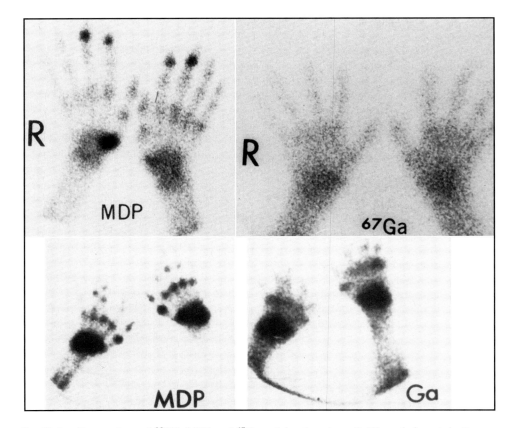

Fig. 12-2. Comparison of ^{99m}Tc-MDP and ^{67}Ga uptakes in osteoarthritis and chronic/active rheumatoid arthritis. *Upper panel:* ^{99m}Tc-MDP manifestations of osteoarthritis of the distal interphalangeal joints of the second and third fingers and trapeziometacarpal joints of both hands. The corresponding ^{67}Ga scans are normal. *Lower panel:* Extensive periarticular uptake of ^{99m}Tc-MDP in the metacarpophalangeal and some of the proximal interphalangeal joints of both hands and both wrists. There is a similar distribution of abnormal ^{67}Ga uptake, but the relative intensities differ at some of the individual joints. This is most likely due to the fact that ^{67}Ga uptake is a reflection of the degree of synovitis, whereas ^{99m}Tc-MDP is a function of inflammation, erosive disease, or both.

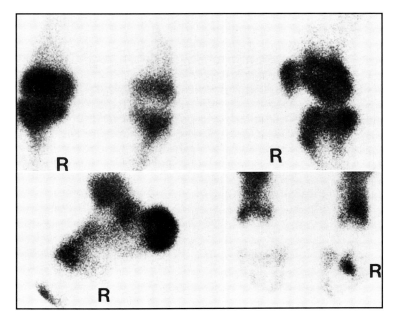

Fig. 12-3. Reiter's disease. A 21-year-old male depicting increased concentration of ^{99m}Tc-MDP about the right knee, right second metatarsophalangeal joint, and both ankles and tarsal bones. It is particularly intense in the right calcaneus, the so-called lover's heel.

fever can show avid radiophosphate and ^{67}Ga uptakes (Fig. 12-4).

The histology of polymyalgia rheumatica features a nonspecific chronic inflammation with infiltration of lymphocytes and plasma cells that extends beyond the synovium to include the capsule and adjacent soft tissues. As in systemic lupus erythematosus, the lack of an acute proliferative synovitis weighs against radiophosphate detection.[65] More success may accrue from inflammatory site markers, but a definitive study has not been done.

The relationship between the temporal radiophosphate joint manifestations and the development of bone erosions in newly diagnosed rheumatoid arthritis has been studied. In 13 patients (387 joints) who were followed for 24 months, only those joints that demonstrated high, persistent radioactive uptakes were prone to

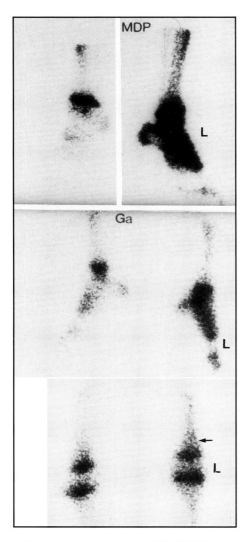

Fig. 12-4.   Rheumatic fever. Increased [99mTc]-MDP periarticular uptake in the left ankle and midfoot in a 9-year-old male. The enhanced ^{67}Ga uptake shows the same localization. There is also an abnormal low-grade uptake of ^{67}Ga in the synovium of the left knee, which flared up clinically a week later (*arrow*).

develop erosions by x-ray, with the toes being earlier than the fingers. Joints that were consistently normal by scan did not develop erosions within the 24-month interval. Computerized measurement of bone uptake had a higher correlation with the incidence of erosion than visual appraisal.[60] In a more chronic stage of rheumatoid arthritis with established radiographic evidence of erosions in the hands, not all of the joints with erosions exhibited increased uptake of radiophosphate.[70] Presumably the absence of abnormal uptake indicated that the erosions were metabolically inactive and stable in size.

Thirty patients with an established diagnosis of rheumatoid arthritis were studied with [99mTc]-IgG. The radiotracer uptake scores were correlated with the scores for joint pain and swelling, radiographic bone destruction, and C-reactive protein levels. Correlation with joint swelling and C-reactive protein levels were good, poor with pain, and not significant with radiography. Among the joints the correlation between swelling and radiotracer uptake was poorest at the shoulders, where uptake was frequently present when swelling was impalpable.[15] This could be anticipated as the clinical assessment of swelling at the shoulder, and especially the hip, are very difficult owing to the overlying muscle mass. Indeed, the radionuclide findings may be more sensitive for active inflammation in those regions.

A crossover clinical trial was reported in two groups of 10 patients, each with active rheumatoid arthritis: [99mTc]-IgG versus [99mTc]-leukocytes in group 1, and [99mTc]-IgG versus [99mTc]-albumin nanocolloid in group 2. In group 1 100% of the clinically active joints had positive [99mTc]-IgG scans, and 92% of the clinically inactive joints had negative scans. This compared with 46% positive [99mTc]-leukocyte scans in clinically abnormal joints and 98% negative scans in the clinically inactive joints. Clinically active joints in group 2 demonstrated 93% positive scans with [99mTc]-IgG and 79% positive [99mTc]–nanocolloid scans, whereas clinically inactive joints had 91% and 95% negative scans, respectively. Shoulders and hips were excluded from the trial. The false-positive frequency was higher for [99mTc]-IgG than either the labeled leukocytes or nanocolloid.[51] It is conceivable that [99mTc]-IgG is more sensitive than the clinical examination. In patients with overt rheumatoid arthritis, histologic proof of inflammation of synovial tissue was found in joints that were not clinically involved.[86] The existence of this subclinical status implies that many of the false-positive radionuclide results may in fact be true-positive results.

In an effort to determine whether the uptake of [99mTc]–anti-CD4 monoclonal antibody in the synovium differed from that of nonspecific [99mTc]–polyclonal human IgG, since both are immunoglobulins, 5 patients with active rheumatoid arthritis were entered into a crossover study. When the uptake in the afflicted joints was expressed as a percentage of total-body activity, there was no significant difference between the two test agents. A different analysis compared the visual grading scores of knee and elbow uptake relative to the adjacent blood vessels at 4 hours postinjection, and they showed that the

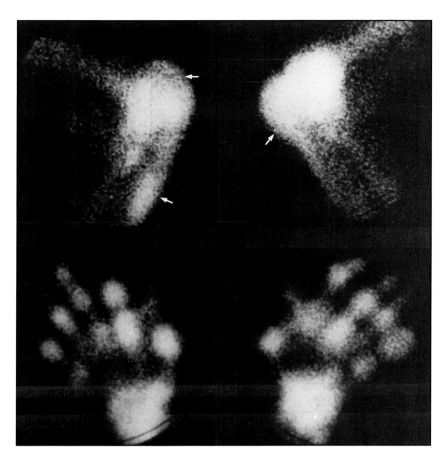

Fig. 12-5. Gout. There is intense periarticular radiophosphate uptake in both wrists, and most of the metacarpophalangeal and proximal interphalangeal joints, and both elbows. Avid uptake by the gouty tophi is seen bilaterally (*arrows*).

anti-CD4 antibody was significantly higher than the polyclonal antibodies in these patients. This indicated that a more specific imaging of the arthritic joints takes place with the anti-CD4 antibodies. It was also speculated that since anti-CD4 antibodies preferentially bind to mononuclear cells infiltrating abnormally inflamed joints, but not polymorphonuclear leukocytes, they may be able to differentiate acute septic arthritis from chronic joint infiltration.[44]

The distinction between septic and aseptic synovitis with ^{67}Ga is not always clearcut. When there is a high-grade intensity in the synovium it favors sepsis, but lower-grade intensity is nonspecific. Rheumatoid joints, for example, may be complicated by sepsis, and it may be difficult to distinguish from reactivation.

Gout is a disorder of uric acid metabolism characterized by hyperuricemia, resulting in the deposition of urates principally in joints, periarticular tissues, and kidneys. This leads to synovitis, and granulation pannus formation and gouty tophi that cause bone erosion. The tophi are composed of crystalline or amorphous urates, which may be seen on the radiophosphate images (Fig. 12-5).

Quantitative Joint Measurement

Quantitative methods have been devised with the aim of removing the subjective indecision related to estimating periarticular radiophosphate accretion. This is usual-

ly addressed by obtaining a ratio of the uptake at the affected joint to that of the adjacent normal bone or soft tissue. Some authors have compared the joint uptake with an in vitro standard source. Measurements of radiophosphate uptake over groups of small joints of the hands, rather than individual joints, and comparing them to the uptake level of an internal reference bone in the form of a ratio has also been advocated to improve sensitivity.[69,98] Another communication related the results of a comparison of four parameters in patients with documented rheumatoid arthritis: ratio of joint-to-nonjoint using count rate per unit area; ratio of joint-to-nonjoint using count rate only; absolute uptake per unit area normalized for body weight and dose; absolute uptake normalized for body weight and dose. The nonjoint reference bone was the combined midradius and midulna when the normal and inflamed hands were measured, and the midfemur served as reference nonjoint bone for the knee measurements. The best separation was achieved with absolute uptake per unit area normalized for body weight and dose, but there was still a considerable overlap between the normals and those with synovitis. The parameter rendering the least discrimination was the ratio of joint uptake to nonjoint uptake.[76]

Many of the studies reported seem to assume that the nonjoint reference bone is unaffected by the inflammatory process, but there is mounting evidence to the contrary. In patients with active rheumatoid arthritis of the hand, the count rates in the midradius and midulna on the same side were on average 35% greater than the contralateral side when the hand was quiescent. No difference was noted between uptakes in the midfemur in patients with active rheumatoid arthritis of the knee and the control side. The existing differences may have been neutralized by the large soft-tissue mass surrounding the femur, which adds to the background and also absorbs and scatters the photons emitted by bone. The lumbar-spine-to-soft-tissue ratio was elevated by 28% in 19 patients with rheumatoid arthritis compared with an age-matched and sex-matched control group of patients. Rheumatoid arthritis usually does not involve the lumbar spine, nor was there evidence of it in this trial.[77] Total-body 24-hour retention measurements of ^{99m}Tc-MDP by two different methods showed that the rheumatoid group was 45% and 33%, respectively, greater than normal.[30,73,88] Although these increases could be attributed to the enhanced periarticular uptake rather than nonjoint uptake, there was no correlation of the 24-hour retention values with the number and size of the joints involved (Landsbury index), sedimentation rate, functional class or rheumatoid factor titer. By inference, the results of the lumbar-spine-to-soft-tissue ratio and total-body 24-hour retention support the thesis of a generalized reaction superimposed on a local articular process. It is not surprising that joint-to-bone ratios have failed to clearly discriminate actively inflamed rheumatoid joints from control joints, because the denominator, representing nonjoint activity, may be elevated. At this time there is no acceptable quantitative parameter for radiophosphate imaging that can be used in a screening procedure. There is merit in these parameters for numerically monitoring the response to treatment, as ratios in the normal range have been shown to decrease with successful inflammatory suppression.[66] Whichever parameter is adopted, the ultimate confirmation of its efficacy will be synovial biopsy, not clinical or radiographic impressions.

An analysis of ^{99m}Tc-pyrophosphate scans in non-pathologic joint pairs showed a significantly higher right-sided concentration in 37%, a left-sided dominance in 21%, and no difference in the remaining 42%. The highest incidence of disparity occurred at the glenohumeral articulation. Some of this discrepancy can be explained by the person's dominant side or handedness.[62]

Normal Radiophosphate Joint Scan

A positive radiophosphate joint scan is not specific for synovitis, and the results must be interpreted within the clinical context. The frequency of false-positive joint scans is unknown, because synovial biopsy verification is rarely performed, and a negative conventional radiograph is not a benchmark for absence of synovitis or some other process that might induce enhanced radiophosphate accretion. An important question is the significance of a negative study in a patient complaining of polyarthralgia, which is a common ailment and usually occurs without causative synovitis. A partial answer to

this question was obtained from a study of two groups of patients. In group A there were 22 patients who had polyarthralgia for at least 3 months. They had normal radiophosphate joint scans, or noninflammatory joint scans typical of osteoarthritis (focal uptake limited to the compartments of the knee joints, focal uptake in the wrists, uptakes limited to one side of a joint, and so forth). Group B had the same number of patients, age-matched and sex-matched, but with abnormal radiophosphate joints portraying diffuse periarticular uptake characteristic of acute synovitis. The patients were reexamined later at 3.6 ± 0.9 and 4.0 ± 1.0 years, respectively. None of the patients in group A with previous normal scans had evidence of inflammatory disease. In contrast, 21 of the 22 patients in group B still had active synovitis by clinical examination. There were 12 cases of rheumatoid arthritis, 5 of psoriasis, and 1 each of Reiter's syndrome, ankylosing spondylitis, mixed connective tissue disease, and undifferentiated connective tissue disease in group B. The one patient who was free of disease on recall was in clinical remission of documented juvenile rheumatoid arthritis. Three patients in group A originally were thought to have clinical synovitis, but two were later shown to have poly-myalgia rheumatica and the other had systemic lupus erythematosus. Both of these conditions are known to render normal radiophosphate joint scans, because they feature a chronic, nonproliferative type of synovitis, unlike the proliferative type of acute rheumatoid arthritis that commands a substantial increase in blood flow.[84] The authors concluded that patients who have polyarthralgia, a negative or low probability rheumatologic examination, and a negative radiophosphate joint scan are unlikely to develop inflammatory polyarthritis. Radionuclide screening of this group of patients is useful.

SACROILIITIS

Sacroiliitis usually presents with bilateral enhanced accretion of radiophosphate. This can be difficult to appreciate visually, because there is normally a relatively higher concentration about the sacroiliac joints, and mild to moderate symmetric increases may escape detection. Various quantitative techniques have been proposed to obviate the subjective interpretation. A ratio of the peak sacroiliac joint count rate to the peak sacral count rate was originally introduced (Fig. 12-6). Early results indicated a clear separation of the controls from an experimental group of patients with ankylosing spondylitis.[81] Modifications were later proposed. One consisted of background-corrected sacroiliac-joint-to-sacrum ratios of the upper, middle and lower thirds of the joint, instead of the full length of the joint as originally described.[61] This maneuver was allegedly more sensitive in revealing the inflammatory process in the synovium, which is located in lower half of the joint. Another suggestion was the ratio of the peak joint count rate to the minimum count rate in the profile slice through the joints and sacrum, as it purportedly rendered a better separation between normal and diseased joints.[3]

To have clinical utility the radionuclide method must possess a high sensitivity at a stage of the disease when the radiographic presentation is normal or equivocal (i.e., grades 0 and 1). It is imperative that the study is performed when the patient is not receiving antiinflammatory drugs and that a standardized procedure is followed. Specifically the same radiophosphate complex test agent must be used in all cases to avoid varying pharmacokinetics. Imaging times should be fixed between 4 and 5 hours, a time when the rate of accumulation of radioactivity has leveled off. Each laboratory should establish its own normal range. The patient should be rested, as physical exertion before the examination induces a hyperemia that may affect the ratio. A prospective study was reported using ^{99m}Tc-MDP in which a tightly standardized technique was followed. It demonstrated a significant difference between controls and ankylosing spondylitis associated with radiographic grades 0 to 1, 2, 3, and 4, respectively. Nevertheless, there was a substantial overlap of the ratios in patients with radiographic grades 0 to 1 disease and the 2 SD range of the ratios in the control group. The absence of a sharp separation militates against this technique for population screening.[23] There was a subset of patients with false-negative ratios in this study who were treated successfully with antiinflammatory drugs, and upon restudy the ratios exhibited a definite decrease. By inference, this is an objective diagnostic sign of preexisting sacroiliitis and may be an indication for monitoring treatment in selected cases. This has been confirmed by others.[21]

A study of the value of the triple profile slice (i.e., upper, middle, and lower thirds of the sacroiliac joint) in 26 patients with ankylosing spondylitis demonstrated no substantive improvement over the single full-length profile slice. Ten more abnormalities were detected with fractionation relative to unfractionation, but nine of these were in radiographic grades 3 and 4, and in grade 0—where it was most needed—only one was uncovered.[22]

Although there is uniform agreement that quantitative sacroiliac scintigraphy is superior to subjective visual appraisal, the lack of absolute separation of the affected and normal groups is well recognized. The degree of overlap in published reports is variable, as is its acceptability for clinical screening.[5,16,20,25,87] False-positive ratios may be caused by osteoarthritis, metabolic bone disease, and previous injury—lowering the specificity of the test. Age, gender, and laterality may also influence the ratios. The normal ratio is on average higher on the right side than the left side in all ages (both female and male), the right ratios are higher in males than females, and there is no variation of the ratio with age in either sex.[97] This contrasts with another communication that related a decrease in the normal ratio values with increasing age in both sexes.[19] To further confound the issue, it is claimed that the normal ratios decreased with age in females, but not males.[3]

The sacrum, the reference bone in these ratios, is assumed to be uninvolved in the inflammatory process. This has been refuted. Significantly higher uptakes of radiophosphate were found in the sacrum of patients afflicted with ankylosing spondylitis and Reiter's disease compared with a control group, perhaps mediated through a concomitant enthesopathy. Also, sacral accretion was normal in patients who had degenerative disk disease and diffuse idiopathic skeletal hyperostosis (DISH) in this control group. This implies that the ratio

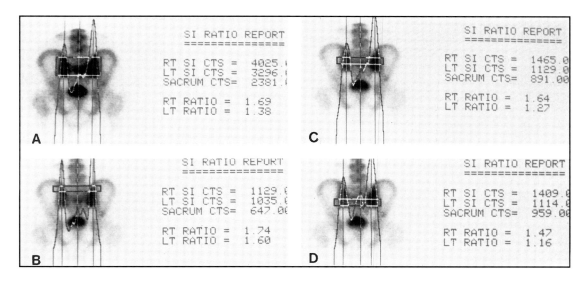

Fig. 12-6. Bilateral sacroiliitis, more prominent on the right. **A,** The profile slice through the full width of the joints registers sacroiliac-sacrum ratios of 1.69 and 1.38 for the right and left, respectively. **B, C,** and **D** These represent the profile slices through the upper, mid, and lower thirds of the joints, respectively.

in sacroiliitis is not just a function of the count rate over the joints (the numerator) but also the sacrum (the denominator). An increase in both leads to a lower than expected value of the ratio and thereby contributes to a loss in sensitivity.[68]

RESPONSE TO TREATMENT

The common clinical criteria for assessing disease include the Ritchie index, grip strength, 50-ft walking time, and morning stiffness, but these are considered by some investigators to be too subjective for a well-designed treatment protocol. Furthermore, the degree of exertional effort volunteered by the patients is variable. To this end, many researchers have resorted to radionuclide methods to measure, either qualitatively or quantitatively, the uptake in the joints before treatment and serially thereafter. Underlying a favorable response to medication is a defervescence of the inflammatory reaction in the synovium, and the radiopharmaceutical manifestation of it is a decreasing concentration of blood compartment markers, radiophosphate, ^{67}Ga, radiolabeled IgG, ^{111}In chloride, and the like. Although this generally occurs with radiophosphate, a persistent high accretion in the face of clinical remission could be due to subclinical synovitis or synovial remission but with ongoing repair of bone erosion. At this juncture blood or inflammatory site compartment markers may be more specific, but a definitive study is yet to be done.

There are a number of reports attesting to the value of radiopharmaceutical joint surveys to assess the efficacy of treatment. Radiopertechnetate measurements before and after corticosteroid medication proved more sensitive than either the grip strength or joint circumference.[63] In another investigation synovial biopsies were performed in 11 patients who presented with knee pain but no definitive evidence warmth or swelling. It was found that increased radiopertechnetate concentration was present only when there were histologic manifestations of hyperemia and cellular infiltration (Fig. 12-7). The radiopertechnetate uptake therefore was considered to be a more sensitive parameter of synovitis than the clinical stigmata.[6] Not many of these histologic correlation studies have been reported, and it is particularly lacking with the newly introduced inflammatory site markers. This is necessary to establish how closely they reflect the underlying pathologic process, which is important for research and drug testing. It is less important in clinical practice when the diagnosis is established, because the goal is to palliate symptoms, not the scan appearance or the numbers generated therefrom.

ANKYLOSING SPONDYLITIS

The ankylosed spine is rigid and osteopenic and therefore susceptible to low-grade traumatic fractures that may

not be symptomatic and which may lead to the development of pseudoarthrosis with continued movement. Proliferation of adjacent bone, ankylosis, and deficient bone mineral may combine to obscure fracture detection by conventional radiography. Other features of ankylosing spondylitis include sternoclavicular, manubriosternal, and sternocostal joint involvement. All of these manifestations can be revealed with radiophosphate imaging (Fig. 12-8).

OSTEOARTHRITIS

The genesis of osteoarthritis, which affects a quarter of the population by age 50 and over half the population by

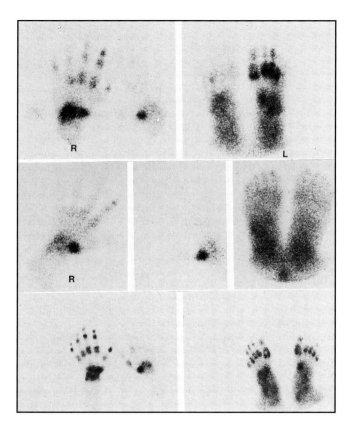

Fig. 12-7. Psoriatic arthritis under treatment. *Upper panel:* Before treatment the right wrist showed a diffuse increased uptake of ^{99m}Tc-MDP, and there was periarticular concentration at four metacarpophalangeal and several proximal and distal interphalangeal joints of the hand. The intense focus at the trapeziometatarsal joint is due to osteoarthritis. High uptakes in the left are present in the tarsus, first four metatarsophalangeal joints, and third toe. *Middle panel:* 9 months after the start of treatment, the right wrist and hand and left foot reverted to normal, except for persistent activity at the right trapeziometatarsal joint. This was due to osteoarthritis that was obscured by wrist synovitis previously. *Lower panel:* Recrudescence of synovitis 1 year later with involvement of both wrists, both feet and the right hand. (*From Rosenthall L: The bone scan in arthritis, in Fogelman I: Bone Scanning in Clinical Practice, Springer-Verlag, Berlin, 1987; with permission.*)

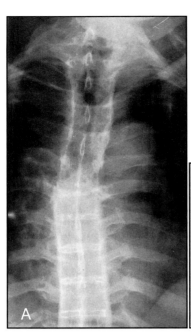

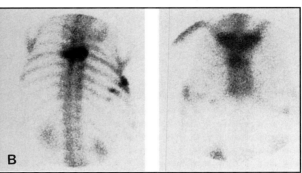

Fig. 12-8. Ankylosing spondylitis. A 57-year-old man with end-stage ankylosing spondylitis. He sustained a fracture in the thoracic spine and several ribs following a minor fall, because of the rigidity and osteopenia of the axial skeleton. **A**, Conventional radiography of the thoracic column failed to show the injury. **B**, Radiophosphate images clearly define the fractures in the thoracic vertebrae and those in the ribs. Augmented uptake at the manubrioclavicular and manubriosternal junctions is also present, which is a feature of ankylosing spondylitis.

age 65, is still uncertain—does it begin in the cartilage or subchondral bone? It afflicts diarthrodial and to some degree amphiarthrodial joints. There is a noninflammatory deterioration of the articular cartilage and reactive new bone formation at joint surfaces and margins. In advanced osteoarthritis the synovium undergoes reactive thickening with increase in the number of cells lining the joint.[96] The induced radiophosphate response can vary from subtle to pronounced, depending on the metabolic activity of the lesions. Osteophytes that are in the process of growing exhibit high uptakes, whereas mature osteophytes tend to have low-grade increases or normal uptake. This was observed in a rabbit model of induced osteoarthritis in the knee and explains the lack of correlation between the radiographic size of the osteophyte and the degree of radiophosphate accretion.[9] This is best illustrated in patients with DISH. Generally they do not have unusual focal or diffuse radiophosphate uptakes in the spine. The lumbar-spine-to-soft-tissue ratios have been found on average to be higher than those with normal spines, but they were not significantly different at the 0.05 probability level.[68] Presumably a high uptake would have been registered at an earlier time during the evolution of these large osteophytes and bony bridges.

Thirty-three patients who had generalized nodal arthritis were subjected to comparative radiophosphate scans and radiography of the hands and wrists. Both methods demonstrated the predominant involvement of the distal interphalangeal, scaphotrapezial, and first carpometacarpal joints, but there were differences between them at many of the sites. Some joints were abnormal either on x-ray or scan alone, whereas others exhibited a marked dissimilarity between the intensity of the focal radiophosphate uptake and severity of x-ray change.[36] The same authors related the results from a group of 14 patients who had generalized nodal osteoarthritis and

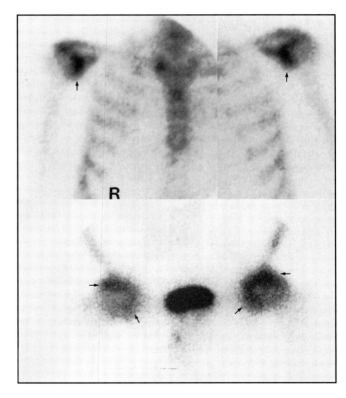

Fig. 12-9. Osteoarthritis of the shoulders and hips (*arrows*).

were followed with x-rays and scintigraphy for 3 to 5 years. The joint scan abnormality appeared to precede the development of x-ray signs, and joints abnormal on scintigraphy showed the most progressive radiographic change. Joints that were x-ray abnormal but normal by bone scan did not show additional deterioration.[37] This

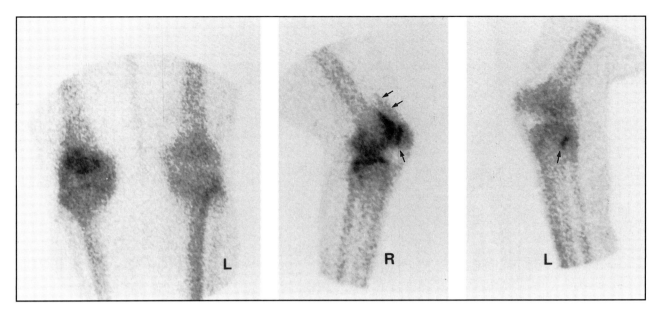

Fig. 12-10. Osteoarthritis of the knees. *Left panel:* Anterior ^{99m}Tc-MDP scan shows increased periarticular uptake at the right knee with accentuation of the patella, whereas the left knee appears normal. *Middle panel:* The right lateral projection clearly depicts a subchondral deposition at the femoral, tibial and patellar (*arrow*) articular surfaces. There is also evidence of a synovitis (*twin arrows*). *Right panel:* Osteoarthritis of the fibulotibial articulation is demonstrated in the left lateral projection (*arrow*).

illustrates the disparity between metabolic activity and morphology, similar to the finding with pannus erosion of bone.

Blood compartment and inflammatory site markers are usually normal in osteoarthritis, because the synovitis is not flagrant (Fig. 12-2). It is impossible to differentiate osteoarthritis and primary synovitis of the small joints of the hands and feet owing to the limited resolution of imaging equipment. In large joint areas such as the wrists, knees, hips, and shoulders the focal nature of the radiophosphate uptake in osteoarthritis can be better appreciated and distinguished from the diffuse juxtaarticular concentration seen in synovitis (Figs. 12-9 and 12-10). SPECT imaging, which renders higher target-to-backgound ratios than planar imaging, further improves the detection of the osteoarthritic lesions.

The patella frequently demonstrates a high uptake of radiophosphate, often without corresponding radiographic abnormalities. The cause of this incidental finding usually is not known because there is no compelling reason to pursue definitive arthroscopy. In 100 consecutive patients it was found to occur bilaterally in 15 patients and unilaterally in 5.[45] Another report of 130 consecutive patients from 4 to 84 years of age found increased patellar radioactivity with normal radiographic findings in 44% and was associated with radiographic evidence of patellar degeneration in 33%.[52]

A number of reports have appeared on the comparison of radiophosphate imaging of the patella and arthroscopy. In 18 patients with proven chondromalacia by arthroscopy, 11 had normal bone scans, and 7 had focal uptakes for a sensitivity of 39%. There was no correlation between the intensity of radiophosphate uptake and severity of chondromalacia.[8] Of 64 knees afflicted with chondromalacia, 39 scans were positive for a sensitivity of 60%, and the proportion of positive scans increased with severity of disease.[29] Fifty patients clinically suspected of having chondromalacia had increased radiophosphate uptake in the patella, but at arthroscopy only 43 patients proved to have chondromalacia. Also, severity of disease varied directly with the intensity of patellar uptake.[47] To be stressed is that a positive scan is not specific for any one condition, but it may be an indication for arthroscopy when the clinical diagnosis is not apparent.

In a comparison of planar imaging and arthroscopy in 119 knees—62 of which were assessments of the patellofemoral surface, 35 of the medial compartment, and 22 of the lateral compartment—the sensitivity and specificity for planar imaging was 90% and 79%, respectively. Eleven false-negative results were obtained; these patients had early softening of the articular cartilage at arthroscopy. There were 14 false-positive results that were attributed to early stress patterns, but could equally be a manifestation of the thesis that subchondral bone change is the initiating factor in degenerative joint disease. In other words they were not falsely positive, but rather they disclosed the first stage of the disease process.[59,71,72]

SPECT has important advantages over planar imaging. It increases the contrast of low-grade subtle uptakes, better defines the location and configuration of the uptake to enhance specificity, and can unravel multiple focal uptakes superimposed on a background of high diffuse activity. An important application is the disclosure of abnormalities in the spine where the overlapping elements of the vertebrae may obscure a low-grade accretion of the radiopharmaceutical. This is particularly useful in the workup of the patient with chronic low back pain and normal or confusing radiographs, wherein the latter may show multiple lesions but not identify the area(s) of active bone remodeling (see Chapter 4). In the knee a comparison of three-phase planar and SPECT radiophosphate imaging, clinical impression, plain film radiography, and arthroscopy was implemented prospectively in 27 patients with chronic pain. Mean duration of pain was 9 months, and no patient had trauma within 1 month of the workup. Sensitivity of SPECT for the patellofemoral, lateral, and medial compartments was 93%, 93%, and 91%, respectively, compared with 57%, 72%, and 86%, respectively, for planar imaging. For radiography the sensitivity was poorer at 22%, 20%, and 71%, respectively. Specificity of SPECT for the lateral compartment was only 50%, but this may be another example of radionuclide detection of subchondral remodeling that purportedly antedates the onset of articular cartilage degeneration. At the patellofemoral and medial compartments, specificity was 100% and 86%, respectively. The authors concluded that the noninvasive and highly sensitive SPECT technique can be used to screen patients for significant internal derangements that could benefit from arthroscopic surgery. Conversely, a normal radionuclide scan might be an indication for continued conservative treatment.[11] Despite the inherent superiority of SPECT over planar imaging, improved identification of focal lesions can be achieved with planar imaging by taking high-resolution images in four projections (i.e., anterior, posterior, and both laterals) as opposed to an anterior and single lateral. This reduced the number of equivocal scans relative to SPECT.[53]

TRANSIENT (TOXIC) SYNOVITIS OF THE HIP

Transient synovitis is an affliction that usually occurs in children under 12 years of age. An association between synovitis and a preceding viral infection of the upper respiratory tract has been alleged, or it may be due to occult trauma. Some authors claim that about 10% of these patients may develop Legg-Perthes disease as a complication.

The anatomic disposition of the vascular supply is such that vessels that feed the femoral epiphysis pass through the joint capsule and are thereby at risk of compression with a critical rise in intracapsular pressure. This may cause an impairment of the blood flow to the epiphysis that will be reflected in the three-phase radiophosphate study.

In a series of 13 patients, the uptake of radiophosphate in the femoral head in the delayed images was normal in 9, increased in 3, and decreased in 3.[32] A well-documented published study of 19 cases of transient synovitis in children related that in 6 the blood pool and delayed phases were normal, 1 patient had increased blood pool, 10 had increased uptake on the delayed images but normal blood pool phases, and 8 had photon deficiency in the blood pool phase. Of the latter 8 patients, 6 had reduced, but not absent, uptake in the delayed views, and all 6 reverted to normal after joint aspiration.[46] In summary, the portrayal of transient synovitis can be decreased, normal, or increased concentration of radiophosphate in the blood pool and delayed images, and the two phases may not parallel each other in a given patient.

REGIONAL MIGRATORY OSTEOPOROSIS

Regional migratory osteoporosis is a syndrome of acute periarticular painful soft-tissue swelling, usually involving the lower extremities, which migrates from joint to joint. There are variants of this disorder that seem to be limited to one joint, but some of them may appear so because the patients were not followed long enough. This condition has been referred to as transient osteoporosis, migratory osteolysis, algodystrophy and partial algodystrophy. It occurs spontaneously in otherwise healthy middle-aged adults, without any precipitating cause. The ratio of males to females is 3:1. About half the reported female cases presented in the last trimester of pregnancy or shortly after giving birth. Episodes of this disorder last 1 year or less and resolve spontaneously without specific therapy. The most frequent site of initial involvement is the hip, but the disease may commence in the knees, ankles, or feet. Once remission occurs in a joint, it is not likely to be affected again. Migration time from one joint the next can be a few months to many years.

An increased number and caliber of the blood vessels, fibrillosis of fatty marrow, and bone remodeling consisting of the formation of lamellar and woven bone are seen in the biopsy specimens. This is somewhat similar to the picture of Sudek's atrophy. Synovial membranes can be normal or show chronic hypertrophic changes.[49,89]

The radiophosphate appearance is that of a high, nonspecific uptake on one or both sides of a joint, affecting the full or partial width of the bone. This portrayal can antedate the conventional radiographic changes, which consist of subchondral osteopenia without loss of cartilage space. Magnetic resonance imaging (MRI) demonstrates focal nonspecific low intensity signals, probably indicative of marrow edema[24,67,79,92,101] (Fig. 12-11).

REFLEX SYMPATHETIC DYSTROPHY

The reflex sympathetic dystrophy syndrome (RSDS) is not well understood and probably encompasses the many other conditions described as causalgia, acute atro-

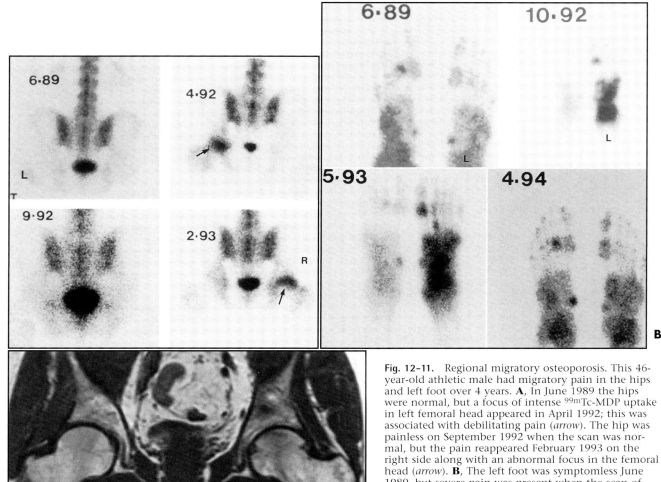

Fig. 12-11. Regional migratory osteoporosis. This 46-year-old athletic male had migratory pain in the hips and left foot over 4 years. **A**, In June 1989 the hips were normal, but a focus of intense ^{99m}Tc-MDP uptake in left femoral head appeared in April 1992; this was associated with debilitating pain (*arrow*). The hip was painless on September 1992 when the scan was normal, but the pain reappeared February 1993 on the right side along with an abnormal focus in the femoral head (*arrow*). **B**, The left foot was symptomless June 1989, but severe pain was present when the scan of October 1992 showed very avid uptake in the ankle, tarsus, and first metatarsophalangeal joint. The pain was aggravated by a stress fracture of the second metatarsal on May 1993. Pain disappeared and the bone remodeling receded to normal by April 1994, at which time the right hip was also normal. **C**, MRI of the hips in February 1993 demonstrated a normal left hip and low signal intensity in the right femoral head and neck, indicating edema.

phy of bone, Sudeck's atrophy, peripheral acute trophoneurosis, traumatic angiospasm, posttraumatic osteoporosis, traumatic vasospasm, reflex dystrophy of the extremities, reflex algodystrophy, shoulder-hand syndrome, reflex neurovascular dystrophy, and reflex sympathetic dystrophy. Signs and symptoms include pain, hyperesthesia, swelling, stiffness, hyperhidrosis, and discoloration of the skin ranging from redness to grayish-blue or a mixture of the two extremes. In the absence of remission, dermal atrophy and contractures may occur. Histologically the synovium demonstrates a proliferation of the lining cells and capillaries and perivascular infiltration with chronic inflammatory cells.

Sudeck's atrophy and shoulder-hand syndrome are most frequently encountered. Shoulder-hand syndrome is bilateral in approximately 30% of the cases and has

been associated with myocardial infarction, trauma, spinal disk disease, neoplasia, cerebrovascular accident, and drugs. A precipitant cannot be found in 35% of cases. In the lower extremity RSDS is usually a sequela to injury and surgery.

In adults the three-phase radiophosphate manifestations of a typical acute stage in the disorder consist of increased perfusion, equilibrium blood pool activity, and uptake in the delayed images about the involved joints (Fig. 12-12). All three phases must be diffusely increased to all portions of the wrist and hand, or entire foot.[33,34] Conventional radiographs depict osteopenia in most patients at this stage, but its appearance is often antedated by the radionuclide abnormalities. With clinical improvement, the accentuated perfusion and blood pool radioactivity are the first to revert to normal, and even-

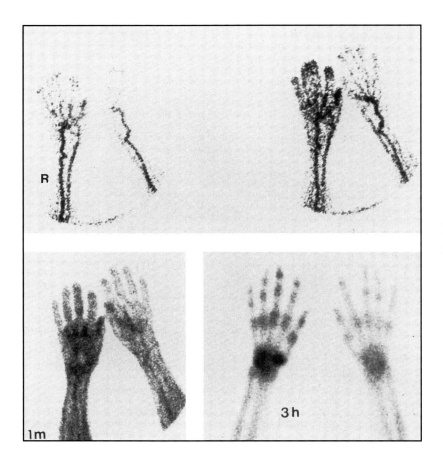

Fig. 12-12. Reflex sympathetic dystrophy of the left upper extremity in a 51-year-old male. The triple-phase ^{99m}Tc-MDP study exhibits increased radioactivity in all three phases.

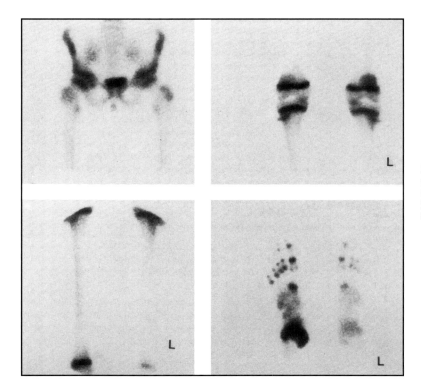

Fig. 12-13. Acute reflex sympathetic dystrophy of the left lower extremity in a 9-year-old female. There is decreased uptake of ^{99m}Tc-MDP in the delayed images, contrary to what is seen in adults.

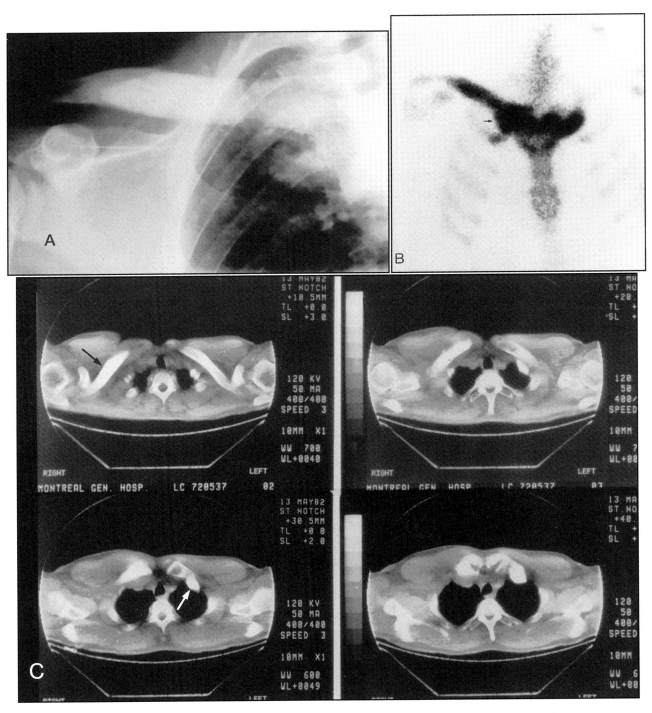

Fig. 12-14. Sternocostoclavicular hyperostosis. **A,** Widening and osteosclerosis of the medial two thirds of the right clavicle. No radiographic evidence of calcification in the intercostal region. **B,** Intense uptake of [99mTc]-MDP in the right clavicle, left first rib anteriorly, and the medial end of the left clavicle. Low-grade accretion in the anterior segment of the right second rib. Arrow points to [99mTc]-MDP concentration in the inflamed soft tissue of the costoclavicular space. **C,** Computed tomographic (CT) scan cuts through the region of interest. A densely sclerotic right clavicle with overlying soft tissue is demonstrated (*black arrow*). There is no evidence of calcium content in the region of [99mTc]-MDP soft-tissue uptake. Osteosclerosis is seen in the left first rib (*white arrow*).

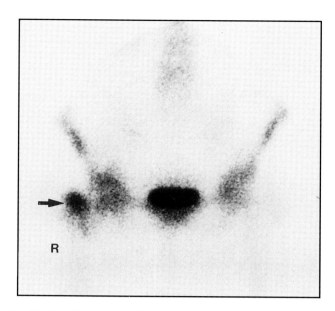

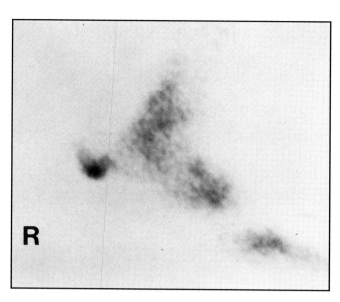

Fig. 12-15. Trochanteric bursitis on the right in a 79-year-old female. Intense focal accretion of radiophosphate in the right greater trochanter, the site of exquisite tenderness to palpation.

Fig. 12-16. Plantar fasciitis. Intense focus of ^{99m}Tc-MDP at the calcaneal insertion of the long plantar tendon. Erosive rheumatoid arthritis may yield a similar depiction.

tually the static images become normal. If the RSDS proceeds toward an atrophic fibrous stage, each of the three phases will abate and may even show radioactivity levels below normal.[55]

Normal asymmetry may exist. It was shown in 61 patients with asymptomatic upper extremities that about a third had distinct asymmetric flow and blood pool images, whereas only a mild difference at most occurred in the delayed images. The authors concluded that a greater reliance should be placed on the delayed images, which had an overall sensitivity of 94%.[64]

Another form of RSDS has been described in which the lesion is localized to the medial femoral condyle, medial tibial plateau, or both, by radiophosphate imaging. It occurred in six women who satisfied the clinical criteria for the disease, and the enhanced uptakes became normal with clinical remission.[12]

In one study of 39 patients with clinically definite, probable, or possible RSDS, the sensitivity was 83%, 40%, and 28%, respectively; overall 60%. Radiographic osteopenia was 81%, 55%, and 57%, respectively. It was also found that patients with an abnormal radionuclide study were more apt to respond to steroid therapy than those with normal images.[48] Radiophosphate scans enabled a diagnosis of RSDS to be made in 13 patients and to be excluded in 5 in another report.[85]

Perfusion and blood pool phases of the radiophosphate study are not as reliable as the delayed images in disclosing RSDS. In 23 patients with RSDS of the hands, positive results were obtained in 10 (45%) by perfusion, 12 (52%) by blood pool, but 22 by delayed images (96%). The specificity of the delayed views was 98%, and the predictive values of positive and negative tests were 88% and 99%, respectively.[34]

Eighty-five patients with cerebrovascular accident were subjected to triple-phase bone imaging. There were 21 patients with RSDS, of which 13 (62%) had increased flow, blood pool, and uptake on delayed images, and 8 (38%) had decreased flow and blood pool but increased uptake on the delayed views. Two of the positive studies antedated the clinical expression. Of the remaining patients, 9 (10%) had normal triple-phase studies, and 55 (65%) depicted decreased flow and blood pool but normal delayed uptake on the side of paralysis. It is postulated that the decreased flow and blood pool radioactivity is caused by the reduced nutrient demands for blood by the muscles of the paralyzed or immobilized limb, whereas blood flow to bone remains unaffected. Thus the delayed images in patients without RSDS are normal but abnormally increased in those with RSDS.[27]

In a combined retrospective and prospective study of the feet, the overall sensitivity and specificity was 100% and 80%, respectively. Positive and negative predictive values were 54% and 100%, respectively. False-positive results were obtained in patients with diabetes, infection, and chronic pain. There were no differences in the radionuclide portrayals as a function of duration of symptoms.[33]

The scan pattern in the pediatric age group may differ from adults. In 11 children aged 7 to 17 years with reflex neurovascular dystrophy, or RSDS, 4 had increases in all three phases of the radiophosphate study, 3 were normal, and 4 had decreases in the three phases.[50] Another report of 8 patients aged 10 to 18 years stated that 4 showed increased uptake in the affected limb, whereas 4 were distinctly decreased[94] (Fig. 12-13). There is no satisfactory explanation for this latter finding in the acute stage of RSDS.

MISCELLANEOUS

Pustulotic Arthrosteitis

Palmoplantar pustulosis or severe acne can be associated with bone disease. The most common site is the chest wall, where it is generally referred to as sternocostoclavicular hyperostosis. On anterior and anterior oblique views, one or both clavicles are enlarged and show a combination of osteoproliferative and osteodestructive changes. Anterior segments of the ribs can demonstrate similar abnormalities, and there may be fusion of the ribs due to enthesopic calcification. Costomanubrial, costochondral, and manubriosternal joints also display a sclerotic reaction, with joint spaces either enlarged by osteolysis, reduced, or completely fused. Other skeletal sites may be afflicted, but with considerable lower frequency, and they include the ilium, scapula, mandible, spine, and long bones (Fig. 12-14). The lesions can resemble infectious osteomyelitis or primary bone tumor radiographically. Radiophosphate manifestations are those of intense, nonspecific accretion. Because of the multifaceted nature of the condition, new terms have been coined such as juxtasternal arthrosteitis and the acronym SAPHO (synovitis-acne-pustulosis-hyperostosis-osteitis).[41,42,43]

Trochanteric Bursitis

Trochanteric bursitis is an inflammation of one or more of the bursa about the gluteus medius insertion on the femoral trochanter of middle-aged or elderly patients. It is a common insidious condition that may be spontaneous or may occur because of excessive frictional forces or trauma. It causes pain on external rotation of the hip and is recognized by exquisite tenderness over the trochanteric area. Radiophosphate imaging may show an increased accretion in the greater trochanter underlying the bursa (Fig. 12-15).

Plantar Fasciitis

Chronic plantar fasciitis is one cause of the painful heel syndrome, wherein pain and tenderness are concentrated at the site of attachment of the long plantar tendon into the base of the calcaneus. The radiophosphate portrayal is that of a focal high accretion in the calcaneus at the point of insertion of the tendon. Radiography may be normal when the radionuclide study is abnormal, or it may exhibit marginal erosions, spur formation, and periosteal new bone formation at the base of the calcaneus[83] (Fig. 12-16).

REFERENCES

1. Ahlstrom S, Gedda PO, Hedberg H: Disappearance of radioactive serum albumin from joints in rheumatoid arthritis. *Acta Rheum Scand* 1956; 2:129.
2. Al-Janobi MA, Jones AKP, Solanski K, et al: Tc-99m labelled leukocyte imaging in active rheumatoid arthritis. *Nucl Med Commun* 1988; 9:987.
3. Ayres J, Hilson JW, Maisey MN, et al: An improved method for sacroiliac joint imaging: A study of normal subjects, patients with sacroiliitis and patients with low back pain. *Clin Radiol* 1981; 32:441.
4. Beckerman C, Genant HK, Hoffer PB, et al: Radionuclide imaging of the bones and joints of the hands. *Radiology* 1976; 118:653.
5. Berghs H, Remans J, Dreiskens L, et al: Diagnostic value of SI joint scintigraphy with Tc-99m-pyrophosphate in sacroiliitis. *Ann Rheum Dis* 1978; 37:190.
6. Boerbooms AM, Buys WC: Rapid assessment of Tc-99m pertechnetate of the knee joint as a parameter of inflammatory activity. *Arthritis Rheum* 1979; 21:348.
7. Breeveld FC, van Kroonenburgh MJPG, Campus JAJ, et al: Imaging of inflammatory arthritis with technetium-99m labeled IgG. *J Nucl Med* 1989; 30:2017.
8. Butler-Manuel PA, Guy RL, Heatly FW, et al: Scintigraphy in the assessment of anterior knee pain. *Acta Orthop Scand* 1990; 61:438.
9. Christensen SB: Localization of bone-seeking agents in developing experimentally induced osteoarthritis in the knee joint of the rabbit. *Scand J Rheumatol* 1983; 12:343.
10. Cohen MD, Lorber A: Avoiding false positive joint scans by the use of labeled albumin. *Arthritis Rheum* 1971; 14:32.
11. Collier BD, Johnson RP, Carrera GF, et al: Chronic knee pain assessed by SPECT: Comparison with other modalities. *Radiology* 1985; 157:795.
12. Cuartero-Plaza A, Martinez-Miralles E, Benito-Ruiz P, et al: Abnormal bone scintigraphy and silent radiography in localized reflex sympathetic dystrophy syndrome. *Eur J Nucl Med* 1992; 19:330.
13. da Sousa M, Dynesius-Trentham R, Mota-Garcia, et al: Activation of rat synovium by iron. *Arthritis Rheum* 1988; 31:653.
14. Davison, Wisham LH: The clearance of ^{24}Na from normal and osteoarthritic knee joints and response to intraarterial Priscoline. *J Clin Invest* 1958; 37:389.
15. de Bois M, Arndt JW, van der Velde EA, et al: ^{99m}Tc human immunoglobulin scintigraphy—a reliable method to detect joint activity in rheumatoid arthritis. *J Rheumatol* 1992; 19:1371.
16. Dequecker J, Goddeeris T, Walravens SM: Evaluation of sacroiliitis: Comparison of radiological and radionuclide techniques. *Radiology* 1978; 128:687.
17. Desaulniers M, Rosenthall L, Fuks A, et al: Radiotechnetium polyphosphate joint imaging: *J Nucl Med* 1974; 15:417.
18. Dick C, Whaley, St. Onge RA, et al: Clinical studies on inflammation in human knee joints: Xenon(^{133}Xe) clearances correlated with clinical assessment in various arthritides and studies on the effect of intraarticularly administered hydrocortisone in rheumatoid arthritis. *Clin Sci (Colchin)* 1970; 38:123.
19. Dodig D, Popovics S, Domljan Z: Influence of age on quantitative sacroiliac joint imaging. *Eur J Nucl Med* 1984; 9:177.
20. Domeij-Nyberg B, Kjallman M, Nylan O, Petterson NO: The reliability of quantitative bone scanning in sacroiliitis. *Scand J Rheumatol* 1980; 9:77.
21. Dunn NA, Mahida BN, Merrick MV, Nuki G: Quantitative sacroiliac scintiscanning: A sensitive and objective method for assessing efficacy of non-steroidal, anti-inflammatory drugs in patients with sacroiliitis. *Ann Rheum Dis* 1984; 43:157.
22. Esdaile J, Rosenthall L: Unpublished data.

23. Esdaile J, Rosenthall L, Terkeltaub R, et al: Prospective evaluation of sacroiliac scintigraphy in chronic inflammatory low back pain. *Arthritis Rheum* 1980; 23:998.

24. Gaucher A, Colomb JN, Naoun A, et al: The diagnostic value of Tc-99m diphosphonate bone imaging in transient osteoporosis of the hip. *J Rheumatol* 1979; 6:574.

25. Goldberg RP, Genant HK, Shimchak D, Shames D: Applications and limitations of quantitative sacroiliac joint scintigraphy. *Radiology* 1978; 128:683.

26. Greyson ND: Radionuclide bone and joint imaging in rheumatology. *Bull Rheum* 1980; 30:1034.

27. Greyson ND, Tepperman PS: Three-phase bone studies in hemiplegia with reflex sympathetic dystrophy and the effect of disuse. *J Nucl Med* 1984; 25:423.

28. Hays MT, Green FA: The pertechnetate joint scan: Timing. *Ann Rheum Dis* 1972; 31:272.

29. Hejgaard N, Diemir H: Bone scan in patellofemoral pain syndrome. *Int Orthop* 1987; 11:29.

30. Helfgott S, Rosenthall L, Esdaile J, et al: Generalized skeletal response to 99mTc-MDP in rheumatoid arthritis. *J Rheumatol* 1982; 9:939.

31. Hernborg J: Elimination of Na^{131}I from joints with degenerative changes. *Arthritis Rheum* 1968; 11:618.

32. Heyman S, Goldstein HA, Crowley W, Treves S: The scintigraphic evaluation of hip pain in children. *Clin Nucl Med* 1980; 5:109.

33. Holder LE, Cole LA, Myerson MS: Reflex sympathetic dystrophy in the foot: Clinical and scintigraphic criteria. *Radiology* 1992; 184:531.

34. Holder LE, Mackinnon SE: Reflex sympathetic dystrophy in the hands: Clinical and scintigraphic criteria. *Radiology* 1984; 152:517.

35. Holopaienen T, Reckonen A: Uptake of radioactive strontium (Sr-85) in joints damaged by rheumatoid arthritis. *Acta Rheum Scand* 1966; 12:102.

36. Hutton CW, Higgs ER, Jackson PC, et al: Tc-99m HMDP bone scanning in generalized nodal osteoarthritis: Comparison of the standard radiograph and four hour bone scan image of the hands. *Ann Rheum Dis* 1986; 45:617.

37. Hutton CW, Higgs ER, Jackson PC, et al: Tc-99m HMDP bone scanning in generalized nodal osteoarthritis. The four hour bone scan image predicts radiographic change. *Ann Rheum Dis* 1986; 45:622.

38. Jeremy R, Cote J, Scott W: Investigation of bone and joint disease using F-18. *Med J Aust* 1969; 1:492.

39. Jones MM, Moore WH, Brewer EJ, et al: Radionuclide bone/joint imaging in children with rheumatic complaints. *Skeletal Radiol* 1988; 17:1.

40. Joseph K, Hoffken H, Bosslet K, et al: Imaging of inflammation with granulocytes labelled in vivo. *Nucl Med Commun* 1988; 9:763.

41. Kahn M-F, Chamot A-M: SAPHO syndrome. *Rheum Dis Clin North Am* 1992; 18:225.

42. Kasperczyk A, Freyschmidt J: Pustulotic arthroosteitis: Spectrum of bone lesions with palmoplantar pustulosis. *Radiology* 1994; 191:207.

43. Katz ME, Shier CK, Ellis BI, et al: A unified approach to symptomatic juxtasternal arthritis and enthesitis. *AJR Am J Roentgenol* 1989; 153:327.

44. Kinne RW, Becker W, Schwab J, et al: Comparison of Tc-99m labelled specific murine anti-CD4 monoclonal antibodies and nonspecific human immunoglobulin for imaging inflamed joints in rheumatoid arthritis. *Nucl Med Commun* 1993; 14:667.

45. Kipper MS, Alazraki NP, Feiglin DH: The "hot" patella. *Clin Nucl Med* 1982; 7:28.

46. Kloiber R, Parlosky N, Porter O, Gartke K: Bone scintigraphy of hip joint effusions in children. *AJR Am J Roentgenol* 1983; 140:995.

47. Kohn HS, Guten GN, Collier BD, et al: Chondromalacia of the patella: Bone imaging correlated with arthroscopic findings. *Clin Nucl Med* 1987; 13:29.

48. Kozin F, Soin JS, Ryan LM et al: Bone scintigraphy in the reflex sympathetic dystrophy syndrome. *Radiology* 1981; 138:437.

49. Lagier R: Partial algodystrophy of the knee. *J Rheumatol* 1983; 10:255.

50. Laxer RM, Malleson PN, Morrison RT, Petty RE: Technetium 99m-methylene diphosphonate bone scans in children with reflex neurovascular dystrophy. *J Pediatr* 1985; 106:437.

51. Liberatore M, Clemente M, Lurille AP, et al: A comparison of technetium-99m human nonspecific immunoglobulins, leukocytes and albumin nanocolloids. *Eur J Nucl Med* 1992; 19:853.

52. Lin D, Alavi A, Dalinka M: Bone scan evaluation of patellar activity. *J Nucl Med Biol* 1981; 8:105.

53. Marks PH, Goldenberg HA, Vezina WC, et al: Subchondral bone infarctions in acute ligamentous knee injuries demonstrated on bone scintigraphy and magnetic resonance. *J Nucl Med* 1993; 33:516.

54. Martinez-Villasenor D, Katona G: Scintigraphy by means of radioisotopes of short half-life for diagnosing disease of the joints, in *Medical Radioisotope Scintigraphy*, Vol 2, International Atomic Energy Agency, Vienna, 1968, p 295.

55. Mattar AG, Hurwitz G, MacGuire C: Reappraisal of bone scintigraphy in reflex sympathetic dystrophy syndrome in adults. *Clin Invest Med* 1988; 1:B10 (abstract).

56. Maxfield WS, Weiss TE, Hidalgo JU: Detection of arthritis by joint scintigraphy, in *Medical Radioisotope Scintigraphy*, Vol 2, International Atomic Energy Agency, Vienna, 1968, p 307.

57. Maxfield WS, Weiss TE, Schuler SE: Synovial membrane scanning in arthritic disease. *Semin Nucl Med* 1972; 2:50.

58. McCall JW, Sheppard H, Haddaway M, et al: Gallium-67 scanning in rheumatoid arthritis. *Br J Radiol* 1983; 56:241.

59. Mooar P, Gregg J, Jacobstein J: Radionuclide imaging in internal derangements of the knee. *Am J Sports Med* 1987; 15:132.

60. Mottonen TT, Hannonen P, Towanen J, et al: Value of joint scintigraphy in the prediction of erosiveness in early rheumatoid arthritis. *Ann Rheum Dis* 1988; 47:183.

61. Namey TC, McIntyre J, Buse M, et al: Nucleographic studies of axial spondyloarthritis: Quantitative sacroiliac scintigraphy in early HLA-27 associated sacroiliitis. *Arthritis Rheum* 1977; 20:1058.

62. Norbjerg M, Heerfordt J, Dissing I, et al: Numerical assessment of asymmetry at scintigraphy of normal joint pairs. *Acta Radiol (Diagn)* 1980; 21:235.

63. Nuki G, Collins KE, Deodar H, et al: Radioisotope study of small joint inflammation in rheumatoid arthritis. *Ann Rheum Dis* 1971; 30:401.

64. O'Donaghue JP, Powe JE, Mattar AG, et al: Three-phase bone scintigraphy: Asymmetric patterns in the upper extremities of asymptomatic normals and reflex sympathetic dystrophy patients. *Clin Nucl Med* 1993; 18:829.

65. O'Duffy JD, Wahner HW, Hunder GG: Joint imaging in polymyalgia rheumatica. *Mayo Clin Proc* 1976; 51:519.

66. Olsen M, Halberg P, Halskov O, Bentzon MW: Scintimetric assessment of synovitis activity during treatment with disease modifying antirheumatic drugs. *Ann Rheum Dis* 1988; 47:995.

67. O'Mara RE, Pinals RS: Bone scanning in regional migratory osteoporosis. *Radiology* 1970; 97:579.

68. Paquin J, Rosenthall L, Esdaile J, et al: Elevated uptake of Tc-99m methylene diphosphonate in the axial skeleton in ankylosing spondylitis and Reiter's disease: Implications for quantitative sacroiliac scintigraphy. *Arthritis Rheum* 1983; 26:217.

69. Park H, Terman SA, Ridolfo AS, et al: A quantitative evaluation of rheumatic activity with ^{99m}Tc-HEDP. *J Nucl Med* 1977; 18:973.

70. Pitt P, Berry H, Clarke M, et al: Metabolic activity of erosions in rheumatoid arthritis. *Ann Rheum Dis* 1986; 45:235.

71. Radin EL, Parker HG, Pugh JW, et al: Response of joints to impact loading. III: Relationship between trabecular microfractures and cartilage degeneration. *J Biomech* 1973; 6:51.

72. Radin EL, Paul IL, Lowry MA: A comparison of the dynamic force transmitting properties of subchondral bone and articular cartilage. *J Bone Joint Surg* 1970; 52A:444.

73. Rajapaksec C, Thompson R, Grennan DM, et al: Increased bone metabolism in rheumatoid arthritis as measured by whole body retention of 99mTc-methylene diphosphonate. *Ann Rheum Dis* 1983; 42:138.

74. Rodnan GP, Machachlan MJ: The absorption of serum albumin and gamma globulin from the knee joint of man and rabbit. *Arthritis Rheum* 1960; 3:152.

75. Rosenspire KC, Blau M, Kennedy AC, et al: Assessment and interpretation of radiopharmaceutical joint imaging in an animal model of arthritis. *Arthritis Rheum* 1981; 24:711.

76. Rosenspire KC, Kennedy AC, Russomanno L, et al: Comparison of four methods of analysis of Tc-99m-pyrophosphate. *J Rheumatol* 1980; 7:461.

77. Rosenspire KC, Kennedy AC, Russomano L, et al: Investigation of the metabolic activity of bone in rheumatoid arthritis. *J Rhematol* 1980; 7:469.

78. Rosenthall, L: Nuclear medicine techniques. *Rheum Dis Clin North Am* 1991; 17:585.

79. Rozenbaum M, Zenman C, Nagler A: Transient osteoporosis of the hip joint with liver cirrhosis. *J Rheumatol* 1984; 11:241.

80. Rubin RH, Fischman AJ, Nedelman M, et al: The use of radiolabeled nonspecific polyclonal human immunoglobulin in the detection of focal inflammation by scintigraphy. *J Nucl Med* 1989; 30:385.

81. Russell AS, Lentle BC, Percy JC: Investigation of sacroiliac disease: Comparative evaluation of radiological and radionuclide techniques. *J Rheumatol* 1974; 2:45.

82. Schmerling RH, Parker JA, Johns WD, et al: Measurement of joint inflammation in rheumatoid arthritis with In-111 chloride. *Ann Rheum Dis* 1990; 49:88.

83. Sewell JR, Black CN, Chapman AH, et al: Quantitative scintigraphy in diagnosis and management of plantar fasciitis. *J Nucl Med* 1980; 21:633.

84. Shearman J, Esdaile J, Rosenthall L, et al: Predictive value of radionuclide joint scans. *Arthritis Rheum* 1982; 25:183.

85. Simon H, Carlson DH: The use of bone scanning in the diagnosis of reflex sympathetic dystrophy. *Clin Nucl Med* 1980; 5:116.

86. Soden M, Rooney M, Cullen A, et al: Immunohistological features in the synovium obtained from clinically uninvolved knee joints of patients with rheumatoid arthritis. *Br J Rheumatol* 1989; 28:287.

87. Spencer AG, Adams FG, Horton PW, Buchanan WW: Scintiscanning in ankylosing spondylitis: A clinical, radiological and quantitative study. *J Rheumatol* 1979; 6:426.

88. Steven MM, Sturrock RD, Fogelman I, Smith ML: Whole body retention of diphosphonate in rheumatoid arthritis. *J Rheumatol* 1982; 9:873.

89. Strashun A, Chayes Z: Migratory osteolysis. *J Nucl Med* 1979; 20:179.

90. Streule K, de Schrijver M, Fridrich R: Tc-99m labelled HSA-nanocolloid vs. In-111 oxine labelled granulocytes in detecting skeletal septic process. *Nucl Med Commun* 1988; 9:59.

91. Sullivan MM, Powell N, French AP, et al: Inflammatory joint disease: A comparison of liposome scanning and radiography. *Ann Rheum Dis* 1988; 47:486.

92. Tannenbaum H, Esdaile J, Rosenthall L: Joint imaging in regional migratory osteoporosis. *J Rheumatol* 1980; 7:237.

93. Tannenbaum H, Rosenthall L, Greenspoon M, et al: Quantitative joint imaging using gallium-67 citrate in a rabbit model of zymosan-induced arthritis. *J Rheumatol* 1984; 11:687.

94. ter Meulen DC, Majd M: Bone scintigraphy in the evaluation of children with obscure skeletal pain. *Pediatrics* 1987; 79:859.

95. Uno K, Matsui M, Notina K: Indium-111 leukocyte imaging in patients with rheumatoid arthritis. *J Nucl Med* 1986; 27:339.

96. Vernon-Roberts B: Advances in the pathology and pathogenesis of osteoarthritis. *Ann RCPSC* 1986; 19:45.

97. Vyas E, Eklem M, Seto H, et al: Quantitative bone scanning of sacroiliac joints: Effect of age, gender and laterality. *AJR Am J Roentgenol* 1981; 136:586.

98. Wallace DJ, Brachman M, Feldman G, et al: Quantitative computerized joint scanning in rheumatoid arthritis. *Mt Sinai J Med* 1989; 56:46.

99. Weisberg DL, Resnick D, Taylor A, et al: RA and variants: Analysis of scintiphotographic, radiologic and clinical examinations. *AJR Am J Roentgenol* 1978; 131:655.

100. Weiss TE, Maxfield WS, Murison PJ, et al: Iodinated human serum albumin (^{131}I) localization studies of rheumatoid arthritis joints by scintillation scanning. *Arthritis Rheum* 1965; 8:976.

101. Wilson AJ, Murphy WA, Hardy DC, Totty WG: Transient osteoporosis: Transient bone marrow edema? *Radiology* 1988; 167:757.

CHAPTER 13

ORTHOPEDIC IMAGING IN TRAUMA AND SPORTS MEDICINE

Lawrence E. Holder

Manuel L. Brown

This chapter will address many of the issues of bone scintigraphy as they relate to traumatic conditions, with an emphasis on sports-related injuries. A section discusses the mechanisms and types of injuries, reviews the fundamentals of imaging, and is followed by a brief discussion of correlative imaging as related to orthopedics and sports medicine. The chapter will then focus on various disorders on a site-by-site basis. Chapter 14 deals with other selected topics in orthopedic bone scanning. Many applications of bone single photon emission computed tomography (SPECT) in orthopedics are covered in Chapter 4. Pediatric trauma and other orthopedic applications of bone scanning in children are addressed in Chapter 16.

TRAUMA

The human musculoskeletal system is designed to contain, protect, and move the various vital organs necessary for the maintenance of life. As a species we have added additional stresses on that system for recreational and fitness purposes.

We can consider the musculoskeletal system in several categories: bones, joints, muscles, tendons, and liga-ments. The skeleton is composed of bone that is formed either by intramembranous ossification or enchondral ossification or a combination of both. Both types of ossification begin with the deposition of an organic matrix on which mineral is deposited. Bone can also be discussed as the compact outer portion, the cortex, and the inner portion, the trabecular or cancellous bone. Bone is enveloped by a membrane, the periosteum, except at joints where synovium and/or cartilage covers the bone. Muscles attach to bone by tendons and ligaments whose fibers intertwine with the periosteum. Throughout life there is a continual process of bone remodeling.

Fractures

Fractures are the results of forces exceeding the ability of bone to deform without disruption of the mineral matrix. In broad categories trauma can result in frank fractures, occult fractures (where the physical examination and radiographs are not diagnostic), fatigue fractures, insufficiency fractures, growth plate injuries (i.e., Salter-Harris injuries) and avulsion fractures. Other forms of injuries include joint dislocation, bone bruising, shin splints, enthesopathy, and a variety of other injuries to muscles, ligaments, and cartilage.

Most common are frank fractures, which are the result

of excess forces leading to a disruption of the normal bone architecture. Fractures are classified in many ways—for example, as complete or incomplete (in which only one side of the bone is broken); by alignment of the distal fragment; by the site or configuration of the fracture; whether it is complex, impacted, or depressed, rotated, open (associated with a defect in overlying tissue), or closed (with intact skin); or in many other ways.[55] Most of these are usually obvious on plain film radiography. Fractures are rarely diagnostic problems unless there is a question of viability as in avascular necrosis of the femoral head or concerns related to healing as in nonunion or delayed union. Occasionally a patient who has suffered trauma will present with pain and a negative or equivocal x-ray. These occult fractures are often very obvious on bone scintigraphy, with increased activity on all three phases of the bone scan. Even in elderly patients the bone scan will usually be positive as soon as the patient presents,[71] although occasionally delayed visualization of a fracture may be seen.[90,135] In the hip this is especially so in patients over 80 years old. Common sites for occult fractures are the proximal femur and the scaphoid.

A stress or a fatigue fracture is one that occurs in normal bone that is subjected to abnormal stress. Fatigue fractures that occur when new activities are undertaken or there is increased repetition or increased intensity of an old activity are often symptomatic. Common causes for fatigue fractures include marching in new military recruits and sports injuries such as jogging. The insufficiency fracture occurs when more normal stress is applied to bones that lack the elastic resilience of normal bone. Insufficiency fractures occur in osteoporotic bone (where there is less quantity of normally mineralized bone), in osteomalacia or rickets (where there is a normal amount of abnormally mineralized bone), in rheumatoid arthritis, in pagetic bone, and in other endocrine disorders. Insufficiency fractures may be painless. A sacral insufficiency fracture, for example, is common in elderly women.

The common cause of obvious fractures, ligament and/or tendon ruptures is excessive direct force or torsion that exceeds the elastic resilience of these normal structures (Fig. 13-1).[28] Excessive force as between opposed tendons such as the plantar and Achilles tendon can lead to stress fractures of the calcaneus. Damage to osteonal units occurs due to repetitive forces that have exceeded the inherent strength of the involved bone. Continued abnormal stress before the completion of the appropriate remodeling response results in fatigue fracture (Fig. 13-2).

Bone Bruise

Direct trauma to bone that does not cause a disruption of the cortex may be described as a bone bruise. There may be minimal intraosseous or periosteal bleeding associated with bone bruises. The bone scan may show focal rounded tracer uptake often in a subchondral location. Magnetic resonance imaging (MRI) may show focal bone marrow abnormalities. Soft-tissue injuries may be focal or regional to muscles, tendons, ligaments, or menisci. Avulsion fractures are due to stresses on ligaments or tendons that avulse cartilage and/or small amounts of bone to which the tendon is attached. They are common in apophyses in the immature skeleton because the tendon-apophyseal junction is stronger than the apophyseal-bone junction.

Biomechanical Stress Lesions/Repetitive Stress Syndrome

Repetitive physical activity, with increasing repetitions and increasing muscle loading, is an acceptable training method.[46] When the biomechanics of such muscle loading is abnormal for any reason, or the biomechanical relationships or movement of the functional musculoskeletal unit is abnormal, the resulting changes on bones and joints may be undesirable. The most well-known untoward repetitive stress-related response is the carpal tunnel syndrome, in which symptoms of nocturnal numbness, burning pain along the median nerve distribution, and parestheses, which are increased by elevation and repetitive activities, are secondary to a compressive neuropathy of the median nerve within the carpal tunnel. The most frequent etiology of carpal tunnel syndrome is a flexor tenosynovitis.[84,139] Because this is primarily a soft-tissue lesion, MRI is the diagnostic modality of choice.[97,98] Equivalent osseous lesions are encountered when radionuclide bone imaging (RNBI) is per-

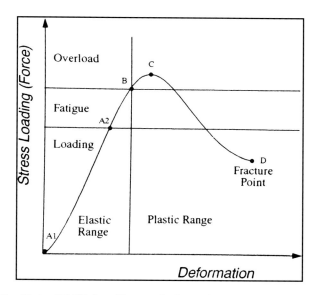

Fig. 13-1. Wolff's law. The graph shows that as the loading forces increase, the deformity on structures also increases. As long as the force does not exceed the amount corresponding to level *B*, the structure will return to its original configuration without evidence of damage; this is also called the *elastic range.* Once the fatigue level has been exceeded, however, further stresses produce permanent deformity. Microfractures begin at point *C* and ultimately failure occurs at point *D*. (*Modified from Daffner RH, Pavlov H: Stress fractures: current concepts. AJR Am J Roentgenol 1992; 159:245; with permission.*)

formed for musculoskeletal pain of unknown etiology.[64,79] One group of such lesions may be primarily related to the sites of insertion of tendons, ligaments, or articular capsules into bone, which are called *entheses*. Inflammation and/or injuries to these areas have been termed *enthesopathy* by Resnick and Niwayama.[115]

Another form of trauma that will often be seen in nuclear medicine practice is that associated with diabetic neuroarthropathy. Because of a loss of pain sensation secondary to peripheral neuroarthropathy, repeated trauma can occur without the diabetic patient's awareness. Diabetics also commonly have peripheral vascular disorders that may play a role in the development of diabetic osteopathy. Diabetic osteopathy occurs frequently in the midfoot and forefoot.

BASICS OF BONE SCINTIGRAPHY AND FRACTURES

Tracer Physiology

Details about the variety of tracers used in skeletal imaging are discussed in great detail in Chapter 2. Localization in marrow disorders and in relation to infectious processes are discussed in Chapters 8 and 11. In traumatic lesions the accumulation of bone-seeking tracers, currently almost exclusively technetium labeled diphosphonates, simply reflects the physiology of nor-

mal bone response and of the many possible posttraumatic sequelae encountered in clinical practice.[65] It is generally accepted that one of the determinants of bone tracer deposition is bone blood flow.[65,129] However, increased metabolism, possibly with a relative increase in the number of smaller crystals and therefore increase in the surface area available for interaction is also a necessary component.[131]

Anatomic Considerations

The primary dictum in orthopedic imaging is to decide where a lesion is located before deciding what that lesion may represent. To that end, creative patient positioning and viewing angles should always be considered. The posterior oblique view of the shoulder will demonstrate the glenohumeral joint structures (Fig. 13-3), a posterior view of the internally rotated knee will separate the fibula head from adjacent tibia, and an arms elevated view, occasionally with oblique angulation, will separate chest wall, humeral, and axillary structures. These views as well as other special views shown in this chapter represent only a few examples.

Images of the lower leg demonstrate the difference between medial and lateral views, as well as the differences between images taken with the legs directly on the collimator surface and those obtained through an interposed imaging table (Fig. 13-4). Although exact localization of tracer on delayed images is usually possible, the

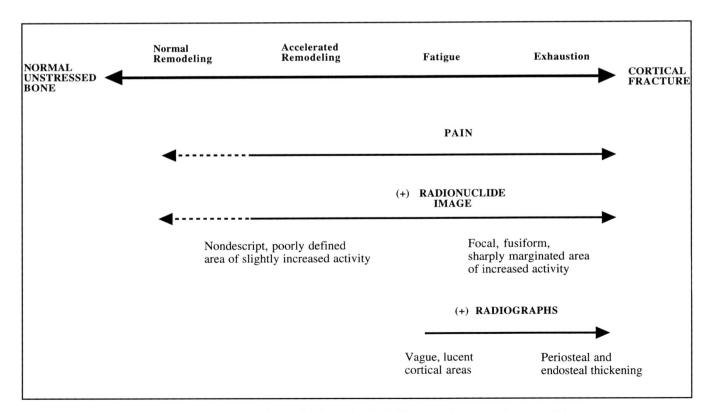

Fig. 13–2.   Stress reactions in bone. *(Modified from Roub LW, et al: Bone stress: A radionuclide imaging perspective,* Radiology *1979; 132:431; with permission.)*

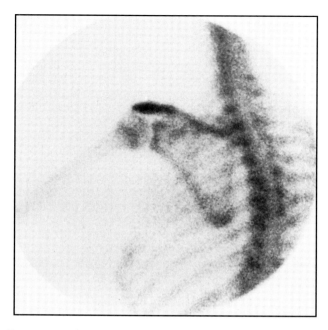

Fig. 13-3. Left posterior oblique (LPO) view of the left shoulder. Delayed image demonstrates the scintigraphic equivalent of the radiographic Grashey view to demonstrate the glenohumeral joint area. Note the separation of the humeral head from the glenoid fossa.

appearance of increased perfusion with radionuclide angiography (RNA), and the increased tracer activity representing increased vascularity on blood pool (BP) or tissue-phase images is usually less well defined. It may only be localized to a more general area, such as the ulnar side of the distal carpal row.

Time to Onset

The physiologic processes associated with fracture healing—hemorrhage, hematoma, inflammatory response, formation of collagen matrix, ossification, and remodeling—are usually demonstrable on RNBI at the time the patient presents to the physician or emergency department, and subsequently to the nuclear medicine department for imaging, no matter how soon after the fracture has occurred.

Matin, in a small study published in 1979,[90] reported that the scans performed on three elderly patients, two with fractures of the hip and one with vertebral compression fracture, and the scan done on a 10-year-old with a third cervical vertebral compression fracture were not abnormal when imaged during the first 24 hours following injury. Holder et al reported on a large prospective and retrospective group of elderly patients with suspected or documented hip fractures imaged within 24, 48, 72 or greater than 72 hours postinjury.[71] Sensitivity was 0.933, specificity 0.950, positive predictive value (PPV)

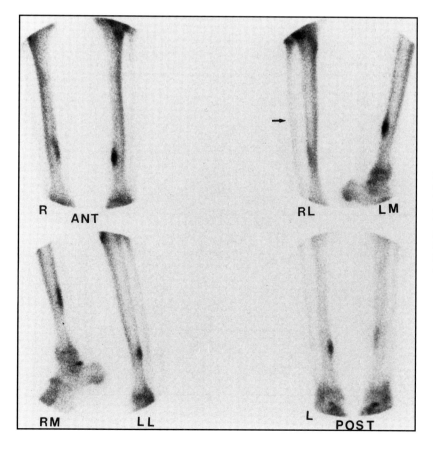

Fig. 13-4. Medial lateral and lateral medial imaging. Delayed images demonstrate the fibula most clearly on the lateral views (*arrow*) as opposed to the medial view. Incidently seen is a stress fracture in the left posteromedial tibial cortex at the junction of the middle and lower third and a shin splint lesion in the middle third of the right posterior tibial cortex. *(From Holder LE: Clinical radionuclide bone imaging.* Radiology *1990; 176:607; with permission.)*

0.918, and negative predictive value (NPV) 0.960 in the entire group, with even greater sensitivity of 0.978 and an NPV of 0.990 in the subgroup of 145 patients with normal or equivocal radiographs. They concluded that imaging could take place any time after injury and that only in patients over 75 years of age with severe pain and normal scans might it be prudent to admit and observe in the hospital and image 48 to 72 hours postinjury.[71] The results are similar to those in younger patients.[123] In the setting of sports-related stress fractures, Rupani et al demonstrated a temporal relationship in the positivity of the three phases of RNBI. In phase 1 the RNA was positive for up to 4 weeks after injury, with a mean of 2.9 weeks. The blood pool (BP) or tissue-phase image was abnormal for up to 8 weeks, with a mean of 5.2 weeks. Phase 3 delayed images were abnormal for up to 36 weeks, with a mean of 11 weeks.[123]

In 1993 Spitz published a retrospective, semiquantitative evaluation (scintimetry) of the bone scans done on 480 patients with fractures, as well as some prospective data on 18 additional patients.[136] He found that in the prospective group all fresh fractures showed increasing accumulation during the first 24 hours after injection. He suggested, only preliminarily because of the small number of patients, that 24- to 4-hour accumulation ratios below 1.1 exclude a fresh fracture. In the larger cross-sectional analysis, he found significant differences between the fracture-to-control-area uptake ratios among the various bones. Fractures near joints had the highest ratios, which were easily detected on the day of trauma. In the spine, pelvis, and midshaft regions of long bones, the ratios were much lower initially and also showed a less steep rise. They did not describe the relationship of these statistical findings to the visual interpretation of scans or

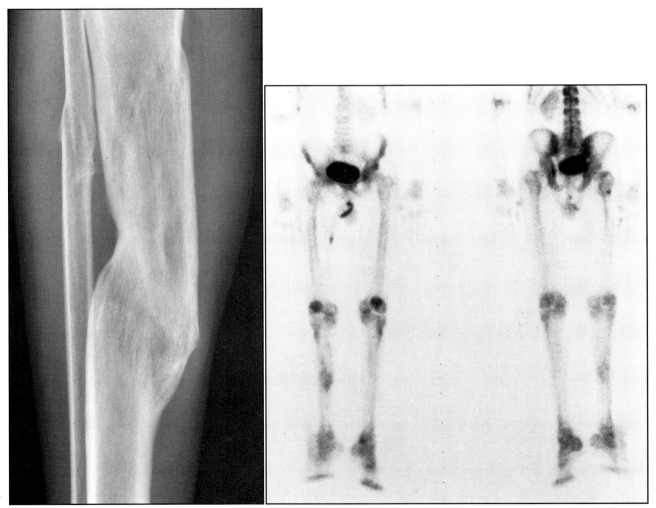

A   B

Fig. 13-5. Healed fracture 27 years postinjury. **A,** Plain radiograph. Note the position of the healed united fragments with development of stress trabecula and buttressing bone. **B,** Delayed anterior and posterior whole-body images demonstrate slight increased metabolic activity associated with minimal continued stress remodeling type of change due to mechanical offset. The patient was being staged for prostate cancer, which accounts for the abnormal uptake in the lumbar vertebra.

the clinical relevance of this interesting semiquantitative data. This report by Spitz does confirm the generally held impression that certain areas in the spine and pelvis are most difficult to evaluate, and that meticulous imaging detail and a strong index of suspicion are important when assessing asymmetric tracer uptake in these areas. Certainly more such quantitative type studies are warranted.

Time to Healing

It is generally accepted that 90% of fractures will show scintigraphic evidence of healing by 1 year and that by 2 years almost all normally healed fractures will be normometabolic on scan.[90] This extended period of continued active metabolism occurs because the remodeling stage of fracture healing involves "the replacement of woven bone with lamellar bone, reconstruction of the medullary canal, and a restoration of the bone diameter to normal," which is required to completely restore the mechanical strength of the fractured bone.[26] The minimum time for normalization of activity is approximately 6 months. Nonaligned fractures in adults may never become scintigraphically normal as remodeling forces continue (Fig. 13-5).

Scintigraphic Appearance of Healing Fractures

The scintigraphic appearance of fractures is directly related to the stage of healing modified by fracture size, the bone involved, and the technical factors of bone scintigraphy. The anatomic detail available on high-resolution delayed images is required to correctly localize the lesion, whereas the RNA and BP images of the three-phase examination aid in dating the injury.[64,90,95,123] During the acute phase, which lasts for 3 to 4 weeks, delayed imaging demonstrates an area of increased tracer that extends away from the fracture line. During the subacute phase, which lasts 8 to 12 weeks, this broader area of activity remains very intense but becomes more focal, often linear in long bones, corresponding more closely to the anatomic fracture site. Over the next 4 to 24 months the intensity diminishes. Acutely the RNA can demonstrate intense, often diffuse and poorly marginated activity in the area of a fracture. This is thought to represent the increased passive diffusion of blood and the development of hematoma associated with the earliest stages of healing. The BP images also reflect these changes (Fig. 13-6). The RNA and BP abnormalities may not be appreciated in cervical spine lesions, and although some authors have suggested a delay in appearance of tracer on all phases in some long bone lesions,[136] that has not been the general experience. After 2 to 3 weeks, the RNA becomes normal, and although BP abnormalities can remain for up to 8 to 10 weeks, the intensity of tracer accumulation relative to delayed images at this period is decreased. During the remodeling phase of repair, only the delayed images are abnormal. This phase usually lasts 3 to 4 months through 2 years. Prolonged BP activity in the appropriate setting may suggest delayed union,

nonunion, or inflammation (Fig. 13-6) (see Chapter 14). Continued abnormal tracer accumulation on RNA may suggest more marked superimposed inflammation or even infection.

Data Manipulation

Especially on delayed images, abnormal increased tracer activity often extends beyond the anatomic fracture line as seen on x-ray. The mechanism of this finding is unclear. It may occur for physiologic reasons such as the recruitment phenomenon described by Charkes[21] or for technical reasons such as Compton scatter. Data manipulation, especially in the era of all digital imaging, is often helpful in accurate localization of the primary focus of abnormal tracer accumulation. Background subtraction alone can be helpful but must often be used with the presubtracted image for anatomic localization (Fig. 13-7). Viewing images on a logarithmic scale will often provide anatomic information from lower count areas for orientation, when a very intense focus of abnormality overwhelms the linear scale. The evaluation of relative intensities of abnormal tracer accumulation, however, should not be performed on most manipulated images. Color scales can be used to detect variations in intensity, while the gray scale is best for delineating structure. Inverse scaling with white dots on a black background is often a helpful variation.

Quantitative Approaches

Quantitative approaches are not routinely used in the practice of orthopedic trauma imaging, despite a variety of "scintimetric" analysis techniques having been reported.[136] Deutsch et al obtained quantitative data from the analysis of flow curves during the 60 seconds postinjection of 99m technetium-MDP (methylene diphosphonate).[34] Resolution limitation necessitated that their evaluation include the activity "…in the vessels that immediately surround and supply these bones, and also the intravascular activity within the bones themselves…" with "no attempt…to separate either system…" Other authors have used region-of-interest analysis of delayed static images to create ratios between areas of clinical concern and other portions of the bone to aid the visual assessment of problems such as posttraumatic growth disturbances[18] or healing tibial fractures.[56] Demangeat evaluated hemovelocity, BP activity, early (3 to 5 minutes) and delayed (2 to 3 hours) bone fixation in patients with reflex sympathetic dystrophy (RSD). He also used Fourier processing of the dynamic acquisition to produce functional images.[33]

CORRELATIVE IMAGING IN TRAUMA

The concept of correlative imaging in some ways implies a primary role for the modality under discussion, with other imaging modalities providing supplemental

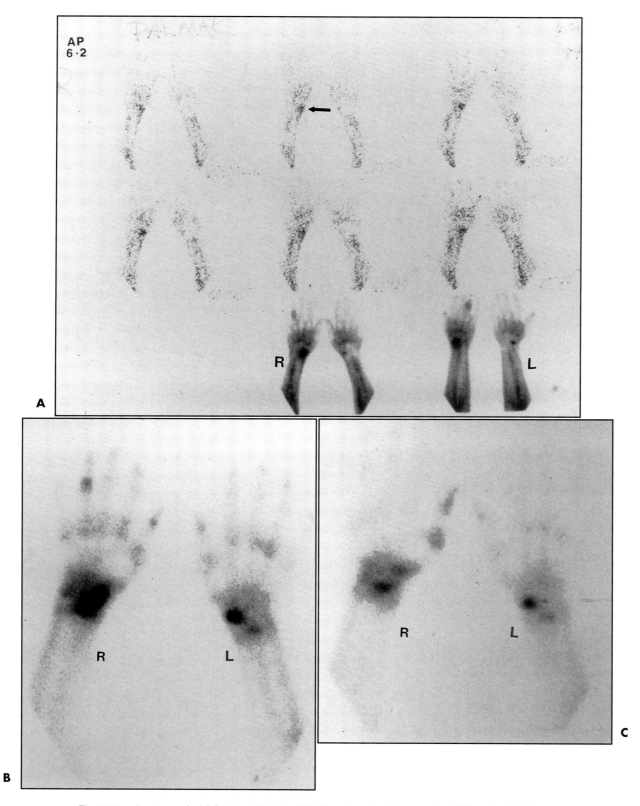

Fig. 13-6. Acute scaphoid fracture (right wrist, *R*) and scaphoid nonunion (left wrist, *L*). **A,** Radionuclide angiogram and blood pool images. In the right wrist, mild-to-moderate focal increased perfusion to the region of the scaphoid (*arrow*). The left wrist is normal. Blood pool images show intense poorly marginated increased activity in the area of the right scaphoid. There is incidental mild activity in the fourth proximal interphalangeal joint region. In the left wrist, there is mild, very focal activity in the scaphoid. **B,** Delayed images. In the right wrist, there is intense abnormal tracer uptake in the region of the right scaphoid but with extended activity. There is also moderately intense focal activity in the left scaphoid. **C,** Two months later activity in the right scaphoid is much less intense and much more focal as healing progresses. In the left wrist the focal activity associated with the nonunion has not changed.

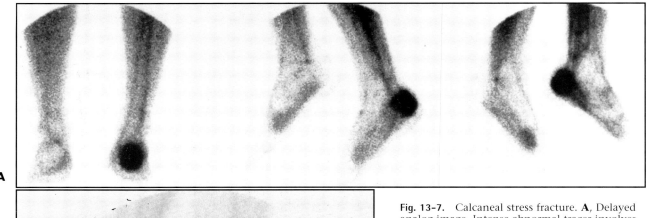

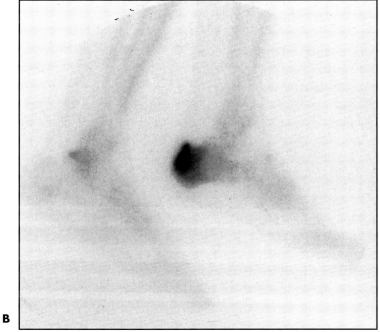

Fig. 13-7. Calcaneal stress fracture. **A**, Delayed analog image. Intense abnormal tracer involves the entire posterior half of the calcaneus. **B**, Digital images. Manipulation of scaling displayed parameters allows visualization of the locus of greatest intensity of tracer accumulation, in this case a somewhat vertically oriented fracture in the superior and posterior two thirds of the calcaneus. *(From Holder LE: Bone scintigraphy in skeletal trauma. Radiol Clin North Am 1993; 31:739; with permission.)*

information for clinicians or diagnosticians. In fact, bone scintigraphy plays a relatively minor, albeit an exceptionally important, role in traumatic and sports injuries.

As a general dictum the imaging approach for the patient with a traumatic or sports-related injury should begin with the least expensive, most widely available imaging modality, the plain film. Plain film radiography has exquisite anatomic resolution and will detect the vast majority of acute fractures. Plain films can also indirectly demonstrate some soft-tissue injuries with swelling, loss of soft tissue or muscle planes, effusions, and so on. However, most soft-tissue injuries such as tendon, ligament, and cartilage injuries will not be seen on plain films. Occasionally plain film tomography, either linear or multidirectional, will be necessary for detection of some disorders such as subtle tibial plateau fractures. Computed tomography (CT) with multiplanar reconstruction is now more commonly used to detect these specific subtle fractures when they are strongly suspected and is even more frequently used for better definition of the location of fracture fragments, such as those involving the acetabulum. When soft-tissue injuries are suspected, MRI has replaced most other forms of imaging such as arthrography for diagnosis and treatment planning.

High-resolution MRI will also detect subtle fractures, stress fractures, bone bruises, and other anatomic abnormalities. Where then does radionuclide imaging fit into the diagnostic armamentarium of the orthopedic surgeons, sports medicine physicians, and other diagnostic imagers? Bone scintigraphy remains a very sensitive technique for detecting the earliest physiologic changes related to osseous injuries (Fig. 13-2). Bone scintigraphy is more often less expensive and is arguably more readily available than MRI. The highest-resolution magnetic resonance (MR) techniques require relatively precise preimaging localization of the suspected lesion site and can assess only a relatively small area of the skeleton. Nuclear medicine techniques on the other hand allow for an easy assessment of larger areas of interest or even of the whole body without any loss of resolution, thus encompassing all possible sources of referred pain.

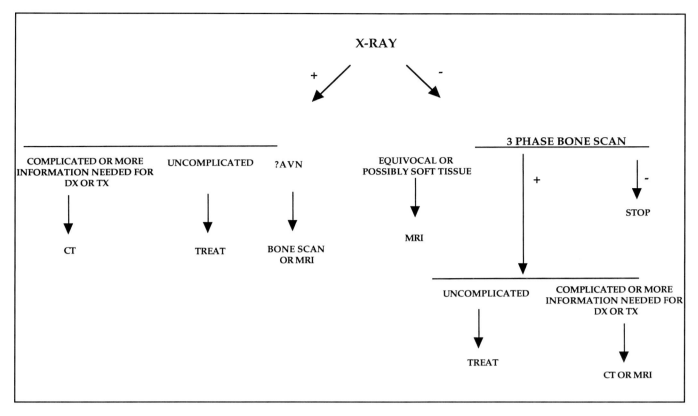

Fig. 13-8. Algorithm for studying patients with pain of potential osseous origin. (*AVN*, avascular necrosis; *Dx*, diagnosis; *Tx*, treatment.)

Figure 13-8 shows one potential diagnostic algorithm for the workup of patients with posttrauma or sports injury pain, which is suspected to be of osseous origin. The patient first has a plain film of the involved area. If that x-ray is positive, appropriate therapy is instituted. If there is a need for more anatomic information about a lesion before therapy is instituted, CT scanning, possibly with multiplanar or three-dimensional reconstruction can be considered. If there is a question of avascularity, MRI or bone scintigraphy is indicated. For acute changes in vascularity, as after an acute femoral fracture, bone scintigraphy is preferred due to the time needed for changes to be detected by MRI.[5]

If the plain film is negative, bone scintigraphy should be performed. The negative predictive value of a bone scan performed even hours or a day or two posttrauma is very high, and therefore if the bone scan is negative, the workup for an osseous etiology can usually be ended.

If the bone scan is diagnostic, as is often the case in a stress fracture of the tibia, shin splints, or plantar fasciitis, for example, treatment can be instituted without further imaging workup. If the bone scan is abnormal and additional information is needed, CT and/or MRI should be performed next depending on whether an osseous or osseous/soft-tissue process is felt clinically to be the most likely cause of the pain.

When a patient presents with pain that is thought to be primarily soft tissue in origin, MRI should be the first

examination, with the exception of some enthesopathies such as plantar fasciitis, where the scintigraphic diagnosis is straight-forward. In these other cases of soft-tissue injury, bone scintigraphy can play a secondary role and may be useful in cases where MRI is not available or where ferrous magnetic devices will degrade the image or where the patient cannot have a MRI study because of metallic surgical clips or pacemakers. Soft-tissue lesions can also be found when radionuclide imaging is performed to detect suspected osseous abnormalities.

LESIONS BY SITE
Differential Diagnostic Considerations

RNBI is most often used when localized signs or symptoms are present, plain radiographs are normal, and an osseous lesion is suspected, but no specific diagnosis is known. To make this section on fractures and other traumatic lesions as clinically relevant as possible, we have chosen to divide it by anatomic site. Even when a specific etiologic diagnosis cannot be made, there is diagnostic, therapeutic planning, and treatment follow-up value in precisely localizing a focus of abnormal increased tracer accumulation and carefully describing its morphologic characteristics and its relative physiologic activity.

Differential diagnostic considerations begin with a

careful history. Knowledge about initial symptoms may lead one to consider a source of referred pain. Knowing exactly what the patient was doing, such as maximum striding, or even less specifically the general activity during which an injury occurred, such as broad jumping, can help in differentiating lesions that may all present with a nonspecific focus of increased tracer accumula-

tion. The time between injury and the patient's first awareness of signs or symptoms can be correlated with the physiology depicted on the scan and the anatomic changes present or absent on the initial plain radiographs, for a more precise differential diagnosis, or to suggest the most appropriate correlative imaging examination.

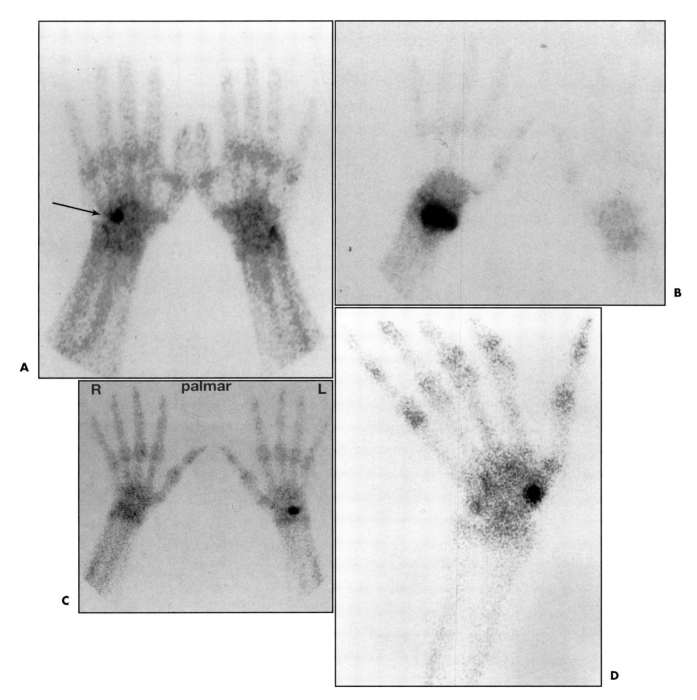

Fig. 13-9. Focal bone uptake. **A**, Osteonecrosis, hook of the hamate. **B**, Impacted fracture, distal radius. **C**, Nonspecific degenerative cyst lunate, left lunate. **D**, Intraosseous cyst, hyalinized wall at surgery, distal pole scaphoid.

Hand and Wrist

Localization of abnormal tracer on delayed images to a specific bone in the wrist or hand is usually possible[66,93,110] (Fig. 13-9). Hawkes et al suggested that registration and combined display of the x-ray image and isotope bone scan was helpful in improving localization,[62] but that is really not necessary in this area of the body which is so amenable to the highest-resolution planar imaging.

In the appropriate setting, abnormal tracer in all three phases of the RNBI such as in an acute occult scaphoid fracture allows for treatment without the need for other testing[70] (Fig. 13-6). Alternatively, activity in the hamate region, with a normal radiograph, may require CT scanning to locate a fracture of the hook or base of the hamate, which may need surgical treatment[50,140] (Fig. 13-9). Activity in a lunate, for example, even with mild sclerosis on the plain radiograph, might suggest in the appropriate setting that T1 and T2 MRI be obtained to diagnose avascular necrosis (Kienböck's disease) or to

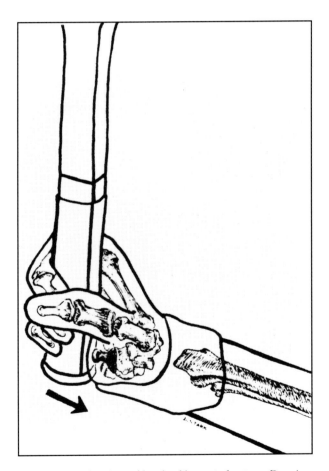

Fig. 13-10. Mechanism of hook of hamate fracture. Drawing of hand grasping a tennis racket shows the relationship of the handle to the hamate. In athletes the hook is fractured by the butt end of a racquet, club, or bat striking it during a swing. *(From Stark HH, et al: Fracture of the hook of the hamate in athletes. J Bone Joint Surg Am 1977; 59A:575; with permission.)*

assess the status of repair[134] (Fig. 13-9). The plethora of specialized imaging now available,[78,81,87,113] makes knowledge of the clinical possibilities associated with particular abnormal areas critical. We believe that in many subacute and chronic situations, symptomatic treatment without more imaging by CT or MRI is appropriate. Isolated degenerative subchondral cysts,[66] which appear radiographically similar to intraosseous ganglia[61] are such lesions. Even when they have intense abnormal tracer uptake on delayed images, a course of conservative therapy is warranted. When less physiologic activity is demonstrated, especially with normal RNA (flow images) and BP (early images), the clinician and patient can be further reassured that any lesion present is most likely benign.

Stark in 1977 reported the association of hook of the hamate fractures in raquet sports[137] (Fig. 13-10), with subsequent authors adding to the literature and emphasizing the value of RNBI.[49] Fractures of the body of the hamate,[107] trapezoid,[128] and other carpal bones have all been reported. Patel reported a variety of techniques for wrist imaging.[110] The pisiform, for example, moves away from the ulnar styloid on radial deviation views and is well seen ventrally on the lateral view. The scaphoid fracture remains by far the most common fracture in the wrist. RNBI is a well-established adjunct in the assessment of the scaphoid when a fracture cannot be confirmed radiographically.[52,70] Stress fractures have also been reported in the scaphoid,[60] with RNBI used for diagnosis when initial radiographs are normal or when a bipartite scaphoid or pseudoarthrosis is in the differential diagnosis.[40] Apple et al reported a painful carpal boss secondary to an os styloideum, an anatomic variant that may occur as an accessory ossicle dorsally between the capitate and trapezoid and the bases of the second and third metacarpals. RNBI was used to confirm this ossicle as the source of the patient's pain.[4] Conway et al reviewed the carpal boss and suggested that it could also represent degenerative osteophyte formation.[25] Occult, often impacted fractures of the distal radius are not uncommon (Fig. 13-9). Stress changes of the distal radial growth plate have also been reported in athletes such as gymnasts.[20] The ulnar impaction syndrome, manifested by focal increased tracer on both sides of the ulnar carpal joint in patients with positive ulnar variance is another cause of wrist pain secondary to the transfer of excessive compressive forces from the ulna to the triquetrum and lunate through the triangular fibrocartilage complex.

Upper Extremity

The upper extremity includes those entities and problems affecting the shoulder girdle, arm, elbow, and forearm. The most distal radius and ulna are discussed in the section on hand and wrist.

SHOULDER

The acromioclavicular (AC) joint is a true synovial joint. There remains debate as to whether degenerative changes occur in asymptomatic patients as a consequence of aging, or whether changes in the AC joint are always pathologic.[146] Bone proliferation along the anterior edge of the acromion can be seen in patients who have impingement symptoms involving the rotator cuff.[146] When the clinical picture is confusing, especially when potential incidental anatomic abnormalities are discovered on plain radiographs, RNBI can be used to demonstrate abnormal increased metabolic activity on either side of the AC joint or at the acromion and coracoid process, thus suggesting that the AC joint or the attachments of the AC ligament are involved and etiologically related.

Although the complex three-dimensional anatomy of the shoulder is ideal for multiplanar CT or MRI for the

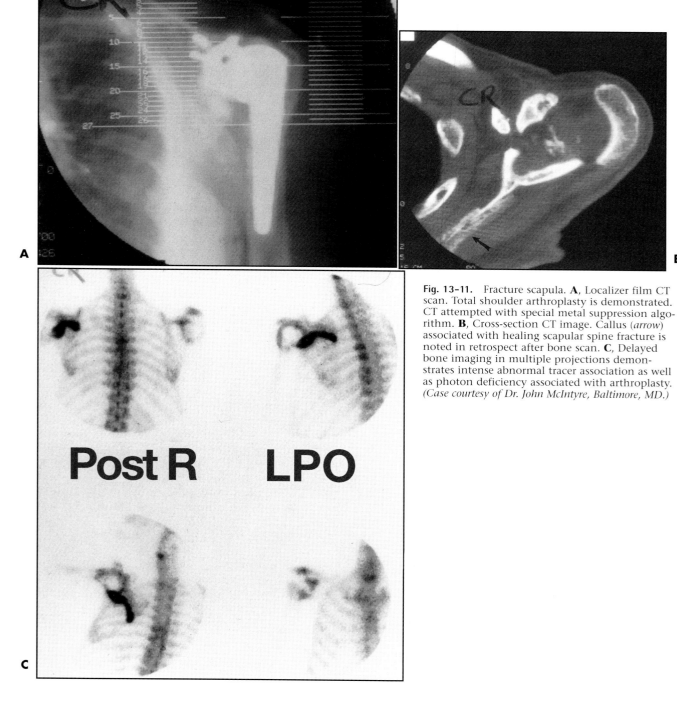

Fig. 13-11. Fracture scapula. **A,** Localizer film CT scan. Total shoulder arthroplasty is demonstrated. CT attempted with special metal suppression algorithm. **B,** Cross-section CT image. Callus (*arrow*) associated with healing scapular spine fracture is noted in retrospect after bone scan. **C,** Delayed bone imaging in multiple projections demonstrates intense abnormal tracer association as well as photon deficiency associated with arthroplasty. (*Case courtesy of Dr. John McIntyre, Baltimore, MD.*)

diagnosis of fracture or soft-tissue abnormality, RNBI can be used when the primary source or etiology of patient's complaints is uncertain. This can be particularly helpful in the postoperative patient who has rearranged anatomy or metal appliances or prosthesis in place (Fig. 13-11). A fatigue fracture of the medial clavicle has been reported,[73] as has the entity of osteolysis of the distal clavicle.[19,92] Both entities, which manifest as focal areas of increased tracer accumulation associated with osseous repair, have been reviewed in the athletic injury context.[64] Condensing osteitis of the clavicle also presents as a focus of increased tracer accumulation of the medial clavicle on delayed images.[108] The significance of this painful lesion lies in knowing of its existence.

ARM

Most humeral fractures as well as tumor and tumorlike lesions associated with pain are discovered by physical examination or routine plain radiographs. Abnormal increased activity associated with stress-remodeling or benign bony proliferation at muscle insertion sites has been reported to involve the pectoralis major[48] and the deltoid muscle.[45] The distal deltoid insertion is on the anterolateral aspect of the proximal third of the humerus. Fink-Bennett illustrated in 1980 a more lateral location of this activity and suggested that an anterior view of the humerus in internal rotation could be obtained to "...show beyond question that the increased tracer accumulation is within the thickened cortex." For reproducibility we routinely obtain whole-body scans with the palms down. This position fully internally rotates the humerus, projecting the tuberosity medially (Fig. 13-12). Thus with the resolution now routinely obtainable with modern gamma cameras, it is important to know the patient's anatomic position during imaging. We have also encountered a midhumeral stress fracture in a weight lifter,[89] and heterotopic ossification, commonly referred to myositis ossificans, in the biceps of a

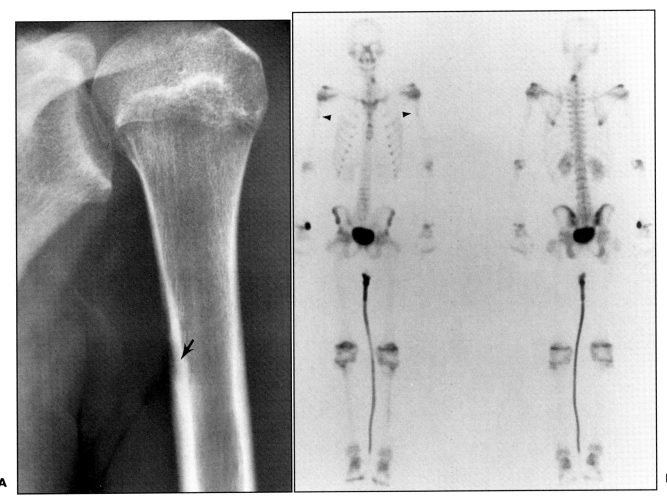

A   **B**

Fig. 13-12. Deltoid insertion. **A,** Plain radiograph, 14-year-old male quadriplegic, incidentally noted cortical irregularity (*arrow*). **B,** Delayed whole-body image. Radionuclide angiogram and blood pool were normal. Bilateral minimal areas of increased activity projected medially with the arms placed in full pronation, projecting the tuberosity medially.

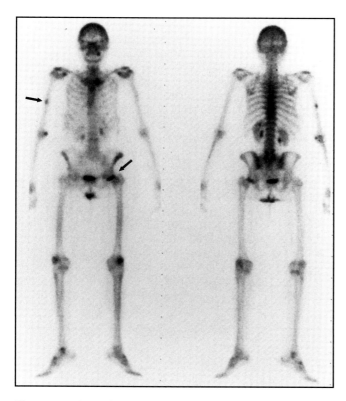

Fig. 13-13. Stress fracture, right humerus and occult left subcapital fracture. Delayed whole-body bone images. Classical horizontal subcapital fracture, left hip. Focal activity, right mid-humerus (*arrow*) represents stress fracture in a patient using a walker for 2 to 3 weeks because of hip pain.

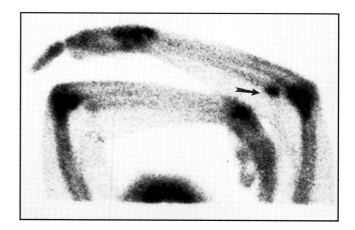

Fig. 13-14. Stress lesion, proximal radius. Delayed lateral spot images. Focal increased tracer at the radial tuberosity (*arrow*), the biceps brachii tendon insertion site, may represent a type of avulsion fracture or stress fracture in a patient who does heavy lifting. The scintigraphic pattern on these images is nonspecific; however, the site of pain is localized and treatment can be undertaken. This patient was referred to evaluate elbow pain.

baseball pitcher. During a search for metastasis, an interesting stress fracture was encountered in the right proximal humerus in a patient using a walker for 2 to 3 weeks because of severe left hip pain (Fig. 13-13). By watching her use the walker, it was clear that the upper extremities were being subjected to significant new biomechanical stress.

ELBOW

The elbow is another area subjected to significant mechanical stress, the complex anatomy of which often creates clinical uncertainty as to the source of the patient's signs or symptoms. Because a specific diagnosis can rarely be made with RNBI, the goal of the examination should be directed toward accurate localization of abnormal activity. To this end, routine oblique and specialized views such as the acute flexion view described by Fink-Bennett and Carichner can be used.[44] It is helpful to the clinician if abnormal activity about the elbow can be localized to one of four regions (lateral, medial, posterior, or anterior) or if within the joint to one of three compartments (posterior, lateral, or medial).[109] The lateral region includes the lateral epicondyle, the site of findings in tennis elbow. The medial area and the medial compartment include the medial epicondyle, the site of findings in Little League elbow. Torg reported a stress fracture through the olecranon epiphyseal plate in an adolescent

pitcher,[141] and Hulkko described stress fractures of the olecranon in javelin throwers.[72]

FOREARM

Acute fractures of the forearm are usually obvious. Since the forearm, as well as the lower leg, consists of two separate bones united by ligaments and joints, they can be thought of as a ring structure similar to the pelvis. Goldberg et al have described the common occurrence of double injuries to the forearm, with many of the less obvious ones diagnosed by RNBI.[53]

Ulnar diaphyseal stress fractures have been reported in athletes participating in a wide variety of sports and are probably best thought of as lifting fractures.[59,104,116] A stress lesion of the proximal radius at the tuberosity, the biceps brachii tendon insertion site, can also be thought of as a lifting injury, with the nonspecific focus of abnormal tracer used to localize the probable source of the patient's pain (Fig. 13-14). A stress fracture of the distal radius, proximal to the wrist, has also been reported in a high-level tennis player.[83] Probably because the bones of the forearm are so easily examined, localized swelling and marked focal tenderness associated with trauma can often be seen. Similarly patients who have osteoporosis associated with rheumatoid arthritis and have sustained insufficiency fractures can present with signs and symptoms suggesting cellulitis.[100]

Chest

Rib fractures and traumatic separations at the costochondral junctions are most often seen during RNBI when a patient with chest pain of uncertain etiology is examined. The typical lesions are round, often multiple, and when oriented one above the other in adjacent ribs are diagnostic. When there is an isolated lesion, careful

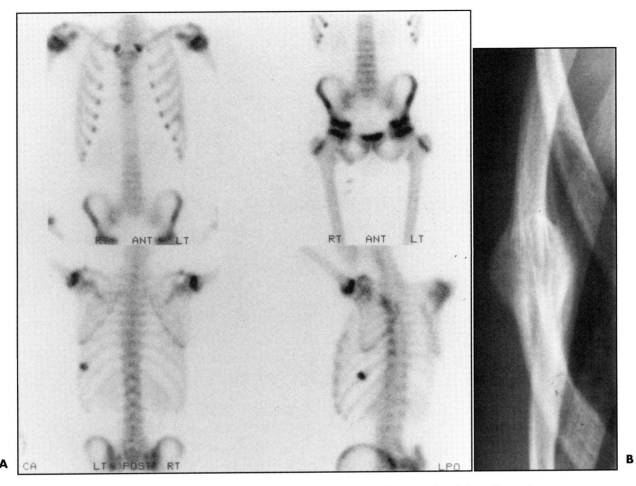

Fig. 13-15. Rib fracture. A 15-year-old football player imaged because the plain radiograph was originally thought suspicious for malignancy. **A,** Delayed bone image—moderately intense, well-defined round area of increased tracer in posterolateral aspect of left tenth rib. **B,** Oblique radiograph—note fusiform appearance of callus associated with healing rib fracture. In retrospect, pain began 5 to 6 weeks previously, the day after a football game during which he had taken a direct hit to this area.

history is particularly essential for correct interpretation of the initial radiographs and the bone scan (Fig. 13-15). Rib stress fractures have been reported in both athletes[58] and nonathletes.[80] Although these often present with a history of a "snap" from the shoulder, the symptoms are variable.[80] Insufficiency fractures of the ribs have been described as a source of pain in elderly osteopenic patients with accentuated kyphosis of the thoracic spine.[22] An interesting normal stress response consisting of cortical thickening of one to four posterior ribs and the articulating transverse processes of the corresponding vertebral bodies has been reported as possibly secondary to the chronic direct pull of the iliocostalis thoracis muscle at its origins and insertions on the posterior angles of the ribs and to indirect motion at the synovial costotransverse articulations.[85] Activity on delayed bone images was only minimally intense and poorly marginated.

Head and Spine

CERVICAL SPINE

RNBI in the evaluation of cervical and thoracic spine trauma has been used primarily to determine if an x-ray abnormality represents an acute process potentially responsible for the patient's pain or to exclude a significant osseous abnormality as the source of patient complaints when plain radiographs are normal. Planar cervical spine imaging has been technically limited. Placing the patient's neck directly on the collimator surface dramatically improves resolution by decreasing distance. Slight posterior oblique images of the cervical spine can also be helpful. Reports[90,136] and anecdotal experience make most nuclear physicians hesitant to exclude an early non-displaced cervical spine fracture even when initial imaging is normal. RNBI has been evaluated in patients with whiplash injury.[6,63] There was no correla-

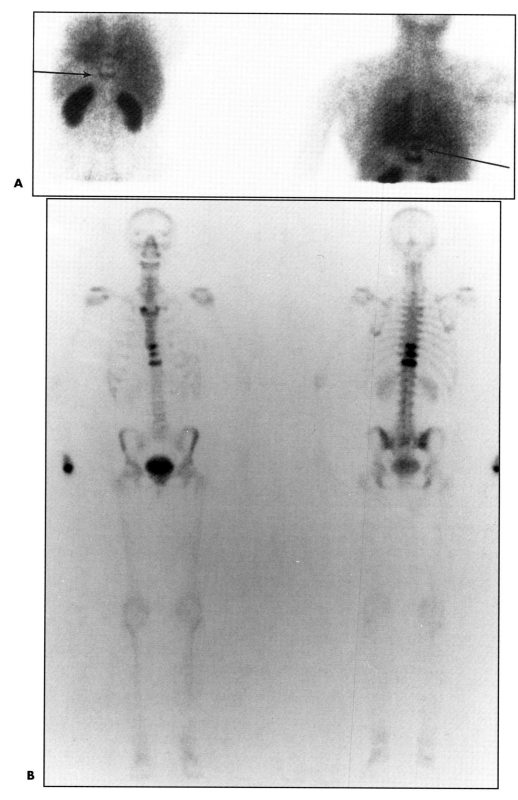

Fig. 13-16. Thoracic vertebral compression fractures, 1 month following trauma. **A,** Blood pool images demonstrate horizontal linear activity in three adjacent lower thoracic vertebrae (*arrows*). **B,** Delayed images demonstrate horizontal linear activity which in upper vertebrae are more suggestive of the superior end plate location. This was better defined on computer subtracted images (not shown).

tion in either study between the symptoms or signs of the injury and the scintigraphic findings. However, in the first, a retrospective study of 35 patients,[63] the authors concluded that a negative RNBS excluded a skeletal injury; and in the second, also a prospective study involving 20 patients with whiplash injury, none were shown to have radionuclide bone scan suggesting fracture, and none were subsequently diagnosed as having a fracture. Similarly, since BP image activity is difficult to delineate in the cervical spine, the differential diagnosis of abnormal increased activity on delayed imaging remains that of nonspecific stress response or degenerative arthritis versus a healing fracture. Recently SPECT imaging has been tried, again with some anecdotal reports of increase in diagnostic accuracy.

THORACIC SPINE

In the thoracic spine, imaging is technically easier than the cervical spine. In addition to visualizing fractures on delayed imaging, the BP images are often abnormal when the fractures are acute (Fig. 13-16). Horizontal linear activity most marked at the superior end plate is very characteristic of traumatic fractures. Even in patients with multiple lesions and severe pain, plain radiographs can be normal. In one study of osteoporotic vertebral fractures, only those vertebrae that had radiographic deformities more than 3 SD below the normal mean could be confidently diagnosed on the plain radiographs.[124] Scoliotic curves are easily visualized, especially with whole-body images produced with newer-generation cameras. Lateral activity, usually focal and on the concave side, but often not sharply marginated, is most often associated with nonspecific degenerative changes or stress changes. Because of the prevalence of vertebral fractures in ejection injuries, RNBI is used routinely by the Royal Air Force in evaluating these airmen.[15] Bury found that almost 50% of those with normal radiographs had abnormal bone images.[15]

LUMBAR SPINE

Almost all of the lesions or syndromes associated with the lumbar spine and presenting with lower back pain can demonstrate RNBI findings, even though those findings alone are not always specific. SPECT imaging techniques, discussed in Chapter 4 may add specificity.[24,51] Degenerative joint disease or osteoarthritis involving the posterolateral aspects of the vertebra, for example, can often be differentiated from isolated central body activity that would suggest a metastasis. Facet arthritis and facet syndrome also have a characteristic appearance

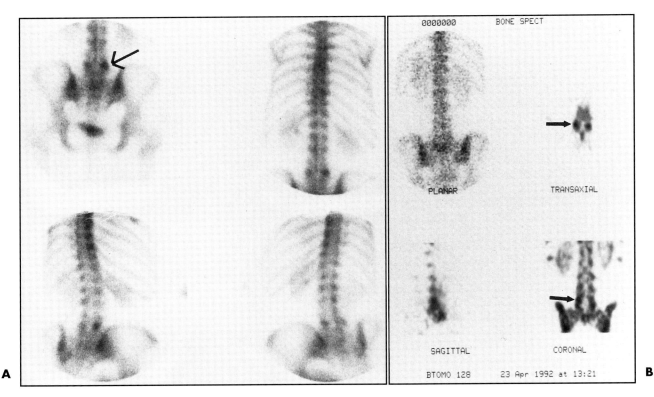

Fig. 13-17. Facet joint uptake (facet syndrome, facet arthritis). **A,** Delayed images. Bilateral facet joint uptake right (*arrow*) more marked than left. Note the orientation of the facet activity on the RPO and LPO views (*lower images*); this orientation is 90 degrees to the orientation of the adjacent pars region. **B,** SPECT imaging. Bilateral abnormal uptake appreciated most clearly in this reproduction on transaxial and coronal images (*arrows*). *(From Holder LE, Machin JL, Asdourian P, et al: Planar and high resolution bone imaging in the diagnosis of facet syndrome.* J Nucl Med *1995; 36:37; with permission.)*

consisting of focal increased tracer accumulation on delayed images corresponding to the facet joint regions (Fig. 13-17). Unfortunately this activity has a better NPV (100% SPECT; 93% planar) than specificity (71% SPECT, 76% planar) for the diagnosis of facet syndrome.[67] Congenital or acquired abnormalities, which can be associated with either ipsilateral or contralateral symptoms,[86] include developmental pars interarticularis defects or other posterior element abnormalities such as defects in neural arch development.[7,145] Correlative imaging techniques, discussed elsewhere in this chapter and in Chapter 5, are usually required for specific diagnosis, after the site of abnormal metabolism has been localized by RNBI. Nonradicular low back pain in adolescents and in older athletes such as football linemen or wrestlers, whose activities place stress on the posterior elements, are candidates for RNBI.[68] Blanda et al have recently proposed a protocol for nonoperative treatment of athletes with defects of the pars interarticularis. They emphasize that bone scans should be obtained "a) when signs and symptoms are suggestive of pars defect but oblique plain films are normal; b) to determine the acuteness of the pars defect; or c) to rule out additional pathology if signs and symptoms are unusual."[8] SPECT imaging can detect abnormal foci when planar studies are normal,[24,51] although the physiologic significance of this activity is still uncertain.

RNBI can also detect foci of activity in patients with low back pain subsequently shown on CT to be due to small fractures in the laminae or apophyseal processes. Without RNBI these patients otherwise would be labeled as having "nonspecific back pain."[132] Similarly, pain from the sacroiliac (SI) joints, other areas of the pelvis, and even the thoracic spine and lower extremities can be referred to the low back,[121] emphasizing again the value of whole-body bone imaging even when symptoms are very focal.[105] Acute lumbar vertebral fractures appear similar to those described for the thoracic spine. Transverse process fractures can also be seen.

A normally healed postoperative fusion mass (Fig. 13-18) is normometabolic without any focal areas of increased activity. When the fusion mass does not heal normally, the scintigraphic findings are similar to any other fracture, as has been discussed earlier in this chapter. Other authors have also suggested a greater sensitivity for SPECT imaging to detect painful pseudoarthrosis.[133] Even-Sapir et al[41] have used SPECT imaging to evaluate painful late effects of lumbar spinal fusion. They emphasize that arthrodesis alters the biomechanics of the spine, creating areas of compensatory increased motion and increased mechanical load associated with the free motion segments adjacent to the fusion.[41]

Pelvis

One of the most common stress fractures of the pelvis encountered in nuclear medicine departments is the insufficiency fracture of the sacrum seen in elderly females. The scintigraphic pattern may vary, but the classic appearance is that of the Honda or butterfly sign, where the fracture involves both sacral alae and crosses the midportion of the sacrum (Fig. 13-19). Variants of sacral insufficiency fractures include only the body of the sacrum, only the alae (Fig. 13-20), or the more extensive fractures that involve other bones in the pelvis. The pelvic insufficiency fracture may be discovered incidentally when a bone scan is done for malignancy or to search for an etiology for low back pain. In a study by Rawlings et al,[114] 16 patients with osteoporotic sacral fractures were studied. The average age was 71 years, and the most common complaint was diffuse back pain accompanied by hip, thigh, or buttock discomfort. Conservative treatments to reduce pain yielded good results in this patient population. In another series[127] most of the 23 patients were osteoporotic and had only minor trauma or no traumatic event. As in other series, plain films were positive in approximately half of the cases, although many fractures were initially overlooked. After bone scan detection, confirmation when occasionally needed can be done by either CT or plain film tomography.

Other insufficiency fractures of the pelvis can occur. Davies[31] reported on 11 postmenopausal women with parasymphyseal insufficiency fractures. Nine of the eleven also had sacral insufficiency fractures (Fig. 13-21). Plain radiographs or CT scans may show mixed lytic and sclerotic zones at the fracture site compatible with delayed healing. However, these radiographic findings may also simulate a pathologic fracture. Multiple sites of insufficiency fractures of the pelvis are common. Davies, in another series,[29] had 25 patients with insufficiency fractures of the pelvic ring, 80% of whom had multiple fractures.

Stress fracture of the pubis can occur in a variety of athletic activities, especially in long-distance running.[111] Runners may also present with pubic symphysitis.[75] Swimmers[74] and ice hockey players[12] have all been reported with pubic symphysitis. The etiology of the symphysitis is thought to be due to mechanical stresses related to the adductor magnus and the rectus abdominal muscles. These athletes may present with vague groin or lower abdominal pain.

Avulsion fractures of the pelvis may also be diagnosed by a characteristic radiographic appearance and knowledge of the typical locations.[43] One area that is prone to avulsion-type injuries is the anterior iliac crest.[119] It is essential when imaging that the patient be positioned symmetrically, as any rotation can cause an asymmetric appearance of the iliac crest. The insertion of the rectus femoris just above the acetabulum and the insertion of the hamstring at the ischial tuberosity are other common sites of avulsion fractures. Because these lesions are in metabolically active areas in young patients, especially when symptoms are acute, there can be increased activity on RNA and on BP images. Activity, however, is generally less intense and less diffuse than when osteosarcoma is encountered. X-ray and clinical correlation is of critical importance in these patients. Enthesopathy of the ischial tuberosity has been reported in a patient who began retrorunning to reduce the symptoms of patellofemoral pain that occurred during forward running.[125]

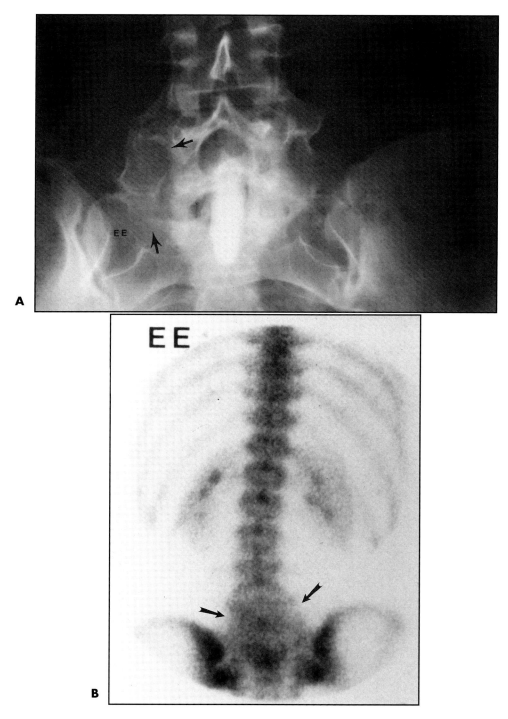

Fig. 13-18. Healed fusion mass. **A**, AP radiograph. Radio-opaque contrast in the lumbar subarachnoid space. Bilateral fusion mass is best seen on the right (*arrow*). **B**, Delayed radionuclide bone image. Posterior view. The fusion mass has the same activity as the adjacent normal bone.

Hip

The hip joint is composed of the acetabulum, the proximal femur and associated cartilage, synovium, and bursa. It is a relatively common location for traumatic injuries and the sequelae of sports-related activities. In an

article on exercise-induced stress injuries of the femur, Clement et al[23] studied 71 symptomatic athletes to identify the signs and symptoms of femoral stress injuries, the sites and the distribution of these lesions. The group was mostly runners, 45% were recreational, 27% were marathon runners, and 18% were other competitive run-

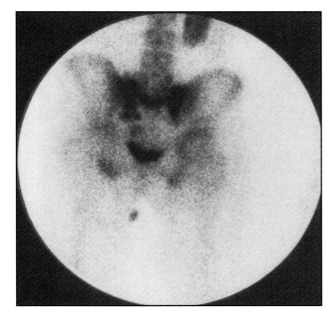

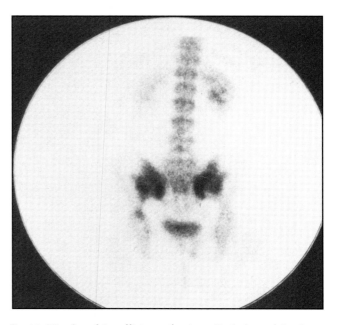

Fig. 13-19. Sacral insufficiency fracture. Posterior view of the pelvis demonstrates the classical "H" or "Honda sign." Note increased activity-oriented vertically in both medial SI joints, with a horizontal component across the upper sacral segments.

Fig. 13-20. Sacral insufficiency fracture. Posterior pelvic view showing increased uptake in both SI joints without the sacral component.

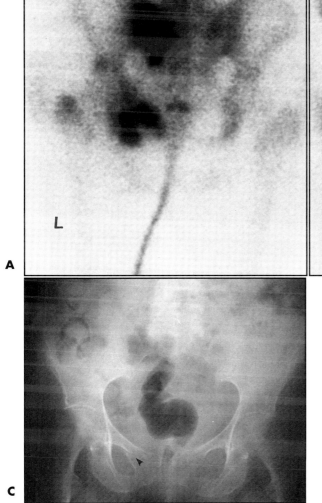

Fig. 13-21. Pubis ramus fracture. **A**, Posterior view of the pelvis. **B**, Anterior view of the pelvis. Bone scan shows intense increased uptake in the left SI joint, left superior and inferior pubic rami, and moderate increased uptake in the left greater trochanter. **C**, AP radiograph demonstrates the subtle fracture in the pubic ramus (*arrowheads*) in this reversed radiograph. This postmenopausal female had minimal trauma. This can be considered either an insufficiency fracture or a subtle fracture of which only one of the components was detected on plain films and where the inferior pubic ramus and SI fractures were radiographically occult.

ners. Most of these subjects complained of anterior thigh pain (46%) followed by hip pain (27%) and groin pain (8%). X-rays were positive in only 11 of the 46 cases (24%). The distribution of the 74 lesions on bone scintigraphy included 39 (53%) in the shaft, 15 in the lesser trochanter, 1 in the greater trochanter, 8 in the neck, and 11 in the intertrochanteric region. To maximize the ability of bone scintigraphy to detect stress-related abnormalities, Ammann[2] demonstrated that the frog-leg view significantly improved the yield, especially for those lesions involving the lesser trochanter.

Avulsion injuries of the hip include those related to the insertion of the gluteus medius at the greater trochanter, the iliopsoas at the lesser trochanter, and the pectineus in the proximal femoral shaft. Three-phase bone scanning will show focal uptake at the site of avulsion injuries. Although acute severe trochanteric bursitis can be seen scintigraphically on all three phases of the bone scan as a focal area of increased tracer in the peripheral aspect of the greater trochanter[1] (Fig. 13-22), it is most often seen in less acute processes only on delayed images. The degree of uptake in greater trochanteric bursitis may simulate a stress fracture.[82] Bursitis may also occur in other locations such as the ischial bursa (Fig. 13-23).

One of the major roles of bone scintigraphy in the hip is in the diagnosis of stress fractures[23] and occult fractures.[71,82] Tountas[142] described 13 insufficiency fractures in elderly women with severe osteoporosis. Most cases

had a delayed diagnosis due to the vague pain and the subtle or absent findings on x-ray. In a prospective study by Fairclough et al,[42] 693 patients with acute hip pain had x-ray evaluation. In 94% of cases x-rays confirmed the diagnosis. In 30 of the 43 patients with negative plain films, the bone scan was normal and none of those patients had a fracture on follow-up. All 13 patients with positive bone scans proved to have a fracture as a cause of their pain (Fig. 13-24).

Holder et al[71] studied 175 patients, 105 retrospective and 70 prospective, to determine features related to the detection of proximal femoral fractures. The study group had 60 hip fractures, 36 fractures at other sites, and 58 cases with other final diagnoses. Bone scintigraphy detected 56 of the 60 hip fractures for a sensitivity of 93% and a specificity of 95%. There was no evidence that the age of the patient or the time between injury and the bone scan made any difference in diagnosis. Three of the four false-negative studies were in clinically and roentgenographically obvious displaced subcapital fractures. Disruption of the blood supply was thought the most likely etiology. There were no false-negative intertrochanteric fractures (sensitivity of 100%) (Fig. 13-25, A). Eighty-six percent of studies in patients over 70 years of age were true-positive for fractures without a difference if the elderly patients were examined within 24 hours after an injury or at a later time. The results of this study suggest that only the occasional patient with severe symptoms with a negative bone scan needs to be studied at 72 hours or later with a repeat scan. This high rate of detection of occult fractures with bone scans was also shown by Rizzo[118] who reported that MRI was as accurate as the bone scan in diagnosing hip fractures.

Lewis et al[82] discussed some of the pitfalls in the bone

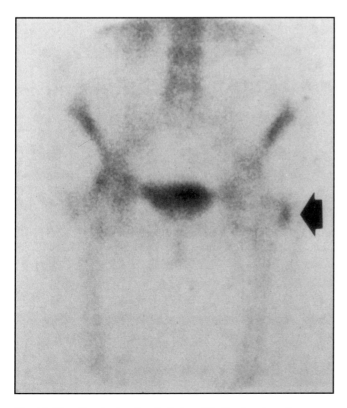

Fig. 13-22. Greater trochanteric bursitis. Predominantly peripheral increased uptake in the greater trochanter.

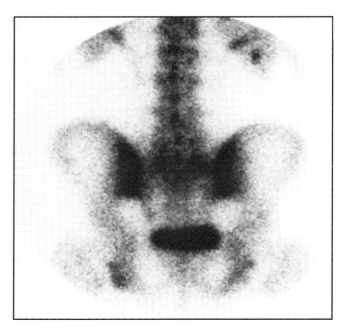

Fig. 13-23. Ischial bursitis. Moderate increased uptake in both ischial tuberosities. *(Case courtesy of Robert Cooper, MD.)*

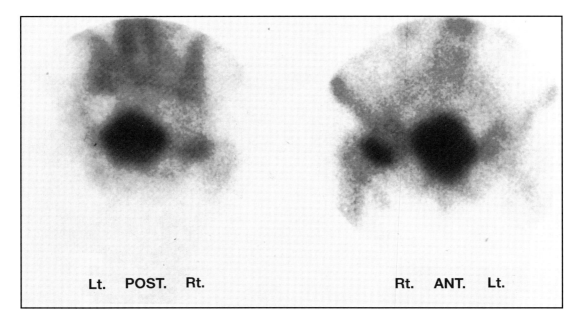

Fig. 13-24. Occult right femoral neck fracture. Delayed posterior and anterior bone scan images.

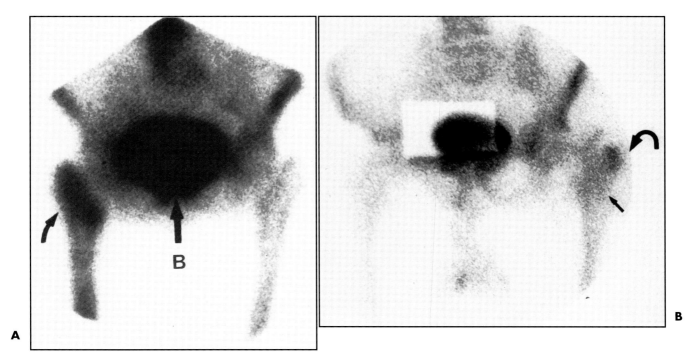

Fig. 13-25. Intertrochanter and greater trochanter fracture. **A,** Note the relatively homogeneous distribution of increased tracer throughout the intertrochanteric region. This contrasts to the more focal increased tracer at the greater trochanter in patients who have fractured only that portion of the hip (**B**).

scan diagnosis of hip fractures. Categorizing uptake in the greater trochanter as a fracture was the major problem they encountered. In retrospect, they felt that the uptake was due to trochanteric bursitis in all cases. Holder et al described a specific scintigraphic pattern of isolated greater trochanter fracture, consisting of increased activity either confined to the greater trochanter or much more intense than any minimal activity extending into the intertrochanteric region[71] (Fig. 13-25, *B*). In Clement's younger population, only 1 of 74 lesions was in the greater trochanter.[23] The potential misclassification of trochanteric bursitis as an isolat-

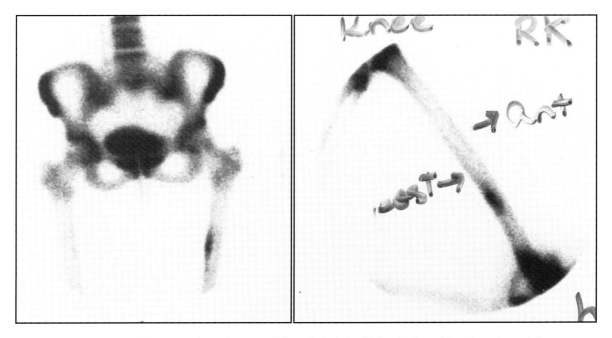

Fig. 13-26. Adductor avulsion fracture. Although slightly thicker in the midportion, the activity in the posteromedial femoral cortex is not classically fusiform.

ed fracture may not be a clinical problem as both conditions are treated conservatively.

Although the spectrum of scintigraphic findings in traumatic and sports-related injuries in the hip are quite varied, bone scintigraphy is quite valuable in the detection of stress fractures, avulsion injuries and bursitis, in detecting occult femoral fractures, and as discussed in Chapter 14, in determining the likelihood of complications in patients with clinically and radiographically evident proximal femoral fractures. Chapter 16 addresses the use of bone scanning in the detection and the evaluation of the child with slipped capital femoral epiphysis (SCFE). The spectrum of scintigraphic findings in children with SCFE can go from increased activity in the physis to the findings of avascular necrosis in the slipped femoral head. Chondrolysis may be predicted by moderate to marked increased periarticular activity and a loss in activity in the greater trochanter.

Lower Extremity

FEMUR

In one study 39 of 74 femoral lesions in athletes[23] were in the shaft. The authors emphasized that symptoms are difficult to localize, and since the femur is surrounded by thick musculature, direct clinical examination is limited. Butler describes subtrochanteric stress fractures, partially attributing them to bounding, an exercise of repetitive jumping.[16] Most seem to occur on the medial side of the femoral shaft and are often fusiform. We have been unable to routinely separate adductor avulsion fractures from true biomechanical stress fractures[64] (Fig. 13-26). In some cases, the clinical history of a sudden pain while stretching and a characteristic location can suggest an adductor avulsion fracture.[120] Davies reported three skeletally immature patients initially referred with a diagnosis of probable sarcoma who had adductor avulsion fracture.[30] There was no hyperemia on RNA or BP images, and the delayed scan activity was fusiform and involved the posteromedial cortex. A midfemoral fracture in an oligomenorrheic athlete with four prior fibular stress fractures has been reported.[37] Her total amenorrheic period was 100 months, and her bone mineral density (BMD) was reported as less than the mean for other amenorrheic athletes. Bilateral femoral lesions have also been reported in an otherwise normal 15-year-old high school runner.[10]

KNEE

Although RNBI has been used to delineate and site abnormalities before arthroscopy in patients with acute knee pain following trauma,[103] acute knee pain is now almost exclusively evaluated with plain radiographs and MRI. Usually incidental to the cartilage and ligament evaluation for which the study was performed, MRI can localize bone marrow changes potentially due to subchondral fracture. RNBI can be used to assess the metabolic activity of such marrow changes and to demonstrate additional subtle lesions.[88] Many authors have studied RNBI in patients with chronic knee pain as a means to identify patients requiring more invasive evaluation, to establish prognosis or to assess the results of therapeutic intervention.[17,38,39,76] A normal scan supports an excellent prognosis for recovery.[17,38] Dye has described two patterns of patellofemoral activity associated with persistence of clinical symptoms that might benefit from earlier intervention. One is inferior pole activity and the other is combined femoral trochlear and patellar uptake. Patients with other patterns of focal uptake or with diffuse uptake usually resolve their symptoms. He therefore cautions against too early surgical intervention in these patients, who may apparently be failing conservative therapy.[39] Inferior pole patella uptake in an adult is often a patella tendonitis associated with injury to the quadriceps mechanism[64] (Fig. 13-27). In children, quadriceps mechanism injury often results in damage and radiotracer uptake at the tibial tuberosity.

Although some authors have described a very high sensitivity for the presence of abnormal increased patellar activity in patients later shown to have chondromalacia arthroscopically,[76] others have reported low sensitivity.[17] Specificity is also low in this application of RNBI.

Osteoarthritic changes, discussed in detail in Chapter 12, are usually recognizable. In our experience they can occur well before any corresponding plain radiographic changes. RNBI can be used to provide objective evidence of disease preoperatively in patients whose pain is incapacitating but out of proportion to plain film anatomic changes.

"Spontaneous" osteonecrosis may occur in the elderly. There is pain and plain films are often normal at presentation.[96,106,122] Abnormal increased activity in these patients is most often intense, sharply defined, and localized to the immediate subchondral region of the medial femoral condyle. The abnormality may also be seen in the proximal tibia.

LEG

The conception of shin splints as any pain between the knee and ankle has given way to a spectrum of entities responsible for leg pain. RNBI remains the diagnostic modality of choice when an underlying osseous lesion is suspected. Stress fractures in the leg occur predominantly at the middle third-lower third junction of the tibia in the posteromedial cortex. Focal, fusiform increased tracer accumulation on delayed images is the hallmark (Fig. 13-28). A similar appearance is present in the lower and upper tibia, the fibula, and in other long bones.[123] Multiple lesions occur, often with the second or incidental lesions relatively asymptomatic. There are usually no differences in type, location or distribution of lesions between males and females or between competitive and non-competitive athletes. Anterior, midshaft tibial stress fractures often have positive radiographs at the time of clinical presentation. Because RNBI frequently demonstrates less intense tracer accumulation than expected for an acute fracture, and the plain radiographs demonstrate anterior cortical thickening and horizontal fissuring, we believe that these findings represent a stress fracture that has extended over time rather than healed and now rep-

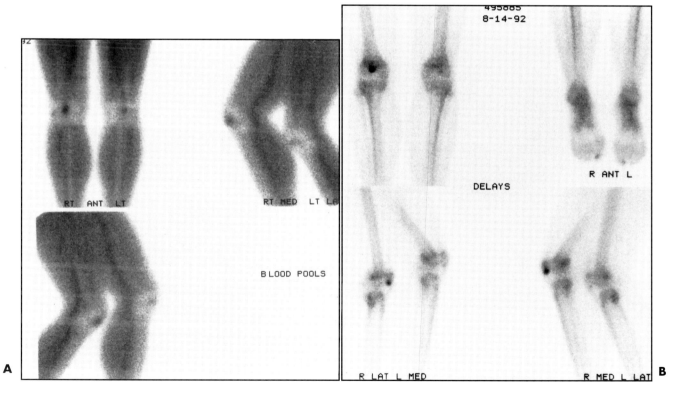

Fig. 13-27. Patellar tendinitis. **A,** Blood pool images. Focal mild to moderately increased tracer in the area of the inferior right patella. There is some minimal activity in a similar location on the left. **B,** Delayed images. Very focal mild to moderately intense increased tracer at the inferior pole of the right patella. *(From Holder LE: Bone scintigraphy in skeletal trauma. Radiol Clin North Am 1993; 31:739; with permission.)*

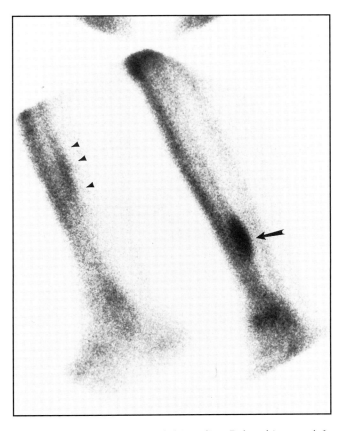

Fig. 13-28. Stress fracture and shin splint. Delayed images, left lateral and right medial. On the left, a focal fusiform area of intense abnormal tracer in the middle third, lower third junction of the posterior tibial cortex (*arrowheads*). This contrasts with the more linear activity with slightly varying intensity of tracer accumulation along its course in the midposterior tibial cortex on the right (*arrow*).

resents a nonunion of an incomplete cortical fracture.[9,117] In children the softer cancellous bone of the most proximal tibia is prone to horizontally oriented stress fractures.[35] Devas feels that these are compression stress fractures occurring because of the greater tendency of young bone to bend and the richer blood supply of a growing bone (Fig. 13-29).

The shin splint lesion, often called the medial tibial stress lesion, is a periostitis-type process.[99,102] Originally described as occurring in the skeletally immature, overweight, flat-footed individual, these lesions are seen in patients of any age and body habitus. Patients usually have some excess pronation with heel valgus. Michael and Holder demonstrated the relationship of shin splints to the soleus muscle tendon complex.[99] The soleus is a bipennate muscle that is active in pronation and supination.

RNA and BP images are almost always normal in patients with shin splints. On delayed images tibial lesions involve the posterior cortex, are longitudinally oriented, are long—involving one third of the length of the bone and often show varying intensities of tracer uptake along its length[69] (Fig. 13-30). It is important to differentiate these lesions from stress fracture, because the therapeutic approach is very different and significant to the athlete in training.[68,123]

The concept of abnormal loading of bone is reinforced by considering patients who cannot transmit forces normally. Kottmeier reported a patient who after an ankle injury developed partial ossification of the normally elastic distal tibiofibular syndesmotic ligament, thus restricting normal stress transference.[77] He then sustained a fibular stress fracture proximal to the superior extent of the ossific mass. Surgical resection of the mass resulted in uneventful fibular healing. Ankle surgery such as fusions may also alter physical and mechanical ankle joint function, create abnormal stress transference, and result in unexpected sites of fracture (Fig. 13-31). Straaton et al

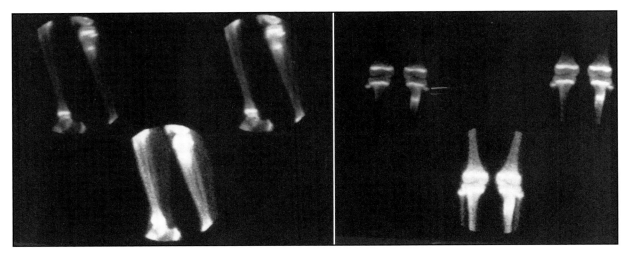

Fig. 13-29. Proximal tibial stress fracture. Delayed images, triple-lens Polaroid display. Anterior view on right, left lateral and right medial views on left. Linear intense increased activity is almost as intense as physes activity.

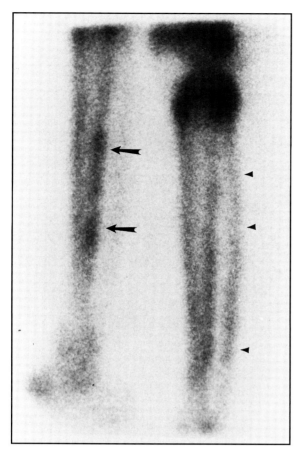

Fig. 13-30. Bilateral shin splints. Left lateral and right medial views. Note the relatively long, linear area of increased activity in the posteromedial tibial cortices with varying intensity along the course. The fibula is well seen on the lateral view; the shin splint activity is better seen on the medial view.

reported insufficiency fractures of the distal tibia in patients with rheumatoid arthritis whose lesions were initially misdiagnosed as cellulitis.[138] We have also seen a similar patient with rheumatoid arthritis, and steroid-induced osteopenia whose distal tibia fracture was originally diagnosed as an exacerbation of her primary joint disease.

FOOT AND ANKLE

Stress fractures occur quite commonly in the foot. In a large series reported by Greaney et al,[54] the distribution of stress fractures in the lower extremity included 21% in the calcaneus, primarily in the posterior tuberosity, 17% in metatarsals, and 3% in the tarsal navicular. In Matheson's review[32] of 320 cases of stress fractures in athletes, the most frequent site was the tibia followed by the tarsals and metatarsals, which accounted for approximately 25% and 9%, respectively. Most metatarsal stress fractures occur in the second and third metatarsals (Fig. 13-32). The tarsal stress fractures occurred more commonly in non-runners than in runners. The difference between the distribution in athletes and in the military is likely due to the type of exercise involved as well as train-

ing of the individuals and the type of footwear used. Stress fractures in the midfoot and forefoot may also occur in sesamoid bones[94] (Fig. 13-33). The classic "march" stress fracture occurs in the body of the metatarsal, although in Greaney's study, the majority of his metatarsal fractures were in the base and head of the metatarsal rather than in the body.[54] In stress fractures involving the fifth metatarsal, the treatment may be different if the fracture involves the tuberosity or when it involves the metatarsal shaft within 1.5 cm of the tuberosity.[32]

Calcaneal stress fractures were very common in Greaney's series.[54] He described a sharp drop in the incidence of calcaneal stress fractures in Marines from 20% to 7% after a change in training routine. Calcaneal stress fractures as other stress fractures may initially present with normal radiographs. The bone scan may show diffuse increased uptake in the posterior portion of the calcaneus, but when imaged and displayed appropriately, one can often demonstrate a linear area of increased activity located in the superior midportion of the calcaneus or involving the main portion of the body of the calcaneus (Figs. 13-7 and 13-34).

Navicular stress fractures can also be diagnosed earlier with bone scintigraphy than with plain films. As with other types of stress-related injuries, these patients may be symptomatic for long periods before the correct diagnosis is considered.[112]

Dislocation and avascular sequelae may occur after severe stress to the ankle region. This can be seen in the talus (Fig. 13-35). With lesser degrees of stress, osteochondral fractures of the talar dome can occur. The osteochondral fracture may be quite subtle and the plain films may be normal. Patients may carry the clinical diagnosis of an ankle sprain. Anderson et al,[3] studied 24 patients who had osteochondral fractures of the talar dome. They demonstrated the value of scintigraphy in assessing these patients when plain films were negative. They concluded that patients with positive bone scans should be further evaluated with MRI, whereas those patients who initially had positive plain films should have CT to adequately stage the fracture. The value of bone scintigraphy was also demonstrated by Burkus et al[14] and Urman et al.[143] Urman reviewed 122 patients with ankle pain, 97 of whose plain films were negative. Bone scintigraphy was performed followed by CT. When the bone scans showed abnormal uptake in the talar dome on one or two views, (intermediate or high probability), the sensitivity and specificity of the bone scan was 94% and 76%, respectively. They concluded that bone scanning was a very good screening procedure in patients who are suspected of having talar dome fractures but present with negative plain films (Fig. 13-36).

Occult fractures that occur in the midfoot region may be easily diagnosed with plain films. The Lisfranc fracture, which often occurs with forced plantar flexion and rotation, is a dislocation injury that may or may not include a fracture. The plain film findings may be very subtle and bone scanning can be important in making the correct diagnosis.

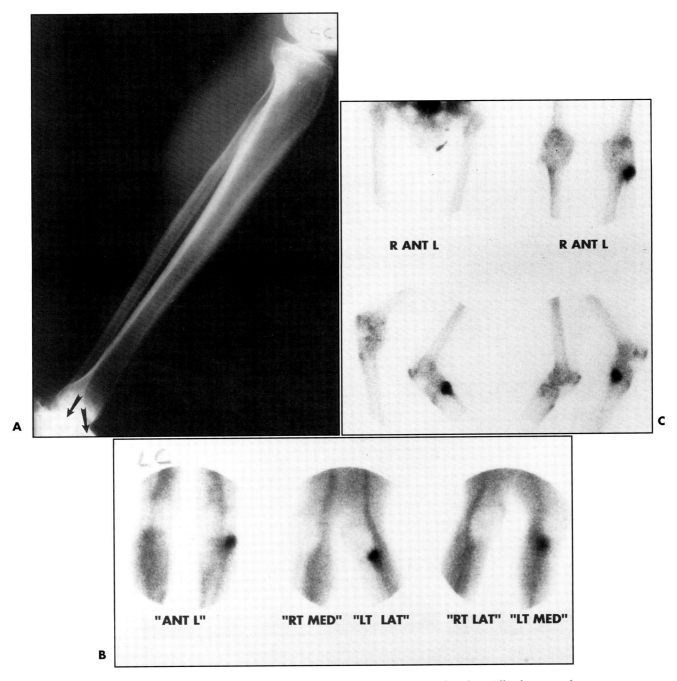

Fig. 13-31. Proximal fibular fracture. **A,** Lateral radiograph centered at the midleg because of nonspecific symptoms. Large staples from prior triple arthrodesis as well as ankle arthritis are noted at the bottom of the film. **B,** Blood pool image demonstrates increased vascularity in the region of the fibular head. **C,** Delayed image demonstrates intense abnormal tracer. The patient had stepped off a curb, with abnormal forces transmitted proximally because of prior ankle surgery. *(Courtesy of Dr. John McIntyre, Baltimore, MD.)*

The os trigonum is an accessory ossicle posterior to the talus. This normal variant can be simulated by a fracture of the posterior process of the talus or by injury to the ossicle. Bone scintigraphy can be helpful when focal increased uptake in this region correlates with the patient's symptoms.[64,147]

Stress fractures also occur in the medial malleolus. As in other locations the pain may be gradual in onset and is often secondary to repetitive activity such as running and jumping. Subtle fractures at the junction of the medial malleolus and tibial plafond can be seen, and bone scans were positive in all seven patients described by Schils.[126]

Abnormal stress forces involving the Achilles tendon

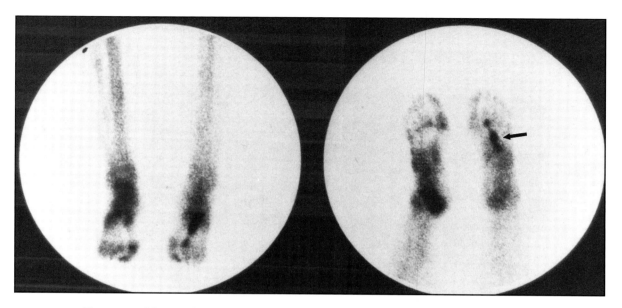

Fig. 13-32.   Metatarsal stress fracture. Focal increased uptake in the left second metatarsal.

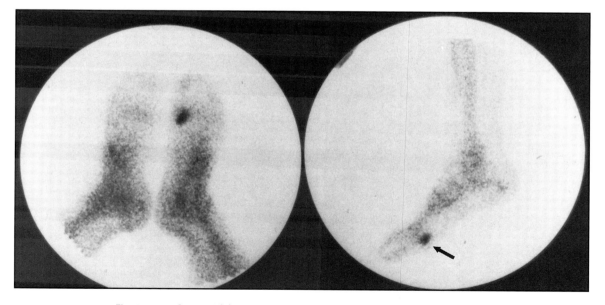

Fig. 13-33.   Sesamoid fracture. Focal uptake in the region of the sesamoid.

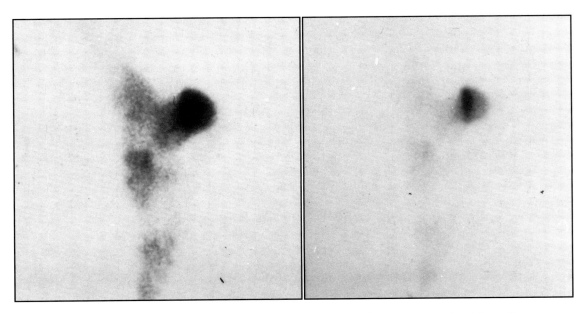

Fig. 13-34.   Calcaneal stress fracture. Left image demonstrates intense increased uptake in the posterior half of the calcaneus. When the bone scan is properly windowed (right image), a very focal area of increased uptake in the midcalcaneus is easily identified.

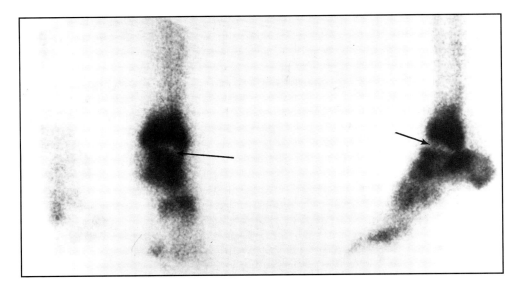

Fig. 13-35.   Avascular talus posttrauma. AP and lateral bone scan views demonstrate intense increased uptake in the distal tibia, superior aspect of the calcaneus, and in the midfoot. There is a relative lack of activity in the region of the talus.

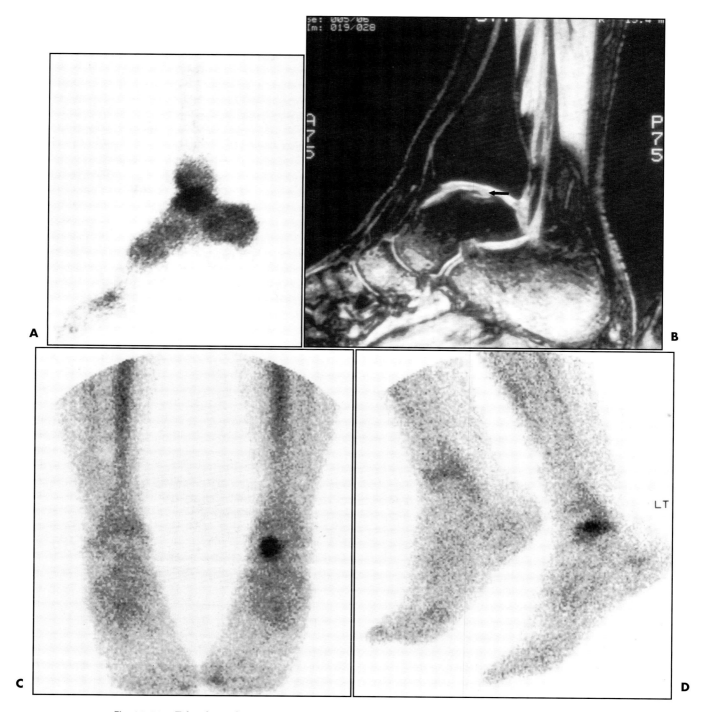

Fig. 13-36. Talar dome fracture. **A,** Lateral bone scan, moderately intense increased uptake in the talus with a more focal area of increased uptake in the region of the talar dome. Initial radiographs were negative. **B,** MRI. Osteochondral fracture is demonstrated (*arrow*). **C** and **D,** Activity in another patient with focal localized uptake in the talar dome secondary to a talar dome fracture. *(Courtesy of Robert Cooper, M.D.)*

and the plantar fascia may result in tendinitis and/or fasciitis, posttraumatic calcification, or rupture.[64,68] Bone scintigraphy will show focal areas of increased uptake in active Achilles tendinitis (Fig. 13-37) and plantar fasciitis (Fig. 13-38). Calcifications at the site of insertion of these

tendons may be present in asymptomatic patients due to prior injury. In these cases the bone scan will be negative. Retrocalcaneal bursitis may show soft-tissue activity in the bursa, or increased activity associated with the subadjacent superior-posterior aspect of the calcaneus.

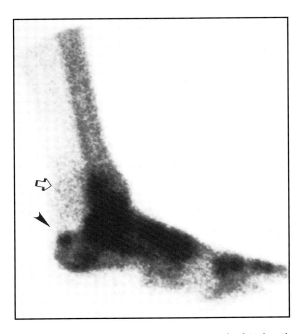

Fig. 13-37. Achilles tendinitis. Moderate increased uptake in the hind and midfoot with a focal area of increased uptake at the site of the Achilles tendon insertion (*arrowhead*). Also note the soft tissue swelling and mild increased soft tissue activity in the posterior distal leg (*open arrow*) due to a posttraumatic rupture of the Achilles tendon. *(Courtesy of Robert Cooper, M.D.)*

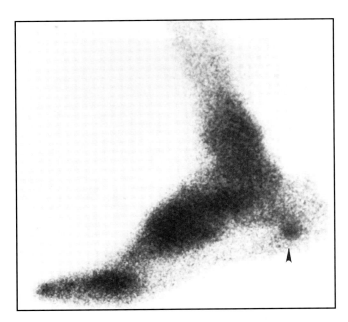

Fig. 13-38. Plantar fasciitis. Lateral bone scan of the foot shows a focal area of moderate increased uptake at the site of the plantar fascia insertion (*arrowhead*).

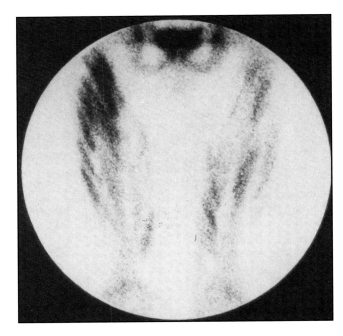

Fig. 13-39. Primary muscle injury.

Ankle diastasis related to the tibiofibular ligament injury can be seen by bone scintigraphy.[77] In the tibiotalar impingement syndrome, the bone scan may show uptake in the osseous spurs that is secondary to the trauma of forced dorsiflexion of the foot onto the leg.[64]

MUSCLE INJURY

Damaged skeletal muscle takes up the technetium phosphate compounds. The exact mechanism of this uptake is uncertain but includes absorption to the denatured proteins or binding to mitochondrial calcium, which is increased in ischemic tissues.[13,36,130] Matin et al[91] performed whole-body bone scintigraphy on 11 runners who ran either a 50- or 100-mile race. The study was initially conceived to assess the possibility of myocardial damage. Blood samples from these ultramarathon runners had shown creatine kinase (CK) levels that were markedly elevated with CK MB isoenzyme levels that suggested myocardial damage. In this report all 11 runners had elevated CK levels and 77% had MB isoenzyme elevations. All but one runner had uptake of Tc-99m pyrophosphate (PYP) in the muscle groups of the lower extremities. The degree of uptake correlated well with the degree of muscle pain. The location of the uptake also correlated with the type of race. Athletes that completed the 100-mile race, primarily downhill, had uptake in the buttocks, hamstrings, and quadriceps groups, whereas those runners in the primarily uphill 50-mile race had increased uptake in the thigh adductor group. As in myocardial infarction, scintigraphy with PYP showed muscle group activity at 1 day after exercise, which was less intense activity after 5 days. Scans returned to normal by 7 to 8 days. There was no uptake in the myocardium in any of the 11 runners.

Muscle localization of bone tracers has also been reported in the upper extremities and abdominal muscles after vigorous exercise.[11,144] We have also seen muscle uptake in the thigh after vigorous training for bicycle racing (Fig. 13-39) and in abdominal muscles following a push-up contest. Bilateral activity accumulating posteriorly in the teres major muscle has been reported in a weight lifter.[57] The cause of muscle localization is thought to be rhabdomyolysis, which occurs with excessive stresses. Frymoyer[47] reported on seven patients with muscle uptake due to a variety of causes. Five of these patients also had myoglobinuria. Crenshaw et al have recently investigated the posterior leg muscles in four ultramarathon runners including scintigraphic, morphologic, and intramuscular pressure analysis of sore muscles after exercise.[27] In the intensive areas of tracer uptake, only 1% of biopsied muscle fibers were necrotic, strongly suggesting that increased uptake reflects changes other than fiber necrosis. They suggested further that tracer uptake was occurring when changes could not yet be detected by morphologic means even at the ultrastructural level. Tissue calcification was not directly visualized, nor was any detected with the alizarin red staining technique. They concluded that some relative ischemia may be playing a role.

Even in four-footed animals bone scintigraphy has played a role in diagnosis. Morris reported on the use of bone scintigraphy to assess horses with a history of inadequate athletic performance and subtle lameness.[101] Of the 109 horses studied, 9.2% showed muscle uptake. A muscle biopsy in one case confirmed rhabdomyolysis.

We have chosen to emphasize in this section the more direct uptake of the phosphorus tracers by injured muscle. In Chapter 14, we discuss heterotopic ossification and the use of the term *myositis ossificans*. The bone scan is rarely needed as a primary method of assessing muscle damage, but the finding of muscle uptake should be recognized as an incidental or primary finding when the patient is imaged because a stress or occult fracture is suspected.

REFERENCES

1. Allwright SJ, Cooper RA, Nash P: Trochanteric bursitis: Bone scan appearance. *Clin Nucl Med* 1988; 13:561.
2. Ammann W, Matzinger J, Lloyd-Smith DR, et al: Femoral stress abnormalities: Improved scintigraphic detection with frog-leg view. *Radiology* 1988; 169:844.
3. Anderson IF, Crichton KJ, Grattan-Smith T, et al: Osteochondral fractures of the dome of the talus. *J Bone Joint Surg Am* 1989; 71A:1143.
4. Apple JS, Martinez S, Nunley JA: Painful os styloideum: Bone scintigraphy in carpe bossu disease. *AJR Am J Roentgenol* 1984; 142:181.
5. Asnis SE, Gould ES, Bansal M, et al: Magnetic resonance imaging of the hip after displaced femoral neck fractures. *Clin Orthop* 1994; 298:191.
6. Barton D, Allen M, Findlay D, Belton I: Evaluation of whiplash injuries by technetium-[99m] isotope scanning. *Arch Emerg Med* 1993; 10:197.
7. Bellah RD, Summerville DA, Treves ST, Micheli LJ: Low-back pain in adolescent athletes: Detection of stress injury to the pars interarticularis with SPECT. *Radiology* 1991; 180:509.
8. Blanda J, Bethem D, Moats W, Lew M: Defects of pars interarticularis in athletes: A protocol for nonoperative treatment. *J Spinal Disorder* 1993; 6:406.
9. Blank S: Transverse tibial stress fractures: A special problem. *Am J Sports Med* 1987; 15:597.
10. Blatz DJ: Bilateral femoral and tibial shaft stress fractures in a runner. *Am J Sports Med* 1981; 9:322.
11. Briele B, Hotze A, Biersack HJ. Incidental visualization of the teres major muscles during bone scanning after vigorous exercise. *Clin Nucl Med* 1992; 17:971.
12. Briggs RC, Kolbjornsen PH, Southall RC: Osteitis pubis, Tc-99m MDP, and professional hockey players. *Clin Nucl Med* 1992; 17:861.
13. Buja LM, Parkey RW, Dees JH, et al: Morphologic correlates of technetium-99m stannous pyrophosphate imaging of acute myocardial infarcts in dogs. *Circulation* 1975; 52:596.
14. Burkus JK, Sella EJ, Southwick WO: Occult injuries of the talus diagnosed by bone scan and tomography. *Foot Ankle* 1984; 4:316.
15. Bury RF: Bone scintigraphy in the evaluation of ejection injuries. *Aviat Space Environ Med* 1989; 60(suppl 7):A16.
16. Butler JE, Brown SL, McConnell BG: Subtrochanteric stress fractures in runners. *Am J Sports Med* 1982; 10:228.
17. Butler-Manuel PA, Guy RL, Heatley FW, Nunan TO: Scintigraphy in the assessment of anterior knee pain. *Acta Orthop Scand* 1990; 61:438.
18. Bylander B, Hansson LI, Karrholm J, Naversten Y: Scintimetric evaluation of posttraumatic and postoperative growth disturbance using [99Tcm] MDP. *Acta Radiol (Diag)* 1983; 24:85.
19. Cahill BR: Osteolysis of the distal part of the clavicle in male athletes. *J Bone Joint Surg Am* 1982; 64-A:1053.
20. Caine D, Roy S, Singer KM, Broekhoff J: Stress changes of the distal radial growth plate: A radiographic survey and review of the literature. *Am J Sports Med* 1992; 20:290.
21. Charkes ND: Skeletal blood flow: Implications for bone-scan interpretation. *J Nucl Med* 1980; 21:91.

22. Chen C, Chandnani V, Kang HS, et al: Insufficiency fracture of the sternum caused by osteopenia: Plain film findings in seven patients. *AJR Am J Roentgenol* 1990; 154:1025.

23. Clement DB, Ammann W, Taunton JE, et al: Exercise-induced stress injuries to the femur. *Int J Sports Med* 1993; 14:347.

24. Collier BD, Johnson RP, Carrera GF, et al: Painful spondylolysis or spondylolisthesis studied by radiography and single-photon emission computed tomography. *Radiology* 1985; 154:207.

25. Conway WF, Destouet JM, Gilula LA, et al: The carpal boss: An overview of radiographic evaluation. *Radiology* 1985; 156:29.

26. Cornell CN, Lane JM: Newest factors in fracture healing. *Clin Orthop* 1992; 77:297.

27. Crenshaw AG, Friden J, Hargens AR, et al: Increased technetium uptake is not equivalent to muscle necrosis: Scintigraphic, morphological and intramuscular pressure analyses of sore muscles after exercise. *Acta Physiol Scand* 1993; 148:187.

28. Daffner RH, Pavlov H: Stress fractures: Current concepts. *AJR Am J Roentgenol* 1992; 159:245.

29. Davies AM, Bradley SA: Iliac insufficiency fractures. *Br J Radiol* 1991; 64:305.

30. Davies AM, Carter SR, Grimer RJ, Sneath RS: Fatigue fractures of the femoral diaphysis in the skeletally immature simulating malignancy. *Br J Radiol* 1989; 62:893.

31. Davies AM, Evans NS, Struthers GR: Parasymphyseal and associated insufficiency fractures of the pelvis and sacrum. *Br J Radiol* 1988; 61:103.

32. Delee JC, Evans JP, Julian J: Stress fracture of the fifth metatarsal. *Am J Sports Med* 1983; 11:349.

33. Demangeat JL, Constantinesco A, Brunot B, et al: Three-phase bone scanning in reflex sympathetic dystrophy of the hand. *J Nucl Med* 1988; 29:26.

34. Deutsch SD, Gandsman EJ, Spraragen SC: Quantitative regional blood-flow analysis and its clinical application during routine bone-scanning. *J Bone Joint Surg Am* 1981; 63-A:295.

35. Devas MB: Stress fractures in children. *J Bone Joint Surg Br* 1963; 45B:528.

36. Dewanjee MK: Correlation of protein binding and the localization of Tc-99m pyrophosphate and other agents in infarcted myocardium. *J Nucl Med* 1977; 18:597.

37. Dugowson CE, Drinkwater BL, Clark JM: Nontraumatic femur fracture in an oligomenorrheic athlete. *Med Sci Sports Exerc* 1991; 23:1323.

38. Dye SF, Boll DA: Radionuclide imaging of the patellofemoral joint in young adults with anterior knee pain. *Orthop Clin North Am* 1986; 17:249.

39. Dye SF, Chew MH: The use of scintigraphy to detect increased osseous metabolic activity about the knee. *J Bone Joint Surg Am* 1993; 75-A:1388.

40. Engel A, Feldner-Busztin H: Bilateral stress fracture of the scaphoid. *Arch Orthop Trauma Surg* 1991; 110:314.

41. Even-Sapir E, Martin RH, Mitchell MJ, et al: Assessment of painful late effects of lumbar spinal fusion with SPECT. *J Nucl Med* 1994; 35:416.

42. Fairclough J, Colhoun E, Johnston D, et al: Bone scanning for suspected hip fractures. A prospective study in elderly patients. *J Bone Joint Surg Br* 1987; 69-B:251.

43. Fernbach SK, Wilkinson RH: Avulsion injuries of the pelvis and proximal femur. *AJR Am J Roentgenol* 1981; 137:581.

44. Fink-Bennett D, Carichner S: Acute flexion of the elbow: Optimal imaging position for visualization of the capitellum. *Clin Nucl Med* 1986; 11:667.

45. Fink-Bennett D, Vicuna-Rios J: The deltoid tuberosity—a potential pitfall (the "delta sign") in bone-scan interpretation: Concise communication. *J Nucl Med* 1980; 21:211.

46. Friedman MJ, Nicholas JA: Conditioning and rehabilitation, in Scott WN, Nisonson B, Nicholas JA (eds): *Principles of Sports Medicine*, Williams and Wilkins, Baltimore, 1984; p 396.

47. Frymoyer PA, Giammarco R, Farrar FM, et al: Tc-99m medronate bone scanning in rhabdomyolysis. *Arch Intern Med* 1985; 145:1991.

48. Fulton MN, Albright JP, El-Khoury GY: Cortical desmoid-like lesion of the proximal humerus and its occurrence in gymnasts (ringman's shoulder lesion). *Am J Sports Med* 1979; 7:57.

49. Futami T, Aoki H, Tsukamoto Y: Fractures of the hook of the hamate in athletes. *Acta Orthop Scand* 1993; 64:469.

50. Ganel A, Engel J, Oster Z, et al: Bone scanning in the assessment of fractures of the scaphoid. *J Hand Surg* 1979; 4:540.

51. Gates GF: SPECT imaging of the lumbosacral spine and pelvis. *Clin Nucl Med* 1988; 13:907.

52. Gelberman RH, Wolock BS, Siegel DB: Fractures and non-unions of the carpal scaphoid. *J Bone Joint Surg Am* 1989; 71-A:1560.

53. Goldberg HD, Young JWR, Reiner BI, et al: Double injuries of the forearm: A common occurrence. *Radiology* 1992; 185:223.

54. Greaney R3, Gerber FH, Laughlin RL, et al: Distribution and natural history of stress fractures in US Marine recruits. *Radiology* 1983; 146:339.

55. Greenspan A: *Orthopedic Radiology. A Practical Approach*, ed 2, Raven Press, New York, 1992.

56. Greiff J: Autoradiographic studies of fracture healing using $^{99}Tc^m$-Sn-polyphosphate. *Injury* 1978; 9:271.

57. Grimm ES, Bekerman C: The bench press mark. *Clin Nucl Med* 1991; 16:56.

58. Gurtler R, Pavlov H, Torg JS: Stress fracture of the ipsilateral first rib in a pitcher. *Am J Sports Med* 1985; 13:277.

59. Hamilton HK: Stress fracture of the diaphysis of the ulna in a body builder. *Am J Sports Med* 1984; 12:405.

60. Hanks GA, Kalenak A, Bowman S, Sebastianelli WJ: Stress fracture of the carpal scaphoid. *J Bone Joint Surg Am* 1989; 71-A:938.

61. Hastings G, Oates E: Bilateral intraosseous ganglia of the lunates: Bone imaging, CT scanning, and plain film correlation. *Clin Nucl Med* 1984; 9:658.

62. Hawkes DJ, Robinson L, Crossman JE, et al: Registration and display of the combined bone scan and radiograph in the diagnosis and management of wrist injury. *Eur J Nucl Med* 1991; 18:752.

63. Hildingsson C, Hietala SO, Tollanen G: Scintigraphic findings in acute whiplash injury of the cervical spine. *Injury* 1989; 20:265.

64. Holder LE: Bone scintigraphy in skeletal trauma. *Radiol Clin North Am* 1993; 31:739.

65. Holder LE: Clinical radionuclide bone imaging. *Radiology* 1990; 176:607.

66. Holder LE: Radionuclide bone imaging in surgical problems of the hand, in Gilula LA (ed): *The Traumatized Hand and Wrist*, WB Saunders, Philadelphia, 1992, p 19.

67. Holder LE, Machin JL, Asdourian P, et al: Planar and high resolution bone imaging in the diagnosis of facet syndrome. *J Nucl Med* 1995; 36:37.

68. Holder LE, Matthews LS: The nuclear physician and sports medicine, in Freeman L, and Weissman H (eds): *Nuclear Medicine Annual 1984*, Raven Press, New York, 1984, p 81.

69. Holder LE, Michael RH: The specific scintigraphic pattern of "shin splints in the lower leg": Concise communication. *J Nucl Med* 1984; 25:865.

70. Holder LE, Mulligan ME, Gillespie TE: Editorial: Diagnosis of scaphoid fractures: The role of nuclear medicine. *J Nucl Med* 1995; 36:48.

71. Holder LE, Schwartz C, Wernicke PG, et al: Radionuclide bone imaging in the early detection of fractures of the proximal femur (hip): Multifactorial analysis. *Radiology* 1990; 174:509.

72. Hulkko A, Orava S, Nikula P: Stress fractures of the olecranon in javelin throwers. *Int J Sports Med* 1986; 7:210.

73. Kaye JJ, Nance EP, Green NE: Fatigue fracture of the medial aspect of the clavicle. *Radiology* 1982; 144:89.

74. Kim SM, Park CH, Gartland JJ: Stress fractures of the pubic ramus in a swimmer. *Clin Nucl Med* 1987; 12:118.

75. Koch RA, Jackson DW: Pubic symphysitis in runners: A report of 2 cases. *Am J Sports Med* 1981; 9:62.

76. Kohn HS, Guten GN, Collier BD, et al: Chondromalacia of the patella: Bone imaging correlated with arthroscopic findings. *Clin Nucl Med* 1988; 13:96.

77. Kottmeier SA, Hanks GA, Kalenak A: Fibular stress fracture associated with distal tibiofibular synostosis in an athlete. *Clin Orthop* 1992; 281:195.

78. Kursunoglu-Brahme S, Gundry CR, Resnick D: Advanced imaging of the wrist. *Radiol Clin North Am* 1990; 28:307.

79. Lawson JP: Not-so-normal variants. *Orthop Clin North Am* 1990; 21:483.

80. Leung HY, Stirling AJ: Stress fracture of the first rib without associated injuries. *Injury* 1991; 22:483.

81. Levinsohn EM: Imaging of the wrist. *Radiol Clin North Am* 1990; 28:905.

82. Lewis SL, Rees JI, Thomas GV, et al: Pitfalls of bone scintigraphy in suspected hip fractures. *Br J Radiol* 1991; 64:403.

83. Loosli AR, Leslie M: Stress fractures of the distal radius. *Am J Sports Med* 1991; 19:523.

84. Mackinnon SE, Dellon AL: Carpal tunnel syndrome, in Mackinnon SE, Dellon AL (eds): *Surgery of the Peripheral Nerve*, Thieme Medical Publishers, New York, 1988, p 149.

85. Macones AJ, Fisher MS, Locke JL: Stress-related rib and vertebral changes. *Radiology* 1989; 170:117.

86. Maldague BE, Malghem JJ: Unilateral arch hypertrophy with spinous process tilt: A sign of arch deficiency. *Radiology* 1976; 121:567.

87. Mann FA, Wilson AJ, Gilula LA: Radiographic evaluation of the wrist: What does the hand surgeon want to know? *Radiology* 1992; 184:15.

88. Marks PH, Goldenberg JA, Vezina WC, et al: Subchondral bone infarctions in acute ligamentous knee injuries demonstrated on bone scintigraphy and magnetic resonance imaging. *J Nucl Med* 1992; 33:516.

89. Martire JR, Levinsohn EM: *Imaging of Athletic Injuries*. McGraw-Hill, New York, 1992.

90. Matin P: The appearance of bone scans following fractures, including immediate and long-term studies. *J Nucl Med* 1979; 20:1227.

91. Matin P, Lang G, Carretta R, et al: Scintigraphic evaluation of muscle damage following extreme exercise: Concise communication. *J Nucl Med* 1983; 24:308.

92. Matthews LS, Simonson BG, Wolock BS: Osteolysis of the distal clavicle in a female body builder. *Am J Sports Med* 1993; 21:150.

93. Maurer AH, Holder LE, Espinola DA, et al: Three-phase radionuclide scintigraphy of the hand. *Radiology* 1983; 146:761.

94. Maurice HD, Newman JH, Watt I: Bone scanning of the foot for explained pain. *J Bone Joint Surg Br* 1987; 69B:448.

95. McDougall IR, Keeling CA: Complications of fractures and their healing. *Semin Nucl Med* 1988; 18:113.

96. Mesgarzadeh M, Sapega AA, Bonakdarpour A, et al: Osteochondritis dissecans: Analysis of mechanical stability with radiography, scintigraphy, and MR imaging. *Radiology* 1987; 165:775.

97. Mesgarzadeh M, Schneck CD, Bonakdarpour A: Carpal tunnel: MR imaging. Part I. Normal anatomy. *Radiology* 1989; 171:743.

98. Mesgarzadeh M, Schneck CD, Bonakdarpour A: Carpal tunnel: MR imaging. Part II. Carpal tunnel syndrome. *Radiology* 1989; 171:749.

99. Michael RH, Holder LE: The soleus syndrome: A cause of medial tibial stress (shin splints). *Am J Sports Med* 1985; 13:87.

100. Mikhail IS, Bernreuter WK, Alarcon GS: Insufficiency fracture of the distal ulna presenting as cellulitis. *Arthritis Rheum* 1994; 36:1027.

101. Morris E, Seeherman HJ, O'Callaghan MW, et al: Scintigraphic identification of skeletal muscle damage in horses 24 hours after strenuous exercise. *Equine Vet J* 1991; 23:347.

102. Mubarak SJ, Gould RN, Lee YF, et al: The medial tibial stress syndrome (a cause of shin splints). *Am J Sports Med* 1982; 10:201.

103. Murray IPC, Dixon J, Kohan L: SPECT for acute knee pain. *Clin Nucl Med* 1990; 11:828.

104. Mutoh Y, More T, Suzuki Y: Stress fractures of the ulna in athletes. *Am J Sports Med* 1982; 10:365.

105. Nagel CE: Cost-appropriateness of whole body vs. limited bone scanning for suspected focal sports injuries. *Clin Nucl Med* 1986; 11:469.

106. Norman A, Baker ND: Spontaneous osteonecrosis of the knee and medial meniscal tears. *Radiology* 1978; 129:653.

107. Ogunro O: Fracture of the body of the hamate bone. *J Hand Surg* 1982; 8:353.

108. Outwater E, Oates E: Condensing osteitis of the clavicle: Case report and review of the literature. *J Nucl Med* 1988; 29:1122.

109. Parkes JC: Common injuries about the elbow in sports, in Scott WN, Nisonson B, Nicholas JA (eds): *Principles of Sports Medicine*, 1984, p 140.

110. Patel N, Collier BD, Carrera GF, et al: High-resolution bone scintigraphy of the adult wrist. *Clin Nucl Med* 1992; 17:449.

111. Pavlov H, Nelson TL, Warren RF, et al: Stress fractures of the pubic ramus: A report of 12 cases. *J Bone Joint Surg Am* 1982; 64-A:1020.

112. Pavlov H, Torg JS, Freiberger RH: Tarsal navicular stress fractures: Radiographic evaluation. *Radiology* 1983; 148:641.

113. Pin PG, Semenkovich JW, Young VL, et al: Role of radionuclide imaging in the evaluation of wrist pain. *J Hand Surg Am* 1988; 13A:810.

114. Rawlings CE, Wilkins RH, Martinez S, et al: Osteoporotic sacral fractures: A clinical study. *Neurosurgery* 1988; 22:72.

115. Resnick D, Niwayama G: Entheses and enthesopathy. Anatomical, pathological and radiological correlation. *Radiology* 1983; 146:1.

116. Rettig AC: Stress fracture of the ulna in an adolescent tournament tennis player. *Am J Sports Med* 1983; 11:103.

117. Rettig AC, Shelbourne KD, McCarroll JR, et al: The natural history in treatment of delayed union stress fractures of the anterior cortex of the tibia. *Am J Sports Med* 1988; 16:250.

118. Rizzo PF, Gould ES, Lyden JP, et al: Diagnosis of occult fractures about the hip. Magnetic resonance imaging compared with bone-scanning. *J Bone Joint Surg Am* 1993; 75-A:395.

119. Rockett JF: Three-phase radionuclide bone imaging in stress injury of the anterior iliac crest. *J Nucl Med* 1990; 31:1554.

120. Rockett JF, Freeman BL: Scintigraphic demonstration of pectineus muscle avulsion injury. *Clin Nucl Med* 1990; 15:800.

121. Rothwell RS, Davis P, Lentle BC: Radionuclide bone scanning in females with chronic low back pain. *Ann Rheum Dis* 1981; 40:79.

122. Rozing PM, Insall J, Bohne WH: Spontaneous osteonecrosis of the knee. *J Bone Joint Surg Am* 1980; 62-A:2.

123. Rupani HD, Holder LE, Espinola DA, Engin SI: Three-phase radionuclide bone imaging in sports medicine. *Radiology* 1985; 156:187.

124. Ryan PJ, Fogelman I: Osteoporotic vertebral fractures: Diagnosis with radiography and bone scintigraphy. *Radiology* 1994; 190:669.

125. Satterfield MJ, Yasumura K, Abreu SH: Retro runner with ischial tuberosity enthesopathy. *J Orthop Sports Phys Ther* 1993; 17:191.

126. Schils JP, Andrish JT, Piraino, et al: Medial malleolar stress fractures in seven patients: Review of the clinical and imaging features. *Radiology* 1992; 185:219.

127. Schneider R, Yacovone J, Ghelman B: Unsuspected sacral fractures: Detection by radionuclide bone scanning. *AJR Am J Roentgenol* 1985; 144:337.

128. Shirazi KK, Agha FP, Amendola MA: Isolated fracture of greater multangular. *Br J Radiol* 1982; 55:923.

129. Siegel B, Donovan RI, Alderson PO, Mack GR: Skeletal uptake of ^{99m}Tc-diphosphonate in relation to local bone blood flow. *Radiology* 1976; 120:121.

130. Siegel BA, Engel WK, Derrer EC: Localization of technetium-99m diphosphonate in acutely injured muscle. *Neurology* 1977; 27:230.

131. Silberstein EB, Brown ML, Rosenthall L, Wahner HW: Skeletal nuclear medicine, in Siegel BA, Kirchner PT (eds): *Nuclear Medicine: Self Study Program I*, Society of Nuclear Medicine, New York, 1988, 93.

132. Sims-Williams H, Jayson MIV, Baddeley H: Small spinal fractures in back pain patients. *Ann Rheum Dis* 1978; 37:262.

133. Slizofski WJ, Collier BD, Flatley TJ, et al: Painful pseudarthrosis following lumbar spinal fusion: Detection by combined SPECT and planar bone scintigraphy. *Skeletal Radiol* 1987; 16:136.

134. Sowa DT, Holder LE, Patt PG: Application of magnetic resonance imaging to ischemic necrosis of the lunate. *J Hand Surg* 1989; 14:1008.

135. Spitz J, Becker C, Tittel K, et al: Die klinische relevanz der ganzkorperskelettszintigraphie bei mehrfachverletzten und polytraumatisierten patienten. *Unfallchirurgie* 1992; 18:133.

136. Spitz J, Lauer I, Tittel K, Weigand H: Scintimetric evaluation of remodeling after bone fractures in man. *J Nucl Med* 1993; 34:1403.

137. Stark HH, Jobe FW, Boyes JH, Ashworth CR: Fracture of the hook of the hamate in athletes. *J Bone Joint Surg Am* 1977; 59-A:575.

138. Straaton KV, Lopez-Mendez A, Alarcon GS: Insufficiency fractures of the distal tibia misdiagnosed as cellulitis in three patients with rheumatoid arthritis. *Arthritis Rheum* 1991; 34:912.

139. Taleisnik J. Compression neuropathies of the upper extremity, in Chapman MW, Madison M (eds): *Operative Orthopaedics*, Vol 1, JB Lippincott Company, Philadelphia, 1988, p 1345.

140. Tiel-van Buul MMC, van Beek EJR, Dijkstra PF, et al: Significance of a hot spot on the bone scan after carpal injury—evaluation by computed tomography. *Eur J Nucl Med* 1993; 20:159.

141. Torg JS, Moyer RA: Non-union of a stress fracture through the olecranon epiphyseal plate observed in an adolescent baseball pitcher. *J Bone Joint Surg Am* 1977; 59-A:264.

142. Tountas AA: Insufficiency stress fractures of the femoral neck in elderly women. *Clin Orthop* 1993; 292:202.

143. Urman M, Ammann W, Sisler J, et al: The role of bone scintigraphy in the evaluation of talar dome fractures. *J Nucl Med* 1991; 32:2241.

144. Valk P: Muscle localization of Tc-99m MDP after exercise. *Clin Nucl Med* 1984; 8:493.

145. Van Den Oever M, Merrick MV, Scott JHS: Bone scintigraphy in symptomatic spondylolysis. *J Bone Joint Surg Br* 1987; 69-B:453.

146. Weissman BNW, Sledge CB (eds): *Orthopedic Radiology*, WB Saunders, Philadelphia, 1986, p 270.

147. Wolff MH, Sty JR: Painful ankle. Os trigonum vs fracture. *Clin Nucl Med* 1985; 10:197.

14

SELECTED TOPICS IN ORTHOPEDIC BONE SCANNING

Manuel L. Brown

Lawrence E. Holder

Radionuclide musculoskeletal imaging has become a critical part of the modern practice of orthopedic surgery. Many imaging applications of interest to the orthopedist including infection, primary and metastatic bone tumors, and pediatric nuclear medicine are covered elsewhere in this book. The selected topics in orthopedic bone scanning covered in this chapter include: evaluation of fractures and other traumatic injuries, joint replacement, concepts of stress loading and orthopedic appliances, limb-lengthening surgery, limb-salvage surgery, spine and pelvis surgery, thermal injuries, and orthopedic vascular problems. Osseous manifestations of systemic disease of interest to the practicing orthopedic surgeon are covered elsewhere in this book.

EVALUATION OF FRACTURES AND OTHER TRAUMATIC INJURIES

In normal fracture healing, bone scintigraphy plays little or no role. It is only when there are complications such as in suspected infection, pain out of proportion to the normal course of healing, delayed union or nonunion that the bone scan may be helpful.

Experimental Aspects of Fracture Healing

Fracture uptake of the bone tracers has been investigated in animal models.[38,39] Gumerman et al[39] studied the pattern of methylene diphosphate (MDP) uptake in a rabbit fracture model. In the uncomplicated fracture group, there was an initial double peak of activity at the osteotomy site, which coalesced into a single peak by 2 weeks. In the delayed healing model, which had undergone periosteal stripping, there was a delay in the biphasic activity peaks and a delay in callus formation. In the nonunion model there was a variable pattern. In Grundnes and Reiker's work,[38] a rat model was used. They showed that fractures treated by closed nailing did better than open nailing in the early postoperative period, but this finding was not related to bone blood flow.

As noted in Chapter 13, the bone scan becomes positive shortly after trauma, although some sites in some patients may take upward of several days to become active.[65,76,111] This may in part be related to the blood supply to these areas.[53,65,128] The normal sequence of bone tracer activity relates to the pathophysiology at the fracture site.[96] Initially there is hematoma formation at the fracture site. During this initial period, which lasts up to 4 weeks, the bone scan will show rather diffuse

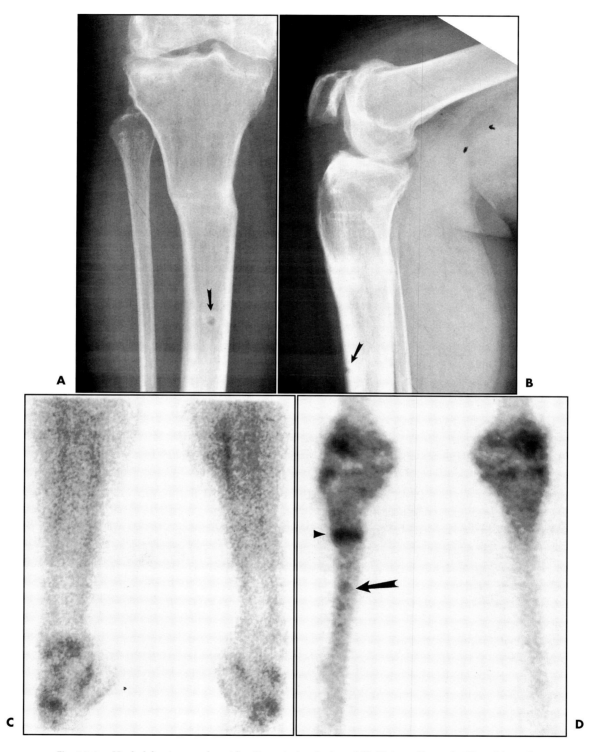

Fig. 14-1. Healed fracture and postfixation pin track. **A** and **B**, Plain radiograph AP and lateral radiograph demonstrate proximal right tibia fracture healed with slight offset. The bull's-eye appearance of the healed pin track showing lucency and sclerosis is identified (*arrows*). **C**, Anterior blood pool image. No increased activity is associated with the pin track. **D**, Delayed images show mild to moderate increased tracer associated with continued stress remodeling at the fracture site (*arrowhead*), and very minimal activity is seen in association with the old pin track (*arrow*). The bull's-eye appearance at the healed pin track does not reproduce well but could be seen on the original image.

increased activity. As the hematoma resolves and is replaced by callus, the bone tracer uptake becomes more focal about the fracture site. This uptake slowly normalizes over time. Matin[76] noted that the bone scan would return to normal in 2 years in about 90% of patients, with the minimum time for normalization being approximately 6 months. Nonaligned fractures in adults may never become scintigraphically normal as remodeling forces continue (Figs. 14-1 and 14-5). In cases of delayed union and nonunion, bone scintigraphy will also show uptake for a prolonged time.

Complications of Fracture Healing and Trauma

PREDICTIVE VALUE OF RADIONUCLIDE BONE IMAGING

Nuclear medicine studies can play a role in the evaluation of fractures to assess the likelihood of complications such as avascular necrosis (AVN) of the head, and delayed union or nonunion. A study using Tc-99m antimony colloid in a rabbit model and also in 30 patients examined within 24 hours of a subcapital hip fracture showed that the lack of activity indicated AVN.[118] Eleven of twelve patients with no activity in the head of the fractured femur developed AVN within 2 years. Fifteen of the sixteen patients with activity healed without evidence of AVN. This was also shown using Tc-99m sulfur colloid scanning by Phillips et al.[94] Magnetic resonance imaging (MRI) is very sensitive for the detection of AVN; however, its value in detecting femoral head viability in the immediate posttraumatic period is not as good. Asnis et al[9] showed that MRI did not detect posttraumatic AVN in hips in the early posttraumatic period. In a canine model of AVN Brody[14] showed that MRI can detect marrow changes of AVN, but not earlier than 1 week posttrauma. However, the use of dynamic contrast MRI may show acute AVN earlier than either spin echo and STIR imaging.[86]

Bone scintigraphy has been used to assess the likelihood of other complications of fracture healing. Segmental collapse of the femoral head as well as redisplacement and pseudarthrosis occurred more commonly in patients with Tc-99m MDP uptake ratios of less than 1.0 (fracture to uninvolved side) in postoperative patients with femoral fracture in a study by Stromquist.[112] In a larger series by Stromquist[113] 306 patients were studied within 2 weeks of surgery. Ninety-one percent of patients with uptake ratios of 1.0 or greater had no complications, whereas ninety percent of those with a ratio of less than 1.0 had postoperative complications. Several recent prospective studies[4,15,66,122] all have shown the value of scintigraphy in predicting complications of fracture healing. Broeng[15] had a sensitivity of 90% to 100% for uncomplicated healing with normal or increased uptake but a specificity of only 50% with decreased activity. Lausten,[66] using visual assessment, and Alberts,[4] using a quantitative ratio, showed preoperative scanning was a very good indicator of those patients likely to have difficulties in fracture healing. Van Vugt[122] found that a preoperative study was more accurate at predicting fracture healing problems such as nonunion, redislocation, and necrosis than a postoperative study.

Wallace et al[124] used the ratio of activity between 5 and 9 minutes after injection of MDP 2 weeks after trauma. There was less activity in the group that had intramedullary nailing compared with the groups that had had either external fixation or merely were casted. However, this technique could not predict which patients would have problems with fracture healing. Reduced uptake at the site of screw fixation in elderly patients with subcapital femoral fractures was predictive of healing failure in a study by Alho et al.[6]

Although these studies show a value in the bone scan done in the immediate posttraumatic period as a means of predicting complications, in practice this is not used to any significant extent.

NONUNION

Nonunion has been defined as that point in time after which spontaneous healing can no longer be expected to occur.[50] The pattern of a photon-deficient separation of activity between the edges or ends of bone has been termed *atrophic nonunion*.[50] When there is only a single focus of increased activity encompassing both sides of a fracture site, the term *reactive nonunion* has been used.[50] Usually on a single scan in time, reactive nonunion cannot be differentiated from delayed union. Nonunion can be caused by synovial, fibrous, or infected tissue interposed between fracture fragments. When infection is suspected, gallium or indium leukocyte studies are often useful. The scintigraphic patterns associated with infection imaging have been reviewed in Chapter 11. Seabold et al[104] studied 49 patients with 50 fracture nonunion sites 4 to 8 months postinjury; 42% of these sites were positive for infection on biopsy. The accuracy of the gallium scan was only 39%, the accuracy of the indium leukocyte study was between 74% and 88%. In a more recent, larger study from that group,[87] 102 sites of delayed union or nonunion were studied. The combined MDP/In white blood cell (WBC) scans had a sensitivity of 86%, a specificity of 84%, and an accuracy of 82% for the diagnosis of osteomyelitis.

The use of labeled leukocyte studies to predict infected pseudarthrosis, which can also be considered a type of nonunion, is usually performed well after the acute fracture. Labeled leukocytes and labeled platelets in the indium-111 WBC preparations are likely to go to hematoma in the acute fracture. Van Nostrand et al[121] prospectively studied In-WBC uptake in 27 sites of noninfected closed fractures in 19 patients. There was indium WBC uptake in 41% of the 27 sites. The degree of uptake was minimal in 55%, moderate in 36%, and marked in only 9%. The 1 patient with marked uptake was only 3 days posttrauma, and of the 4 patients with moderate uptake, 3 were within the first 2 weeks following trauma. Therefore it is important not to use leukocyte uptake in acute and early subacute fractures to diagnose osteomyelitis.

The use of bone scintigraphy to stratify patients with nonunion into those likely to benefit from electrical stimulation has been reported by Desai[28] and Gunalp.[40] In both studies the sites of nonunion were categorized as group I: intense increased activity at the fracture site;

group II: intense uptake of both sides of the fracture with a photon deficient area between the fragments; and group III: categorized neither as group I nor group II. In both series 90% of group I patients had healing of the nonunion following pulsed electromagnetic stimulation.

About half of group III patients had successful treatment, and none of the group II patients had successful healing of their fractures. The reason for the failed treatment in both series were true pseudarthrosis, those patients with synovial lined cavities, soft-tissue interposition and/or

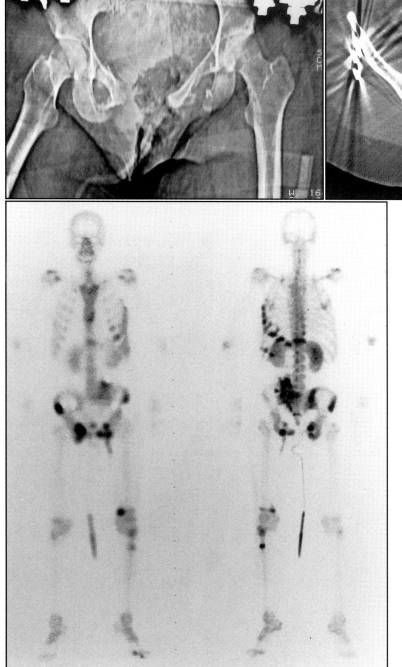

Fig. 14-2. Massive skeletal trauma. **A**, Computed tomography (CT) scan 17 days following trauma. Localizer image demonstrates the placement of two sacral bars, external fixator hardware in place, continued diastasis of the symphysis, and fractures of all four pubic rami. **B**, Transaxial CT slice demonstrates the large left sacral fracture as well as the type of streak artifacts associated with metal (*arrows*). Soft-tissue windows confirmed posttraumatic hematoma anterior to the sacral fracture. **C**, Delayed whole-body image demonstrated abnormal uptake associated with the multiple fractures involving the pelvis and at other sites. The diastasis of the symphysis pubis is again noted. Areas of photon deficiency are associated with the metallic hardware.

infections at the site of fracture. Although bone scanning is not used frequently in the assessment of patients with fractures, it can play a role in those patients who have delayed union or nonunion; the use of indium WBC studies has also been shown to be very helpful in determining which cases of nonunion are secondary to infection.

POSTTRAUMATIC COMPLICATIONS

In this section we address the use of radionuclide bone imaging (RNBI) in a variety of posttraumatic situations for which the referring clinician is usually asking a specific question. We limit the discussion to problems affecting the musculoskeletal system. It should also be remembered that RNBI is ideal for evaluating the patient with massive skeletal trauma, often directing the clinician to sites of more occult trauma, after primary stabilization has occurred. When patients continue to have unexplained pain, pain out of proportion to the recognized injuries, or there is concern about superimposed infection, whole-body bone scanning is appropriate (Fig. 14-2).

AVASCULAR NECROSIS. In the setting of known acute trauma, the development of avascular necrosis (AVN) occurs after the blood supply to a segment of bone has been interrupted by fracture.[80] The most commonly

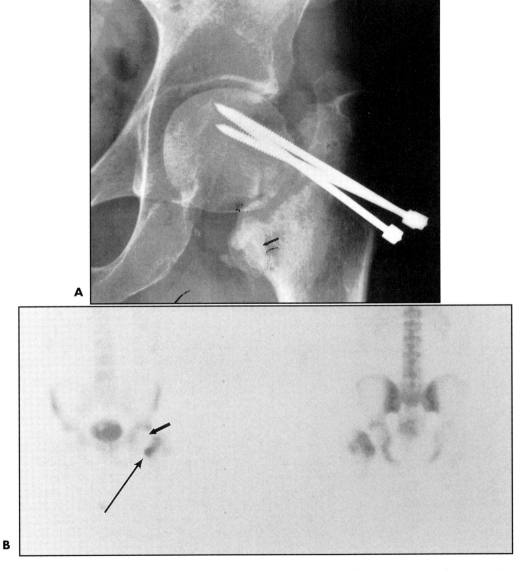

Fig. 14-3.   Avascular necrosis, femoral head. **A,** Plain radiograph 2 years status postfracture and Knowles pinning. The nonunited fracture, Knowles pins, and a tiny focal area of sclerosis in the region of the lesser trochanter (*arrow*) is noted. **B,** Delayed images demonstrate that the photon-deficient femoral head is well seen (*short arrow*). There is a tiny focal area of increased metabolic activity associated with continued efforts at healing of the lesser trochanteric fragment (*long arrow*).

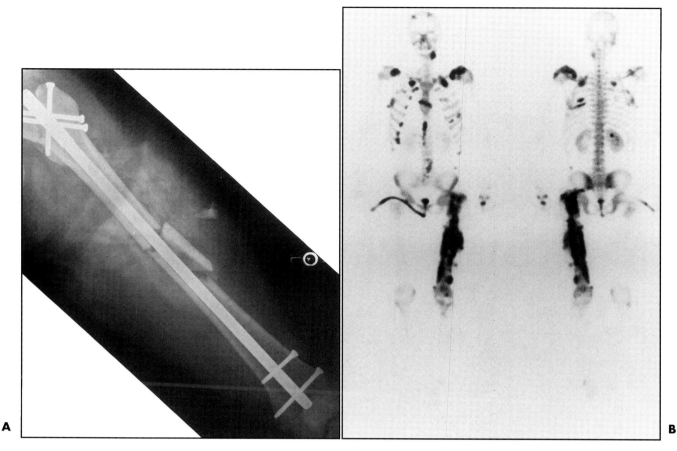

Fig. 14-4. Heterotopic ossification. **A**, Radiograph 23 days after a moderately comminuted fracture of the mid-shaft of the left femur and 16 days after intramedullary rod with proximal and distal interlocking screw placement, in a patient who had multiple trauma. **B**, Whole-body delayed image 1 day later demonstrates healing at craniotomy sites, multiple healing fractures throughout the appendicular skeleton, and significant activity about the femur that was thought to represent a combination of reparative bone at the fracture site as well as marked metabolically active heterotopic bone formation.

affected bones are the femoral head[66] and the proximal pole of the carpal scaphoid.[34]

Preoperative RNBI in displaced fracture of the hip has been reported to have a positive predictive value of 0.92 (confidence interval [CI] of 0.62 to 1.00) and a negative predictive value of 0.93 (CI of 0.66 to 1.00) for the prediction of the late complication of femoral head AVN.[66] When patients with non-displaced fracture were included in the analysis, the positive predictive value was only 0.63 if visually reduced femoral head uptake on delayed images was diagnosed as AVN. On this basis Lausten recommends RNBI be used to select those patients with displaced fractures who will benefit from primary arthroplasty instead of fixation of the fracture. In the scaphoid, scintigraphy has been less successful in detecting AVN in the early avascular phase and in guiding early therapy. Fractures of the proximal pole therefore are considered inherently unstable, with some authors recommending open reduction and internal fixation.[29,34] Postoperative AVN after hip pinning is often the query in patients with pain, in whom the differential diagnosis is the develop-

ment of heterotopic ossification (HO), nonunion, progressive arthritis, or simply a low pain threshold and unrealistic expectations. Absent tracer in the femoral head is usually obvious[46] (Fig. 14-3).

AVN of other carpal bones such as the lunate (Kienböck's disease)[11,109] or the hook of the hamate[33] has been reported. Carpal bone AVN often presents as non-specific increased tracer accumulation relatively localized to the involved bone.[46,109] In adolescents this often suggests the revascularizing phase with healing potential,[21] whereas in adults abnormal increased tracer on blood pool (BP) and delayed images is also associated with mechanically unstable fragments that may need surgical treatment.[82] A photon-deficient area with a rim of increased activity was reported in Freiberg's disease, a traumatic lesion of the head of the second metatarsal, thought to be AVN.[74] Other aspects of AVN are discussed in Chapters 4, 5, 8, and 15.

HETEROTOPIC OSSIFICATION. Although recent literature suggests that the term *myositis ossificans* be used when new bone arises as the result of inflammation in

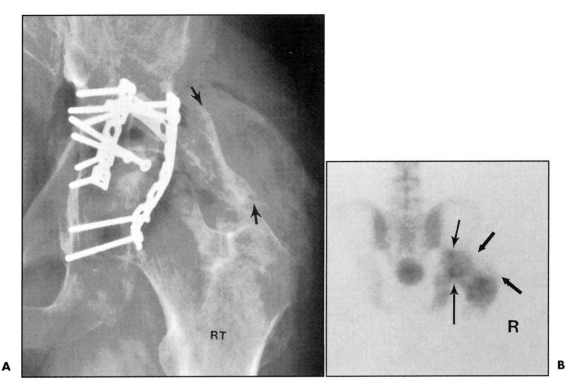

Fig. 14-5. Heterotopic ossification. **A**, AP radiograph 6 months following complex acetabular fracture with posterior dislocation of the right femoral head and 5 months following postsurgical hardware placement (oriented to correspond to bone scan image). Radiographically mature heterotopic ossification lateral to the inferior acetabulum and neck region (*arrow*). **B**, Delayed image posterior view 1 day following radiograph. The heterotopic bone is normometabolic (*thicker arrows*). There is some minimal stress remodeling type of change associated with the medial aspect of the most superior fixation screw and one of the screws at the inferiormost part of the acetabulum (*thin arrows*).

muscle tissue, with heterotopic ossification (HO) or heterotopic bone formation (HBF) reserved for new bone formed in soft parts in the absence of a well-defined cause,[117] this differential is probably artificial. The deposition of bone tracer as a result of primary soft-tissue injury has been discussed in Chapter 13. Thomas, in a recent review of HBF after total hip arthroplasty, emphasizes the concept that primordial mesenchymal cells may differentiate into osteoblasts with the deposition of osteoid matrix, which then calcifies and ossifies.[117]

HO is visualized radiographically from 4 to 12 weeks after injury[3,88] (Fig. 14-4). Maturation has been reported to continue for up to 5 years, with the majority occurring within 1 year[3] or even 6 months.[117] Reflecting the physiology of increased blood flow, calcium deposition, and bone formation, radionuclide angiography (RNA), BP, and delayed bone scan images will demonstrate abnormal increased tracer accumulation. Orzel and Rudd reported that the RNA and BP phases became abnormal before the delayed images, which in turn were abnormal before the radiographs.[88] Once bone has become mature, activity on delayed images appears similar to other bone, a level of activity we describe as normometabolic (Fig 14-5). The recurrence rate associated with resection surgery

to free ankylosed joints or entrapped nerves can be reduced or eliminated if surgery is delayed until maturation is documented[88,117] (Fig. 14-5). In all types of HO local features may mimic cellulitis or deep vein thrombosis so that in the appropriate setting, this diagnosis should be considered.[88,117] Some centers use low-level external beam radiation therapy from 600 to 1000 rads as prophylaxis following hip surgery. Since radiation can cause decreased bone metabolism, it is important that there be careful shielding of any porous arthroplasty surfaces.

SYMPATHETIC MAINTAINED PAIN SYNDROME (SMPS). The term *sympathetic maintained pain syndrome* (SMPS) covers a broad grouping of clinical conditions in which pain and autonomic dysfunction are intimately related.[7,64] These signs and symptoms occur during the recovery period following a traumatic episode, often but not exclusively following surgical treatment or other nonsurgical intervention. Reflecting the variety of symptoms associated with these conditions are the many terms used such as causalgia, sympathetic dystrophy, Sudeck's atrophy, traumatic arthritis, minor causalgia, posttraumatic spreading neuralgia, posttraumatic osteoporosis, posttraumatic edema, posttraumatic angiospasm, shoulder-hand syndrome, algodystrophy, and algoneurodystrophy[2,64] (Fig. 14-6). Although neither the etiology of the condition nor the underlying mechanisms of pain production or autonomic changes are clearly known or understood, a variety of successful therapies has been developed.[2,30,64] RNBI has become the most accepted objective method for diagnosing at least one of these disorders (if one is a splitter) or one of the specific clinical presentations (if one is a lumper).* On delayed images, diffuse increased tracer throughout the hand and wrist, or similarly throughout the foot, with juxtaarticular accentuation, is the most consistent finding in the reflex sympathetic dystrophy (RSD) variant (Figs. 14-7 and 14-8).[27,47,49] In the hand the sensitivity is 96% and specificity 97%. In the foot the sensitivity reaches 100%, with a much lower specificity, because of "falsely" abnormal scans in the presence of diffuse infection, particularly in patients with underlying diabetes mellitus.[47] RNA and BP images can also be abnormal, with diffuse increased perfusion (RNA) and relative vascularity (BP) (Fig. 14-7). Although some authors have reported abnormal RNA and BP with normal delayed

*References 10, 26, 35, 49, 70, 126.

images,[64] that has not been our experience.[49] Furthermore, the distinctive pediatric patterns of RSD are discussed in detail in Chapter 16. The condition is also discussed from the point of view of the rheumatologist in Chapter 12.

Patients present for imaging either when recovery is prolonged or pain is increased out of proportion to the extent of trauma, or at any point following trauma when signs or symptoms suggesting RSD are present. These might include pain, tenderness, allodynia, hyperpathia, swelling with or without pitting edema, dystrophic skin and nail changes, hyperhidrosis and hypertrichosis, vasomotor changes including color and temperature, as well as limitations of movement and function.[30,64,69] In areas other than the hand or foot such as around the knee, focal pain usually without x-ray changes or with localized osteoporosis has been given a variety of names and, usually as a diagnosis of exclusion, has been called, for example, algodystrophy,[101] RSD,[60] or transient migratory osteoporosis.[72] Many such patients have had focal areas of increased tracer accumulation on delayed images. Kline has reported a more specific patient population with a segmental RSD pattern in the hands[63] (Fig. 14-9). As specifically defined for the hand,[70] RSD is not seen in

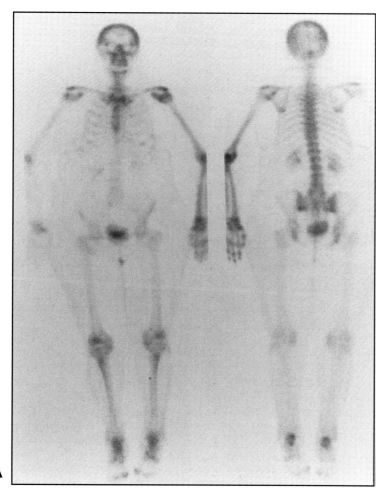

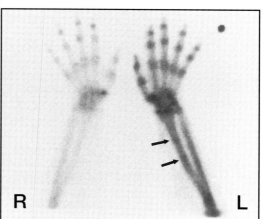

Fig. 14–6. Shoulder-hand syndrome in a 60-year-old individual 3 months following internal plate and external fixation of a comminuted distal radial fracture with continued pain after healing. **A,** Whole-body scan demonstrates diffuse increased tracer accumulation in the left shoulder, arm, elbow, forearm, wrist, and hand region. **B,** Delayed palmar spot images. In better detail, the diffuse increased tracer throughout the forearm, wrist, and hand with juxtaarticular accentuation is noted. The minimal foci of activity remaining at the fixation pin sites (*arrows*) can be seen normally.

children or adolescents. In children[73] and in some adults,[58] a relative decrease in tracer uptake in the lower extremities on delayed images has been reported in association with pain and autonomic symptoms. The differences in these groups are uncertain. It should also be noted that the finding of diffuse increased tracer accumulation on delayed images is also seen following sympathetic blockade,[44,107] even though such treatment results in alleviation of patient symptoms. Greyson and others have shown that disuse of an extremity usually results in normal metabolic activity on delayed images

and thus the superimposition of RSD can still be diagnosed in this setting.[37,125]

JOINT REPLACEMENT

A common request in nuclear medicine departments is to evaluate the patient with a painful arthroplasty. The total hip arthroplasty is the most common reconstructive joint procedure performed in the United States. Harkess

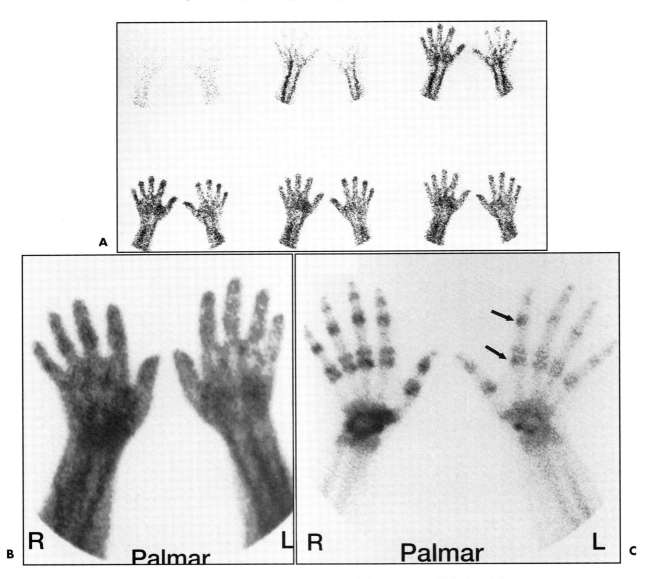

Fig. 14-7. Reflex sympathetic dystrophy. **A,** Radionuclide angiogram. Right hand demonstrates minimum increased activity compared with that of the entire left hand, which persists throughout all frames. Grades I/III diffusely positive (for details of grading system, see reference 49). **B,** Blood pool or tissue-phase image. Right hand demonstrates mild to moderate increased activity throughout the hand. This is best appreciated in the carpal region and shafts of the digits, as well as the proximal interphalangeal joint juxtaarticular regions. **C,** Delayed image. Easily seen differences in the abnormal right hand involving the wrist as well as all of the metacarpophalangeal and interphalangeal joints. A few areas of noninflammatory arthritis (*arrows*) in the left hand contrast with the diffuse increased juxtaarticular activity in all of the joints of the right hand.

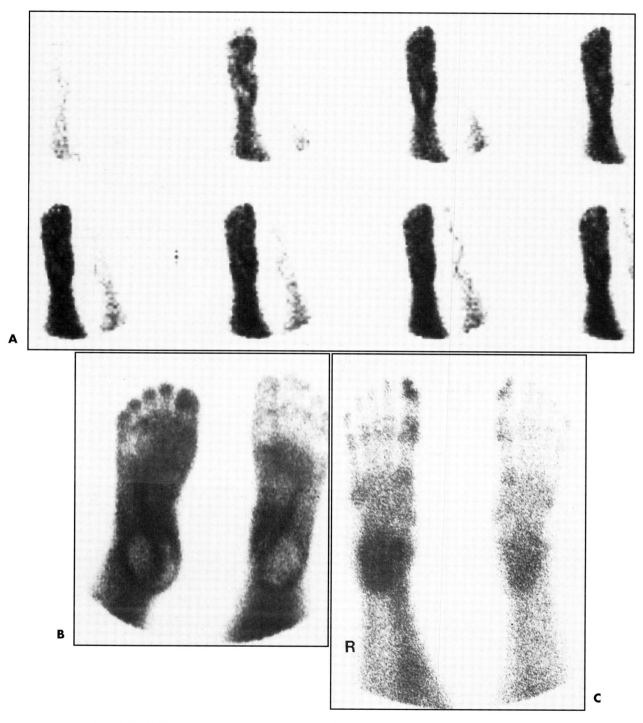

Fig. 14–8. Reflex sympathetic dystrophy in the foot. **A**, RNA, plantar view. Intense increased perfusion throughout the right distal leg and foot. **B**, Plantar blood pool image. Note diffuse increased relative vascularity throughout the hindfoot, midfoot, and forefoot. **C**, Delayed image, different patient than (**A**) and (**B**). Note mild diffuse relative increase in activity in the distal leg, ankle, hindfoot, midfoot, and forefoot. Clear differentiation between the right side uptake (*R*) and the left side with juxtaarticular accentuation.

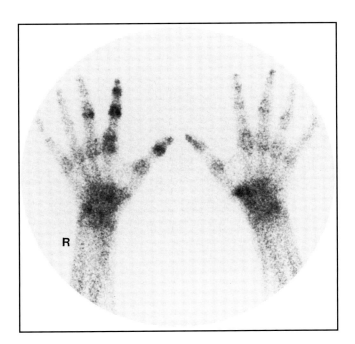

Fig. 14-9. Segmental reflex sympathetic dystrophy. Delayed images palmar view. Isolated ray involvement with mildly intense diffuse increased tracer in the right second ray, with juxtaarticular accentuation at the metacarpophalangeal and interphalangeal joints. Incidental mild focal activity was thought to be nonspecific biomechanical stress response (noninflammatory arthritis) at right first interphalangeal and third proximal interphalangeal and left first carpometacarpal joints. *(From Kline SC, Holder LE: Segmental reflex sympathetic dystrophy: clinical and scintigraphic criteria.* J Hand Surg [Am] *1993; 18A(5):853; with permission.)*

discusses the history of hip arthroplasties and provides an excellent review of the biomechanics and many of the complications involved in this procedure.[41] Charnley made major advances in total hip arthroplasties after Thompson and Moore developed the hip endoprosthesis. Most total hip arthroplasties depend on polymethylmethacrylate as a cement used to fix the component securely in the bone, although it has no adhesive properties. More recent developments in arthroplasties include the use of porous materials that allow for bone ingrowth. The hope is that bone ingrowth will provide stability above and beyond that which occurs with the cement. There can be many complications with arthroplasties including implant wear, loosening, fractures of the component, and infections. In total knee arthroplasties, noninfected loosening of the tibial component is perhaps the most common cause of arthroplasty failure.

Loosening

The biomechanics of total hip arthroplasties and an understanding of the selection of components are important to better appreciate the development of complications. As suggested by Harkess[41] "to describe the force acting on the hip joint, the body weight may be depicted as a load applied to a lever arm extending from the

body's center of gravity to the center of the femoral head." The load on the femoral head equals the sum of forces of the body weight and those forces created by abductor muscles and varies from 3 times body weight at rest up to 10 times body weight when running, jumping, or lifting. Forces on hip joints occur not only in the coronal plane but also in the sagittal plane bending the stem posteriorly. These forces can lead to aseptic loosening. Failure of cemented prostheses appeared to be at the prosthesis-cement interface and attempts to decrease this complication include modifying the surface of the components. Loosening may be diagnosed radiographically by detecting a space between the cement and bone of greater than 2 mm. Loosening of the femoral and acetabular components of a total hip arthroplasty is the most serious long-term complication and the most common indication for revision arthroplasties. The radiographic diagnosis of loosening of bone ingrowth arthroplasties is more difficult where subsidence is the primary finding. The incidence of loosening of the femoral component has decreased with component improvement. Initial reports of component loosening were in the range of 24% at 5 years, with little additional loosening occurring in the years beyond that time. More recent series have reported loosening rates of less than 2% at 6 years, again with little additional loosening. Acetabular loosening tends to be a rather late finding and increases with time.

Loosening can be detected by progressive plain film findings, contrast arthrograms, which are improved by subtraction techniques, or with the use of bone scintigraphy or RNA. The nuclear medicine techniques are discussed in the following material.

Postoperative infections in total hip arthroplasties are uncommon, ranging from 1% or less. These infections may occur early or may be low grade and not detected for years. Plain film findings that suggest infected arthroplasties include endosteal scalloping, periosteal new bone formation, and with arthrograms the detection of large pseudocapsules and fistulae. The nuclear medicine studies that have been used for defining arthroplasty infections include bone scintigraphy, gallium scanning, indium and technetium leukocyte scanning, and more recently scanning with radiolabeled polyclonal antibodies. These are discussed in the following material. Another complication that occurs with arthroplasties is HO, which has been discussed earlier in this chapter.

Pain is the major symptom that brings patients with arthroplasties to the nuclear medicine department. The differential diagnosis of that pain, especially in the hip, includes infection and aseptic loosening. The workup of these patients usually begins with plain films and occasionally joint aspiration and/or an arthrogram. Bone scintigraphy may show intense increased uptake when an arthroplasty is loose or infected[55,93] (Fig. 14-10). A negative scan is strong evidence that loosening or infection is not present.[93] One of the problems of most of the early published studies was that the natural history of the uncomplicated arthroplasty was not evaluated. Sonne-Holm et al[108] prospectively studied 14 cemented and 15 noncemented Moore arthroplasties. Both groups showed

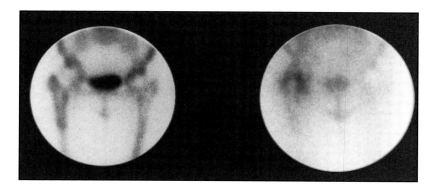

Fig. 14-10. Loose and infected total hip arthroplasties. *Left panel*: Delayed bone scan demonstrates moderately intense increased uptake in the acetabular and femoral component of the right total hip arthroplasty and intense increased uptake in the acetabular component of the left total hip arthroplasty, with normal activity about the femoral component of the left total hip arthroplasty. *Right panel*: Delayed gallium scan shows intense increased uptake about the acetabular component of the right total hip arthroplasty and mild increased uptake about the femoral component of the right total hip arthroplasty. No abnormal gallium localization in the left total hip arthroplasty. At surgery this patient had an infection of the acetabular component and loosening of the femoral component of the right total hip arthroplasty. Left hip symptoms did not warrant surgery.

increased uptake throughout the first postoperative year with little change over time. In this group there was no correlation between bone scan uptake and functional hip assessments. Utz et al[120] reviewed 267 bone scans in 97 asymptomatic patients with previously implanted hip prosthesis. One hundred and ninety-three scans in 59 patients were obtained prospectively, and the others were performed for reasons other than hip pain. There was a good distribution of time postsurgery in these patients varying from 1 month to greater than 3 years. Their study concluded that in most patients the bone scan will return to normal approximately a year after surgery. Twenty percent of patients will have some area of modestly increased activity and ten percent will have definite persistent activity, most commonly in the greater trochanter or in association with the tip of the femoral component. By recognizing this normal postoperative distribution one can avoid a certain number of false-positive diagnoses. Aliabadi[5] combined radiographic and scintigraphic criteria for prosthetic loosening with a sensitivity of 84% and a specificity of 92%. Rosenthall and the group from Montreal General Hospital[98] studied 55 patients with 62 asymptomatic arthroplasties. They developed quantitative ratios of uptake and showed relative stability of most of the uptakes except for the tip and lesser trochanter area. The ratio of the tip and lesser trochanter to either the sacroiliac (SI) joint or the stem decreased between 1 and 5 years. They reported that too few of their patients had any complications to draw conclusions on whether this quantitative assessment was useful. They also stated that the different designs of prosthesis may have different temporal uptakes. It is therefore important to understand that areas of uptake on the bone scan in either cemented or porous coated prostheses may not be related to loosening, but rather may be the natural history of that arthroplasty.

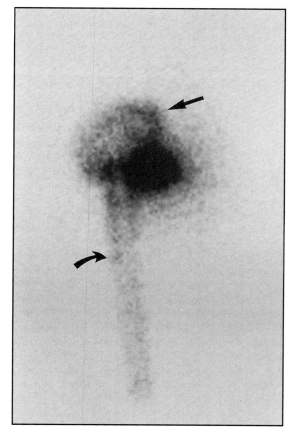

Fig. 14-11. Loose total hip arthroplasty. Delayed arthroscintigraphy image of the right total hip arthroplasty following injection of Tc-99m sulfur colloid into the joint capsule. Focal intense increased uptake in the capsule with mild to moderate increased activity is seen surrounding both the acetabular (*straight arrow*) and femoral (*curved arrow*) components in this patient with a loose right total hip arthroplasty. *(Case courtesy of Robert A. Cooper, M.D., Sydney, Australia.)*

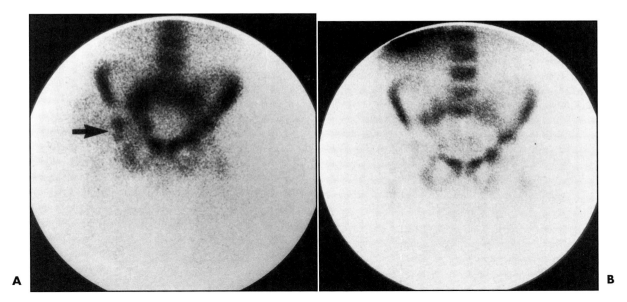

Fig. 14-12. Infected arthroplasty. **A,** Indium leukocyte scan at 24 hours demonstrates a focal area of moderately intense increased uptake in the region of the proximal femoral component (*arrow*) and mild increased uptake in the surrounding soft tissues (*immediately above arrow*). **B,** Sulfur colloid scan does not demonstrate any area of activity corresponding to the white cell localization.

Another means of using nuclear medicine to determine whether an arthroplasty is loose is the scintigraphic arthrogram.* During radiographic arthrography various radiopharmaceuticals including Tc-99m sulfur colloid, Tc-99m DTPA (diethylenetriamine pentaacetic acid), indium-111 DTPA, or gallium-67 can be injected into the joint. From 0.5 to 1.0 mCi of Tc-99m SC in a volume of 4 to 6 ml can be injected alone or in a volume of 1 ml if the radiotracer is injected following a routine contrast arthrogram. Immediate and 1- to 4-hour delayed images after ambulation can be obtained. Loosening is diagnosed when the tracer is seen outlining the component (Fig. 14-11). Abdel-Dayem[1] performed scintigraphic arthrography in a group of patients, five of whom had total hip prostheses and one had a total knee prosthesis. A scintigraphic arthrogram showed both the tibial and femoral components in the knee prosthesis to be loose. They described various findings in the patients with hip prostheses. Uri et al[119] studied 29 hips. Of the 13 hips with surgical confirmation, the radionuclide arthrogram was 100% sensitive for loosening, whereas the radiographic arthrogram was only 55% sensitive. Maxon's group[79] had 13 of their 15 patients confirmed at surgery. Both the radiographic and radionuclide techniques had an 80% accuracy, but in their series the x-ray technique was more sensitive, whereas the radionuclide arthrogram was more specific. Miniaci et al[83] had 65 cemented femoral components assessed surgically. In this group 16 were thought not to be loose, 12 were minimally loose, 37 were grossly loose. Both the radionuclide arthrogram and radiographic arthrogram were equally specific (88%),

*References 1, 42, 79, 83, 114, 119.

but the radionuclide arthrogram was significantly better than the radiographic study with a sensitivity of 86% versus 53%. For the acetabular component, however, the radionuclide study was significantly less sensitive, 48% versus 68%, and less specific, 67% versus 90% when compared with the radiographic arthrogram. The work of Herzwurm[42] and Swan[114] confirms that the radionuclide arthrogram is a specific technique especially for the femoral component. An advantage of the nuclear technique is that the patient can ambulate and the images can be delayed for hours. Why this particular study has not received greater clinical acceptance is uncertain, except that diagnosis of acetabular component loosening is very difficult due to the normal activity within the capsule.

Infection

The evaluation of arthroplasties for infection is covered in more detail in the chapters on infection (see Chapter 6) and bone marrow imaging (see Chapter 7). Some comments are appropriate here, however, because patients are often initially evaluated for pain of uncertain etiology.

The three-phase bone scan is very sensitive for the detection of infected arthroplasties, although not specific. In the review by Magnuson et al,[71] bone scanning was 100% sensitive for osteomyelitis in a group of 98 patients with painful hip arthroplasty, all of whom had surgical confirmation. However, the specificity of the bone scan was 18% for an overall accuracy of only 53%. To improve the specificity of bone scanning, gallium scintigraphy[68,81,127] or indium-111 labeled leukocyte imaging[71,85] should be done, either with or without the bone scan. The criteria for an infected arthroplasty using gallium-67 is that the gallium should be more intense than the comparative bone scan (Fig. 14-10), or there should be spatially incongruent gallium activity. For indium leukocyte scans the indium should be again more intense or spatially incongruent compared with a bone scan.

Oswald[89,90] showed in two prospective studies in asymptomatic patients with hip arthroplasty that indium leukocyte activity could be seen in 48% of prostheses tips at 24 months, and 37% of patients had significant uptake in the acetabular component at 24 months. They conclude that the scintigraphic pattern in uncomplicated porous coated hip arthroplasties was different from cemented prostheses. This "normal" finding may simply have been due to residual or compacted marrow at these sites. Palestro,[91,92] Seabold,[105] and King[62] all demonstrated that the addition of a Tc-99m sulfur colloid scan to define areas of active marrow in hips, knees, and in areas where there are postoperative bone marrow alterations can significantly improve the specificity of the indium labeled leukocyte scan (Fig. 14-1 The sulfur colloid technique is discussed in more de l in Chapters 8 and 11, where other examples of infected arthroplasties also are provided. Other agents used for imaging sites for infection such as radiolabeled human immunoglobulin, radiolabeled nanocolloid, and technetium labeled WBCs have all been used successfully to evaluate suspected areas of infection in patients with arthroplasties.

CONCEPTS OF STRESS LOADING AND ORTHOPEDIC APPLIANCES

Motion in long-bone fractures treated with closed techniques stimulates callus formation, which stabilizes the fracture and adds strength during remodeling. Too much motion, however, blocks healing. Cyclic loading of bone is most effective in promoting bone hypertrophy. Compressive loading, which results when plates or other devices are used to improve mechanical stability, is less effective than cyclic loading in promoting repair. Therefore the rate of healing is slower, the healing fracture is weaker, and osteopenic and weakening effects of shielding the bone from stress (the concept of stress shielding) are evident.[24] The physiologic changes in bone healing of the callus or secondary healing type, compared with osteonal or primary healing, as well as the complications that occur are also reflected in the radionuclide bone images. Chapman quotes White et al, who have described the four biomechanical stages of fracture repair as opposed to the histologic and morphologic phases mentioned in the introduction of this chapter. In stage 1 the union is usually fibrous, there is little stiffness, and the original fracture can break down. In stage 2, although there is ossification, the fracture site is still not as strong as surrounding bone, and refracture may occur at the original fracture site. In stage 3 callus and bone strength are similar and when refracture

occurs, it does so partly through the fracture and partly through intact bone. In stage 4 the callus is stronger than normal bone and refracture may occur in the adjacent bone.[126]

Advances in the overall understanding of fracture healing, and more specifically, the importance of mechanical stability have led to an increase in the various types of internal fixation and have also contributed to the development of limb-lengthening and aggressive limb-salvage surgery. The onset of pain during both normal healing and when complications develop often leads to a referral for RNBI. Methods of internal fixation include screws, plates, wires, fixation nails, and intramedullary nails. Good basic reviews of these concepts can be found in comprehensive orthopedic textbooks, such as Chapman's *Operative Orthopedics.*[22]

Screw Fixation

Screws are used to attach implants, to fix bone to bone, or to fix tendons or ligaments to bone. Bray and Templeton state that the most important aspect of screw fixation is interfragmentary compression to minimize motion between fragments.[13] Lag screws purchase or grip into the far cortex, with holding ability most dependent on the density and quality of the patient's bone. There has been little published information concerning the scintigraphic appearance of either the normally functioning screw during the various stages of the healing process; or of the abnormal screw, which is loose, broken, or is simply causing an abnormal focus of stress remodeling change. Minimal amounts of activity on delayed images up through 12 to 18 months can be associated with normal healing (Figs. 14-13 and 14-5). More intense abnormal tracer, often with increased BP activity, can suggest movement or persistent abnormal stress (Fig. 14-14). The presence of such activity, however, does not of itself demand clinical attention.

Plate Fixation

Compression plating of a fracture often leads to healing without visible external callus. Plates are designed so that shape and function match both the bone involved and the type and location of the fracture. Static compression (axial loading), dynamic compression (tension band), neutralization (protection of lag screw fixation from bending, torsion, and shearing forces during early active movement or partial weight-bearing), or buttressing (for fixation of articular fragments to the shaft and support of the metaphyseal area) can be emphasized in the surgeon's choice of appliance depending on the need.[99] Scintigraphically there may be minimal increased activity on delayed images associated with plates and the screws or wires used to apply them to bone (Figs. 14-14 and 14-15). This makes sense if one remembers that healing is taking place very slowly without any visible callus formation. When activity is present, it is usually eccentric or associated with one or more of the fixation screws. This increased activity may alert the surgeon to possible

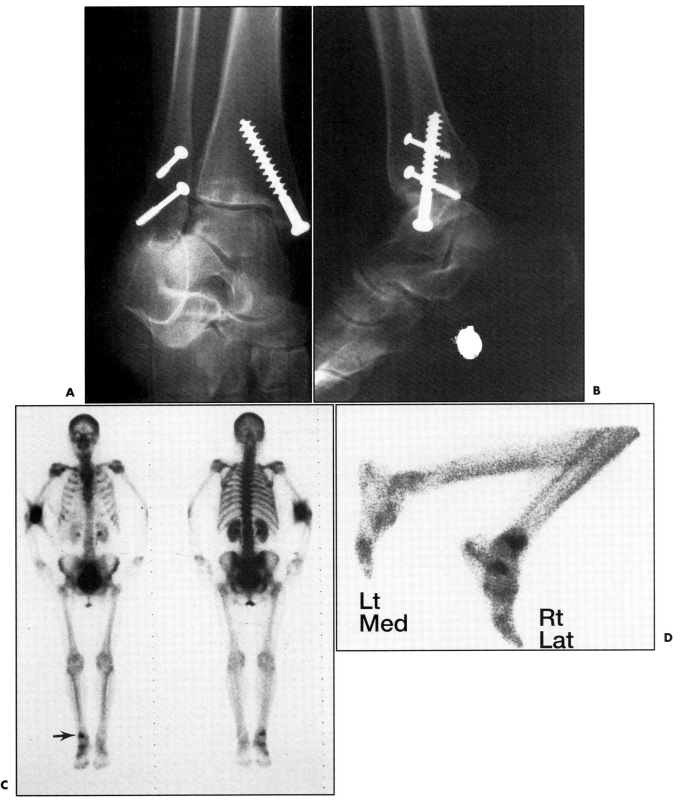

Fig. 14-13. Right bimalleolar ankle fracture, 20 years postscrew placement. Oblique (**A**) and lateral (**B**) radiographs demonstrate two distal fibular and one medial malleolar distal tibial screws and degenerative changes at tibiotalar joint. **C**, Delayed whole-body image in this patient, currently being evaluated for metastatic cancer, demonstrates very well defined focal area of moderate increased tracer accumulation in the distal tibia (*arrow*) as well as a portion of the midfoot. **D**, Delayed right lateral image demonstrates the abnormal increased activity located primarily at the tibiotalar joint and in the anterior calcaneal cuboid articulation. There is no significant activity associated with the purchase points of the screws with the cortex. The abnormal activity is most likely due to degenerative arthritic change.

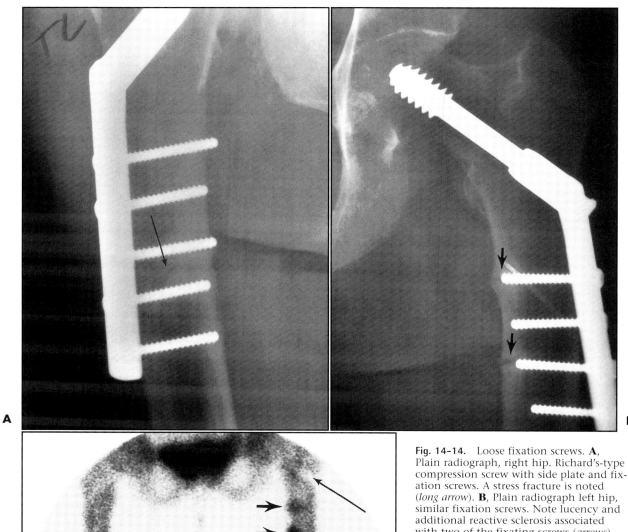

Fig. 14–14. Loose fixation screws. **A**, Plain radiograph, right hip. Richard's-type compression screw with side plate and fixation screws. A stress fracture is noted (*long arrow*). **B**, Plain radiograph left hip, similar fixation screws. Note lucency and additional reactive sclerosis associated with two of the fixating screws (*arrows*). **C**, Delayed bone image. On the right side there is abnormal activity associated with the stress fracture. Bilaterally there is photon deficiency associated with the screw in the femoral neck (*long arrow*). On the left there is moderate focal activity associated with the two loose screws (*short arrows*). *(A and C, from Holder LE: Bone scintigraphy in skeletal trauma, Radiol Clin North Am 1993; 31:739; with permission.)*

focal increased stress or loosening of a screw, but in our experience it is not specific, especially when visualized on a single scan in time. The combination of possible increased flow on the radionuclide angiogram, increased vascularity on the BP images, and more intense, more focal activity on delayed images is again nonspecific, but can be seen in superimposed infection, refracture or new fracture, loosening or nonspecific focal stress remodeling, which should lead to an additional review of correlative radiographs.

Wire Fixation

Fine Kirschner wires, commonly called K-wires, are used for provisional intraoperative fracture fixation or definitive fixation where subsequent loading on the fractured bone is going to be small, such as in the bones of the hands and feet. Larger Steinmann pins are often used for traction, and other flexible wires are made of stainless steel.[36] Tension band wires are commonly used to immobilize patella, greater trochanter, comminuted medial

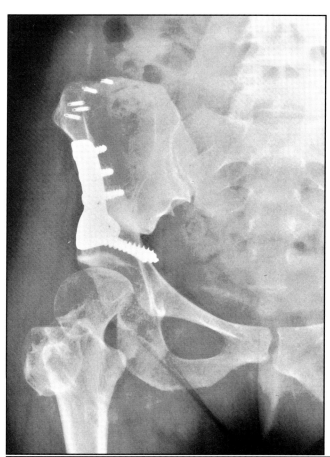

A

B

Fig. 14–15. Post–iliac osteotomy with plate fixation; history of CDH with hip surgery. **A,** Plain radiography. Deformity of the femoral head and previous surgical change involving the greater trochanteric region are identified. The plate and screws immobilizing the iliac osteotomy are also seen as is a minimal area of sclerosis in the supraacetabular region. **B,** Delayed bone images. Photon deficiency associated with the plate (*arrow*). Only the most minimal increased metabolic activity associated with the ilium just above the metallic plate and in the immediate supraacetabular region (*arrowheads*). There is also some minimal increased tracer associated with continued remodeling at the greater trochanteric region.

malleolar, and distal clavicular fractures. Cerclage wires are used to aid in the fixation of long-bone fractures. Scintigraphically there is little activity associated specifically with wires or pins when normal healing is taking place. As with other forms of fixation, foci of increased tracer activity, especially 6 or more months after surgery, should alert the nuclear physician to communicate with the orthopedic surgeon to determine if the visualized activity represents increased bone turnover associated with normal healing, nonunion, or is an indication of an abnormal biomechanical stress response of the bone (Fig. 14-16).

Intramedullary Nailing

Intramedullary nails, which can often be placed using percutaneous closed techniques, are load-sharing devices that give excellent axial alignment of fractures and allow early weight-bearing. A variety of reamed and non-reamed nail designs are used. Reaming of the intramedullary canal provides a precise fit for the nail. Overreaming can thin the cortex and results in comminution during nail placement.[23] Eccentric placement of nails can cause more focal areas of stress and lead to later fracture. Cross-screws can be placed to control angulation and rotation. Most intramedullary nails associated with normal healing appear as well-defined central photon-deficient areas within the medullary canal. On delayed images minimal areas of increased tracer can be associated with the cortex at its junction with the distal tip of the nail (Fig. 14-16). We have occasionally seen diffuse increased activity throughout on the bone on delayed images with normal RNA and BP phases. We have associated this with bone turnover or healing associated with the reaming process but have not discovered any adverse clinical correlation or effect on overall healing (Fig. 14-17). As with other orthopedic hardware, more focal areas of increased tracer uptake must be correlated with the entire clinical picture including the original fracture, the surgery performed, the resultant position and alignment, and the plain radiographs to determine the physiologic significance of any focal increased tracer accumulation in each individual patient.

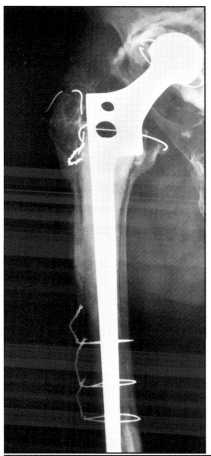

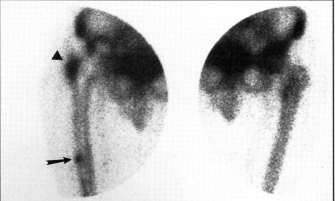

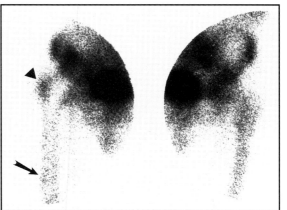

Fig. 14-16. Total hip arthroplasty. Cerclage wire fixation. **A**, AP radiograph demonstrates total femoral arthroplasty. Cerclage-type wires are associated with the greater trochanteric and lesser trochanteric fragments as well as the distal portion of the femoral stem component. **B**, Delayed bone images 6 months following surgery. Photon deficiency associated with the prosthesis, moderate activity associated with healing greater trochanteric fragment (*arrowhead*), and minimal activity at the tip of the femoral component lateral cortex interface (*arrow*). **C**, Delayed bone image 10 months after (**B**). There is less metabolic activity associated with the greater trochanteric fragment, and there is much less activity associated with the tip of the prosthesis lateral cortical interface. **B** and **C**, There is no significant activity associated with the cerclage wires. (*Study courtesy of Randall Winn, M.D., Reading, Pa.*)

External Fixation

Behrens provides a concise tutorial with beautifully drawn schematics about the terminology, basic equipment, and basic concepts of external fixation.[12] Pins fix the bony fragments. They are connected by rods via a variety of articulations and held in place by a three-dimensional structure called a fixator frame, which maintains the set alignment under varying loading conditions.[8]

If a fixator stays in place for 3 to 4 weeks, one or more pin tracks may be contaminated.[12] The scintigraphic differential diagnosis between an infected pin track and an area of focal stress remodeling change is often difficult. When the RNA and BP are abnormal and the increased activity on delayed images is increased and less well defined, infection should be given strong consideration.

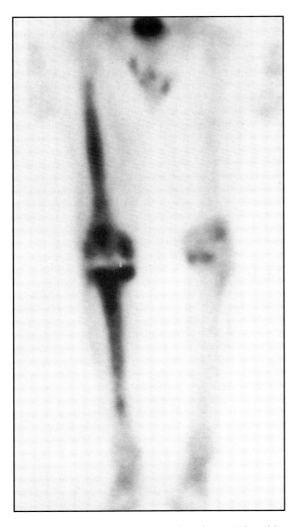

Fig. 14–17. Status post–total knee arthroplasty. Delayed bone image. Abnormal intense increased tracer in the distal two thirds of the right femur and proximal two thirds of the tibia extend proximally and distally to the metallic components of the photon-deficient prosthesis, corresponding to areas in which intramedullary reaming was undertaken as part of the arthroplasty procedure.

The minimally intense, bull's-eye–appearing activity on delayed images often years after pins have been removed in an area of a totally asymptomatic pin track, may represent normal metabolism associated with a relatively greater volume of residual bone that developed around the pin as a response to stress (Fig. 14-1).

Smith–Petersen Nails/Knowles Pins

Among the most common types of orthopedic hardware encountered are those larger nails, pins, or screw devices used for internal fixation of hip fractures. Knowles pins and Richard's-type compression screws have replaced the Smith-Petersen triflange nail introduced in 1931, with internal fixation now the standard of reference in femoral neck fracture treatment. Scintigraphically the normal healing pinned fracture demonstrates a photon deficiency associated with a large pin or screw, with minimal if any focal increased tracer accumulation (Fig. 14-14). A loose or displaced screw results in increased tracer localized to the site of abnormal stress response.

LIMB–LENGTHENING SURGERY

When one lower extremity is longer than another, the longer leg can be shortened by epiphysiodesis or epiphyseal stapling to stop or retard its growth, or alternatively the shorter leg can be lengthened by osteotomy and distraction techniques.[115] RNBI evaluation of the physes is discussed in Chapters 3 and 16. Shortening procedures, which usually involve transverse or oblique osteotomy, segmental resection, and intramedullary rod fixation or internal fixation with a plate and screws can be considered physiologically analogous to fracture fixation. Ilizarov's name is connected with the controlled mechanical distraction osteogenesis. His work has been summarized by Tachdjian.[115] Bone grafting techniques can be incorporated into distraction osteotomy procedures. Many of the problems and complications of limb-lengthening surgery can be evaluated with RNBI. They include disruption of the blood supply, fracture at the osteotomy site, soft-tissue necrosis at the surgical site, RSD, pin movement with vessel erosion, erosion of the pins, and stress fractures at the ends of plates.

LIMB SALVAGE SURGERY

The development of adjuvent chemotherapy, preoperative radiation therapy, and modern orthopedic appliances has dramatically reduced the use of primary amputation in the treatment of malignant extremity tumors. Allografts are also used alone or in combination with prostheses. An allograft is transplanted between genetically nonidentical members of the same species. Some authors use the term *implant* for nonviable bone such as

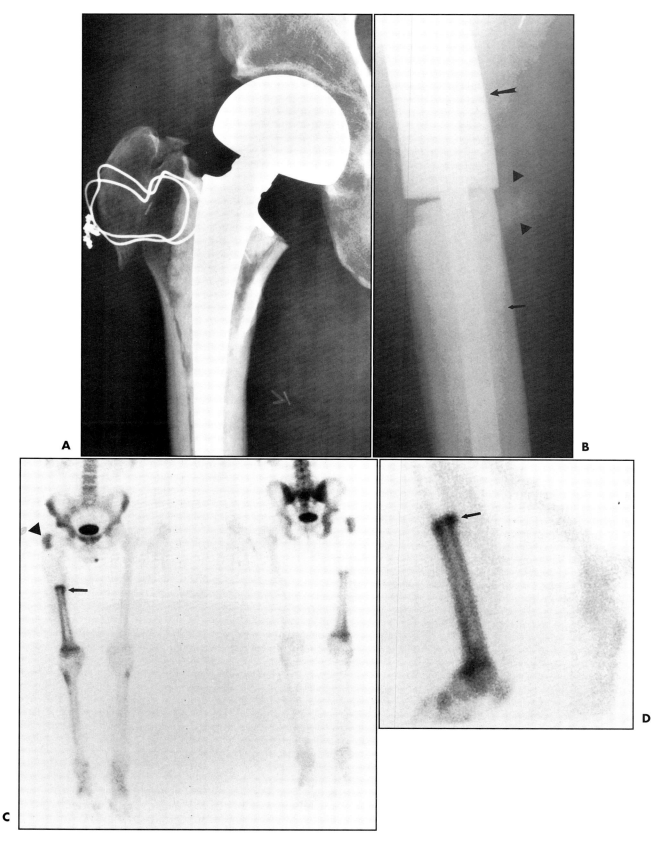

Fig. 14-18. Limb-salvage surgery. **A**, Plain radiograph, upper femur. Metallic femoral prosthesis, cerclage wires immobilizing greater trochanteric fragment. **B**, AP radiograph, lower femur. Intramedullary stem of metallic prosthesis is noted bridging the upper proximal allograft (*larger arrow*) and native femur distally (*small arrow*). A small amount of cancellous autograft is used (*arrowheads*). **C**, Delayed bone scan. Mild to moderate activity associated with the greater trochanteric fragment (*arrowhead*), photon deficiency associated with the metallic prosthesis and the allograft, minimal increased focal activity associated with the cancellous autograft (*arrow*), and mild activity associated with the native bone surrounding the metallic stem. **D**, Lateral spot view, lower femur. Delayed bone image demonstrates the lip of anterior activity associated with the cancellous autograft (*arrow*) at the junction between the photon-deficient proximal allograft and distal native bone.

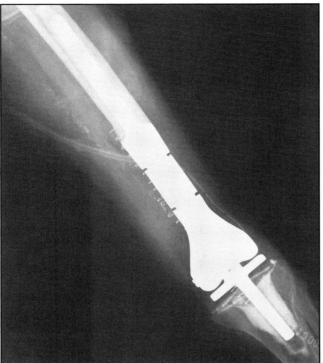

A

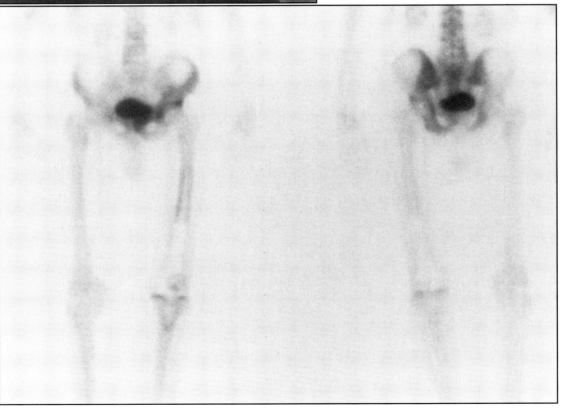

B

frozen, freeze-dried, sterilized bone from tissue banks. An autograft by contrast is bone transplanted from one part of the body to another. Autogenic is the preferred adjective.

Johnson has reviewed the principles of limb-salvage surgery[59] and Rodrigo and Prolo the concepts of allograft use.[97] It has been our experience[48] and others[102] that initially allografts are photon deficient on delayed bone images. Over time, during the incorporation process, the allograft weakens with fatigue fractures first occurring 18 to 36 months after implantation. Earlier authors[20] reported fractures as early as 6 to 8 months, but that has not been the experience at our institution. Focal well-defined activity at the junction of allograft and normal bone most often represents normal healing of autogenic cancellous graft or normal stress remodeling changes and not recurrent tumor or loosening (Fig. 14-18). Over many

Fig. 14–19. Customized implant following limb-salvage surgery. **A,** Plain radiograph demonstrates a metallic implant replacing bone in the lower half of the femur. **B,** Delayed bone scan. Photon deficiency associated with the distal femoral metallic component. Minimal nonspecific stress change surrounds the proximal stem in the femur. This does not represent definite loosening. There is also some mild nonspecific stress surrounding the proximal tibial component. This does not represent loosening, especially on a single scan in time.

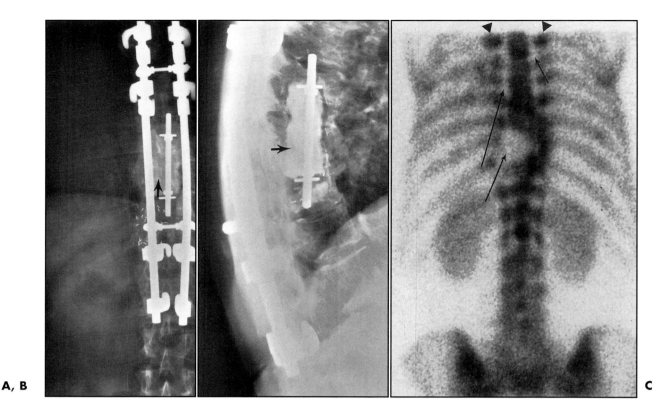

A, B
C

Fig. 14-20. Harrington distraction and compression rod and hook system. AP (**A**) and lateral (**B**) radiographs demonstrate the hook and rod system placed for spine stability. Methacrylate spacer at T9 vertebral body resection (*arrows*) is also noted as are small implanted radium seeds, in this patient with squamous cell carcinoma metastasis. **C**, Delayed bone image magnified posterior view demonstrates photopenia associated with the spacer and metallic rods (*thin arrows*). The uppermost hooks show the greatest area of nonspecific stress remodeling change (*arrowheads*). This is normal healing.

years of resorption and growth of new bone, the photon-deficient allograft becomes first more metabolically active and then normometabolic. New foci of activity that develop, when associated with pain, should prompt further evaluation and more frequent temporal follow-up. Large customized implants with strong intra-medullary stems allow for juxtaarticular limb-salvage surgery in young patients with expected higher levels of activity[59] (Fig. 14-19).

Vascularized bone grafting, most often using the fibula with the peroneal artery, can be combined with both autografts and allografts, as well as prosthesis. Since this bone can be hypermetabolic with increased activity on delayed images, or normometabolic versus the photon deficiency of allografts, the nuclear medicine physician must be knowledgeable about the use of such grafts.[84]

SPINE AND PELVIS SURGERY

An excellent review of the orthopedic aspects of spine and pelvic trauma can be found in the text *Skeletal Trauma* edited by Browner et al.[17] A variety of surgical

techniques and instrumentation systems have been developed for achieving stability and promoting healing. It is beyond the scope of this chapter to review the principles and goals of each individual system. However, to understand whether focal increased tracer uptake on an RNBI study is a normally expected response of the bone to the transfer of forces, or whether abnormal or unexpected forces are present and possibly related to the patient's complaint of pain, it is important to know what instrumentation has been used, for what purpose, and with what expected result. Close consultation with a referring physician is therefore invaluable. The orthopedic surgeon can also explain his choice of instrumentation, which is based on his knowledge about the mechanism of injury and the nature of the instability.

The Harrington distraction and compression rod and hook system used for reducing anterior vertebral body fractures and for the treatment of scoliosis is well known (Fig. 14-20). Hook problems include dislodgement with fracture of the lamina and the development of neurologic complications secondary to angulation into underlying neural tissue.[31]

Pedicle screws, which provide segmental fixation, have also become popular in a variety of systems. There

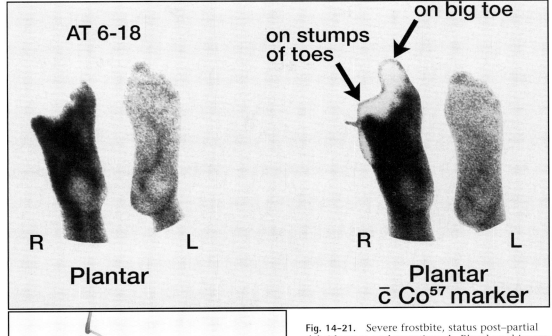

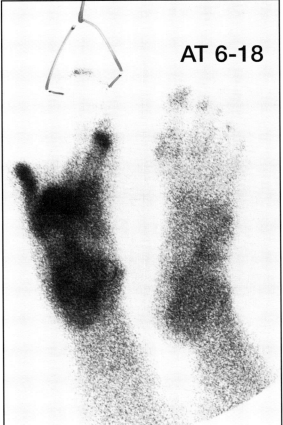

Fig. 14-21. Severe frostbite, status post–partial debridement and resection. **A,** Blood pool image shows absent tracer accumulation in the distal aspect of the right foot. Cobalt-57 string marker outlines the distal tip of great toe as well as the anatomic extent of other digits postsurgery. **B,** Delayed plantar image confirms absent perfusion to the distal aspects of foot. Cobalt marker again used to define anatomic extent of injury.

are many sizes and configurations, and many mechanisms for linking the screws. Pedicle screws can loosen with resulting loss of correction. Other problems include incorrect anatomic placement of the screw or pedicle fracture.[31] Knowledge of the patient's surgery is also required since surgical decompression is often per-

formed, which can explain both foci of photon deficiency and focal increased activity on delayed images (Fig. 14-20).

Stabilization in the lumbar spine and sacrum is more difficult than for the thoracic or thoracolumbar spine, primarily due to anatomic and motion considerations.

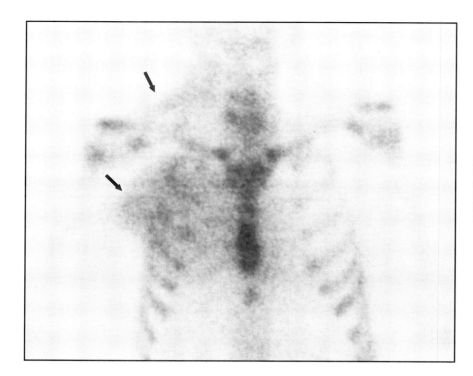

Fig. 14-22. Minimal burn injury, right anterior chest and neck muscles (*arrows*) of a 27-year-old individual with a lightning injury. Significant muscle necrosis would have activity much more intense than the ribs.

The lumbar lordosis must be restored and movement allowed. Pedicle screws are particularly used in the lumbar spine because they reduce the number of levels that need instrumentation to achieve adequate reduction or rigid fixation.[67]

Repair of pelvic ring fractures is directed toward creating stability. The specific instrumentation used depends on the combination of injuries present.[61,129] External fixation with the placement of pins is common as are plates with multiple fixation screws. Especially when there is concomitant soft-tissue infection through which fixation pins must traverse, the nuclear physician should have a high index of suspicion for pin track infection. Later SI joint nonunion may also cause leg length discrepancy, and pain can occur associated with abnormal biomechanics. RNBI can be done to detect occult fracture of the lumbar spine in patients who complain about localized SI joint pain despite anatomic reduction and satisfactory healing. In the imaging literature, RSD in the lower extremity was first reported after lumbar surgery.[106]

Complications of acetabular fracture treatment seen by the nuclear physician include infection, periarticular HBF, and especially as a late sequela, posttraumatic arthritis.[77]

THERMAL INJURIES

Electrical or direct flame burns generate heat[16] and freezing temperatures cause intracellular ice crystal formation.[100] These processes not only produce direct cellu-

lar death and tissue necrosis, but also are thought to damage blood vessels resulting in additional cellular damage and death in areas whose blood supply is disrupted. The early detection of nonviable tissue is crucial for successful early management of these injuries.[95] Imaging with thallium-201 or technetium-labeled MIBI[103] has been used to evaluate muscle viability following thermal injury. In addition, the three-phase bone scan provides useful prognostic information about the location of irreversibly damaged bone and soft tissue that will ultimately require surgical resection[100] as well as the extent of damaged yet viable tissue.[54,57] The RNA and BP phases reflect progressive macrovascular involvement, with absent bone uptake on 3-hour delayed images suggesting severe microvascular damage and dead bone that will not recover[57] (Fig. 14-21). If there is an intact blood supply to areas of tissue infarction that will require subsequent debridement, there can be intense soft-tissue tracer accumulation on delayed images. Minimal soft-tissue tracer accumulation often reflects minimal burn injury that can be treated conservatively (Fig. 14-22). A variety of reports has suggested that zones of irreversibly damaged or nonviable tissue can be identified as early as 2 to 5 days after injury by RNBI, well before clinical or radiologic demarcation of such zones occurs. Although we have used this technique with success as soon as the patient presented to our emergency department, if an immediate answer is not necessary for a management decision, it is preferable to support the patient for several days before imaging so as to increase uptake at sites of injury. HBF is a late sequela of tissue injury secondary to a thermal burn.[32]

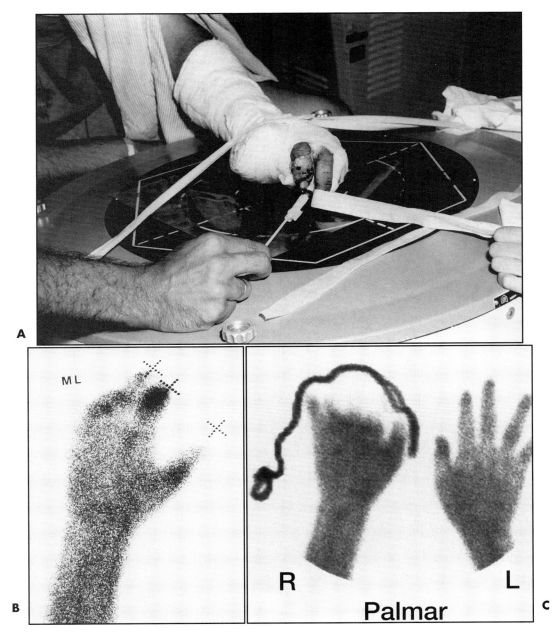

Fig. 14-23. Postreplant, extent of the viability. **A**, Heavily bandaged patient after replantation. Note creative positioning to isolate the digit or area of interest. Marker (in this case a cobalt-57 point source) indicates the physical, anatomic extent of the digit. **B**, Blood pool image shows vascularity extending to the tips of the fingers with reactive hyperemia associated with the replantation site. *X*'s are the marker points. **C**, In another patient postfrostbite, the physical extent of the digits is marked by a cobalt-57 gel string marker. Perfusion is clearly discordant. *(From Holder LE: Radionuclide bone imaging in surgical problems of the hand, in Gilula LA (ed): The Traumatized Hand and Wrist: Radiographic and Anatomic Correlation, Philadelphia, WB Saunders, 1991, p 19; with permission.)*

ORTHOPEDIC VASCULAR PROBLEMS

Three-phase RNBI is only rarely used by the orthopedist for the evaluation of most acute or chronic vascular problems,[51] having been supplanted by color Doppler sonography (CDS)[56] and magnetic resonance angiography (MRA).[51] However, when CDS and MRA are inappropriate or unavailable, the technique is still an accurate noninvasive method for addressing the vascular concerns confronting the orthopedic or hand surgeon.[45,78]

As is the case following thermal injuries, both the macrocirculations and microcirculations following

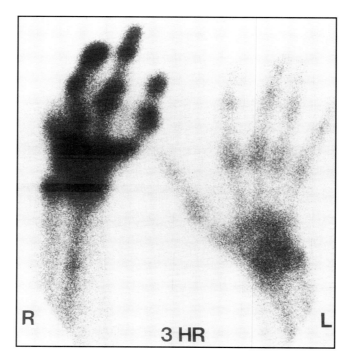

Fig. 14-24. Posttraumatic RSD, same patient as in Fig. 14-23, **A** and **B**. Delayed images. Diffuse increased activity throughout the entire wrist and hand.

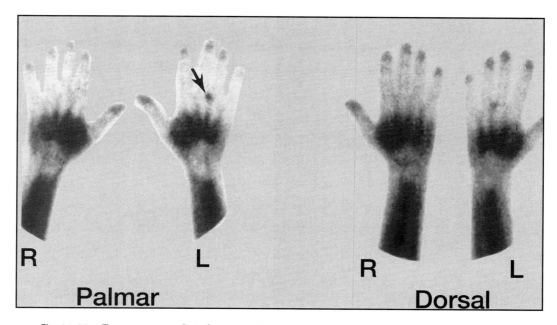

Fig. 14-25. True aneurysm digital artery. RNA was normal. Blood pool image demonstrates focal area of increased vascularity in the third web space of the left hand (*arrow*). Delayed image was normal. *(From Ho PK, Dellon AL, Wilgis EFS: True aneurysms of the hand resulting from athletic injury: report of two cases. Am J Sports Med 1985; 13:136; with permission.)*

replantation can be assessed with RNBI. It is important to mark the physical extent of the limb or ray to accurately assess the extent of viability (Fig. 14-23).[45] Because the trauma leading to re-implantation is often associated with major nerve injury, it is not surprising that RSD is present in many of these patients (Fig. 14-24).

Traumatic aneurysms appear as foci of increased tracer on BP images and often correspond to either a palpable mass or the site of the patient's deep pain. Most aneurysms seen in orthopedic practice occur following penetrating injuries and are often unrecognized during initial debridement. A true aneurysm of the hand has been reported resulting from repetitive trauma in a volleyball player[43] (Fig. 14-25).

REFERENCES

1. Abdel-Dayem HM, Barodawala YK, Papademetriou T: Scintigraphic arthrography, comparison with contrast arthrography in future applications. *Clin Nucl Med* 1982; 7:516.

2. Abrams S: Incidence-hypothesis-epidemiology, in Stanton-Hicks M (ed): *Pain and the Sympathetic Nervous System*, Kluwer Academic Publishers, Boston, 1990, p 1.

3. Ahrengart L: Periarticular heterotopic ossification after total hip arthroplasty: Risk factors and consequences. *Clin Orthop* 1991; 263:49.

4. Alberts KA: Prognostic accuracy of preoperative and postoperative scintimetry after femoral neck fracture. *Clin Orthop* 1990; 250:212.

5. Aliabadi P, Tumeh SS, Weissman BN, et al: Cemented total hip prosthesis: Radiographic and scintigraphic evaluation. *Radiology* 1989; 173:203.

6. Alho A, Benterud JG, Muller C, et al: Prediction of fixation failure in femoral neck fractures. Comminution and avascularity studied in 40 patients. *Acta Orthop Scand* 1993; 64:408.

7. Amadio PC, Mackinnon SE, Merritt WH, et al: Reflex sympathetic dystrophy syndrome: Consensus report of an ad hoc committee of the American Association for Hand Surgery on the definition of reflex sympathetic dystrophy syndromes. *Plast Reconstr Surg* 1991; 87:371.

8. Aro HT, Chao EYS: Biomechanics and biology of fracture repair under external fixation. *Hand Clin* 1993; 9:531.

9. Asnis SE, Gould ES, Bansal M, et al: Magnetic resonance imaging of the hip after displaced femoral neck fractures. *Clin Orthop* 1994; 298:191.

10. Atkins RM, Tindale W, Bickerstaff D, Kanis JA: Quantitative bone scintigraphy in reflex sympathetic dystrophy. *Br J Rheumatol* 1993; 32:41.

11. Beckenbaugh RD, Shives TC, Dobyns JH, Linscheid RL: Kienböck's disease and consideration of lunate fractures. *Clin Orthop* 1980; 149:98.

12. Behrens A: External fixation: General principles and application in the lower leg, in Chapman MW (ed): *Operative Orthopaedics*, JB Lippincott, Philadelphia, 1988, p 161.

13. Bray TJ, Templeton DC: Principles of screw fixation, in Chapman MW (ed): *Operative Orthopaedics*, JB Lippincott, Philadelphia, 1988, p 125.

14. Brody AS, Strong M, Babikian G, et al: Avascular necrosis: Early MR imaging and histologic finding in a canine model. *AJR Am J Roentgenol* 1991; 157:341.

15. Broeng L, Bergholdt Hansen L, Sperling K, et al: Post-operative Tc-scintimetry in femoral neck fracture: A prospective study of 46 cases. *Acta Orthop Scand* 1994; 65:171.

16. Browne BJ, Gaasch WR: Electrical injuries and lightning. *Emerg Med Clin North Am* 1992; 10:211.

17. Browner BD, Mast J, Mendes M: Principles of internal fixation, in Browner BD, Jupiter JB, Levine AM, Trafton PG (eds): *Skeletal Trauma*, WB Saunders, Philadelphia, 1992, p 243.

18. Buja LM, Parkey RW, Dees JH, et al: Morphologic correlates of technetium-99m stannous pyrophosphate imaging of acute myocardial infarcts in dogs. *Circulation* 1975; 52:596.

19. Buja LM, Tofte AJ, Kulkarn PV, et al: Sites and mechanisms of localization of technetium-99m phosphorus radiopharmaceuticals in acute myocardial infarcts and other tissues. *J Clin Invest* 1977; 60:724.

20. Burchardt H, Eneking WF: Transplantation of bone. *Surg Clin North Am* 1978; 58:403.

21. Cahill RB, Berg CB: 99m-Tc phosphate compound joint scintigraphy in the management of juvenile osteochondritis dissecans of the femoral condyles. *Am J Sports Med* 1983; 11:329.

22. Chapman MW (ed): *Operative Orthopaedics*, JB Lippincott, Philadelphia, 1988.

23. Chapman MW: Principles of intramedullary nailing, in Chapman MW (ed): *Operative Orthopaedics*, JB Lippincott, Philadelphia, 1988, p 151.

24. Chapman MW, Loo SLY: Principles of fracture healing, in Chapman MW (ed): *Operative Orthopaedics*, JB Lippincott, Philadelphia, 1988, p 115.

25. Charkes ND, Siddhivarn N, Schneck CD: Bone scanning in the adductor insertion avulsion syndrome ("thigh splints"). *J Nucl Med* 1987; 28:1835.

26. Constantinesco A, Brunot B, Demangeat JL, et al: Three phase bone scanning as an aid to early diagnosis in reflex sympathetic dystrophy of the hand. *Ann Chir Main* 1986; 5:93.

27. Demangeat JL, Constantinesco A, Brunot B, et al: Three-phase bone scanning in reflex sympathetic dystrophy of the hand. *J Nucl Med* 1988; 29:26.

28. Desai A, Alavi A, Dalinka M, et al: Role of bone scintigraphy in the evaluation and treatment of nonunited fractures: Concise communication. *J Nucl Med* 1980; 21:931.

29. Duncan DS, Thurston AJ: Clinical fracture of the carpal scaphoid—an illusionary diagnosis. *J Hand Surg Br* 1985; 10B:375.

30. Dzwierzynski WW, Sanger SR: Reflex sympathetic dystrophy. *Hand Clin* 1994; 10:29.

31. Eismont FJ, Garfin SR, Abitbol J: Thoracic and upper lumbar spine injuries in skeletal trauma, in Browner BD, Jupiter JB, Levine AM, Trafton PG (eds): *Skeletal Trauma*, WB Saunders, Philadelphia, 1992, p 729.

32. Evans EB: Heterotopic bone formation in thermal burns. *Clin Orthop* 1991; 263:94.

33. Failla JM: Osteonecrosis associated with nonunion of the hook of the hamate. *Orthopedics* 1993; 16:217.

34. Gelberman RH, Wolock BS, Siegel DB: Fractures and nonunions of the carpal scaphoid. *J Bone Joint Surg Am* 1989; 71-A:1560.

35. Gellman H, Keenan MAE, Stone L, et al: Reflex sympathetic dystrophy in brain-injured patients. *Pain* 1992; 51:307.

36. Gershuni DH: Principles of wire fixation, in Chapman MW (ed): *Operative Orthopaedics*, JB Lippincott, Philadelphia, 1988, p 141.

37. Greyson ND, Tepperman PS: Three-phase bone scans in hemiplegia with reflex sympathetic dystrophy and the effect of disuse. *J Nucl Med* 1984; 25:423.

38. Grundnes O, Reiker O: Closed versus open medullary nailing of femoral fractures: Blood flow and healing studies in rats. *Acta Orthop Scand* 1992; 63:492.

39. Gumerman LW, Fogel SR, Goodman MA, et al: Experimental fracture healing: Evaluation using radionuclide bone imaging: Concise communication. *J Nucl Med* 1978; 19:1320.

40. Gunalp B, Ozguven M, Ozturk E, et al: Role of bone scanning in the management of non-united fractures: A clinical study. *Eur J Nucl Med* 1992; 19:845.

41. Harkess JW: Arthroplasty of the hip, in AH Crenshaw (ed): *Campbell's Operative Orthopaedics*, ed 8, Mosby–Year Book, 1992.

42. Herzwurm PJ, Ebert FR: Arthroscintography for detection of femoral component loosening. *J Arthroplasty* 1991; 6:327.

43. Ho PK, Dellon AL, Wilgis EFS: True aneurysms of the hand resulting from athletic injury: Report of two cases. *Am J Sports Med* 1985; 13:136.

44. Hoffman J, Phillips W, Blum M, et al: Effect of sympathetic block demonstrated by triple-phase bone scan. *J Hand Surg Am* 1993, 18A:860.

45. Holder LE: Radionuclide bone imaging in surgical problems of the hand, in Gilula LA (ed): *The Traumatized Hand and Wrist: Radiographic and Anatomic Correlation*, Saunders, New York, 1991, p 19.

46. Holder LE: Bone scintigraphy in skeletal trauma. *Radiol Clin North Am* 1993; 31:739.

47. Holder LE, Cole LA, Myerson MS: Reflex sympathetic dystrophy in the foot: Clinical and scintigraphic criteria. *Radiology* 1992; 184:531.

48. Holder LE, Levine A: Evaluation of orthopedic appliances using radionuclide bone imaging (in preparation).

49. Holder LE, Mackinnon SE: Reflex sympathetic dystrophy in the hands: Clinical and scintigraphic criteria. *Radiology* 1984; 152:517.

50. Holder LE, Matthews LS: The nuclear physician and sports medicine, in Freeman L, Weissman H (eds): *Nuclear Medicine Annual 1984*, Raven Press, New York, 1984, p 81.

51. Holder LE, Merine DS, Yang A: Nuclear medicine, contrast angiography, and magnetic resonance imaging for evaluating vascular problems in the hand. *Hand Clin* 1993; 9:85.

52. Holder LE, Schwartz C, Wernicke PG, et al: Radionuclide bone imaging in the early detection of fractures of the proximal femur (hip): Multifactorial analysis. *Radiology* 1990; 174:509.

53. Holmberg S, Dalen N: Intracapsular pressure and caput circulation in nondisplaced femoral neck fractures. *Clin Orthop* 1987; 219:124.

54. Hunt JL: The use of technetium 99m stannous pyrophosphate scintigraphy to identify muscle damage in acute electrical burns. *J Trauma* 1979; 19:409.

55. Hunter JL, Hattner RS, Murray WR, et al: Loosening of the total hip arthroplasty: Detection by radionuclide bone scanning. *AJR Am J Roentgenol* 1980; 135:131.

56. Hutchinson DT: Color duplex imaging: Applications to upper-extremity and microvascular surgery. *Hand Clin* 1993; 9:47.

57. Ikawa G, dos Santos PAL, Yamaguchi KT, et al: Frostbite and bone scanning: The use of 99m-labeled phosphates in demarcating the line of viability in frostbite victims. *Orthopedics* 1986; 9:1257.

58. Intenzo C, Kim S, Millin J, Park C: Scintigraphic patterns of the reflex sympathetic dystrophy syndrome of the lower extremities. *Clin Nucl Med* 1989; 14:657.

59. Johnson JO: Principles of limb salvage surgery, in Chapman MW (ed): *Operative Orthopaedics*, JB Lippincott, Philadelphia, 1988, p 893.

60. Katz MM, Hungerford DS: Reflex sympathetic dystrophy affecting the knee. *J Bone Joint Surg Br* 1987, 69-B:797.

61. Kellam JF, Browner BD: Fractures of the pelvic ring, in Browner BD, Jupiter JB, Levine AM, Trafton PG (eds): Saunders, Philadelphia, 1992, p 849.

62. King AD, Peters AM, Stuttle AWJ, et al: Imaging of bone infection with labeled white blood cells: Role of contemporaneous bone marrow imaging. *Eur J Nucl Med* 1990; 17:148.

63. Kline SC, Holder LE: Segmental reflex sympathetic dystrophy: Clinical and scintigraphic criteria. *J Hand Surg [Am]* 1993; 18A:853.

64. Kozin F: Reflex sympathetic dystrophy syndrome: A review. *Clin Exp Rheumatol* 1992; 10:401.

65. Lahtinen T, Alhava EM, Karjalainen P, Romppanen T: The effect of age on blood flow in the proximal femur in man. *J Nucl Med* 1981; 22:966.

66. Lausten GS, Hesse B, Thygesen V, et al: Prediction of late complication of femoral neck fractures by scintigraphy. *Int Orthop* 1992; 16:260.

67. Levine AM: Lumbar and sacral spine trauma, in Browner BD, Jupiter JB, Levine AM, Trafton PG (eds): *Skeletal Trauma*, Saunders, Philadelphia, 1992, p 805.

68. Lisbonna R, Rosenthall L: Observation on the sequential use of ^{99m}Tc-phosphate complex and 67-Ga imaging in osteomyelitis, cellulitis and septic arthritis. *Radiology* 1977; 123:123.

69. Mackinnon SE, Dellon AL: Carpal tunnel syndrome, in Mackinnon SE, Dellon AL (eds): *Surgery of the Peripheral Nerve*, Thieme Medical Publishers, New York, 1988, p 149.

70. Mackinnon SE, Holder LE: The use of three-phase radionuclide bone scanning in the diagnosis of reflex sympathetic dystrophy. *J Hand Surg [Am]* 1984; 9A:556.

71. Magnuson JE, Brown ML, Houser MF, et al: In-111-labeled leukocyte scintigraphy in suspected orthopedic prosthesis infection: Comparison with other imaging modalities. *Radiology* 1988; 168:235.

72. Mailis A, Inman R, Pham D: Transient migratory osteoporosis: A variant of reflex sympathetic dystrophy? Report of 3 cases and literature review. *J Rheumatol* 1992; 19:758.

73. Majd M: Bone scintigraphy in children with obscure skeletal pain. *Ann Radiol (Paris)* 1979; 22:85.

74. Mandell GA, Harcke HT: Scintigraphic manifestations of infarction of the second metatarsal (Freiberg's disease). *J Nucl Med* 1987; 28:249.

75. Marymont JV, Lynch, MA, Henning CE: Acute ligamentous diastasis of the ankle without fracture: Evaluation by radionuclide Imaging. *Am J Sports Med* 1986; 14:407.

76. Matin P: The appearance of bone scans following fractures, including immediate and long-term studies. *J Nucl Med* 1979; 20:1227.

77. Matta JM: Surgical treatment of acetabular fractures, in Browner BD, Jupiter JB, Levine AM, Trafton PS (eds): *Skeletal Trauma*, Saunders, Philadelphia, 1992, p 899.

78. Maurer AH, Holder LE, Espinola DA, et al: Three phase radionuclide scintigraphy of the hand. *Radiology* 1983; 146:761.

79. Maxon HR, Schneider HJ, Hopson CN, et al: A comparative study of Indium-111 DTPA radionuclide and iothalamate meglumine roentgenographic arthrography in the evaluation of painful total hip arthroplasty. *Clin Orthop* 1989; 245:156.

80. McDougall IR, Keeling CA: Complications of fractures and their healing. *Semin Nucl Med* 1988; 18:113.

81. Merkel K, Brown ML, Fitzgerald RH: Sequential technetium-99m-HMDP-Gallium-67 citrate imaging for the evaluation of infection in the painful prosthesis. *J Nucl Med* 1986; 27:1413.

82. Mesgarzadeh M, Sapega AA, Bonakdarpour A, et al: Osteochondritis dissecans: Analysis of mechanical stability with radiography, scintigraphy, and MR imaging. *Radiology* 1987; 165:775.

83. Miniaci A, Bailey WH, Bourne RB, et al: Analysis of radionuclide arthrograms, radiographic arthrograms, and sequential plain radiographs in the assessment of painful hip arthroplasty. *J Arthroplasty* 1990; 5:143.

84. Moore JR, Weiland AJ: Vascularized bone grafts, in Chapman MW (ed): *Operative Orthopaedics*, JB Lippincott, Philadelphia, 1988, p 1041.

85. Mulamba L, Ferrant A, Leners N, et al: Indium-111 leukocyte scanning in the evaluation of painful hip arthroplasty. *Acta Orthop Scand* 1983; 54:695.

86. Nadel SN, Debatin JF, Richardson WJ, et al: Detection of acute avascular necrosis of the femoral head in dogs: Dynamic contrast-enhanced MR imaging vs spin-echo and STIR sequences. *AJR Am J Roentgenol* 1992; 159:1255.

87. Nepola JV, Seabold JE, Marsh JL, et al: Diagnosis of infection in ununited fractures: Combined imaging with indium 111-labeled leukocytes and technetium-99m methylene dignosphosite. *J Bone Joint Surg Am* 1993; 75-A:1816.

88. Orzel JA, Rudd TG: Heterotopic bone formation: Clinical, laboratory, and imaging correlation. *J Nucl Med* 1985; 26:125.

89. Oswald SG, Van Nostrand D, Savroy CG, et al: Three-phase bone scan and Indium white blood cell scintigraphy following porous coated hip arthroplasty: A prospective study of the prosthetic tip. *J Nucl Med* 1989; 30:1321.

90. Oswald SG, Van Nostrand D, Savroy CG, et al: The acetabulum: A prospective study of 3-phase bone and Indium white blood cell scintigraphy following porous-coated arthroplasty. *J Nucl Med* 1990; 31:274.

91. Palestro CJ, Kim CK, Swyer AJ, et al: Total-hip arthroplasty: Periprosthetic Indium-111-labeled leukocyte activity and complementary technetium-99m-sulfur colloid imaging in suspected infection. *J Nucl Med* 1990; 31:1950.

92. Palestro CJ, Swyer AJ, Kim CK, et al: Infected knee prosthesis: Diagnosis with In-111 leukocyte, Tc-99m sulfur colloid and Tc-99m MDP imaging. *Radiology* 1991; 179:645.

93. Pearlman AW: The painful hip prosthesis: Value of nuclear imaging in the diagnosis of late complications. *Clin Nucl Med* 1980; 5:133.

94. Phillips TW, Aitken GK, MacKenzie RA: Sulfur colloid bone scan assessment of femoral head vascularity following subcapital fractures of the hip. *Clin Ortho* 1986; 208:52.

95. Purdue GF, Lewis SA, Hunt JL: Pyrophosphate scanning in early frostbite injury. *Am Surg* 1983; 49:619.

96. Resnick D, Niwayama G: *Diagnosis of Bone and Joint Disorders*. WB Saunders, Philadelphia, 1988.

97. Rodrigo JJ, Prolo DJ: Allografts, in Chapman MW (ed): *Operative Orthopaedics*, JB Lippincott, Philadelphia, 1988, p 911.

98. Rosenthall L, Gahazal ME, Brooks CE: Quantitative analysis of radiophosphate uptakes in asymptomatic porous-coated hip endoprostheses. *J Nucl Med* 1991; 32:1391.

99. Ruedi TP: Principles of plate fixation, in Chapman MW (ed): *Operative Orthopaedics*, JB Lippincott, Philadelphia, 1988, p 135.

100. Salimi Z, Vas W, Tang-Barton P, et al: Assessment of tissue viability in frostbite by ^{99m}Tc pertechnetate scintigraphy. *AJR Am J Roentgenol* 1984; 142:415.

101. Sarangi PP, Ward AJ, Smith EJ, et al: Algodystrophy and osteoporosis after tibial fractures. *J Bone Joint Surg Br* 1993; 75-B:450.

102. Saltiel AA, Petasnick JP, Charters JR, Gitelis S: Allograft transplantation in skeletal reconstructive surgery: Poster exhibit. *Radiology* 1990; 177:368.

103. Sayman HB, Urgancioglu I, Uslu I, Kapicioglu T: Prediction of muscle viability after electrical burn necrosis. *Clin Nucl Med* 1992; 17:395.

104. Seabold JE, Nepola JV, Conrad GR, et al: Detection of osteomyelitis at fracture nonunion sites: Comparison of two scintigraphic methods. *AJR Am J Roentgenol* 1989; 152:1021.

105. Seabold JE, Nepola JV, Marsh JL, et al: Post-operative bone marrow alterations: Potential pitfalls in the diagnosis of osteomyelitis with In-111-labeled leukocytes scintigraphy. *Radiology* 1991; 180:741.

106. Simon H, Carlson DH: The use of bone scanning in the diagnosis of reflex sympathetic dystrophy. *Clin Nucl Med* 1980; 5:116.

107. Smith FJ, Powe JE: Effect of sympathetic blockade on bone imaging. *Clin Nucl Med* 1992; 17:665.

108. Sonne-Holm S, Dyrbye M, Walter S, et al: Bone scintigraphy in Moore hemiarthroplasty with and without cement following femoral neck fractures: A controlled study. *Acta Orthop Scand* 1983; 54:194.

109. Sowa DT, Holder LE, Patt PG: Application of magnetic resonance imaging to ischemic necrosis of the lunate. *J Hand Surg* 1989; 14:1008.

110. Speer KP, Spritzer CE, Harrelson JM, et al: Magnetic resonance imaging of the femoral head after acute intracapsular fracture of the femoral neck. *J Bone Joint Surg Am* 1990; 72-A:98.

111. Spitz J, Becker C, Tittel K, et al: Die klinische relevanz der ganzkorperskelettszintigraphie bei mehrfachverletzten und polytraumatisierten patienten. *Unfallchirugie* 1992; 18:133.

112. Stromqvist B, Brismar J, Hansson LI, et al: Tc-99m methylenediphosphonate scintimetry after femoral neck fracture: A 3 year follow-up study. *Clin Orthop* 1984; 182:177.

113. Stromqvist B, Hansson LI, Nilsson LT, et al: Prognostic precision in postoperative 99m-Tc MDP scintimetry after femoral neck fracture. *Acta Orthop Scand* 1987; 58:494.

114. Swan JS, Braunstein EM, Wellman HN, et al: Contrast and nuclear arthrography in loosening of the uncemented hip prosthesis. *Skeletal Radiol* 1991; 20:15.

115. Tachdjian M: *Pediatric Orthopedics*, ed 2, Saunders, Philadelphia, 1990, p 2850.

116. Tencer AF, Johnson KD, Kyle RF, Fu FH: Biomechanics of fractures and fracture fixation. *Instr Course Lect* 1993; 42:19.

117. Thomas BJ: Heterotopic bone formation after total hip arthroplasty. *Orthop Clin North Am* 1992; 23:347.

118. Turner JH: Post-traumatic avascular necrosis of the femoral head predicted by preoperative Tc-99m antimony-colloid scan: An experimental and clinical study. *J Bone Joint Surg Am* 1983; 65-A:786.

119. Uri G, Wellman H, Capello W, et al: Scintigraphic and x-ray arthrographic diagnosis of femoral prosthesis loosening: Concise communication. *J Nucl Med* 1984; 25:661.

120. Utz JA, Lull RJ, Galvin EG: Asymptomatic total hip prosthesis: Natural history determined using Tc-99m MDP bone scans. *Radiology* 1986; 61:509.

121. Van Nostrand D, Abreu SH, Callaghan JJ, et al: In-111-labeled white blood cell uptake in noninfected closed fractures in human: Prospective study. *Radiology* 1988; 167:495.

122. van Vugt AB, Oosterwijk WM, Goris RJ: Predictive value of early scintimetry in intracapsular hip fractures: A prospective study was regarding the femoral head necrosis, delayed union and non-union. *Arch Orthop Trauma Surg* 1993; 113:33.

123. Villareal DT, Murphy WA, Teitelbaum SL, et al: Painful diffuse osteosclerosis after intravenous drug abuse. *Am J Med* 1992; 93:371.

124. Wallace AL, Strachan RK, Blane A, et al: Quantitative early phase scintigraphy in the prediction of healing of tibial fractures. *Skeletal Radiol* 1992; 21:241.

125. Weiss L, Alfano A, Bardfeld P, et al: Prognostic value of triple phase bone scanning for reflex sympathetic dystrophy in hemiplegia. *Arch Phys Med Rehabil* 1993; 74:716.

126. White AA, Panjabi MN, Southwick WO: The four biomechanical stages of fracture repair. *J Bone Joint Surg Am* 1977; 59-A:188.

127. Williams F, McCall IW, Park WM, et al: Gallium-67 scanning in the painful total hip replacement. *Clin Radiol* 1981; 32:431.

128. Wilson MA: The effect of age on the quality of bone scans using technetium-99m pyrophosphate. *Radiology* 1981; 139:703.

129. Young J, Burgess A: *Radiologic Manifestations of Pelvic Ring Fracture*, Urban & Schwartzenberg, Baltimore, 1987.

CHAPTER 15

BONE INFARCTS AND OSTEONECROSIS

Robert J. Boudreau

Harry J. Griffiths

The introduction of magnetic resonance imaging (MRI) has profoundly affected the use of nuclear medicine for the diagnosis of bone infarcts and osteonecrosis. With the possible exception of Legg-Calvé-Perthes disease (LCPD), MRI has largely supplanted the scintigraphic examination of these diseases at many institutions in the United States. However, such ready access to MRI devices for musculoskeletal problems is not routinely available throughout the world, and nuclear medicine continues to be commonly used in many countries. Vascular problems of bone are also frequently noted in scintigrams done for other purposes. Thus an appreciation of the appearance of these lesions on scintigrams is required by all those who interpret them. At our institution we rarely perform bone scintigraphy for avascular necrosis (AVN), despite having a very large patient population at risk for the disease. With that statement as our starting point, we begin with a general description of the disease process.

PATHOGENESIS AND CLINICAL FEATURES

General

The etiology of AVN includes such posttraumatic causes as fractures, dislocations, and microfractures, and certainly fractures of the femoral neck are the most common cause of secondary AVN seen anywhere in the body. However, there are nontraumatic causes as well, of which one group is due to emboli or infarcts. This would include the hemoglobinopathies, sickle cell disease, sickle cell trait, and sickle cell thalassemia. Various decompression states such as deep sea diving, caisson disease, and high-altitude flying or ballooning can also lead to both AVN and bone infarcts. Similarly pancreatitis and alcoholism can be associated with fat emboli and fat necrosis, and hence secondary AVN may occur.

The collagen vascular diseases involve the small vessels and are associated with AVN. These are mainly the connective tissue disorders such as systemic lupus erythematosus, polyarteritis nodosa, giant cell arteritis, and Fabry's disease. Another common etiologic factor is the presence of abnormal cells in the marrow; the disease that is best known in this category is Gaucher's disease. However, steroid therapy and Cushing's disease are also both associated with rather bulky cells, as well as with vasculitis, and steroid therapy is today by far the most common cause of AVN in the nontraumatic group.

AVN has been described in association with many other conditions. For instance, both radiation therapy as well as multiple injuries and burns can lead to AVN. Pathologists find a common association between degenerative arthritis and the presence of AVN. AVN of the hip has also been described in association with gout and hyperuricemia, as well as prolonged immobilization and pregnancy. There is a definite association between AVN

and both primary and secondary hyperparathyroidism as well as with metastases, lymphoma and inflammatory bowel disease, even in the absence of a history of steroid therapy.[12]

Another way of viewing these different causes is to look at the underlying pathogenesis of the disease, which can conveniently be subdivided into five main categories.[1] Emboli and infarcts, including fat emboli in pancreatitis and alcoholism as well as nitrogen emboli in caisson disease, can cause both intramedullary bone infarcts and AVN of an epiphysis. Infarcts also occur as a result of sickle cell anemia and its variants.[2] Of the various vascular causes, obviously the small-vessel collagen vascular diseases are the largest group in this category.[3] Mechanical causes, though, are by far the most common cause of AVN, particularly following fractures of the femoral neck as well as after dislocations of the hip joint.

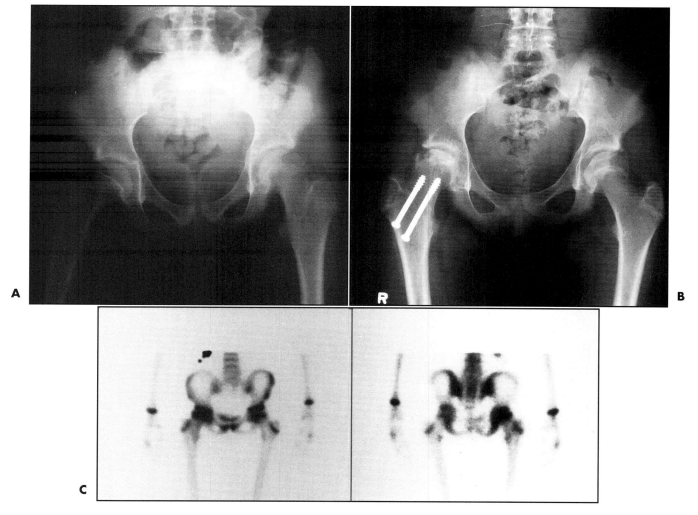

Fig. 15-1. This 11-year-old male patient suffered an intertrochanteric fracture of the right femur (**A**) which was pinned (**B**). Note the femoral head flattening and sclerosis, which are typical changes of avascular necrosis. Corresponding bone scans (**C**) done in the anterior (*left*) and posterior (*right*) projections show increased uptake of tracer in the right femoral epiphysis and also, to a lesser degree, the acetabulum. The uniform uptake in the epiphysis corresponds with the late reparative phase of avascular necrosis.

As a rule of thumb, if a dislocated hip is replaced within 4 hours of dislocation, the incidence of AVN is extraordinarily low, whereas if the femoral head remains dislocated for longer than 24 hours, there is a 100% incidence of secondary AVN.[4] There is a category of infiltration with abnormal cells, and this includes both steroid therapy and Cushing's disease as well as Gaucher's disease.[5] Finally, fat necrosis, which is classically seen in patients with either pancreatitis or alcoholism, is another cause of infarcts and AVN.

Avascular Necrosis in Association with Femoral Neck Fractures

Subcapital fractures are associated with approximately a 33% incidence of secondary AVN, transcervical fractures of the femoral neck with a 20% incidence, intertrochanteric fractures with a 15% incidence, and subtrochanteric fractures of the femur with a 10% incidence of AVN (Fig. 15-1). The reason for this disparity is that although the main blood supply enters via the long nutrient artery supplying the whole shaft of the femur, there is a secondary blood supply carried by both capsular and the gubernacular vessels just below the capsule. Thus a subcapital fracture inherently removes virtually all sources of major blood supply to the femoral head, whereas following an intertrochanteric fracture, a collateral blood supply can easily open up through the capsular and gubernacular vessels.

Legg-Calvé-Perthes Disease

Although the exact cause of Legg-Calvé-Perthes disease (LCPD) is unknown, it is undoubtedly related to transient synovitis and can also be seen in children who have recurrent trauma to the hip with effusions. LCPD is a disease of white male children under the age of 7 years in the United States, although it can be seen in somewhat older children elsewhere. The children are usually short and have high intelligence quotients. LCPD is bilateral in 20% and interestingly goes on to secondary AVN in adult life in 20% of patients. The etiology of LCPD is thought to be due to compression of the capsular arteries as well as the artery in the ligamentum teres as a result of a long-standing or recurrent effusion. The incidence of LCPD coincides with the time that the blood supply alters from

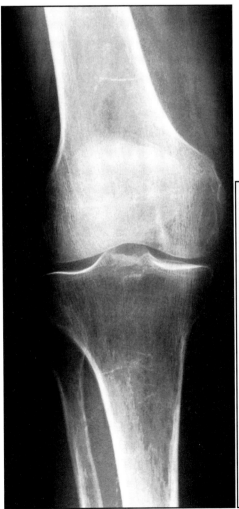

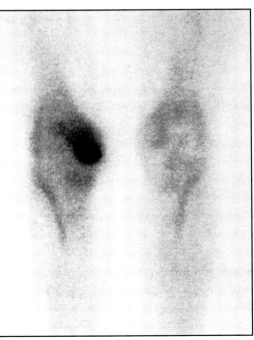

Fig. 15-2. This 92-year-old female presented with the sudden onset of acute knee pain without a history of trauma. Radiographs (**A**) show moderately severe osteoporosis but no other abnormality. Associated bone scan (**B**) shows intense increased uptake of tracer in the mediofemoral condyle of the right knee. Note that the bone scan is intensely positive even though the pain had only started 24 hours earlier. The patient had no predisposing cause for avascular necrosis. This combination of findings is typical of spontaneous osteonecrosis.

A

B

being virtually 100% supplied by the artery of the ligamentum teres to virtually zero blood supply coming in by that route.

The classical radiologic changes of LCPD start with the finding that there is an increased medial joint space on the affected side, and that the femoral head is somewhat smaller than on the other normal side. As the disease progresses, subchondral fissures as well as irregularities and widening of the metaphyseal plate occur. The disease progresses slowly: within 3 to 6 months some sclerosis appears within the epiphysis associated with some typical physeal plate cysts or erosions, widening, and fragmentation. From 6 to 9 months the metaphyseal cysts enlarge and then start to ossify, although this can be associated with widening of the growth plate. At 12 months the epiphyses may appear very fragmented and be much smaller than normal, although by now the metaphysis is actually beginning to heal. From 15 to 18 months the epiphysis continues healing, with reossification and new bone formation, although there is often continued flattening and distortion of the femoral head. At 3 years reossification is continuing within the femoral head, but the metaphyseal bone may remain widened or splayed.

Spontaneous Osteonecrosis

The etiology of spontaneous osteonecrosis is unknown. It is equally common in men and women and occurs in the middle years. The clinical presentation is that of a middle-aged patient who suddenly feels the knee snap and develops an acute bloody painful effusion. On the initial film there are no radiographic findings, although a bone scan will be positive, frequently showing a localized area of increased uptake in the medial femoral condyle, which represents an infarct (Fig. 15-2). The underlying bone is weakened, so ultimately synovial fluid will be forced up through any cracks in the hyaline cartilage and will flow in between the living subchondral bone and the dead cancellous bone, causing an oval area of lucency and a "crescent" sign. It is of interest that three quarters of these patients also have medial meniscus tears. The radiograph becomes positive only at 3 to 6 months, whereas the bone scan is often positive within 24 hours of the spontaneous osteonecrosis. AVN of the knee classically occurs on the most distal weight-bearing surface of the medial femoral condyle, where it can appear similar to AVN in the femoral head with a crescent sign and fragmentation. However, on the lateral view of the knee it usually lies somewhat more anterior to the true weight-bearing surface of the distal femur.

Avascular Necrosis Elsewhere

Because the shoulder joint is non–weight-bearing, AVN of the humeral head may often not produce any major radiographic changes until after there has been marked collapse of the humeral head. AVN can also be seen in such bones as the lunate, capitellum, tarsal navicular, and in the talar dome.

IMAGING OF AVASCULAR NECROSIS

Radiographic Appearance of Classical Avascular Necrosis

The initial radiographic appearance of AVN of the femoral head occurs relatively late in the pathogenesis of the disease. The crescent sign is by far the most characteristic early sign, although this does not appear until 6 months after the infarct has occurred (Fig. 15-3). This is best seen on a frog-leg or tube-lateral view of the femoral head. The crescent sign actually represents a fracture that occurs between the living subchondral bone and the dead infarcted cancellous bone (Fig. 15-4). The subchondral cortical bone and hyaline cartilage receive their nutrients directly from the synovial fluid and hence remain alive. The infarct occurs at the junction of the deeper cancellous bone with the more peripheral cancellous bone and is often triangular, radiating out to what appears to be the outer weight-bearing surface of the femoral head.

Another, albeit later, radiologic finding can be cyst formation, which occurs at the inferior junction between the proximal living bone and the more distal surface of the infarct. Again a fracture may occur through this point

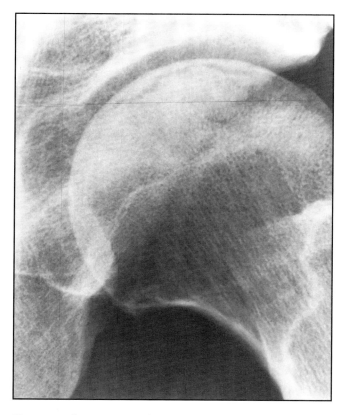

Fig. 15-3. Crescent sign. This is a classical, but rare, finding in avascular necrosis and represents a fracture between the living subchondral bone and the dead infarcted area. Note the step-off on the lateral aspect of the femoral articular surface. Indelible line on radiograph is courtesy of an anonymous orthopedic surgeon.

of weakness and then sclerosis, cyst formation, and bone destruction can be seen radiologically. One of the earliest signs of AVN of the femoral capital epiphysis in some patients is small patchy areas of increased density deep within the femoral head and neck, representing localized infarcts. In the femoral head this may be seen as a somewhat triangular area on the posterolateral surface. As the AVN progresses, an increasing subchondral lucency becomes apparent, often in association with some surrounding sclerosis (Fig. 15-5). At this stage the femoral head becomes flatter and loses its normal contour. If unchecked, the process will progress so that ultimately fragmentation and collapse of the femoral head occurs,

often with some buttressing and bony sclerosis at the interface between the infarct and the underlying bone. This will ultimately lead to secondary degenerative arthritis with loss of joint cartilage space, particularly on the most lateral aspect of the hip joint.

Although we have discussed the radiographic appearance of AVN in the femoral head itself, AVN does occur at other sites, including the medial femoral condyle of the knee and the humeral head. The radiographic appearances are similar for the epiphyses of all the long bones. Obviously there are methods other than radiographs for diagnosing AVN since radiologic findings are present only in the later stages of the disease. Steinberg[24]

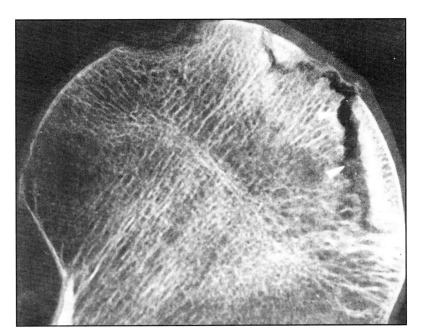

Fig. 15-4. This radiograph of a pathologic specimen shows the somewhat triangular area of the infarct (*arrowhead*) as well as the fracture or crescent sign between the living and the dead bone.

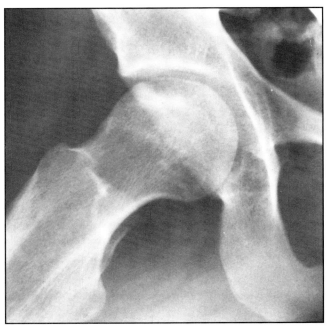

Fig. 15-5. Avascular necrosis of the femoral head. Some patchy areas of sclerosis can be seen in the femoral head and neck. There is also a clearly seen area of sclerosis underlying a relatively lucent subchondral region of bone, typical of a well-established infarct.

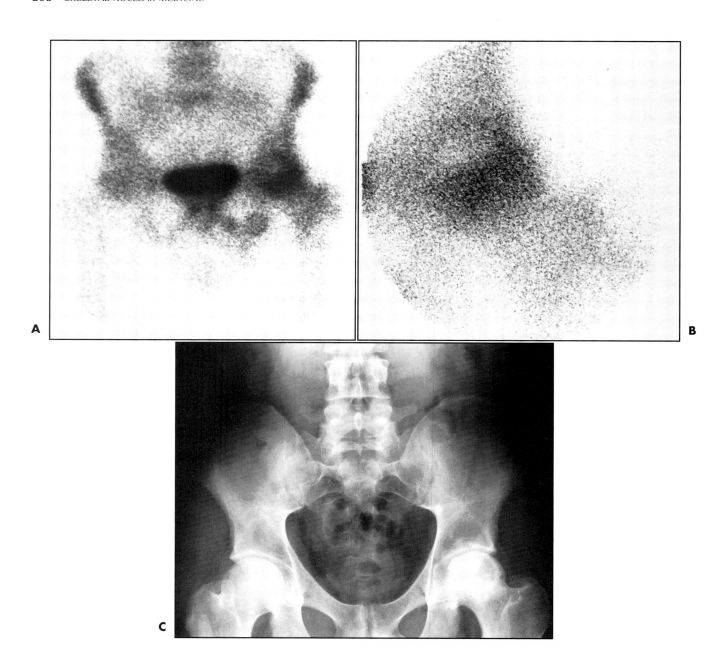

Fig. 15-6. Delayed anterior pelvis images from a 32-year-old alcoholic who had left hip pain (**A**). Intense uptake of tracer is noted in the left femoral head with an associated area of photopenia at its superior aspect, best appreciated on pinhole image of left femoral head (**B**). These findings are pathognomonic of avascular necrosis. These images were acquired in the early 1980s. The associated radiograph (**C**) shows subchondral lucency and peripheral sclerosis, again consistent with avascular necrosis of the left hip.

reviewed his findings in 14 early cases of AVN in whom the radiographs were normal: 54% of these had positive computed tomography (CT) scans, 71% had characteristic bone scans, and 86% had positive MRI findings. In an overall group of 55 patients at various stages in the disease process, he reported that radiographs were positive in 78%, bone scans in 87%, CT scanning in 92%, and MRI in 96%. He also mentioned that in the 40 cases of AVN that were apparent radiologically, flattening of the femoral head occurred in 100%; there were associated degenerative changes in 95%, and the crescent sign was present in 84%.

Bone Scanning in Avascular Necrosis

Although many tracers have been used to investigate AVN of bone, the only commonly used agents today are the technetium 99m labeled diphosphonates. Bone marrow imaging has also been employed, but its role can now be considered of historical interest only.[1,19] There is

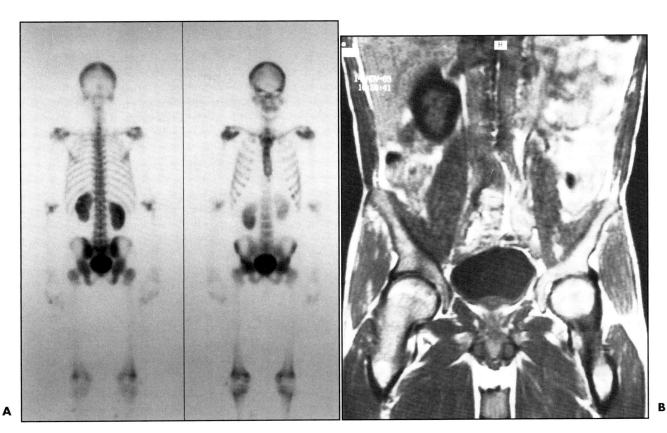

Fig. 15-7. A portion of a total-body bone scan is shown in the posterior and anterior projections from a 30-year-old male who is homozygous for sickle cell disease (**A**). The patient had a history of multiple infarcts to bone and lung. The bone scan shows increased uptake of tracer in multiple joints, particularly the shoulders, knees, and possibly the hips. Since the hip uptake is diffuse and symmetric, one cannot be definitive about the diagnosis of avascular necrosis of the hips. The posterior abdominal view of the bone scan (*left set of images*) shows focal filling defects in the kidney consistent with renal infarcts. The patient had complained of low back pain before this bone scan. **B**, MRI study of the pelvis shows patchy decreased intensity in the right femoral head and femoral neck consistent with infarcts and AVN. Note that the right innominate bone also shows similar findings, which are typical of sickle cell anemia.

perhaps a use for marrow scans in patients with sickle cell disease, but it is expected that MRI will totally supplant nuclear medicine techniques for the assessment of bone marrow. Accordingly we only discuss the use of technetium 99m diphosphonate bone scans in this chapter.

Much of the reported literature involves the use of a pinhole collimator and older gamma cameras.[8,17,25] It would appear that pinhole imaging had definite advantages when using older equipment; an example of a case from the early 1980s is shown in Fig. 15-6. Whether this holds true for modern equipment capable of zoom magnification is not known. We would expect that the results would be at least as good as those obtained with the older gamma cameras and pinhole collimators, due to the significant advances in gamma camera technology that have occurred over the years. The bone-scanning technique is straightforward and is no different from other uses of the test. The patient is imaged 3 to 4 hours following injection, and in many instances localized spot views will suffice. However, sickle cell disease and AVN associated with renal transplantation are often multicen-

tric and best imaged on whole-body scans with selected spot views (Fig. 15-7). If LCPD is suspected, both hips should be imaged in full medial rotation with magnification.

Single photon emission computed tomography (SPECT) imaging can also be performed, and this procedure is discussed at length in Chapter 4. Collier et al[5] found SPECT imaging to be more accurate than planar imaging in a series of 21 adult patients with AVN of the femoral head. They reported a sensitivity of 85% for SPECT, whereas planar imaging was positive in only 11 of 20 hips affected. However, it should be noted that due to problems with bladder filling degrading the SPECT studies, 5 of 25 patients were excluded from the investigation. In a clinical setting these patients would not have been diagnosed by SPECT imaging and should therefore be included in the analysis. Also, the criteria used were strict, since the planar bone scans were called positive only if a photon-deficient lesion was seen in the femoral head. Because SPECT imaging is considerably more expensive and time consuming than its planar counterpart, it is difficult to justify its routine use based on the preceding data. At our institution the cost of a SPECT bone scan is only slightly less than that of an MRI. Therefore it probably would be more appropriate to compare the SPECT scan with MRI imaging, rather than its planar counterpart. It would be reasonable to use planar imaging as a screening procedure and then proceeding to MRI in cases where the bone scan was negative. However, if MRI is not available, and if adequate images can be obtained, SPECT is likely to provide information superior to the planar images. An example of a tomographic study of the hips is shown in Fig. 15-8.

Accuracy of Bone Scanning

All series published to date have confirmed the superiority of bone scanning to radiographs in the early diagnosis of AVN. Numerous authors have described the pattern of bone scan changes seen in AVN.[2,4,7,8,17] Initially the scan shows decreased uptake of tracer that is then followed by a "hot", or reparative, phase. After healing has occurred, the uptake returns to normal. The most specific bone scan finding of AVN is a photopenic defect, which implies that we must catch the disease early to have any degree of specificity. Unfortunately the accuracy of bone scanning for the diagnosis of AVN is probably lower than generally appreciated. Zizic et al[29] in *Arthritis and Rheumatism* studied 169 patients with known AVN of 288 bone sites. Radiologically 58 (20%) of these appeared normal. Qualitative scintigraphy was used to evaluate 249 sites of which 91 (37%) were positive, 29 locations (12%) were equivocal, and 129 (52%) were falsely negative. Quantitative scintigraphy was done in 56 bones, and it was correct in 57% of the bones involved, with 5% equivocal results, and a 38% false-negative rate. In spite of these results, it was the authors' opinion that the first step in evaluating patients with normal radiographs and suspected AVN should be a radioisotope scintigram, since qualitative bone scans helped identify 14 (40%) of 35 bones with AVN and normal radiographs. The authors did not address the role of MRI in this chapter.

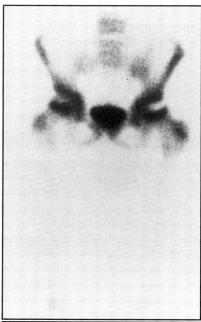

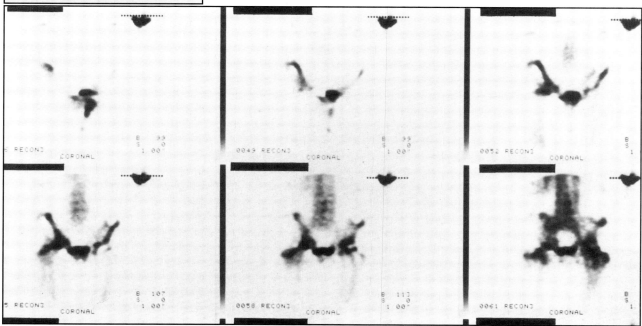

Fig. 15-8. **A**, Anterior view of the pelvis showing a photopenic defect of the left femoral head. **B**, A series of coronal SPECT images through the pelvis from anterior to posterior. The lower left and lower middle images clearly show the photopenic defect in the left femoral head. *(From Lull RJ et al, eds:* Bone Scintigraphy Kit, *ACNP information module I, ACNP, Washington, 1988, p 11; with permission.)*

Conklin et al[6] prospectively studied 36 patients with systemic lupus erythematosus. All patients underwent radiography and 10 had interosseous pressure determinations. Interosseous pressure measurements[28] were occasionally used in patients with normal radiographs to establish the diagnosis of AVN. Sensitivity of the bone scan was 89% in these patients, although the specificity was only 50%. Only 11 of 27 joints had abnormal radiographs for a sensitivity of 41%. Sutherland et al[25] found that the radionuclide bone scan reliably diagnosed LCPD with a sensitivity of 98% and a specificity of 95%. We discuss LCPD in further detail later in this chapter. Gregg and Walder[14] showed in an experimental model of caisson disease that the scintigram had increased activity in 12 of 14 animals by 3 weeks postinsult, whereas the radiograph was positive in only 2 of 13 cases.

The bone scan has also been shown to be helpful in the diagnosis of postradiotherapy osteonecrosis of the jaw. Epstein et al[10] found it to be more sensitive than the radiographs. However, the authors noted that the degree of uptake in the mandible following irradiation is quite variable. Fig et al[11] used bone scanning to evaluate the survival of revascularized composite flap grafts of the mandible. They found that a uniform uptake pattern was indicative of viability, whereas a "cold" defect was associated with necrosis of the graft. These authors found that SPECT imaging was more helpful than planar imaging. This was due to the importance of finding the cold defect and the considerable overlap of bony detail in the mandible on planar images.

By the mid 1980s scintigraphy had established itself as being more sensitive than radiography for the diagnosis of AVN, and it was thought to be of value in the clinical management of selected patients. Following the publication of a comparative study of MRI, radionuclide bone scanning, and CT in the diagnosis of AVN of the hip by Mitchell et al,[20] the situation changed. These authors retrospectively analyzed the images of 188 hips by MRI, 141 by radionuclide imaging, and 106 by CT. Hip images of patients with no disease were added as controls so that the number of normal and abnormal hips for each technique was about equal. The results were analyzed by receiver operating characteristic (ROC) analysis. MRI was shown to be better than both techniques over the entire case pool with the difference between MRI and radionuclide scanning exceeding 2 SE. In the subsample of patients with early disease, MRI was better than CT by over 2 SE and better than radionuclide scanning by over 3 SE. The authors concluded that MRI is the most sensitive imaging technique for the early diagnosis of AVN. Since that time it has been widely accepted that MRI is superior to the radionuclide bone scan for the diagnosis of AVN, with the possible exception of LCPD. Accordingly we now discuss the role of MRI.

Magnetic Resonance Imaging in Avascular Necrosis

Since both plain film radiography and planar scintigraphy are not particularly accurate in the diagnosis of AVN, MRI has become the imaging method of choice at many institutions in the United States. There are a number of patterns of AVN in MRI, depending on the age of the infarct. In the initial T1-weighted findings, the femoral head shows an area of low intensity that is fairly homogenous and is usually situated in the superior lateral aspect of the femoral capital epiphysis in the form of a triangle (Fig. 15-9). As the condition advances and the infarct becomes more obvious, this area becomes more inhomogeneous with patches of both increased and decreased density (Fig. 15-10). Ultimately it may separate out from the underlying bone as an area of high signal running beneath the infarct and the normal underlying bone (Figs. 15-11 and 15-12). In an interesting study of beagles, Brody et al[3] showed that there were four stages of avascular necrosis. Up to 7 days there was increased T2 signal in the area of the infarct, and then from 7 to 14 days there were linear areas of low signal; from 14 to 23 days there were patchy areas of decreased signal, and finally after 23 days there were mixed areas of both low and intermediate signal. Also recently a clinicopathologic radiologic study was reported by Vande Berg and Malghein,[27] who showed that a high T1 and an intermediate T2 signal represented early AVN with mummified fat. At the other end of the spectrum a low T1 signal and a low T2 signal basically represented dead bone with necrotic marrow and an old established infarct (Fig. 15-13). A low T1 with an intermediate T2 signal represented viable mesenchyme but with some surrounding sclerosis. Finally a low T1 and a high T2 signal represented viable mesenchyme with either edema or bleeding.

In another article correlating pathophysiologic changes and MRI signals, Lang et al[18] found that low signal on T1 and T2 represented dead bone and necrotic bone marrow and tissue, low T1 and high T2 was associated with thick intratrabecular bone with mesenchymal infiltration, and low T1 and intermediate T2 indicated normal trabeculation with high vascularity—which was best seen in the healing stages of the process. Glickstein and Dalinka[13] looked at 23 patients with proven AVN, 22 patients with hip disease without AVN, and 10 normals. The specificity of MRI was 98% in the patients with AVN versus the normal group (97%) versus the group with other types of hip disease (85%). These authors point out that one of the problems with the diagnosis of very early avascular necrosis is that in patients with severe degenerative change, it is conceivable that the subchondral sclerosis can resemble AVN.

IMAGING OF SPECIFIC DISEASE STATES

Legg–Calvé–Perthes Disease

There is still some debate about which imaging modality is superior for the diagnosis of Legg-Calvé-Perthes disease (LCPD). The radionuclide bone scan has been shown to reliably diagnose LCPD with a sensitivity of 98% and a specificity of 95%.[25] Comparable figures for radi-

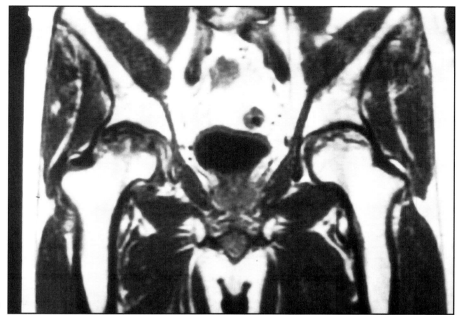

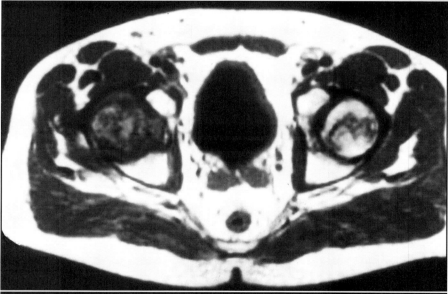

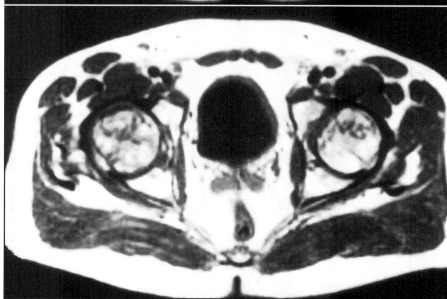

Fig. 15-9. MRI of avascular necrosis. On the left side there is an obvious crescent sign; on the right there is more advanced AVN with collapse and fragmentation. **A**, Coronal T1 view shows these changes clearly. **B**, Axial T1 view shows that more superiorly through the upper part of the femoral head there is a "crescent" line on the left and there are more advanced subchondral changes on the right. **C**, A somewhat lower axial slice shows similar serpiginous lines bilaterally but note the loss of normal contour on the right due to collapse of the femoral head.

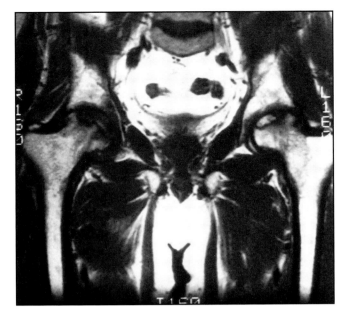

Fig. 15-10. More advanced AVN (MRI). This proton density image shows a triangular area of decreased intensity in the left femoral head with a fracture line typical of early AVN. On the right the whole femoral head and neck appears to be involved with several separate areas of infarction. On the right, though the whole femoral head and neck appears to be involved, there are several separate areas of infarction in the head itself.

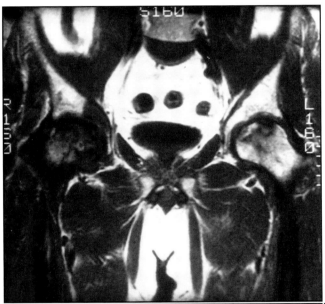

Fig. 15-11. MRI AVN. In a different patient some localized areas of infarction can be seen on the left with some separation of the subchondral bone. **A**, Coronal view. **B**, A sagittal view through the left femoral head shows a typical serpiginous infarct with separation of the subchondral bone from the infarct. **C**, A sagittal view on the right shows more involvement with some separate areas of high signal intensity inferring viable marrow.

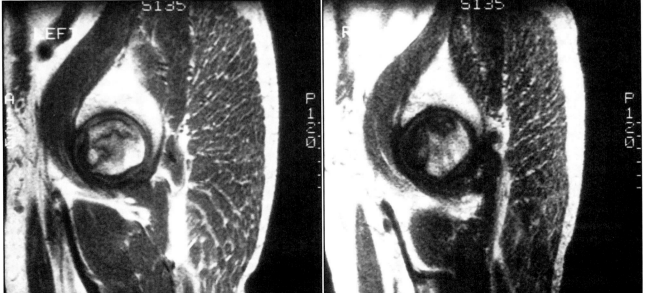

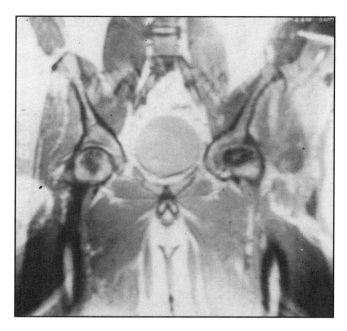

Fig. 15-12. MRI. Congenital hip dysplasia with AVN. This 56-year-old professor had hip dysplasia as a child and developed secondary AVN on the left with marked distortion of the femoral head. However, the changes on the right are due to secondary degenerative arthritis with sclerosis and are not due to AVN. This was confirmed by a core biopsy and shows some of the difficulties of interpreting the MRI scan without plain films.

ographic examinations were sensitivity of 92% and specificity of 78%. These figures come from a large-scale investigation of 131 children, of which 48 were assigned a final diagnosis of LCPD, 79 transient synovitis, and the remainder miscellaneous conditions. The radionuclide investigation was actually more accurate than these numbers reflect, since there were several cases of transient synovitis with definite reversible ischemia of the capital epiphysis, which were called false-positives on the bone scan. In another investigation by Danigelis,[8] all 59 LCPD patients studied had an uptake defect of variable size in the proximal femoral epiphysis. Given accuracy figures such as these, it is hard to envision the need for another more expensive test for the workup of these patients.

Conway et al[7] studied 107 children with LCPD and bone scintigraphy. They reported that early LCPD presents as absent radioactivity throughout the epiphysis associated with normal radiographs. Radiographic changes do not appear until many months after the onset of the condition. One to two years following the onset of the disorder, there is complete revascularization of the bone, which first appears as a peripheral column of epiphyseal radioactivity. There is little published information comparing MRI with the bone scan in the LCPD patient population. Hendersen et al[15] evaluated the role

of MRI in LCPD in a prospective blinded study. However, all 22 of their patients had positive radiographs for LCPD. Even at this advanced stage of disease, 1 patient failed to show MRI changes indicative of necrosis. Although MRI can provide additional anatomic information about femoral head viability and containment, we believe it is up to MRI investigators to prove that MRI is as sensitive as the bone scan for the diagnosis of this disease before promoting its preferential use.

Renal Transplantation

In a review of AVN in a group of 600 renal failure and renal transplant patients, we found AVN in the hips in 112 patients, in the distal femoral condyles in 12 patients, in the shoulder in 8 patients, in the talus in 3 and in the elbow in 1. Spencer and Maisey[23] prospectively followed 42 consecutive renal transplant patients with routine 6-month whole-body scans for 2 to 3 years. They found 7 patients with AVN that would have otherwise remained undetected without bone scans. The incidence of AVN in this group was 17%. The bone scan was only useful if it showed a pattern of grossly increased or decreased uptake at the end of a long bone (Fig. 15-14). Due to the presence of metabolic bone disease in these patients, symmetric increased uptake throughout the skeleton was not a reliable indicator of AVN. Similarly, equivocal areas of increased uptake had a low predictive value of disease. Of the 7 patients found to have AVN, only 2 would have remained undetected without the use of the bone scans. Given the high expense of screening patients frequently for such a low yield, it would be hard to justify doing routine bone scans every 6 months to follow these patients. Another recent study[16] looked at 104 patients following renal transplantation. MRI was extremely helpful in diagnosing early AVN by finding crescentic areas of decreased signal in the weight-bearing portion of the femoral head, often with rings of low intensity, suggesting bone marrow edema. A later appearance was of dark bands of high signal intensity, ultimately with a margin or a "double-line" sign before the collapse of the femoral head.

Similarly, Tervoronen and Amin[26] from the Mayo Clinic looked at 100 asymptomatic renal transplant patients and used a short T1 sequence to ascertain if AVN was present. All the patients had been on steroids for 6 months or longer, and the authors found 6 patients with evidence of early asymptomatic AVN. Siddiqui et al[22] studied 72 renal allograft recipients over 24 months with both MRI and SPECT. Only 3 patients developed hip pain and required joint arthroplasty. These patients had positive findings by both MRI and SPECT. Surprisingly another group of 16 patients had positive results on one study only (nine SPECT, seven MRI) without any clinical evidence of disease. This was likely related to either a self-limited form of AVN or some other temporary drug-induced osteopathy. Again, it would appear that neither modality was particularly helpful in the clinical management of these patients, and routine screening was not justifiable

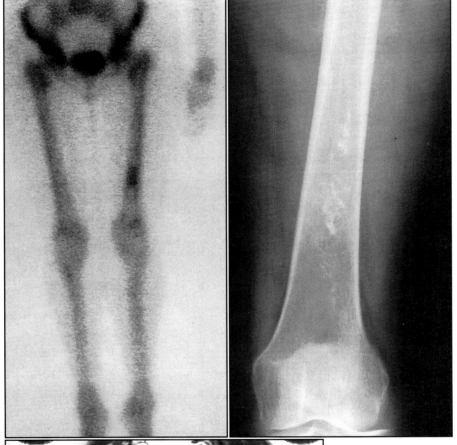

Fig. 15–13. Bone infarct. This 69-year-old patient suffered from lymphoma. A Tc-99m MDP bone scan was done to assess possible bone involvement. An anterior view shows intense increased uptake of tracer in the distal one third of the femur (**A**). Plain radiographs (**B**) of the distal left femur show the typical intramedullary calcifications of a bone infarct. **C**, MRI shows multiple areas of reduced to absent signal intensity in the left femur, both proximally and distally, consistent with infarcts.

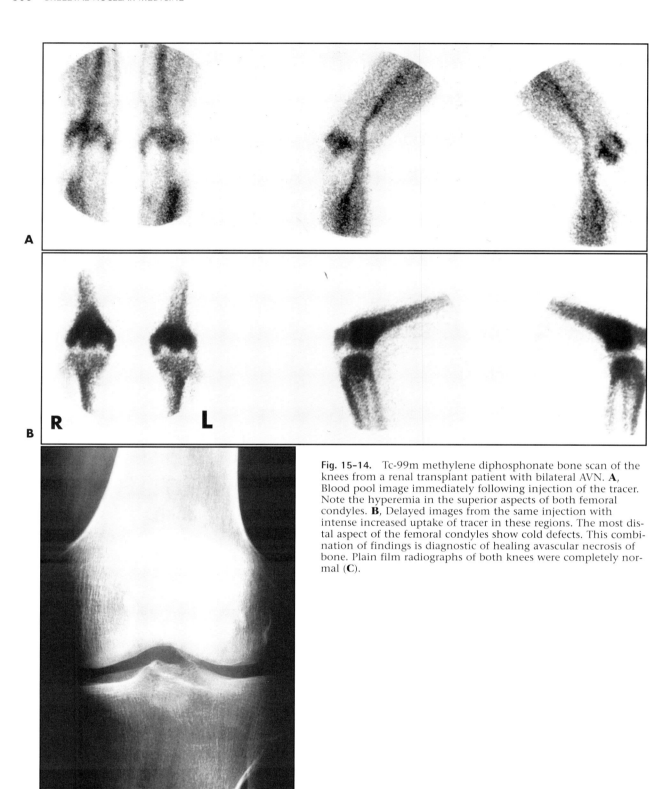

Fig. 15–14. Tc-99m methylene diphosphonate bone scan of the knees from a renal transplant patient with bilateral AVN. **A,** Blood pool image immediately following injection of the tracer. Note the hyperemia in the superior aspects of both femoral condyles. **B,** Delayed images from the same injection with intense increased uptake of tracer in these regions. The most distal aspect of the femoral condyles show cold defects. This combination of findings is diagnostic of healing avascular necrosis of bone. Plain film radiographs of both knees were completely normal (**C**).

MANAGEMENT

There is no totally effective management for AVN, although the hope of the orthopedic profession is that the process can be slowed. Of the various methods used, core decompression, which was introduced some 30 years ago, fell out of favor but is now back in use. The rationale for core decompression is that in many patients with AVN, the intraosseous intravascular pressure appears to be elevated. The most recent advances in performing core decompression include removing the core and replacing two-thirds as a powdered form of homograft. This can be associated with the use of a vascularized fibular implant or by inserting an osteoblast-stimulating device. Pure bone grafting results do not appear to be as effective. In the past varus and valgus osteotomies were used, and since these do not work, the rotational osteotomy of Sugioka[9] was introduced but found to produce poor results. Electrical bone stimulation devices can be used in association with any of these procedures.

At an advanced stage of AVN, it is often necessary to replace the femoral head, which can be done either by using a femoral endoprosthesis or by total hip arthroplasty. Both of these modes of therapy appear to be successful. Steinberg,[24] however, tried to moderate the inexorable process of AVN of the femoral head before this late stage by doing a core decompression, returning two thirds of the core using both internal and external electrical stimulation of bone growth. He appears to have quite promising results.

Saito[21] looked at the results of different joint-preserving operations for AVN of the femoral head. The natural history of AVN without treatment is that 84% of the femoral heads will go on to collapse. These authors reported excellent results in 53% of patients who had core decompression, 44% of patients who had bone grafting, and 33% of patients who had femoral neck osteotomies.

SUMMARY

In general, MRI has supplanted the bone scintigram as the method of choice for evaluating AVN of bone or bone infarcts. MRI is very sensitive and also provides additional information about the joint, cartilage, and marrow, which are only indirectly appreciable on a bone scan. The bone scan is not as accurate as widely believed in the diagnosis of AVN in most clinical settings. However, LCPD seems to be an exception, with a very high published sensitivity and specificity for the radionuclide study. A strong case can be made for using the bone scan for patients with suspected LCPD and normal radiographs. AVN of bone is a common clinical condition, and it is important that we are able to recognize its features, even if the finding is incidental to the primary reason for performing a bone scan.

ACKNOWLEDGMENTS

We wish to acknowledge Charla Zaccardi and Clem Wait for their help with the manuscript, Dr. Tom Gilbert for supplying some of the MRI scans, and David Priest for researching some of the MRI references.

REFERENCES

1. Alavi A, McCloskey JR, Steinberg ME: Early detection of avascular necrosis of the femoral head by 99m technetium diphosphonate bone scan: A preliminary report. *Clin Orthop* 1977; 127:137.
2. Bauer G, Weber DA, Ceder L, et al: Dynamics of Tc-99m methylene-diphosphonate imaging of femoral head after hip fracture. *Clin Orthop* 1980; 152:85.
3. Brody AS, Strong M, Babikian G, et al: Avascular necrosis: Early MR imaging and histologic findings in a canine model. *AJR Am J Roentgenol* 1991; 157:341.
4. Burt RW, Matthews TJ: Aseptic necrosis of the knee: Bone scintigraphy. *AJR Am J Roentgenol* 1982; 138:571.
5. Collier BD, Carrera GF, Johnson RP, et al: Detection of femoral head avascular necrosis in adults by SPECT. *J Nucl Med* 1985; 26:979.
6. Conklin JJ, Alderson PO, Zizic TM, et al: Comparison of bone scan and radiographic sensitivity in detection of steroid-induced ischemic necrosis of bone. *Radiology* 1983; 147:221.
7. Conway JJ, Weiss SC, Maldonado V: Scintigraphic patterns in Legg-Calvé-Perthes disease. *Radiology* 1983; 149P:102.
8. Danigelis JA: Pinhole imaging in Legg-Perthes disease: Further observations. *Semin Nucl Med* 1976; 6:69.
9. Dean MT, Cabanella ME: Transtrochanteric anterior rotational osteotomy for AVN of the femoral head. *J Bone Joint Surg Br* 1993; 75B:797.
10. Epstein JB, Wong FL, Dickens A, et al: Bone and gallium scans in postradiotherapy osteonecrosis of the jaw. *Head Neck* 1992; 14:288.
11. Fig LM, Shulkin BL, Sullivan MJ, et al: Utility of emission tomography in evaluation of mandibular bone grafts. *Arch Otolaryngol Head Neck Surg* 1990; 116:191.
12. Freeman HJ, Kwan WCP: Brief report: Non-corticosteroid-associated osteonecrosis of the femoral head in two patients with inflammatory bowel disease. *N Engl J Med* 1993; 329:1314.
13. Glickstein MR, Burk DL Jr, Schiebler ML, et al: Avascular necrosis versus other disease of the hip: Sensitivity of MR imaging. *Radiology* 1988; 169:213.
14. Gregg PJ, Walder DN: Scintigraphy versus radiography in early diagnosis of experimental bone necrosis: With special reference to caisson disease of bone. *J Bone Joint Surg Br* 1980; 62B:214.
15. Henderson RC, Renner JB, Sturdivant MC, Greene WB: Evaluation of magnetic resonance imaging in Lee-Perthes disease: A prospective, blinded study. *J Pediatr Orthop* 1990; 10:289.
16. Kopecky KK, Braunstein EM, Brandt KD, et al: Apparent avascular necrosis of the hip: Appearance and spontaneous resolution of MR findings in renal allograft recipients. *Radiology* 1991; 179:523.

17. LaMont RL, Muz J, Heilbronner D, et al: Quantitative assessment of femoral head involvement in Legg-Calvé-Perthes disease. *J Bone Joint Surg Am* 1981; 63A:746.

18. Lang P, Jergesen HE, Moseley ME, et al: Avascular necrosis of the femoral head: High-field-strength MR imaging with histological correlation. *Radiology* 1988; 169:517.

19. Lutzker LG, Alavi A: Bone and marrow imaging in sickle cell disease: Diagnosis of infarction. *Semin Nucl Med* 1976; 6:83.

20. Mitchell MD, Kundel HL, Steinberg ME, et al: Avascular necrosis of the hip: Comparison of MR, CT, and scintigraphy. *AJR Am J Roentgenol* 1986; 147:67.

21. Saito S, Inoue A, Ono K: Intramedullary hemorrhage as a possible cause of avascular necrosis of the femoral head. *J Bone Joint Surg Br* 1987; 69B:346.

22. Siddiqui AR, Kenyon KK, Wellman HN, et al: Prospective study of magnetic resonance imaging and SPECT bone scans in renal allograft recipients: Evidence for a self-limited subclinical abnormality of the hip. *J Nucl Med* 1993; 34:381.

23. Spencer JD, Maisey M: A prospective scintigraphic study of avascular necrosis of bone in renal transplant patients. *Clin Orthop* 1985; 194:125.

24. Steinberg ME, Brighton CT, Corces A, et al: Osteonecrosis of the femoral head. Results of core decompression and grafting with and without electrical stimulation. *Clin Orthop* 1989; 249:199.

25. Sutherland AD, Savage JP, Paterson DC, et al: The nuclide bone scan in the diagnosis and management of Perthes' disease. *J Bone Joint Surg Br* 1980; 62B:300.

26. Tervonen O, Mueller DM, Matteson EL, et al: Clinically occult avascular necrosis of the hip: Prevalence in an asymptomatic population at risk. *Radiology* 1992; 182:845.

27. Vande Berg S, Malghem J, Labaisse MA, et al: Avascular necrosis of the hip: Comparison of contrast-enhanced and nonenhanced MR imaging with histologic correlation. *Radiology* 1992; 182:445.

28. Zizic TM, Lewis CG, Marcoux C, Hungerford DS: The predictive value of hemodynamic studies in preclinical ischemic necrosis of bone. *J Rheumatol* 1989; 12:1559.

29. Zizic TM, Marcoux C, Hungerford DS, Stevens MB: The early diagnosis of ischemic necrosis of bone. *Arthritis Rheum* 1986; 29:1177.

CHAPTER 16

PEDIATRIC BONE SCANNING

Gerald A. Mandell

H. Theodore Harcke

The general use of bone-seeking tracers to evaluate the skeleton in pediatric patients became feasible with the introduction of technetium-99m phosphates in 1971. Since that time the bone scan has been relied on for evaluating children and has maintained its usefulness even with the introduction of other imaging modalities. This relates to its sensitivity for physiologic change. In some respects this is more important in pediatrics than in adult scintigraphy, because the normal growing skeleton will appear different from one age group to another. On the other hand, interpretation of bone images in children becomes a challenge because increased activity at a growth center can obscure adjacent lesions or injury to the physis itself. Chapter 3 provides an in-depth discussion of skeletal maturation and its scintigraphic appearance.

PERFORMING PEDIATRIC MUSCULOSKELETAL SCINTIGRAPHY

The technetium-99m phosphate compounds generally behave the same way in children as in adults. Currently pediatric nuclear medicine laboratories favor the use of methylene diphosphonate (MDP) because it

seems to produce the best-quality images. Although this is somewhat subjective, it may relate to a little faster blood clearance and a greater rate of bone adsorption than the other bone-seeking tracers.

A prime consideration in all pediatric imaging is to minimize absorbed radiation dose. In bone scintigraphy, technetium-MDP is administered on the basis of 200 µCi/kg of body weight with a minimum total dose of 0.5 to 1.0 mCi. Good hydration and frequent voiding are important because they will help to reduce the dose, particularly to gonadal tissue.

Gallium imaging of the skeleton is done principally for detecting infection. It is most common to use gallium in conjunction with a technetium-MDP bone scan in situations where a preexisting abnormality causes the phosphate scan to be positive. Gallium is also used when there is a strong suspicion of infection and the technetium phosphate scan is normal. There is logic in doing two studies because of the different mechanism for gallium localization (relating to leukocytes and inflammatory proteins). The usual dose of gallium is 0.5 to 3.0 mCi. It does present a higher radiation dose than the phosphate scan and so it is reserved for problem cases.

Bone imaging with labeled white blood cells is becoming popular as a technique for detecting infection in pediatric patients. Labeling with indium-111 or technetium-hexamethylpropyleneamine oxide (HMPAO) is possible in children. The technetium label produces higher-quality images and gives less radiation. These studies require a blood sample of 20 to 50 ml (depending on patient size and white blood cell count), and so the technique is not used for infants and small children. We find the labeled white blood cell doses to be in the 0.075 to 0.5 mCi range with indium (15 µCi/kg) and the 2 to 15 mCi range (200 µCi/kg) with technetium-99m HMPAO. Thallium is used for tumor imaging in a dose of 50 µCi/kg (0.25 to 3.0 mCi).

To obtain satisfactory images, it is essential that the child remain still during the examination. As a rule, sedation is not necessary in the older child. Infants and young children, however, are not always able to cooperate and sedation needs to be considered. With the gamma camera there is less need to sedate a child than if a whole-body scanner is used. The complete study can be divided into a series of large-field-of-view images and because the time for each image is relatively short, the child is able to relax briefly between successive images. Experienced nuclear medicine technologists have developed techniques for swaddling and taping and also know that feeding young infants has a sedating effect. We have purchased a mobile television and videocassette recorder combination to be positioned by each camera so that children are entertained during the course of the scan. Still, there are instances where an adequate study cannot be obtained without a sedative. Sedation may be necessary in young children when lengthy procedures such as single photon emission computed tomography (SPECT) and pinhole views are performed. The choice and time of administration of the sedative depends on a number of factors, particularly the length of the procedure. Oral sedation with chloral hydrate is a popular technique because of the drug's relative safety. We recommend doses in the range of 80 to 100 mg/kg (maximum, 2.5 g) and could use this in the child to obtain delayed bone images and/or a SPECT examination. Intravenous sedation is another option used in pediatric centers because it is reliable, rapid acting, and can be controlled. Pentobarbital at a dose of 2.5 to 7.5 mg/kg (maximum, 200 mg), is a standard regimen. We advise sedation only when it is absolutely necessary because proper precautions must be taken when administering either an oral or intravenous medication. We use nursing personnel and monitoring equipment to ensure the safety of the child during and after the procedure. There are now definitive sedation guidelines published by the American Academy of Pediatrics.[61]

Although the basic principles of scintigraphy apply to both children and adults, there are important variations in the approach to children that are essential to quality imaging. With technetium phosphate in skeletal scintigraphy, multiphase imaging is required when dealing with potential conditions that are infectious or inflammatory. We consider the second and third phase of four-phase scintigraphy to be mandatory in these circumstances. The first (flow) phase has not shown us any significant information that was not present on the second (soft-tissue) phase. Also, we have not found 24-hour imaging to be helpful. We image both phases with a high-resolution collimator and acquire images of the trunk for 400,000 to 800,000 counts and images of the extremities for 200,000 counts. Magnification views can be obtained either electronically or with pinhole collimation. In studying the hips, we always include pinhole images in anterior and frog-leg projections for 150,000 to 300,000 counts. We use the 1.5-mm insert to obtain highest resolution. There are also times when a lesion is identified on large-field-of-view images and additional pinhole views contribute important detail. Our routine tomographic (SPECT) imaging parameters are 64×64 byte matrix, 30-second acquisition per station and 64 stations.

In those instances where special isotopes are used to search for infection, we vary imaging sequences. With gallium it is sometimes helpful to image about 4 hours after injection (with medium-energy collimation). We always image at 24 hours and prefer to do our total-body and SPECT images at this time. Imaging at 48 and 72 hours is done on a case by case basis, based on the results of earlier images, the site of abnormality, and if bowel activity is affecting interpretation. The labeled white blood cell studies involve different protocols, depending on whether indium or technetium is the labeling agent. With indium, 24- and 48-hour imaging is done with 100,000 count images and shielding of the liver. Labeled white blood cell imaging is done at 15 minutes and 3 hours. Here images of 400,000 to 800,000 counts are possible to obtain. Later images are not always reliable because of tagging breakdown and bowel activity. Thallium imaging is done 30 minutes postinjection and images of the trunk are 300,000 counts; extremities are 150,000 counts.

INFECTION AND INFLAMMATION

General Concepts

Childhood osteomyelitis can be characterized by location: epiphyseal, metaphyseal, diaphyseal, and metaphyseal equivalent. Foci of infection can be unifocal or multifocal. Certain age groups (i.e., infantile, preadolescent, and adolescent) have a predilection for multifocal presentations. The earliest radiographic sign of osteomyelitis (first few days) is deep soft-tissue swelling adjacent to the bone.[51] Lysis of bone cannot be appreciated on standard radiographic images until the lesion is 1.0 to 1.5 cm or has destroyed 30% to 50% of the bone matrix. Frank osseous destruction and periosteal reaction may not become visible until 10 to 14 days after the onset of symptoms. Early diagnosis and treatment is especially critical in pediatrics to maximize the chances of favorable long-term results, prevent deformities (leg length discrepancy and angulation), and avoid limitations of joint motion (ankylosis).

Acute and Chronic Osteomyelitis

Bone scintigraphy lends itself to the detection of acute and subacute osteomyelitis because the bone-seeking radiopharmaceuticals avidly concentrate in the local area of hyperemia and bone resorption induced by the infectious process. Bone repair also contributes to the increased bone activity in subacute and chronic infections. The multiphase bone scan (two or three phases) has been invaluable in differentiating cellulitis from osteomyelitis in the proper clinical setting.[261] We recommend it as the second step in imaging children suspected of having osteomyelitis (the first study should be radiographs). The scintigram demonstrates diffuse or discrete increased uptake on the two early phases (angiographic and soft tissue) and increased uptake localizing to the infected focus in bone on the delayed phase (Fig. 16-1). Cellulitis may show diffuse increased uptake in the soft tissues on the early phase images, with disappearance or lessening on the delayed images. The multifocality of infection of the skeleton in infants and preadolescent/ adolescent children has prompted the recommendation to study the whole body in phases two and three of the bone scan.[112]

Other hyperemic pathologic processes of bone such as neoplasm, trauma, and fibrous dysplasia, can produce scintigraphic patterns similar to osteomyelitis. However, bone scans have been found to have a sensitivity of 95% and a specificity of 92% for osteomyelitis, compared with 32% sensitivity and 89% specificity for radiographs.[285] In the early avascular or thrombotic phase of medullary infection, the bone scan may be normal or "cold." Subsequent bone scintigraphy following therapy or surgical intervention may show conversion from a normal or photopenic image to increased concentration of the bone-seeking radiopharmaceutical. When infection is suspected, the presence of a photopenic lesion is compatible with osteomyelitis; confusion over this appearance should not delay therapy.

Other imaging techniques (gallium and tagged white blood cells) are more specific for infection than conventional bone scintigraphy. We advocate their use when phosphate scans are not diagnostic (Fig. 16-2). Combined gallium and bone scanning increases the accuracy of the scintigraphic diagnosis of osteomyelitis.[139,218] Gallium can at times give false-positive results in juvenile rheumatoid arthritis (JRA), fracture, and in some neoplasms.[32] Early scanning with gallium (3 or 4 hours after intravenous injection) has an accuracy of 91% in the detection of septic arthritis and osteomyelitis in children. More specificity in the detection of acute bone infection has been achieved by the introduction of indium-111 and technetium-99m tagged white blood cell studies. There is some controversy over the sensitivity of these agents in chronic infection, which consists mainly of macrophages, lymphocytes, and plasma cells. Schauwecker reported in chronic osteomyelitis a 60% sensitivity with indium-111 imaging. In chronic osteomyelitis sensitivity also varied with location: 94% for peripheral bones, 80% for middle bones, and 53% for the central skeleton. In acute osteomyelitis the sensitivity was 90% to 95%, regardless of location of the bone in the body.[333]

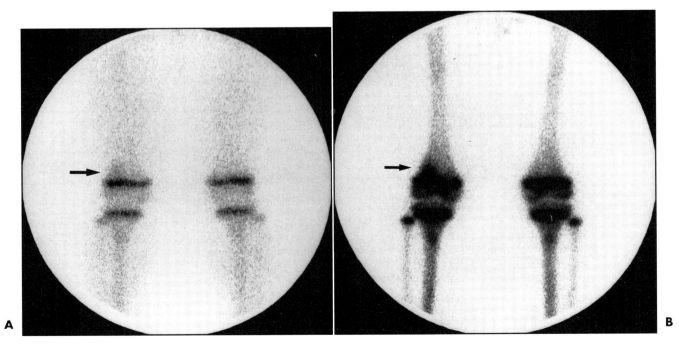

Fig. 16–1. Osteomyelitis of the distal femur in a 5-year-old female. Focally increased uptake in the right femoral metaphysis is present on both the tissue phase (**A**) and bone phase (**B**) (*arrows*).

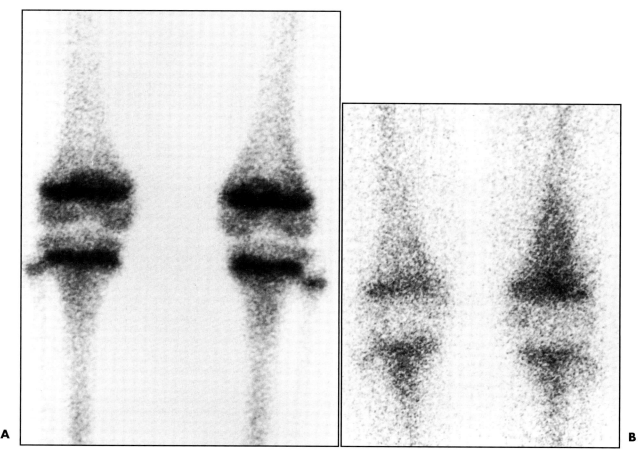

Fig. 16-2. Osteomyelitis of the distal left femur in a 9-year-old male. The initial study with technetium-99m MDP was equivocal (**A**), so a follow-up scan with technetium-99m HMPAO labeled white blood cells (**B**) was performed. This was strongly positive.

Technetium-99m HMPAO labeled leukocytes have been popularized because of the ability to obtain higher count images that result in better resolution of the infectious process, faster and earlier (within 4 hours) imaging time, and less radiation burden. This agent also favors the use of SPECT. Labeling of white blood cells requires extensive and careful separation. The labeling procedure usually takes about 2 hours and requires skills to ensure that the cells are not damaged. Preliminary results with technetium-99m HMPAO cells have been encouraging, although some false-negative results have been reported.[133,206] The presence of marrow uptake in children may interfere with interpretation. Additional experience will be necessary to determine the specific role of this agent in imaging of pediatric bone infection.

METAPHYSEAL OSTEOMYELITIS

Seventy-five percent of cases of hematogenous osteomyelitis involves the metaphyses of tubular bones.[288] The predominance of metaphyseal locations in childhood osteomyelitis is based on the vascular anatomy. The terminal artery ramifications of the nutrient artery are thought to form loops adjacent to the physeal germinal layer of cartilage. These empty into a system of large venous sinusoids in the metaphyseal intramedullary portions of the long bone. The sluggish circulation of the sinusoids is an ideal medium for collecting and proliferating circulating bacteria.[376] The most common sites include the femur and tibia. Hematogenous metaphyseal osteomyelitis frequents children under 6 years of age. In one series 46% of acute osteomyelitis occurred between 6 weeks and 3 years of age.[165]

METAPHYSEAL-EQUIVALENT INFECTIONS

The pediatric skeleton between 6 and 16 years of age is susceptible to infection at skeletal locations that physiologically resemble the long-bone metaphyses. A *metaphyseal-equivalent location* is defined as the portion of a flat or irregular bone that borders cartilage (apophyseal growth plates, articular cartilage, or fibrocartilage).[289] Diagnosing pelvic osteomyelitis or septic arthritis in children is often difficult because of the vagueness and lack of specificity of the symptoms.[155] The sacroiliac joint, the ischiopubic synchondrosis, and pubic rami are common sites of involvement. Other metaphyseal-equivalent locations, in order of decreasing frequency, include the

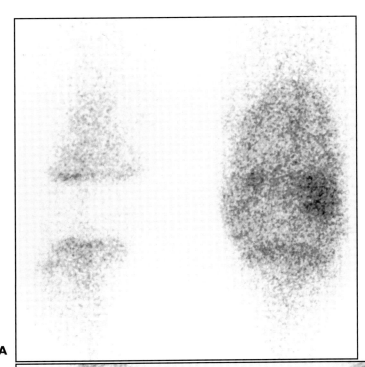

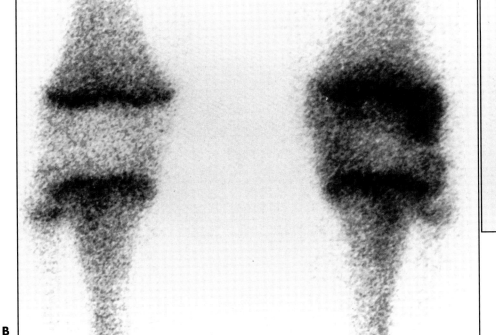

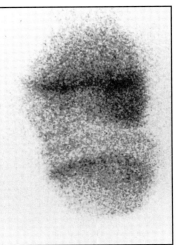

Fig. 16-3. Epiphyseal osteomyelitis of the distal left femur in a 15-year-old female. The tissue phase (**A**) and bone phase (**B**) show generally increased uptake on both sides of the knee. The focal increase is in the lateral aspect of the femoral epiphysis, which is confirmed by a magnification (pinhole) view of the left knee (**C**). The bone infection has produced a secondary arthritis in the knee joint.

vertebrae, calcaneus, apophyseal center of the greater trochanter, ischium, tibia tubercle, scapula, and talus.[289]

The vascular anatomy of metaphyseal-equivalent regions is similar to the ends of the long-bone metaphyses and also results in sluggish end-arterial blood flow. The most common organism causing the suppurative process in the adolescent is *Staphylococcus aureus*. Before 10 years of age the site usually manifests by a subacute infectious process with no identifiable organism. Diagnosis of infection is difficult at metaphyseal-equivalent locations, usually devoid of early radiographic changes, and lends itself to bone scintigraphy. Computed tomography (CT) is usually used to identify the precise anatomic changes in the cortex and adjacent soft tissues, especially when diagnostic or therapeutic intervention is being considered.

EPIPHYSEAL OSTEOMYELITIS

Isolated epiphyseal infection in the older child is a recognized entity. Most of the lesions are sterile, affecting children between 2 and 4 years of age.[130] The transphyseal arterial connections were thought to disappear as a child approached 1 year of age. However, subsequent identification of the vascular architecture of the epiphysis has demonstrated multiple branches of a large encircling artery perfusing the peripheral portions of the metaphysis and the entire epiphysis.[325] The epiphyseal branches are radially oriented to supply the articular and physeal cartilages and empty into radially oriented venous sinusoids that drain to the center of the epiphysis. A hemodynamic pattern of relatively slow flow in the epiphyseal sinusoids is similar to what occurs in the metaphysis. The epiphyses of the lower extremities are most frequently affected.

Bone scintigraphy with magnification imaging (e.g., pinhole collimation) can readily identify the focus of epiphyseal infection because it permits resolution of the metaphysis and the epiphysis from the very active physis (growth plate) (Fig. 16-3). Recognition of focally increased epiphyseal uptake is almost impossible with routine planar scintigraphy.

NEONATAL OSTEOMYELITIS

Neonatal infection (infants < 6 weeks of age) is characterized as multifocal and bacterial in origin. The infection is typically difficult to recognize because of the lack of specific systemic signs and symptoms. This virulent type of osteomyelitis (*S. aureus* and group B beta-hemolytic streptococci), when not readily detected, can destroy the physis and joint, leaving a child with permanent musculoskeletal deformity. Neonatal osteomyelitis usually originates as a hematogenous metaphyseal process at the end of a long bone or in the iliac portion (acetabular or body) of the osseous pelvis. The infection usually crosses the growth plate by traveling along transphyseal blood vessels to reach the epiphysis.[295] Direct destruction of the growth plate is another factor that allows bacterial penetration into the epiphysis with resulting joint involvement (Fig. 16-4).

The sensitivity of bone scintigraphy for the detection of neonatal osteomyelitis has been variable. From an initially poor sensitivity of 31.5%,[9] the detection of neonatal osteomyelitis has improved to 87%[36] with the use of higher-resolution gamma cameras and magnification techniques. The practice of safe sedation in young and mentally/physically disabled children has virtually eliminated most problems of motion during prolonged imaging. Sedation permits the acquisition of high-count, high-resolution (magnification) images that increase the accuracy of interpretation. The bone scan can be cold (photopenic) in the neonate. The purulent material is assumed to accumulate in the marrow, causing increased intraosseous pressure and diminution of the blood supply. With surgical drainage and decompression of the subperiosteal or intraosseous pus, the cold area can convert to a "hot" focus.[183,278,281] Sometimes gallium is required in the evaluation to increase sensitivity and specificity.[156] The volume of blood needed for labeling of white blood cells precludes usage of this study in neonates.

DISKITIS AND VERTEBRAL OSTEOMYELITIS

Two patterns of spine infection are recognized in children: diskitis and osteomyelitis. Diskitis is an inflammatory process that arises in the intervertebral disk space. Usually the process is indolent and the patient is not particularly ill. There are two peak age periods of incidence: young children age 6 months to 4 years and older children age 10 to 14 years.[386] Positive cultures of blood or biopsy material are found in only approximately one third to one half of patients. Infection may reach the intervertebral disk space via subchondral vascular channels that arise in the marrow of the vertebral body and perforate the vertebral end plate. This vascular system which extends into the nucleus pulposus and ultimately courses between the fibers of the annulus fibrosus has been noted in children up to the age of 8 years but can persist up to 30 years of age.[67] Other reports claim the blood supply to the disk is independent of the end plate.

Bacterial osteomyelitis of the spine is less common in the pediatric population than in adults. It appears predominantly in the first decade of life, usually accompanied by systemic illness. A coexisting pyogenic focus at another site is not unusual. Positive blood cultures are generally not found in patients who have had symptoms more than 6 weeks.[362] In contradistinction to diskitis, an organism, usually *S. aureus*, is recovered in a high percentage of cases of vertebral osteomyelitis. It is presumed that a septic embolus lodges in the metaphyseal artery, an end arteriole in the vertebral body metaphysis. The clot propagates into the metaphyseal anastomosis and results in septic infarction producing osteomyelitis.[318]

Initial radiographs of the spine may be normal in both vertebral osteomyelitis and diskitis. The most common site of diskitis is from L2 to L4.[100] The mid and lower thoracic spine are the most common sites of osteomyelitis. The first radiographic sign of disk space infection is diminution in the width of the space. Positive findings in bone scintigraphy, as early as 7 days after the onset of symptoms,[135] can predate radiographic changes in both diskitis and osteomyelitis by weeks.

The usual scintigraphic pattern in diskitis is increased uptake in the disk space and the contiguous ends of the adjoining vertebrae.[110] The increased radiotracer activity is noted on both the tissue-phase and delayed bone images (Fig. 16-5). SPECT imaging and pinhole collimation appear to be helpful in localizing site and extent of involvement.[362] In children we recommend the technetium bone scan as the study to follow radiographs because it permits a comprehensive body survey. If it is normal and there is a high clinical suspicion for diskitis, magnetic resonance imaging (MRI) or gallium imaging can be considered. MRI has comparable sensitivity to scintigraphy. Gallium has demonstrated diskitis in adults with 86% accuracy.[10] The gallium study should be extended to 72 hours when imaging diskitis.

With vertebral osteomyelitis, bone scintigraphy usual-

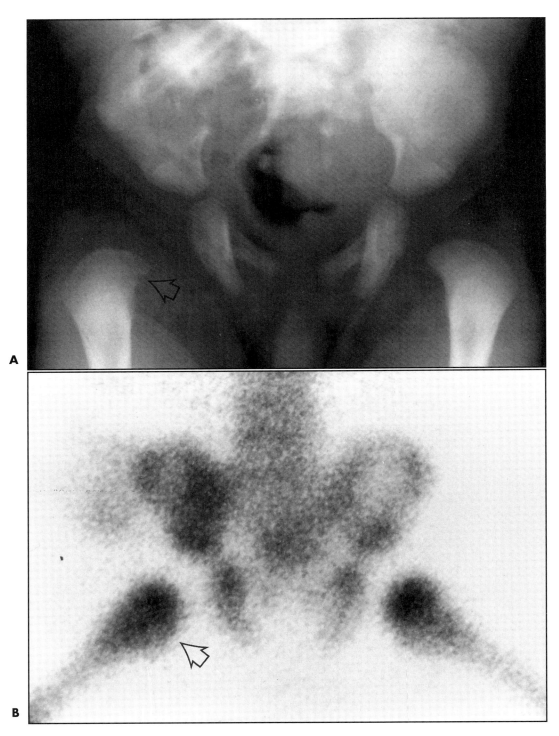

Fig. 16-4. Neonatal osteomyelitis and septic arthritis in a 19-day-old male. The radiograph (**A**) shows displacement of the right hip secondary to the septic arthritis. Destructive changes are present in the medial femoral metaphysis (*arrow*). Bowel gas and stool obscure the right iliac bone. The bone scan (**B**) shows increased activity in the proximal right femur (*arrow*) as well as in the right iliac and pubic bones.

ly shows diffuse uptake of the radiopharmaceutical within the involved vertebra in both blood pool and delayed images.[135] A "butterfly" pattern of uptake on gallium scintigraphy has been described in vertebral osteomyelitis.[43] White blood cell imaging of osteomyelitis of the spine has been disappointing. Although the focus of infection has typically increased activity, photopenia has been reported fairly frequently in osteomyelitis of the spine.[303] It has been postulated that this photopenia results from occlusion of the microcirculation of the involved bone by the acute inflammation and necrosis. Skeletal photopenia with leukocyte imaging is nonspecific: it is also observed in avascular necrosis (AVN), fracture, and fibrous dysplasia.

MULTIFOCAL OSTEOMYELITIS

Thirty-seven percent of multifocal inflammatory/infectious involvement of bone presents in the latter half of the first decade and the first half of the second decade.[206] These infections are characterized by an indolent sometimes recurrent course, lack of an identifiable pathogen, rare systemic manifestations, and a paucity of significant laboratory results (elevated white blood cell count or erythrocyte sedimentation rate). Many of the sites are initially asymptomatic but become painful with chronicity.[253] Chronic recurrent multifocal osteomyelitis (CRMO) can involve the epiphyses, metaphyses, diaphyses, or metaphyseal-equivalent locations of the skeleton. The patient may present initially with either a single

lesion followed by the development of subsequent foci or may present with many concurrent lesions in different phases of activity.

The lack of specific clinical, laboratory, and radiographic criteria for diagnosis forces the biopsy of one or more lesions in each patient. Histology reveals an abundance of plasma cells. In the more acute lesions there may be a greater amount of polymorphonuclear cells. In the older lesions there can be an admixture of inflammatory cells consisting primarily of plasma cells and lymphocytes, multinucleated giant cells, and fibrosis.[23]

The radiographic changes vary from lytic (acute/subacute) to mixed (subacute/chronic) to completely sclerotic (chronic) and can be different at each anatomic site. Flat bones and the short tubular bones of the extremities, distal radius and ulna, distal fibula, and clavicle and ribs usually present as small radiolucent metaphyseal lesions surrounded by more extensive periosteal reaction, sclerosis, and soft-tissue swelling. Many of the lesions, especially in the clavicle, distal radius, and ulna have the appearances of primary bone marrow malignancy; and histologic diagnosis is required to rule out malignancy, especially in monostotic presentation. Lesions in large-diameter bones, such as the metaphyses of the femur and the tibia, usually present as focally destructive lucent metaphyseal lesions with little soft-tissue swelling or periosteal reaction. The process can be bilateral (so-called chronic symmetric osteomyelitis) with almost symmetric changes abutting the growth plates, or each focus can

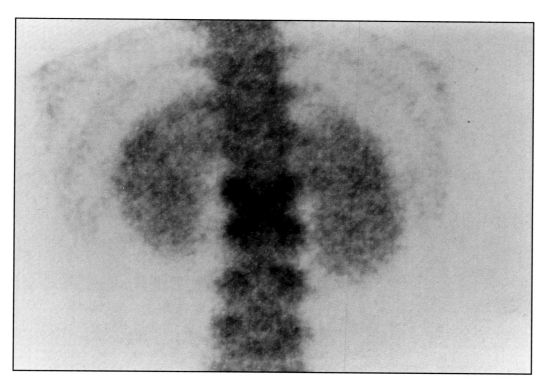

Fig. 16–5. Diskitis in a 6-year-old male. The delayed bone images show increased uptake in two contiguous lumbar vertebral bodies (L1 and L2). This reflects the response to infection in the L1-2 disk space.

show a different phase. Complete sclerosis and slow regression of the lesions with ultimate healing may occur, but the healing process may take several years. The most commonly affected sites are the proximal tibial, distal tibial, and femoral metaphyses, followed by the clavicle and forearm bones (radius and ulna). Other reported skeletal sites have included the mandible, ribs, humerus, radius, metacarpals, metatarsals, talus, pelvis, and sternum.[42] The greater trochanteric apophysis is a common metaphyseal-equivalent site.[108]

Scintigraphic evaluation of the skeleton in childhood for infection or tumor should never be limited to one portion of the skeleton. Positive findings on bone scintigraphy can predate the onset of clinical symptoms and radiographic changes at many metaphyseal sites in both chronic symmetric osteomyelitis and CRMO. Lesions in the healing phase will also be very active on bone scan.

CHRONIC CLAVICULAR INFLAMMATION

Chronic inflammatory clavicular abnormalities (inflammatory clavicular hyperostosis, chronic recurrent osteomyelitis) produce an expanded sclerosis reaction (sometimes bilateral) usually surrounding some areas of lysis. These processes have no clear etiology and occur mainly in children and adolescents.[185] True isolated chronic or acute osteomyelitis of the clavicle with an underlying bacterial or fungal etiology is unusual, with practically no occurrence in adults and an incidence of

7% in children.[129,355] The symptoms of pain and swelling in the involved regions are prolonged. The most lateral part of the clavicle is usually less frequently involved. The lesion on radiographs can be predominantly lytic or mixed in appearance.[114]

The bone scan exhibits extreme intense activity[369] (Fig. 16-6). Biopsy reveals a nonspecific chronic osteomyelitis. CRMO may be clinically indistinguishable from isolated inflammatory hyperostosis of the clavicle. It is often associated with pustulosis palmoplantaris, a skin disease characterized by recurrent sterile pustules on the palms or soles or both.[377]

Inflammatory/Infectious Arthritides

SEPTIC ARTHRITIS

Septic arthritis in children is a surgical emergency. It may be a primary infection or co-exist with osteomyelitis that has seeded the joint. Approximately 75% of cases of septic arthritis involve the lower extremities with the most common joint being the hip.[162,189] In infants more than 75% of cases ultimately result in some degree of joint destruction. Avascular necrosis and hip dislocation can occur concomitantly, leading to chronic orthopedic disability. In the older pediatric population, it is less likely that septic arthritis will cause the same degree of joint damage that it does in neonates. Early in the course of septic arthritis, radiographs can be normal, exhibit soft-

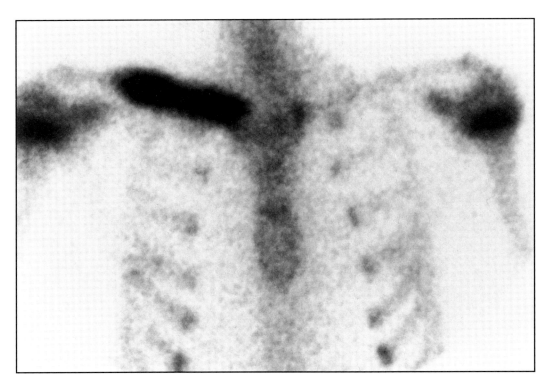

Fig. 16–6. Chronic recurrent osteomyelitis of the clavicle in a 12-year-old female. Markedly increased uptake in the right clavicle corresponds to radiographic sclerosis with extensive periosteal reaction.

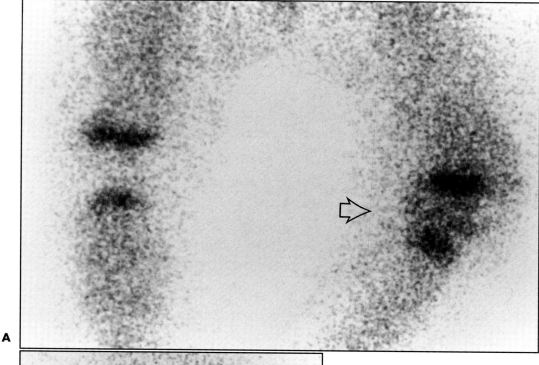

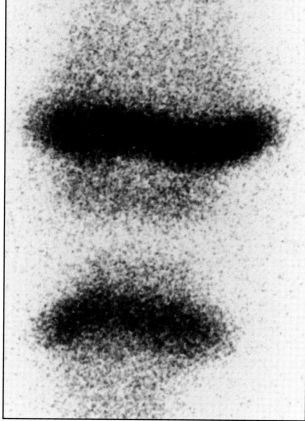

Fig. 16–7. Septic arthritis in an 8-month-old female. The tissue-phase images (**A**) show increased activity in the left knee joint as well as the adjacent growth plates and overlying soft tissue (*arrow*). Delayed bone imaging (**B**) reveals no focal bone uptake (pinhole view). The pattern is similar for any inflammatory arthritis.

tissue derangement, or show subluxation/dislocation of the femoral head. Bone destruction is usually not evident until late in the course of the disease unless the septic arthritis is secondary to osteomyelitis.

On bone scintigraphy, periarticular concentration of the radiotracer is present on the tissue phase. The delayed images show a decrease in the soft-tissue uptake, and bone activity is either normal or mildly increased on both sides (symmetric pattern) of the joint.[364] Other aseptic causes of synovitis (e.g., rheumatoid arthritis, transient synovitis) can produce a similar appearance. Abnormal focal concentration of uptake occurring in an adjacent bone (i.e., in the region of the hip, the proximal femoral epiphysis, innominate bone, or acetabulum) indicates concurrent osteomyelitis (Fig. 16-7).

Photopenia of the femoral head can be found in septic hips secondary to transient ischemia induced by fluid pressure in the joint. The photopenia accompanying septic arthritis is usually manifested by uniformly diminished epiphyseal uptake, whereas with transient synovitis, some scattered epiphyseal uptake is still discernible.[194] Early recognition of septic arthritis and removal of the purulent fluid can reverse the ischemia and prevent permanent necrosis of the femoral head.[393] If saline washings and/or arthrography during arthrocentesis are performed before bone scintigraphy, it is advisable to wait at least 45 minutes before performing the nuclear medicine examination.[241]

TRANSIENT SYNOVITIS

Transient synovitis (toxic synovitis, "irritable hip syndrome") is the most common cause of hip pain in children. The condition is usually self-limited and causes no significant sequelae. Prior viral illness, trauma, and allergy have all been considered as possible etiologies for this benign hip disorder. The male-to-female ratio is 1.9:1.[150] Three fourths of patients are younger than 7 years of age. The ages range from 3 months to 15 years of age. The aspirated joint fluid is sterile.[150] The increased volume of joint fluid creates an elevation of the intraarticular pressure. Maintenance of an elevated pressure for greater than 12 hours has been shown experimentally to produce permanent infarction of the femoral head.[396] Approximately 2.5% of patients with transient synovitis progress to avascular necrosis (Legg-Perthes disease).[150]

Plain radiography reveals no osseous changes at acute presentation. Joint space asymmetry of 2 mm or more on a straight anteroposterior radiograph is suspicious for the presence of synovitis. Scintigraphy is used to differentiate the irritable hip syndrome from early Legg-Perthes disease.[53] The bone scan appearance in transient synovitis is variable. The immediate tissue-phase images may be normal or may exhibit slightly increased activity, reflecting the hyperemia associated with synovial inflammation. Delayed scans may be normal or may display slightly increased uptake on both sides of the joint.

JUVENILE RHEUMATOID ARTHRITIS

The most common cause of polyarthropathy in children is rheumatoid arthritis. Approximately 80% of chil-

dren with JRA are symptomatic by 7 years of age. Joint destruction probably occurs secondary to the chronic synovitis. The synovial proliferation results in a highly cellular pannus that erodes the osteochondral junction, destroys the articular cartilage, and invades the marrow. Mono-oligo forms of arthritis must be differentiated from hematogenous osteomyelitis and septic arthritis as well as some neoplasms. Also, children with neuroblastoma and leukemia (who have splenomegaly and lymphadenopathy) may present with arthritic symptoms secondary to marrow infiltration of the metaphyses, periosteum, and joint capsule.

The knees are the most commonly affected site followed by the wrists and carpus, then the ankles and tarsus. The first radiographic signs of JRA are soft-tissue swelling and effusion. Periostitis can appear early in the course of the disease (dactylitis), and when this occurs with osteopenia and soft-tissue swelling, the findings are similar to osteomyelitis.[255] A bone scan is most useful for excluding serious infection or neoplastic disease in a child with nonspecific arthritic symptoms. A negative study does not exclude active arthritis in children. An abnormal pattern of uptake consistent with arthritis/synovitis consists of increased tissue-phase activity in a synovial distribution (periarticular), with a normal or similarly distributed mild increase on delayed images.[184] Gallium uptake has been reported to be increased in active rheumatoid arthritis presumably due to synovial leukocyte concentration (the number of leukocytes in the synovial fluid parallels the severity of the inflammation of the synovial membrane). In uncomplicated rheumatoid arthritis, the uptake of the radiopharmaceutical is usually mild and polyarticular, whereas superimposed infection demonstrates one of the joints with an inordinate amount of increased uptake.[192] Tagged white blood cell studies are sensitive but not specific for rheumatoid inflammation. Increased accumulation in joints is reported 93% of the time when both pain and swelling are present.[378]

LYME ARTHRITIS

Lyme disease is the most common tick-borne disease in the United States.[68] It is caused by the spirochete *Borrelia burgdorferi*, which is carried by the deer tick, *Ixodes dammini*. The disease begins appearing in the summer. The acute arthritis usually has joint swelling out of proportion to the pain and lasts approximately 8 days. Children generally have acute arthritis, which if left untreated, can evolve into a chronic form.[366] The disease generally starts with a characteristic skin lesion, erythema chronicum migrans. This rash is usually accompanied by headache.

Radiographic changes are typical of inflammatory arthritis. In children the abnormality typically involves one or more joints, especially the knees. Radiographic findings include joint effusion, osteoporosis, and absence of significant cartilage destructions and bone erosions.[209] The bone scan shows increased uptake in the affected joints on blood pool and delayed images similar to the other arthritides.[41]

SPONDYLOARTHROPATHIES

The inflammatory arthropathies affect the joints of the axial skeleton as well as the peripheral joints. The absence of rheumatoid factor and rheumatoid nodules help differentiate the spondyloarthropathies from JRA. It is difficult to differentiate seronegative JRA from the spondyloarthropathies.

Childhood spondyloarthropathies include juvenile ankylosing spondylitis, psoriatic arthritis, postinfectious arthritis (Reiter's syndrome), and arthritis associated with inflammatory bowel disease (regional enteritis, ulcerative colitis). Common characteristics of spondyloarthropathies include a family history of the disease, the presence of HLA-B27 antigen, onset in late childhood, predominance in males, a high incidence of sacroiliitis and enthesitis (inflammation of muscular or tendinous insertions on bone), and negative immunoglobulin M (IgM) rheumatoid factor.[311]

Sacroiliitis is usually bilateral and symmetric in ankylosing spondylitis and asymmetric in the other spondyloarthropathies. Early in the course of ankylosing spondylitis, however, joint involvement may be asymmetric or unilateral.[191] Radiographic changes most commonly occur on the iliac side of the joint. The earliest changes are periarticular demineralization and blurring. The lower half of the sacroiliac joint is diarthrodial and can be involved in the synovial inflammatory processes. Pseudowidening can occur due to erosions on one or both sides of the joint, and over time a reactive osteoblastic repair process with joint space narrowing can evolve. Late changes include fusion of the sacroiliac joints and osteoporosis.

The difficulties associated with recognizing early radiographic disease have prompted the use of bone scintigraphy to detect the sacroiliac abnormalities. Quantitative analysis comparing sacroiliac joint uptake with the sacrum is superior to qualitative assessment.[284] The sum of the right and left joints, divided by two times the central sacral counts, produces the final ratio. An alternative method determines the ratio for each joint by dividing activity in the sacroiliac joint region by activity in the sacral region.[327] Generally, positive cases have ratios greater than 1.3:1 or 1.45:1, respectively (depending on the methodology). The validity of the sacroiliac joint-to-sacrum ratios rests on the unproven assumption that patients with inflammatory sacroiliac disease do not have increased uptake in the sacrum. The epiphyses forming the sacroiliac joints fuse around age 25 years and so, in general, the ratios in children are higher.[383] Any increase in uptake from trauma, metabolic disease, or anatomic variations will make the quantitative technique for radionuclide diagnosis of sacroiliitis unreliable. Quantitative SPECT imaging may offer a more accurate way of assessing the presence of inflammatory disease in the sacroiliac joints. The normal values have been reproducible.[106] A preliminary report compared transaxial MRI with radiography and bone scintigraphy.[373] Seventy-six percent of patients with no radiographic signs of early sacroiliitis had changes on MRI. This is compared with detection rates of 57% for SPECT bone imaging and 9% for conventional planar bone scintigraphy.

CHONDROLYSIS

Chondrolysis, or cartilage necrosis, is the destruction or degeneration of the hyaline articular cartilage. It occurs most commonly in the hip. In idiopathic chondrolysis there is usually an insidious onset of pain in the anterior part of the hip, sometimes associated with a limp and stiffness. The laboratory tests including HLA-B27, white blood cell count, erythrocyte sedimentation rate, rheumatoid latex agglutination test, and antinuclear antibody test are usually normal. Idiopathic chondrolysis is much less common than chondrolysis associated with slipped capital femoral epiphysis (SCFE). In SCFE the onset of cartilage necrosis varies widely, ranging from onset before treatment to appearance 8 months after surgery. Chondrolysis in these patients is characterized clinically by increasing stiffness of the hip joint and muscle spasm causing flexion and adduction contractures. Fibrous ankylosis is an end result in severe cases.[222] Secondary chondrolysis has also been described in association with protrusio acetabuli[154] and with Legg-Perthes disease.[83]

Synovial fluid is the main source of nutrition for articular cartilage. The histologic findings of chondrolysis are nonspecific, with fibrillated degeneration of the cartilage, increased vascular formation subchondrally, and a chronic inflammatory response consisting of mild infiltration of plasma cells and fibrosis.[173,182]

The incidence of chondrolysis varies from 1.8% to 55% in patients with SCFE.[171] The more severe the slip and the longer its duration, the more likely the development of secondary chondrolysis.[148] Cartilage necrosis can develop following in situ pinning, closed reduction, and open reduction. Prolonged immobilization may induce chondrolysis secondary to reduction in the production of synovial fluid. Early restoration of regular exercise such as swimming in a heated pool will restore range of motion and can restore lost cartilage with return to normal in as early as 3 months to a year.

The early radiographic signs of chondrolysis include reduction in joint space, subchondral line blurring, and periarticular osteoporosis.[123] Late stages can be associated with ankylosis, subchondral cysts, osteophytes, and deformity. The joint space narrowing in secondary chondrolysis can involve the entire articulation, or it may be isolated to the superior aspect of the joint. Superior joint space diminution is especially common when osteonecrosis is also present. AVN is present in about 14% of patients with secondary chondrolysis. Late in the course of chondrolysis, the growth plates of the proximal femoral epiphyses and the greater and lesser trochanters can close prematurely,[91] presumably secondary to the chronic contiguous hyperemia.

Early phase bone scintigraphy shows increased regional joint uptake, just like any form of synovitis. On delayed images periarticular increased uptake is seen, indicative of the inflammatory process in the joint. The scintigraphic combination of periarticular hyperemia and premature closure of the physis of the greater trochanter was found indicative of chondrolysis complicating SCFE[248] (Fig. 16-11). The degree of periarticular activity in chondrolysis is usually more intense in the active phase of the disease than the usual reactive synovitis that can accompany an uncomplicated SCFE. In certain instances the presence of positive bone scan findings in patients presenting with SCFE has been predictive of subsequent radiographic narrowing of the joint space.

TRAUMA

Fractures

OCCULT FRACTURES OF THE TODDLER

A toddler's fracture has historically been considered a nondisplaced spiral fracture of the tibia in preschool children, characteristically 1 to 3 years of age.[87] Other occult fractures of the toddler, in particular of the calcaneus and cuboid bone, have been recently recognized.[301] They were identified as a consequence of the scintigraphic evaluation of preschool children with lower extremity pain or limp.[8,94] Increased tarsal bone uptake accounted for over 50% of the scintigraphic abnormalities in preschool children with gait disturbances. Correlative radiographic imaging is not usually available because of the tradition of imaging only from the hip to the ankle. Certainly awareness of the frequency of tarsal abnormalities should prompt the inclusion of radiographic images of the feet in the screening examination of the limping preschool child. The toddler's fractures are difficult to identify on plain radiographs. The fracture line in the tibia is thin and the bony elements non-displaced or minimally displaced. The fractures of the small bones of the feet (the cuboid bone and calcaneus) are of the compression type where radiographs show sclerosis, the condensation of trabeculae. The visibility of periosteal reaction along the tubular bones occurs approximately 10 days to several weeks after the acute traumatic event. Radiographic detection of fractures of the feet is most successful in the metatarsal region, where it is possible to observe the cortical infraction.[248] Usually the causative event leading to the toddler's fracture is unwitnessed and not well documented; these fractures probably result during the usual play activities. Jumping from heights and sliding, followed by a difficult landing, can create enough twisting force to cause either the spiral fracture of the tibia or the compression fracture of a foot bone.

Skeletal scintigraphy should be reserved for children with signs or symptoms that suggest inflammation, accompanied by refusal to walk, or unexplained leg pain. Fractures of the tibia typically express increased uptake in the distal two thirds of the bone or diffuse uptake throughout the entire diaphysis[276] (Fig. 16-8). Fractures of the calcaneus and cuboid are readily detected by scintigraphy; in most cases the entire bone manifests increased activity.[27,353,374] Pinhole (high-resolution magnification) imaging can be helpful in resolving the loca-

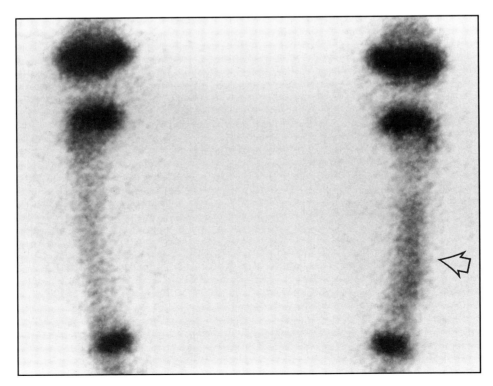

Fig. 16-8.   Toddler fracture of the left tibia in a 15-month-old female. Increased radionuclide uptake is present in a long segment of the diaphysis (*arrow*).

tion of the increased radiotracer uptake in the small bones of the feet.

OCCULT FRACTURES OF THE CARPUS

Occult, or hidden, fractures often involve the carpus, and particularly the scaphoid (navicular) bone in adolescents. Carpal fractures usually result from direct blows. Children have doors close on their hands or are struck by falling objects. These fractures are difficult to detect on conventional radiography when they are nondisplaced. Sclerosis at the fracture site may not be apparent for weeks after the traumatic episode. Some clinicians place the wrist in plaster and if symptoms persist after 3 weeks of immobilization, use bone scintigraphy to prove the presence of the fracture.

Ninety-five percent of closed fractures are scintigraphically positive within 24 hours of the injury.[326] Absence of increased radiotracer concentration at a site of injury 72 hours after the trauma virtually excludes a fracture. In several large series of patients with scaphoid fractures, no false-negative scintigraphic examinations were reported.[324,398] More intense uptake actually is seen in the wrist

at the tenth day following trauma, and maximum activity appears 3 to 5 weeks following trauma.[259] Acute AVN, a well-known complication of scaphoid fractures, is signified by a photopenic proximal segment.[319] This observation is best made on high-resolution magnification (pinhole) images.

PLASTIC BOWING

The radius and ulna of the forearm can exhibit a change in architecture, termed "plastic deformation," as a result of invisible microfractures. Plastic bowing is most common in the forearm[30,70] but also has been reported in less common sites such as the clavicle,[34] the humerus,[323] the mandibular condyle, the femur,[400] the fibula,[257] the tibia,[126] and ribs in children.[52] Plastic bowing of the radius and/or ulna typically occurs when a child falls on the outstretched hand while the wrist is extended. Applied longitudinal compressive forces of low magnitude cause the bone to bend. With removal of the transient force, the bones can return to normal positioning (elastic deformation).[30] Forces greater than maximal bone strength cause obvious fractures. Intermediate forces result in plastic deformation or a bowing that persists when the force is removed.

With plastic bowing, radiographs will show no evidence of new bone formation during the first few weeks after the trauma. There has been report of periosteal reaction occurring 5 weeks after injury.[71] Because bowing occurs in the forearms as a result of falling on the outstretched hand, bowing is usually directed dorsally. In the fibula the bowing can occur posteromedially or anterolaterally depending on the forces involved in the injury. In plastic bowing the scintigram shows diffuse activity along the curvature, allowing differentiation of

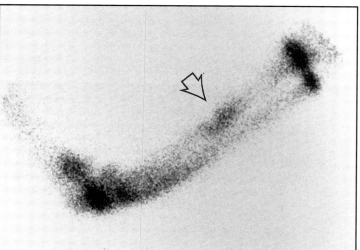

Fig. 16–9. Plastic bowing of the ulna associated with a radial fracture in a 5-year-old male. The radiograph (**A**) shows a midshaft radial fracture (*arrow*) and lateral bowing of both the radius and ulna. The bone scan (**B**) shows focal uptake at the radial fracture site (*arrow*) and diffusely increased uptake in the proximal ulna.

A

B

developmental bowing from a traumatic bend[275] (Fig. 16-9). Scintigraphy may confirm questionable cases of bowing and allow appropriate therapy for relief of pain.

In patients less than 10 years of age, a deformity angulated less than 20 degrees can remodel without intervention. However, correction should be considered in children over 11 years of age and in any child with a deformity greater than 20 degrees.[225]

THE ABUSED CHILD (BATTERED CHILD SYNDROME)

Child abuse is defined as the willful assault of children by their caretakers. Manifestations of child abuse can include intentional physical violence, sexual assaults, neglect, and adverse psychologic situations. This discussion concentrates on injury to the musculoskeletal system, with an emphasis on fracture detection. The majority of physical trauma occurs in children less than 3 years of age.

Radiography has been instrumental in defining mechanisms of abuse and documenting them for medical, legal, and social uses. The osseous skeleton of infants and children has an inherent weakness in the metaphyseal growth complex of the long bones that is vulnerable to injury during violent shaking and hyperextension of the joints. Resulting bone lesions are unique to this age group because of the fragile anatomy of the growing skeleton. Radiographically the skeletal lesions in child abuse tend to be multiple and nearly symmetric. When there have been repeated episodes of trauma, fractures in various phases of healing are identified. The periosteum of the diaphysis is frequently elevated by subperiosteal hemorrhage, and the metaphysis at the zone of provisional calcification is fragmented (corner sign) from twisting or hyperextension of joints, especially the knee and shoulder.

Radionuclide imaging has been successful in identifying bone lesions in the abused child because of its increased sensitivity (25% to 50% over radiography) for detecting occult trauma. Additional information can be garnered from the multiphase bone scan by performing early angiographic images of the calvarium to identify the mass effect of a subdural hematoma (from head trauma) and obtaining 20 minutes of tissue phase imaging of the renal beds to recognize urinary extravasation or obstruction secondary to soft-tissue trauma. The bone scan has been advocated by some as the best screening method for child abuse.[117,361]

On the other hand, there are those who advocate a skeletal survey as the primary study for child abuse. They point out that the characteristics of metaphyseal fracture can be difficult to demonstrate on bone scans because of the proximity of the growth plate.[142] With the improved resolution and sensitivity of current gamma cameras, the likelihood of missing corner or "bucket handle" fractures can be reduced. Trauma can distort the configuration of the growth plate, giving it a spheric or elongated appearance.[368] Sometimes high-resolution pinhole imaging of the metaphyses will detect growth plate fractures. The injuries of the rib cage occur at three principal sites: (1) paraspinal, usually between T4 and T9[348]; (2) axillary,

predominantly in the lower rib cage; and (3) along the costocartilaginous junctions from the second to ninth ribs. Thoracic spine compression injuries are characteristic of a shaking type of trauma. Periosteal injuries occur in the diaphyses of the extremities and can result from holding the child while performing the shaking maneuvers. There are reports documenting the insensitivity of bone scanning in the detection of skull fractures.[312] For this reason, plain radiographs of the skull should be included when scintigraphy is used to screen for child abuse.[136] The inability to detect skull fractures is attributed to the spheric shape of the skull, superimposed activity of the contralateral side, minimal bone displacement, and lack of periosteal reaction. At least four projections of the skull should be obtained on the scintigram to screen for child abuse. The radionuclide bone survey has some other potential limitations from a legal standpoint: inability to be specific in determining stages of healing, inability to detect completely healed fractures, and difficulty in identifying minimal symmetric metaphyseal injuries.

Because it is more readily obtainable, the radiographic skeletal survey is often the initial skeletal screening method. In the presence of obvious acute soft-tissue or skeletal injuries, the radiographic survey should be performed immediately. Bone scintigraphy is added when more information is required. If the physical signs are minimal, there is a high index of suspicion for abuse, and the radiographs are negative (or equivocal), bone scintigraphy is indicated. If the bone scan is normal, no further imaging is required. If there are positive foci on bone scintigraphy, additional correlative radiographs should be obtained. Radiography and scintigraphy are complementary techniques for localizing all of the lesions of child abuse. Bone scintigraphy has increased sensitivity for recognizing periosteal trauma of the extremities, and trauma of traditionally difficult areas to evaluate radiographically such as the spine, scapula, pelvis, and ribs.[348,361] In one series,[180] 50 children had both bone scans and radiographs. Among these children, there were 41 fractures. The skeletal survey detected 52% and bone scans detected 88%. Because both radiography and bone scintigraphy have false-negative results, it follows that the two studies together are more effective than either one alone. This is especially important in children less than 2 years of age, and Conway suggests that both studies may be needed.[63]

STRESS FRACTURE AND "SHIN SPLINTS"

The incidence of stress fractures has increased in recent years with the growing participation of both young girls and boys in sports. Most injuries affect the lower extremities (tibiae, fibulae, and metatarsals) of athletic children 10 years of age or older. In recent times stress fractures are more common in girls than boys.[299]

A fatigue fracture is the result of secondary forces such as vigorous muscular contractions rather than direct trauma. When the bone-muscle system is stressed, changes of bone and muscle hypertrophy result in increased tone or strength of the system. Fatigue fractures occur when bones with normal elasticity undergo stress overload because bone hypertrophy occurs at a slower rate than the muscular system. Shin splints pathophysiologically are either considered to be a musculotendinous irritation or periosteal inflammation and not a stress fracture.[79] The most common definition of the *shin splint* invokes the focal periostitis at the insertions of soleus muscle and its fascia. The tendinous portion of the soleus makes up the anterior half of the Achilles tendon. The aponeurotic fascia envelopes the soleus muscle and extends along the posterior medial border of the tibia for three quarters of its length, where it attaches, presumably through Sharpey fibers.[271]

In the acute fracture phase (lasting 3 to 4 weeks), bone scintigraphy shows a poorly defined area of mildly increased uptake.[62,384] Similar bone scan patterns can be seen in cases of osteomyelitis, metastasis, periostitis, osteoid osteoma, bone infarct, bone tumor, and fibrous dysplasia. Confirmatory roentgenographic changes should not be expected with acute stress fractures. In the subacute phase, which lasts approximately 8 to 12 weeks, there is linear collection of increased radiotracer activity at the fracture location. The third, or healing, phase shows gradual diminution and dissipation of the increased activity. In a recent study a four-grade scintigraphic classification of stress fractures was developed.[401] Grade I lesions showed an ill-defined cortical increase in uptake. Grade II lesions exhibited a larger, well-defined cortical area of moderately increased activity. Grade III fractures consisted of a wide fusiform corticomedullary region of increased activity. In grade IV lesions there was an extensive transmedullary area of increased uptake. Grade I and II fractures healed more completely and in shorter intervals. Partial or incomplete regression occurred most often in grade III and IV fractures. Ninety-six percent of grade I and seventy-nine percent of grade II lesions were negative on radiography. Conversely, 76% and 100% of Grade III and IV fractures, respectively, showed positive roentgenograms. All three phases (angiographic, tissue phase, and delayed phase) can be very active in a stress fracture, particularly in the higher grades.[304]

The scintigraphic pattern of a shin splint has been varied and nonspecific. Spencer et al reported shin splints with four types of abnormalities: focal tibial lesions, diffuse tibial and fibular lesions, and fibular lesions with increased uptake in the bones of the feet.[351] The "double-stripe" sign of parallel cortical bands of activity along the midshaft of the tibia,[220] increased activity posteromedially, in the upper third of the tibia,[277] and increased uptake in the posteromedial cortex of the middle third of the tibia have been described as more specific signs of shin splints.[161]

INSUFFICIENCY FRACTURES

Insufficiency fractures occur in patients with underlying disorders (e.g., osteoporosis, osteogenesis imperfecta, steroid therapy, scurvy, osteomalacia, rheumatoid arthritis, radiation) that weaken bone to the point where focal physiologic stress exceeds the decreased elastic resistance of the underlying bone. The lower extremities are particularly vulnerable in patients with neuromuscular deficiencies such as meningomyelocele, muscular dystrophy, and congenital insensitivity to pain. Patients who have undergone surgery for osteosarcoma can develop stress lesions in the bones of the contralateral extremity, pelvis, ipsilateral leg, and arms. Factors that lead to concentration of excessive forces include shift of weight-bearing to the contralateral leg, leg preservation surgery resulting in shortening or loss of effective joint motion, the use of leg-lengthening devices, osteotomies, and the use of crutches.[2]

Insufficiency fractures are difficult to see on plain films because they occur in an environment of undermineralization or deficient osteoid matrix. A cortical break as a manifestation of an insufficiency fracture is the easiest to detect. Looser zones are incompletely mineralized stress infractions that are usually symmetric and occur in the bowed bones of osteomalacia and deformities of fibrous dysplasia. The bilaterally symmetric looser zones are most common in the axillary borders of the scapulae, pubic rami, and femoral necks.

Bone scintigraphy is often required to identify insufficiency fractures. In osteoporotic individuals the detection of an acute fracture may take longer than in the normally mineralized individual (72 hours as opposed to 24 hours). It is better to delay imaging to 3 or 4 hours after the injection with radiopharmaceutical to allow sufficient accumulation of activity in the bone matrix.

SPONDYLOLYSIS

The term *spondylolysis* refers to a lytic cleft in the pars interarticularis of the vertebral neural arch. In most instances the lesion occurs at L4 to L5 and is more commonly bilateral than unilateral. When bilateral involvement occurs, spondylolisthesis, the displacement of one vertebra forward on another (particularly L5 on S1) can occur. In most instances the development of the defect is assumed to be related to trauma because the abnormality has never been demonstrated in the fetus and rarely in the young child.[31] The defect has been classified as isthmic or dysplastic. In the dysplastic type there is an associated congenital developmental abnormality (hypoplastic pedicles, spina bifida) of the neural arch of L5 or upper sacrum. Defects of the pars interarticularis have been reported to be greater in athletes (e.g., gymnasts, wrestlers, ballet dancers) than in the general pediatric population and the spondylolytic defect has been classified as a fatigue fracture. However, there may be a congenital weakness in the osseous matrix of the pars interarticularis that predisposes some individuals with varying degrees of expressivity to the development of the spondylolysis.[392] This theory is supported by the increased incidence of spondylolysis found in Alaskan Eskimos and in some families.[338,356] Abnormal forces or stresses generated in idiopathic scoliosis,[336] Scheuermann's disease,[297] and posterior spinal fusions[24] are implicated in the increased associations.

Stress-induced osseous changes in the pars interarticularis can result in microfractures that cannot be detected radiographically during the earliest stage of spondylolysis. This response to stress may be manifested on the radiograph, during this early stage, as reactive bone formation. Continued stress results in further bone exhaustion, inadequate reinforcement, and eventual fracture or lysis.

Sometimes a patient with unilateral lysis will show normal scintigraphic activity at this site, but have increased activity on the contralateral side where an area of stress has been created. The sclerosis and bone formation can occur in the pars interarticularis, or the pedicle and lamina on the side of the increased radiotracer uptake. The response in bone density and overgrowth of

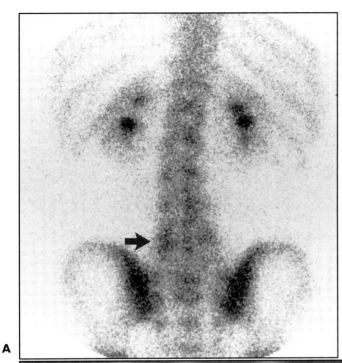

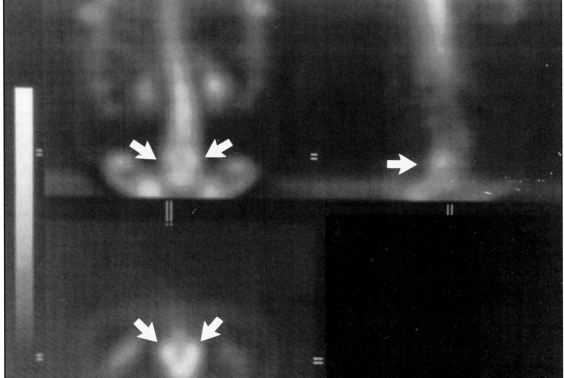

Fig. 16-10. Bilateral spondylolysis in a 13-year-old female with back pain. The posterior planar images (**A**) show mildly increased uptake at L5 on the left (*arrow*). The SPECT images (**B**) indicate bilateral abnormality and clarify the pars location (coronal, sagittal, and prone axial reconstructions) (*arrows*).

the pedicle and lamina in the presence of a defective pars interarticularis on the opposite side probably represents a physiologic response or stress fracture in the presence of an unstable neural arch.[340] Unless the inciting physical activity is discontinued, this site will ultimately develop a fracture.[293] Unilateral sclerosis in association with pain has to be differentiated from osteoid osteoma and osteoblastoma, the usual causes in children and young adults.

Bone scintigraphy plays an important role in the early detection of stress fractures of the pars interarticularis. Posterior oblique views of the lumbar spine help localize abnormal uptake and should be done in addition to anterior and posterior images.[92] In the early stages of spondylolysis when conventional radiographs are normal, there is a poorly defined, slightly increased region of radioactivity that occurs when rapid osteoclastic resorption exceeds the osteoblastic response. Bone scintigraphy may be normal even when lytic changes are evident on radiography. The intensity of uptake depends on the degree of bone repair. It is assumed that the lack of uptake means the lesion is old or stabilized. SPECT, with its propensity to demonstrate small foci of increased radiotracer accumulation, is advocated in patients with low back pain.[29] A tomographic study reconstructed in the transaxial, coronal, and sagittal planes through the area of pain permits detection of very mild increases in activity that are not evident on routine planar views or high-resolution magnification studies (Fig. 16-10). A negative SPECT study seems to exclude the diagnosis of spondylolysis as the etiology of back pain. In a recent study 56% of positive bone scans for low back pain in adolescent athletes were revealed only by SPECT.[15]

PSEUDARTHROSIS IN SPINAL FUSION

Posterior spinal fusion is performed in the pediatric population to stabilize spondylolisthesis, to arrest curve progression in scoliosis, and to stabilize "burst" fractures of the spine. Thirty to forty percent of patients report recurrent back pain after fusion. Pseudarthrosis is the most common postsurgical complication in the first years after spinal fusion. Arthrodesis can alter the biomechanics of the spine and create a compensatory increase in motion in segments adjacent to the fusion, even many years after the initial surgery. A deficiency in the fusion can allow progression of spinal curvature or further spondylolisthesis.

Defects in the fusion mass appear as linear lucencies on radiographs. Typically these are horizontal and do not have sclerotic margins. It is difficult to confidently diagnose pseudarthrosis before bone graft has completely matured. This usually requires at least a year.

Bone scans show focally increased uptake for 6 months to a year after surgery, as the fusion graft material is incorporated into new bone. The most accurate scintigraphic results are obtained 1 year or more after surgery, when the graft has matured. Without the diffuse activity of reparative new bone, the local osteoblastic response of pseudarthrosis becomes obvious. The accumulation of the bone radiotracer depends on sufficient

motion or stress at the site of pseudarthrosis. There have been inconsistent results in planar scintigraphy with a high false-positive rate in one series[144] and a false-negative rate in another series.[140] One exception is when the increased uptake occurs at the site of insertion of a rod hook or the distal limbs of a Luque apparatus anchored in the iliac bones. Because of micromotion and/or stress, it is not unusual to find increased activity at these locations. On planar images it may be difficult to differentiate increased activity in the fusion mass from localized osteoblastic responses of another etiology. Separation of the thin layers of bone in the spinal fusion from the remainder of the vertebrae can be accomplished with SPECT and enhances the detection of foci of mildly increased uptake.[345] In patients with chronic pseudarthrosis, the bone scan may revert to normal in a few years. There are late painful effects of spinal fusion surgery, and previously normal SPECT can revert to positive many years after the fusion. The increased uptake occurs in the vertebral bodies and apophyseal joints in the free motion segments adjacent to the fused segments. This has been observed as early as 8 months and as long as 30 years after the surgery.[96]

Slipped Capital Femoral Epiphysis

Slipping of the capital femoral epiphysis, sometimes referred to as epiphysiolysis, is the most common hip disorder in adolescents during their period of rapid growth. It occurs while the physis is still open, and involves progressive displacement of the femoral head in relation to the neck. Often the onset is insidious, and the patients do not seek medical help until significant slipping has occurred. The incidence of slipped capital femoral epiphysis (SCFE) is reported to be 2 cases per 100,000 and is twice as common in adolescent boys (median, 13 years) as girls (median, 11 years).[44] Black children are affected more frequently than white children.[22]

The epiphyseal slip is often difficult to diagnose on a single film in the frontal projection. It mimics a Salter type I fracture with a slightly widened epiphyseal plate. The addition of a film in frog-leg lateral projection aids in the detection of minor grades of slip. With further slipping the epiphysis moves posterolaterally in reference to the femoral neck, and there is no difficulty in identifying advanced grades radiographically.

Bone scintigraphy is usually not needed to make the diagnosis of SCFE. A small percentage of patients may undergo scintigraphy when the radiologic examination is equivocal, incomplete or incorrectly interpreted, or if a complication such as AVN and/or chondrolysis is suspected. High-resolution (pinhole) anterior magnification views of the hip in neutral and frog-leg lateral positions should be performed to correlate any area of photopenia (representing AVN) with anatomic position of the femoral head on the radiograph (Fig. 16-11). The abnormal posteromedial relationship of the femoral head to the femoral neck is readily visible when there is major displacement. There is usually increased uptake in the physis and in the adjacent proximal femoral metaphyses.[113] This pattern is thought to reflect the increased metabolic activity at the site of cartilage plate disruption. Almost all scans of SCFE show increased periarticular activity, which represents an associated reactive synovitis: this may eventually evolve into chondrolysis.[248]

Management after treatment (traction, cast immobilization, pinning, operative manipulation) can be guided by knowledge of the physiologic status of the femoral head and physis. The use of scintigraphy in assessment of adequacy of treatment (fusion of growth plate) and assessment of persistent pain (complications of AVN and chondrolysis) is helpful. In the patient with a chronic slip and continued pain, knowledge of activity in the growth plate can help determine the necessity of continued immobilization or pinning. The scintigraphic closure of the growth plate predates the radiographic fusion by many weeks[367] and may be helpful in directing subsequent activities or even pin removal.

Reflex Neurovascular Dystrophy

Reflex neurovascular dystrophy (RND) is an extremity pain syndrome of unknown etiology. The syndrome has many synonyms including causalgia, reflex sympathetic dystrophy, posttraumatic pain syndrome, algoneurodystrophy, painful osteoporosis, shoulder-hand syndrome, and Sudeck's atrophy.[160] It has been reported after nerve injury, trauma, surgery, and central neurologic damage in children, but a recognizable antecedent event is rare. In children the lower extremity is predominantly affected,[210]

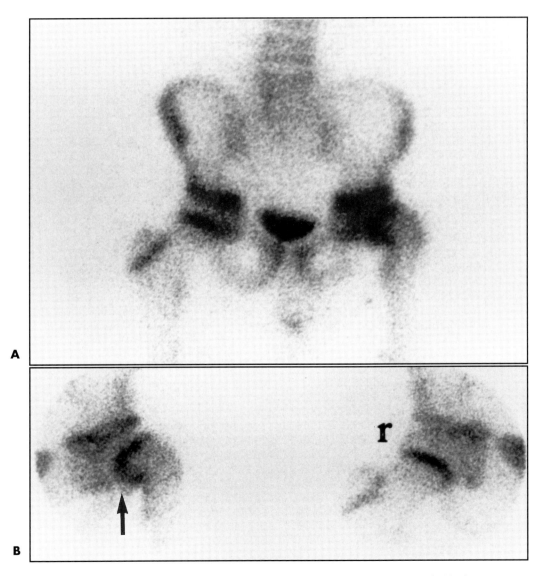

Fig. 16–11.   Slipped capital femoral epiphysis in a 14-year-old male. The large-field-of-view image (**A**) shows generally increased activity around the left hip joint. The pinhole image (**B**) confirms uptake in the slipped epiphysis. Note the vertical orientation of the growth plate uptake in the left femur (*arrow*). Note as well the lack of activity in the greater trochanter on the left. This reflects the presence of chondrolysis at the time of diagnosis.

and girls are more often affected than boys. The clinical features of RND in the pediatric population include burning pain and tenderness, vasomotor instability (mottled blush or erythematous discoloration, hypothermia, hyperhidrosis, and decreased peripheral pulses), and sometimes swelling. Trophic skin changes are usually absent.[19] Radiographs in children are usually normal.

Bone scintigraphy in adults with RND have classically demonstrated increased activity in the extremity.[78] Different stages of RND in adults could be defined on the basis of three-phase bone scintigraphy: the early stage (up to 20 weeks) with increased activity in all three phases, the middle stage (20 to 60 weeks) with flip-flop phenomenon of decreased early phase and increased delayed phase activity, and the last stage with (60 to 100 weeks) with reduced early phase and normalization of the delayed phase.[210] In many reports in children, decreased activity has been observed as soon as a week and up to 14 months following the onset of symptoms.[78,124,212,286] In children the RND appears to represent a different neurovascular event than in adults. The cause of the diffuse decreased tracer uptake is uncertain. Care must be taken in making the diagnosis of RND, because this finding is also noted with decreased use of an extremity and occurs with lack of weight-bearing and immobilization. The bone scan is more sensitive than the radiograph in showing the abnormality of RND in children (72% vs. 36%).[287] Treatment in children is usually conservative and supportive, ranging from mild analgesics and outpatient counseling therapy to oral steroids, vasodilators, and inpatient physical therapy.

Posttraumatic Growth Plate Aberrations

In children injury to the physis (traumatic, infectious, or vascular) may be complicated by growth arrest. This is manifested by premature ossification (fusion) of part or all of the cartilage gap between the epiphysis and the metaphysis (partial and total epiphysiodesis, respectively). The most common cause of partial physeal (growth plate) arrest is a fracture.[310] Partial growth plate arrest is produced when an osseous or cartilaginous bridge forms across the plate. If the bar is located laterally in a physis and the normal physis continues to grow medially, a progressive valgus deformity results. If the bar is medially or anteriorly located, varus and recurvatum, respectively, occur in a similar process. The Salter type IV injury, which crosses both the metaphysis and epiphysis, has the greatest potential for bar formation, even when the fragments are properly reduced. Salter type III and IV fractures may affect only the central portion of the plate, leading to central tethering, a cupped metaphysis, and shortening. Salter type V compression injuries result in complete rather than partial closure of the physis and no angular deformity.[47]

Radiographic, conventional tomographic studies, CT, and MRI of the physis yield useful anatomic information. However, scintigraphy is the one imaging technique that provides direct physiologic information (Fig. 16-12). Scintigraphic images can be stored in a computer and analyzed quantitatively for growth plate activity. A band of increased tracer uptake is quite evident in the active, normal physis. This accumulation of the bone-seeking agent actually occurs at the margin of the cartilage plate in the zone of provisional calcification. Growth plate disturbances are represented by alterations in plate uptake. Initially the insult causes increased uptake (stimulation), which is followed by progressively decreasing uptake until closure.[146] A study of the growth plates should include tissue-phase and delayed images in anterior and posterior views. Magnification should be performed either electronically or with pinhole collimation (100,000 to 150,000 counts) when looking for partial arrest. Qualitative assessment is made by comparing the affected growth plate with the contralateral normal side. The extremities must be symmetrically positioned. Assessment of plate activity becomes quite subjective when there is systemic or metabolic disease that produces changes in the physes. Inactivity in an extremity (secondary to casting or lack of weight-bearing) will lead to some decrease in growth plate activity, but this is accompanied by a proportional decrease throughout the limb. Quantitative techniques applied to the growth plate employ regions-of-interest profiles and ratios. An apex view of the distal femoral growth plate can be generated with the pinhole collimator directed at the flexed knee joint. For this one physis, histograms have been created to provide a functional map showing the size and location of abnormalities.[164] Bone SPECT has been reported as useful in the mapping of the distribution of plate activity in several planes.[395]

Para–osteoarthropathy

Heterotopic or ectopic bone formation (para-osteoarthropathy, myositis ossificans, or ossifying fibromyopathy) represents ossification in soft tissues where bone formation does not normally occur. Pediatric patients at risk include the child and adolescent with spinal cord injuries, cranial trauma, central nervous system lesions, and hip replacements. In one study 15% of head-injured children and adolescents were reported to develop ectopic bone.[37] Myositis ossificans circumscripta is localized to a single muscle and occurs in patients without underlying neurologic impairment. These patients present with a soft-tissue mass, consisting of muscle being replaced by ossifying fibrous tissue; this may represent a diagnostic dilemma.[291] Malignancy can be suspected radiographically and histologically if a biopsy is performed at an early stage or away from the center of the lesion.

The etiology of heterotopic ossification is uncertain. It is believed that primitive cells of mesenchymal origin located in the soft tissue transform into bone-forming cells as a result of trauma. Heterotopic bone formation from rapidly progressive metaplastic osteogenesis is associated with some chondrogenesis. Gross pathologic studies have shown the ectopic bone is most often located in the periphery of muscles and originates in connective tissues between muscle fascicles.

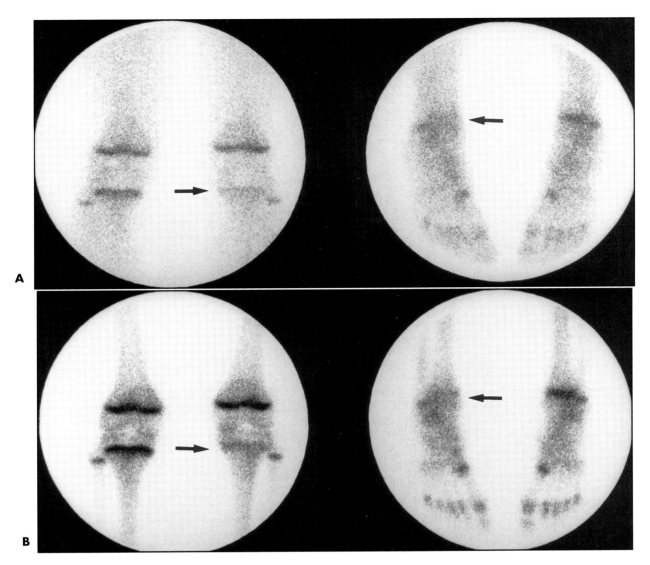

Fig. 16-12. Traumatic and surgical growth plate closure in a 14-year-old male. Tissue-phase images (**A**) and delayed bone images (**B**) of the knees and ankles show absent growth plate activity in the distal right tibia and proximal left tibia (*arrows*). After premature closure of the distal tibial plate secondary to fracture, the contralateral proximal tibial plate was closed surgically to prevent progressive leg length discrepancy. *(From Harcke HT and Mandell GA: Scintigraphic evaluation of the growth plate.* Semin Nucl Med, *1993; 23:266; with permission.)*

In the acute phase of para-osteoarthropathy, plain radiographs may show no abnormality. The appearance of immature heterotopic bone is characterized by indistinct margins between nontrabeculated ossified tissue and the surrounding soft tissue. Mature areas of ossification are characterized by well-defined trabeculae and distinct margins. The roentgenographic appearance of the ossifying process cannot accurately predict the maturity. The most frequent location for heterotopic ossification is in the iliac and iliopsoas muscles adjacent to the hip. Ossification in the vastus medialis and vastus intermedius muscles tends to be bulky, encircling the femoral shaft. Underlying bone may be unremarkable except for demineralization.

Heterotopic ossification in the active phase shows increase in radiotracer uptake on the bone scan. In the early stage the increased activity is present in all three phases of the bone scan. Theoretically, increased uptake of the isotope should be detectable within a week of the initial trauma.[300] The first two phases (angiographic and tissue phase) can be active, and delayed phase can be normal. If only delayed images were obtained, the soft-tissue abnormality would be missed. Conversely, delayed images with soft-tissue uptake reflects a process different from osteomyelitis and cellulitis where early images are also positive. When heterotopic bone is excised before maturity, there is a high recurrence rate. Serial bone scintigraphy has been used to determine the maturity of heterotopic bone. Decreasing activity and uptake equal to normal bone indicates maturity, implying that it is appropriate to schedule the surgical removal of the ectopic ossification.[375] Gallium scintigraphy can be misleading in paraplegics, quadriplegics, and comatose patients when searching for infection because heterotopic ossification can accumulate the radiotracer even before radiographically detectable calcification occurs; the site can be mistaken for an abscess.[86,328]

Osgood-Schlatter Disease

Osgood-Schlatter disease is a common disorder in active adolescents, characterized by pain and swelling at the tibial tuberosity. Boys are noted to have a higher incidence, and in 25% to 50% of all cases the lesions are bilateral. The etiology is attributed to a traumatic insult to the tendon at its insertion into the tibial tuberosity. A shearing force and abnormal stresses applied to the patellar tendon result in ligamentous tearing, hemorrhage, and cartilage avulsion. In long-standing cases, bone production occurs in the contused tendon.

On plain radiography there is swelling and indistinctness of the patellar tendon acutely. Irregular ossification can occasionally be visualized at the site of attachment of the tendon to the tibial tubercle. The soft-tissue changes are always present, and the bone pathology is present in approximately one third of cases. Scintigraphy is not used in the diagnosis but the process might be encountered on scans done for other reasons. The tissue phase and/or delayed images demonstrate accumulation of soft-tissue activity in the patellar tendon region. The mechanism of radiopharmaceutical deposition is not known but probably depends on hyperemia and microscopic calcification in the tendon.

VASCULAR DISEASE AND RELATED CONDITIONS

Idiopathic Femoral Head Necrosis (Legg-Perthes Disease)

The AVN is probably related to the interruption of blood supply to the proximal femoral epiphysis. Multiple or repetitive ischemic events have been postulated. Contributing local factors, such as prior trauma and inflammation (synovitis), have also been implicated. Because bone maturation is significantly delayed in the majority of children, some constitutional factor may contribute to the evolution of the ischemia. The exact etiology of this disorder is difficult to define because it appears to be clinically silent initially. The symptoms of pain and limited motion become prominent later, weeks to months after the onset of the AVN. Radiographic examination is insensitive and nonspecific for vascular changes in bone. Eighty percent of affected children are males between 4 and 8 years of age. The peak incidence is between 5 and 7 years of age.[13] From 10% to 13% of

patients have bilateral disease.[102]

The changing pattern of the vascular supply to the femoral head during growth may explain the vulnerability of the proximal epiphysis to AVN. The major blood supply to the infant femoral head and neck is derived from the multiple small branches of the medial and lateral femoral circumflex arteries, which either pass through or around the physis.[58] By the time the child has reached 2 or 3 years of age, the femoral neck has become elongated and the physis is intraarticular.[294] Major femoral head perfusion now comes from the superior capsular branches (superior retinacular and lateral epiphyseal arteries) of the medial circumflex artery, and compromise of the circulation to the epiphysis is theoretically more likely. With regression of the lateral circumflex system and development of the medial circumflex artery, the blood supply in the child between 4 and 9 years of age preferentially perfuses the posterior half of the femoral head and predisposes the anterior lateral half to ischemia. Later when the physis starts closing, the barrier to metaphyseal-epiphyseal anastomoses is removed and idiopathic AVN does not occur.[294]

There are no pathognomonic radiographic changes in the early stage of the disease, and for up to 4 to 6 weeks the only abnormal findings are those of synovitis: lateral displacement of the femoral head, widening of the medial joint space, and perhaps bulging of the lateral capsular fat/muscle planes. This is followed by the avascular state with an increase in density of part or all of the femoral epiphysis. The increased density most likely relates to lack of removal of mineral from the epiphysis secondary to the loss of normal blood supply. Sclerosis of the femoral head may also be due to osteoblastic new bone formation during early revascularization. When a subchondral fissure develops, the diagnosis is certain. This most likely represents a fracture secondary to the softened avascular epiphysis. The femoral head then fragments into relatively dense regions of osteoid and new bone, interspersed among areas of rarefaction and resorption (the fragmented stage).

Positive bone scintigraphy predates plain radiographic changes by 4 to 6 weeks.[17] The earliest scintigraphic sign is decreased uptake (photopenia) in either part or all of the femoral head (Fig. 16-13). Bone scans will reliably diagnose Legg-Perthes disease; there is a sensitivity of 98% and a specificity of 95%.[365] The bone scan clarifies radiographic femoral head sclerosis with dead bone depicted as cold areas and new bone characterized with increased activity. It is essential that the hips are evaluated with anterior neutral and frog-leg lateral views using a pinhole collimator or high-resolution magnification. Small areas of photopenia are not adequately resolved on routine planar images. The size of the photopenic defect often corresponds to the extent of subchondral fissure or fracture.[102] Revascularization or increased activity on scintigraphy also can predate radiologic evidence of new bone formation (average, 5.5 months).[81] There are two principal mechanisms of revascularization: the recanalization of existing vessels (occurring within minutes to days of the ischemic event), and neovascularization via

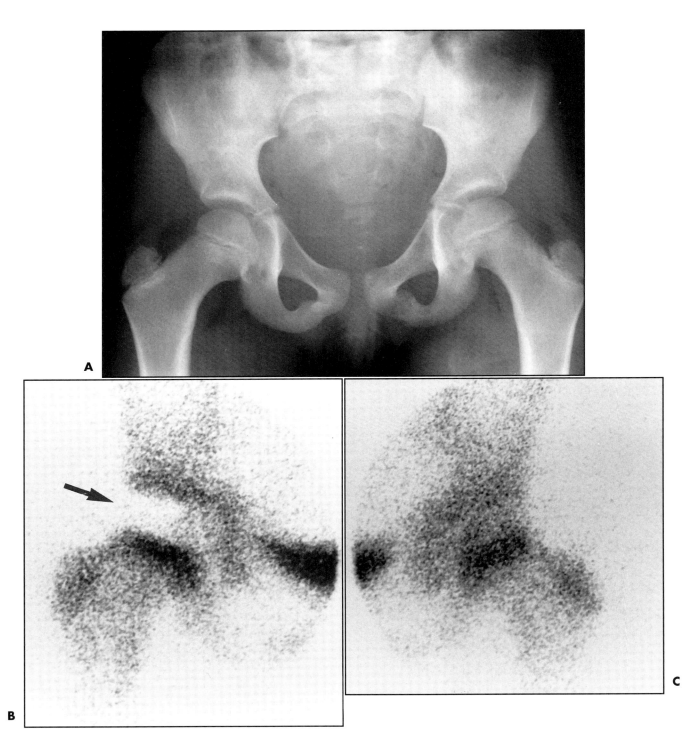

Fig. 16-13. Idiopathic avascular necrosis of the femoral head (Legg-Perthes disease) in a 5-year-old male. The radiograph (**A**) shows no bone abnormality. The pinhole image of the right hip (**B**) reveals no uptake in the capital femoral epiphysis (*arrow*). The normal left hip image (**C**) is provided for comparison.

small branches of the lateral circumflex artery (occurring over months to years).[62] The appearance of a lateral column of activity on the anterior projection that disappears on the frog lateral view is characteristic of recanalization of already existing vessels (medial circumflex cir-

culation). The epiphysis is eventually revascularized from the lateral column medially and anteriorly. A markedly delayed revascularization process indicates absence of recanalization. Initially there is widening of the band of physeal activity, indicating extension of radiotracer deposition through the growth plate into the base of the epiphysis as new vessels form (lateral circumflex circulation). As neovascularization continues, there is extension of uptake into the dome of the epiphysis, described as "mushrooming." With either or both revascularization processes, the entire femoral head eventually achieves complete perfusion and this results in a less voluminous epiphysis with diffusely increased (new bone) activity that matches the pattern of radiographic ossification. Scintigraphs can become normal as early as 10 months after the onset of the disease.

Sickle Cell Hemoglobinopathy

Patients with sickle cell hemoglobinopathies have one factor in common: the presence of the sickle form of hemoglobin (hemoglobin S).[382] A genetic mutation results in the autosomal recessive inheritance of the capability to synthesize abnormal hemoglobin S in erythrocytes. When subjected to hypoxemia, these erythrocytes manifest increased viscosity and sickling. The skeleton in S-S and S-C disease is affected by marrow hyperplasia, infarction, AVN, and osteomyelitis.[335] Osteomyelitis, an uncommon complication of sickle cell disease, can be difficult to distinguish clinically and radiographically from bone infarction or bone crisis without infarct.

From 6 months to 7 years of age, predominantly the long bones (femur, tibia, and humerus)[82] are affected by either infarction or osteomyelitis. Segments of the osseous pelvis and sternum may also be affected in the toddler age bracket.[14,250] In children under 1 year of age, sickle cell dactylitis, or the hand-foot syndrome, occurs and involves the metacarpals, metatarsals, and phalanges most often with infarction. Necrotic bone marrow, however, is often a fertile site for secondary infection, so pathophysiologically both sterile and infected areas of infarction can be present. *S. aureus* is the usual infecting organism, but *Salmonella* (an unusual etiology in the normal population) is a frequent pathogen in cases of osteomyelitis in sickle cell patients. The epiphyses of the femoral and humeral heads are frequently affected by compromised blood supply in S-S and S-C disease.

In the long bones plain films usually are not helpful in differentiating acute osteomyelitis from infarction. Swelling is usually the initial radiographic finding in both infarction and infection. With infarction after approximately 2 weeks, patchy radiolucency in the shaft and a fine periosteal reaction may be seen surrounding the bone. There are many late radiographic signs of subacute or chronic infarction including periosteal reaction, endosteal sclerosis, central vertebral end plate depression, and sternal segment cupping.[14] Expressions of marrow hyperplasia in children 7 to 13 years of age consist of widening of the diploic space of the skull with inner and outer table thickening, increased trabeculation and broadening of ribs, and cortical thinning of the metaphyses of long bones. In children older than 13 years of age, bone marrow hyperplasia can result in osteopenic vertebrae with concavities of the upper and lower margins ("fish vertebrae"). Ischemia to the end plates results

in "H-type" vertebrae.

Bone scintigraphy, even when performed with three-phase technique, can be inconclusive in differentiating osteomyelitis from infarction in the patient with hemoglobinopathy. Increased activity, in general, is nonspecific and can represent either an older healing sterile infarct or bone reaction to osteomyelitis. Foci of decreased activity can be seen in acute infarctions (impaired blood supply) as well as early osteomyelitis (purulent material under pressure in the marrow). Only when there is precise documentation of clinical course and the scan manifests a typical metaphyseal area of increased uptake can osteomyelitis be accurately diagnosed. Subacute sterile infarction can mimic osteomyelitis on bone scan with increased reparative uptake in the metaphyses. The spleen takes up the bone-seeking agent in patients with functional asplenia secondary to the microcalcifications in multiple infarctions.[101] Accumulation of the bone radiotracer in enlarged kidneys has also been described in sickle cell anemia secondary to circulating iron complexes and repeated transfusions.[359]

As the bone scan alone is usually not diagnostic, the addition of other tracers or imaging modalities (CT and MRI)[352] is employed to improve the accuracy of differentiating infection from infarction. The combined use of technetium-99m bone imaging and gallium imaging can successfully differentiate healing infarction from osteomyelitis.[3,7] In bone infarction, gallium accumulation is slightly increased, reduced, or absent when matched to an area of increased, reduced, or absent uptake on bone scintigraphy. Gallium accumulation is noticeably increased in the area of infection, regardless of whether the bone scan shows slightly increased, normal, or decreased activity.[7] Gallium can also be used in combination with marrow scanning using technetium-99m sulfur colloid.[335] When the colloidal radiopharmaceutical is injected intravenously, the reticuloendothelial (RE) cell system including the cells in the red marrow (10% to 15% of the RE system) accumulates the tracer by phagocytosis. There is always decreased uptake of this radiotracer in the case of infarction. Both gallium and marrow scintigraphy can be photopenic in acute infarction. Older infarcts, which are photopenic on marrow scans, exhibit normal gallium uptake. Osteomyelitis at a site of infarction results in increased gallium uptake in the area of photopenia on the marrow scan.

The addition of white blood cell tagging should be effective in differentiating infection in a patient with previous bone infarcts and equivocal areas on bone scan.[98] The tagged leukocyte study can be specific because it does not reflect bone osteogenesis and reflects only the accumulation of white blood cells into an infectious process. A limited number of cases have been presented in the literature.[391] The tagged white blood cell study seems to overcome the problem with gallium localization in healing bone, where increased uptake does not necessarily imply infection. In children a tagged white blood cell study probably should be reserved for instances when the diagnosis of osteomyelitis is strongly suspected but cannot be established by the usual methods (Fig. 16-14).

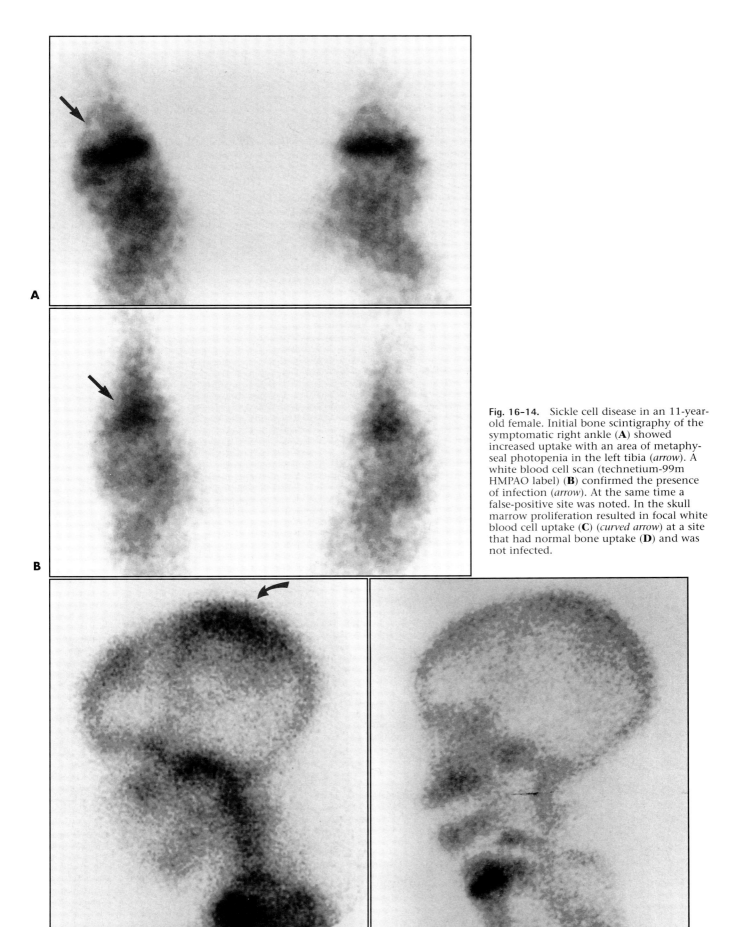

Fig. 16-14. Sickle cell disease in an 11-year-old female. Initial bone scintigraphy of the symptomatic right ankle (**A**) showed increased uptake with an area of metaphyseal photopenia in the left tibia (*arrow*). A white blood cell scan (technetium-99m HMPAO label) (**B**) confirmed the presence of infection (*arrow*). At the same time a false-positive site was noted. In the skull marrow proliferation resulted in focal white blood cell uptake (**C**) (*curved arrow*) at a site that had normal bone uptake (**D**) and was not infected.

Vascular Related Conditions

OSTEOCHONDROSES

The osteochondroses are a group of idiopathic conditions characterized by disordered enchondral ossification occurring at an otherwise normal site. The process can lead to both chondrogenesis or osteogenesis abnormalities. Osteochondroses fall into three categories: normal variation, growth disturbance with no evidence of necrosis, and osteonecrosis.[39]

The irregular, normally dense apophysis of the calcaneus has been referred to as Sever's disease. The pain is in actuality associated with the attachment of the plantar aponeurosis, along the Achilles tendon above its insertion, and at the posterosuperior angle of the calcaneus. Sever's disease is a soft-tissue condition without osseous manifestations.[337] Sometimes a retrocalcaneal bursitis causes the symptoms. Meyer dysplasia represents irregular, delayed ossification of the proximal femoral epiphysis.[269] Köhler's disease is a controversial normal variant with sclerotic fragmentation of the navicular bone of the developing foot. The variation can be seen in 30% of males and 20% of females. Pain, tenderness, and swelling develop over the navicular bone; however, the correlation of the radiographic changes in comparison to the duration of clinical symptoms is not compatible with true AVN.

Only a few of the osteochondroses actually develop osteonecrosis. Kienböck's disease is an osteonecrosis of the lunate bone.[111] Freiberg's infraction is an osteonecrosis of the distal end of the metatarsal, most commonly the second. Seventy percent of cases occur in females. The cause is believed to be chronic, repeated stress placed on the head of the second metatarsal, leading to subchondral fracture and osteonecrosis.

Van Neck's disease is only the normal swollen, irregularly mineralized ischiopubic synchondrosis in which there is an irregular bubbly appearance.[54] A focal increase in radionuclide uptake at the ischiopubic synchondrosis can be normal, the intensity of this focal accumulation is variable and frequently asymmetric. When osteomyelitis is present, a more diffuse pattern of uptake centered on the synchondroses but also involving the adjacent ramus is seen.[179] The extended pattern reflects the associated hyperemia from the infection. In Sever's disease soft-tissue uptake can sometimes be seen at the place of insertion of the Achilles tendon or the plantar fascia. In Kienböck's disease the small size of the lunate bone generally prevents the normal bone from being distinguished on the scan. Increased uptake can be seen in the reactive phase of Kienböck's disease. Usually the patient does not present early enough to recognize photopenia of the avascular bone, but with Freiberg's disease, a patient may present early enough to see photopenia in the metatarsal head.[238] With later presentation the scintigraphic appearance will show increased activity because the bone has revascularized and is in the healing phase. In all of the preceding conditions, diagnosis is enhanced by high-resolution magnification views.

OSTEOCHONDRITIS DISSECANS (KNEE AND ANKLE)

Osteochondritis dissecans is the term used to describe subchondral fragmentation of bone in the knee or ankle joint. It is possible for the articular surface to be intact or for the fragment to separate from the joint surface. Osteochondral lesions of the talus and femoral condyles are similar. There are many theories about the etiology. These include ischemic necrosis, trauma, ossification aberration, or a combination of these. The medial femoral condyle is involved four times more often than the lateral. Osteochondral lesions of the dome of the talus that occur laterally are usually sequelae to inversion or dorsiflexion-inversion trauma. When the lesion is medial, either a traumatic or posttraumatic etiology can be invoked.

A focal increase in activity at the site of the osteochondritis is found on delayed images. The viability of the osteochondral fragments may not be ascertained from the vascularity of the lesion. In one series the greater the focal hyperemia on blood pool image and the greater the degree of uptake on late-phase image, the greater the severity of the disease and the greater the likelihood of a loose fragment.[268] In another series duration of disease (early, intermediate, or late phase) was characterized according to scintigraphic pattern. Early disease manifested focally increased blood flow in the area of the abnormality. Intermediate-stage disease demonstrated a generalized increase in flow, whereas late-stage (stable disease) showed normal blood flow.[262] Scintigraphic severity should be judged from high-resolution pinhole views. Findings vary from focal abnormal uptake in the lesion to additional involvement in the condyle, as well as extension of activity from the femur to inclusion of the ipsilateral transarticular tibial plateau. No prognostication can be given for any stage of the disease at time of presentation. With serial scanning no reduction in activity correlates with poor prognosis and a likelihood of fragment detachment.[48] Scintigraphy of osteochondritis dissecans of the talus usually demonstrates the increased radiotracer uptake of the reactive repair process.

TUMOR AND TUMORLIKE CONDITIONS

Cystic Lesions

UNICAMERAL (SIMPLE) BONE CYSTS

The origin of the simple bone cyst remains obscure. Most cysts are located in the metaphysis of the proximal humerus or femur. These lesions are thought to involute because of their absence in the adult population. After pathologic fracture, a small percentage of patients have subsequent healing and resolution. Multiple unicameral bone cysts occasionally occur in the same patient.[190] Recognition of the unicameral bone cyst usually leads to treatment by curettage and bone grafting, or steroid (methylprednisolone acetate) injection. Eight percent of patients have a satisfactory result from steroid injection.[50] Multiloculation of the cyst diminishes the success rate for injection therapy.

The lesion is characterized by a central, expanding radiolucency with geographic margins and no periosteal reaction or obvious internal ossification. The cyst is often located in the diaphysis but can be metaphyseal and even adjacent to the growth plate. Periosteal reaction and/or an internal vertical fragment ("fallen fragment" sign) usually indicates pathologic fracture.[358]

Scintigraphically a slightly reactive margin frequently surrounds a photopenic center, the so-called "doughnut" sign. On the other hand, a small untraumatized lesion may not be visible within the normal pattern of activity. Usually aneurysmal bone cysts, giant cell tumors, and infected or traumatized cysts have thicker, uneven rims of higher-level activity around their photopenic centers.

ANEURYSMAL BONE CYST

Aneurysmal bone cysts are benign, lytic lesions noted for their expansile nature. Seventy-eight percent of patients with aneurysmal bone cysts are younger than 20 years of age.[74] The tumor can have an aggressive radiographic appearance and may be confused with malignant neoplasms and the giant cell tumor (usually occurs after epiphyseal closure). The lesion consists of an eccentric lytic focus with its center in the metaphysis. The margins are usually well circumscribed, with or without a sclerotic rim. There is a ballooned aneurysmal appearance to the lesion, sometimes with periosteal reaction, but no internal calcifications. The pathogenesis of this tumor is still unknown. Surgical excision of the entire lesion or as much as possible is usually the treatment of choice. Embolization of aneurysmal bone cysts has been performed in lesions where the site (spine, pelvis) makes surgical treatment hazardous.[77] Grossly, the aneurysmal cyst usually contains anastomosing cavernous spaces filled with unclotted blood. Some tumors contain friable fibrous or granular tissue that may compromise half or more of their bulk. Benign giant cells are usually present in large numbers, which accounts for the confusion with a genuine giant cell tumor.

Two thirds of aneurysmal bone cysts show increased uptake around the periphery of the cyst, with less activity in the center[166,230] (Fig. 16-15). The "doughnut" pattern is not specific for an aneurysmal bone cyst, and a high percentage of giant cell tumors and unicameral bone cysts show a similar pattern, although the periph-

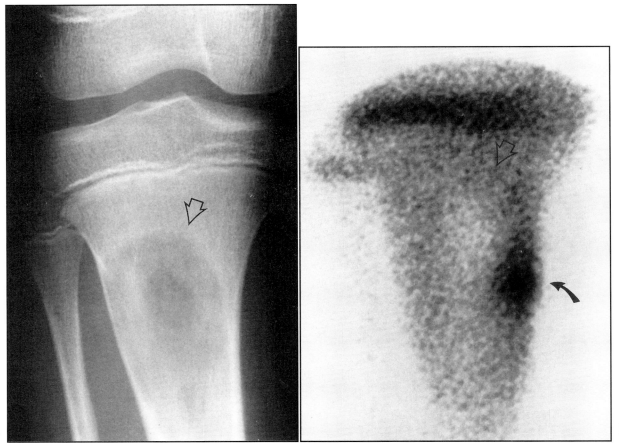

Fig. 16–15. Aneurysmal bone cyst of the tibia in a 9-year-old female. The destructive bone lesion seen radiographically (**A**) produces a scintigraphic "doughnut"; photopenia surrounded by increased uptake (**B**) (*open arrows*). The focal area of higher intensity is attributed to a pathologic fracture at the tumor margin (*curved arrow*).

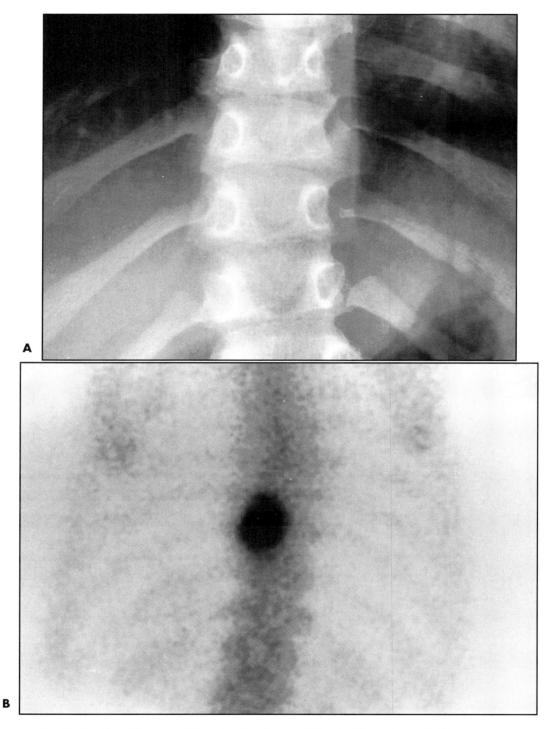

Fig. 16–16. Osteoblastoma of the spine in a 9-year-old female. The radiograph (**A**) shows absence of the pedicle at T10 on the left. There is expansion and sclerosis in the transverse process. The scan (**B**), a posterior image, reveals intense focal uptake at the site. This was a solitary lesion.

eral margin is usually less intense in the uncomplicated unicameral bone cyst. The "doughnut" sign can also be seen in an abscess, hematoma, bone infarct, surgical defect, congenital fenestrations, and in malignant tumors. There is no correlation between the scintigraphic pattern, homogeneously active uptake versus central photopenia, and a specific histologic pattern. The physiologic mechanisms for abnormal accumulation of the bone radiotracer include hyperemia, periosteal new bone formation, and osteoblastic activity.

Osteoid–Containing Lesions

OSTEOID OSTEOMA AND OSTEOBLASTOMA

Painful lesions smaller than 1.5 to 2.0 cm characterized radiographically by a lucent nidus surrounded by reactive sclerosis are regarded as osteoid osteomas. Osteoblastomas are expansile lesions with an admixture of lysis and sclerosis, typically larger than 1.5 to 2.0 cm and can mimic an aneurysmal bone cyst.[176] Osteoid osteomas are about 10 times as common as osteoblastomas. Histology of the two lesions may be similar, but a much higher proportion of osteoid osteomas are painful, with relief afforded by analgesics.[201] Osteoid osteomas are benign bone tumors most commonly found in the metaphyses or diaphyses of lower extremity long bones in children and adolescents. Synovitis can accompany the tumor when it arises in the proximal femur[256] or talus. Both osteoblastomas and osteoid osteomas frequent the spine (36% to 40% of osteoblastomas and 10% of osteoid osteomas). Seventy-five percent of osteoid osteomas are located in the neural arch in the following order of frequency: laminae, facets, pedicles, and spinous processes.[221] Most occur in the lumbar spine. Osteoblastomas usually occur in the posterior elements (the laminae, pedicles, and spinous processes) of the spine.

The lesions of the small bones of the carpus and tarsus, the proximal femur, or the vertebrae can be difficult to identify radiographically. Bone scintigraphy is extremely helpful in locating the nidus of these lesions. Osteoid osteoma and osteoblastoma are scintigraphically very visible bone lesions because of the avid uptake of the radiotracer by the nidus and the accompanying osteoid formation[363] (Fig. 16-16). Twenty-five percent of positive bone scans are associated with normal radiographic examinations.[152] The bone scan usually reveals an osteoid osteoma to be a well-demarcated focal area of intensely increased activity (the nidus) surrounded by less intensely increased activity (reactive sclerosis). This has been characterized as the "double-density" sign.[347] The hyperemia of the tumor is reflected by its increased uptake on early angiographic and tissue-phase images.[93] Pinhole collimation with high-resolution magnification of the lesion is very helpful in identifying the sometimes minute oval nidus. Scintigraphic differential diagnoses include chronic osteomyelitis (Brodie's abscess), aneurysmal bone cyst, tumors, metastasis, and fracture—all of which may be very active and may not be differentiated on skeletal scintigraphy.

Bone scintigraphy can accurately localize the lesion for correlative anatomic imaging (CT, laminography, or MRI) in the spinal column, proximal femur, hand, or foot. The location of the nidus can be marked on the surface of the body during scintigraphy to limit the field of examination for CT (requiring thin slices). Even when the lesions are obvious on plain radiography, however, the nidus sometimes is difficult to find at surgery when tremendous bone overgrowth and reaction is present. Scintigraphy is useful in controlling the extent of surgery in any part of the skeleton by directing the surgeon intraoperatively to the exact site of the nidus, either by portable gamma camera[115,360] or scintillation probe.[119,143] These techniques are effective because the nidus is the most active portion of the lesion. Ratios of activity of the nidus to normal bone and reactive bone can be generated by computer before operation for guidance of intraoperative probe localization. Postoperatively one can confirm successful removal of the nidus by the absence of the focal central uptake. When extirpation results in multiple fragments, the different pieces can be monitored at surgery to confirm nidus removal, and the pathologist can be directed to those high count fragments most likely to contain the nidus.[174]

OSTEOSARCOMA

Osteosarcoma (osteogenic sarcoma) is the most common malignant primary tumor in children and adolescents. Fifty percent of lesions occur in the second decade. Males are affected more commonly than females. Most commonly the intraosseous tumor arises in the metaphyses of the long bones, usually the distal femur (44%), proximal tibia (22%), and proximal humerus (9%).[25] It is not uncommon for the lesion to extend into the diaphysis and/or epiphysis. The tumors are characteristically large at presentation. Two thirds of patients present with a large metaphyseal tumor as the primary focus.

Radiographically the lesion may be predominantly osteosclerotic (25%), osteolytic (25%), or osteosclerotic/osteolytic (50%). There is usually a coexistent soft-tissue mass characterized by the production of osteoid or bone by the tumor cells. The lesion consists of mixed lytic and blastic changes accompanied by a variable amount of extraosseous soft-tissue mass containing calcified osteoid matrix. Periosteal reaction, either of the interrupted or spiculated type, is frequently present.

Any patient with a solitary site of osteosarcoma should undergo bone scintigraphy before initiation of therapy to detect skip lesions and other skeletal foci of tumor (multicentric osteosarcoma or primary lesion with multiple metastases).[372] Multicentric osteosarcoma consists of simultaneous presentation of several sclerotic lesions of comparable size.[229] The presence of multiple osseous lesions radically changes the course of therapy, with limb amputation no longer being appropriate.[263]

Distant metastases are found at initial staging in only 2% of cases.[125] With the advent of adjuvant chemotherapy, the natural course of the disease has been altered, with bone metastases appearing before pulmonary metastases in 15% to 16% of cases.[120,265]

On bone scan osteosarcoma shows very avid accumulation of the bone radiotracer with or without extension into the soft tissues adjacent to the bone (Fig. 16-17, *A*). Occasionally on bone scan an inhomogeneous or even photopenic component (necrosis) is seen in a lytic or sclerotic tumor.[343] In some series the comparison of bone scan with extent of tumor has been fairly accurate.[121] However, an "extended" or "augmented" pattern may imply more extensive marrow extension or even transarticular involvement.[57] At times the intramedullary spread can be confused with increased physiologic uptake secondary to marrow hyperemia, medullary reactive bone, or periosteal new bone. Bone scintigraphy is notoriously poor in defining intraosseous tumor length. The extended pattern is attributed to circulatory changes in the bone that stimulate regional osteoblastic activity. Preoperative assessment of extent and planning for length of resection is now based on MRI. Thallium-201 imaging is now being used as a radionuclide method of defining the actual extent of the tumor and response to

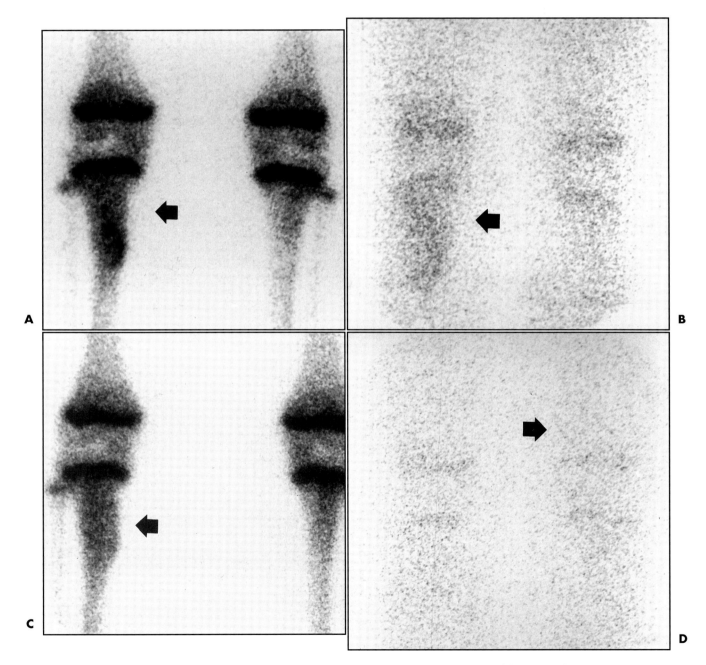

Fig. 16-17. Osteosarcoma of the tibia in a 12-year-old female. At the time of diagnosis, the bone scan (**A**) and thallium scan (**B**) were positive (*arrows*). Preoperative chemotherapy was administered, and after 4 months the bone scan remained positive (**C**) but the thallium scan (**D**) became negative, reflecting tumor response (*arrows*).

treatment. The tumor cells of osteosarcomas have an affinity for the potassium analog, thallium.[316] Thallium uptake correlates with viable tumor tissue. The disappearance of the thallium activity from the tumor site posttreatment usually means at least 95% of the tumor burden has been eradicated (Fig. 16-17). Both thallium-201 and technetium-99m MIBI imaging of primary bone tumors are discussed in greater detail in Chapter 7.

Chondroid Lesions

CHONDROSARCOMAS, EXOSTOSES, ENCHONDROMAS

Chondrosarcoma accounts for fewer than 5% of primary bone malignancies in childhood.[6] Chondrosarcomas may arise within either the medullary portion of bone or the cartilaginous cap of an osteochondroma. An osteochondroma is a protrusion of mature cortical bone (either sessile or pedunculated) with a central segment continuous with the medullary canal. It usually projects away from the nearest joint and its distal tip is covered with a cartilaginous cap. Ninety percent occur as solitary lesions. Multiple hereditary exostoses (osteochondromatosis) is inherited by males as an autosomal dominant condition with complete penetrance.[116] The medullary chondrosarcoma can arise in skeletal enchondromatosis (Ollier's disease) or Maffucci's syndrome, an uncommon congenital mesodermal dysplasia that is characterized by multiple enchondromas, as well as soft-tissue hemangiomas and/or lymphangiomas.[219] Enchondromas may possess a calcified cartilaginous matrix but typically are lytic lesions located in the metaphyses of growing long bones in the extremities. Often the short tubular bones of the hands and feet are affected.

Most chondrosarcomas arise without an antecedent condition. In childhood primary chondrosarcoma is considered a variant of osteosarcoma, and it usually follows a very aggressive course.[254] Primary chondrosarcoma typically arises in the trunk or proximal ends (metaphyses) of the femur or humerus. It may rarely be encountered as a primary soft-tissue mass. Lucent lesions with internal rings or arcs of calcification strongly suggest chondroid lesions. Cartilaginous matrix can be seen in both benign and malignant tumors. When a large lesion has destroyed the cortex and invaded soft tissue, malignant change must be suspected. Central or medullary chondrosarcomas exhibit increased bone tracer uptake. Increased activity on the early phases of the bone scan may identify extension of the chondrosarcoma. Delayed bone scan images show either homogeneous or patchy patterns of activity in the osseous portions of the tumor.[175]

Radiographically it can be difficult to distinguish a benign exostosis from a low-grade chondrosarcoma. The differentiation of benign exostoses (osteochondromas) from peripheral exostotic chondrosarcomas on the basis of scintigraphic activity also may be difficult.[204] The extent and intensity of radiopharmaceutical uptake depends on the amount of enchondral ossification occurring in the exostosis. The most intense exostoses occur in the growing child. In the exostotic chondrosarcoma the distribution and intensity of tracer activity relate to the combination of hyperemia and osteoblastic activity. A

scintigraph in which the lesions show only normal or mildly increased activity usually excludes the possibility of malignant degeneration. The efficacy of serial scanning of patients with hereditary multiple exostoses (only 0.5% of these lesions undergo malignant degeneration) is questionable because increased activity is not specific for malignant degeneration. Trauma with or without fracture as well as sudden intensified growth can cause increased activity.

Benign enchondromas show normal or slightly increased uptake on bone scan. The intensity and uniformity of uptake of the bone-seeking radiopharmaceutical cannot be used to differentiate benign enchondromas from enchondromas degenerating into malignancy (Fig. 16-18).

CHONDROBLASTOMA

These lesions which predominantly occur in the epiphyses of children and young adults (average age, 16 years old) are concentrated at the ends of the proximal femur, distal femur, and proximal humerus.[25] The calcaneus and talus are flat bones occasionally involved. Forty percent of chondroblastomas are located entirely in the epiphysis, and fifty-five percent involve both epiphysis and metaphysis.

These round, lytic lesions (usually 1.5 to 4.0 cm in diameter) are usually visible on conventional radiographs in eccentric epiphyseal locations. Bone scintigraphy is occasionally reported to have normal uptake but in the majority of instances increased uptake.[168,172] When chondroblastoma elicits adjacent soft-tissue inflammation (synovitis), there is usually an extended pattern of very active uptake. The usual treatment is curettage and packing of the osseous defect with bone chips. Local recurrence is greater among patients with an open physis probably because the surgeon limits the resection to avoid damaging the growth plate.

Fibrous Lesions

NONOSSIFYING FIBROMAS, CORTICAL DEFECT

Fibroxanthoma, nonossifying fibroma, and fibrous cortical defect are all terms used to describe the most common benign bone lesions in childhood. These are histologically similar lesions that occur in growing bones of healthy children and adolescents between 2 and 20 years of age. The fibroxanthoma typically consists of spindle-shaped fibroblasts, scattered giant cells, and foam (xanthoma) cells. Thirty-three percent of the pediatric population is said to have one or more of these lesions. Most are encountered as incidental radiographic findings. Small lytic lesions with scalloped margins that occur eccentrically in a metaphysis and disappear spontaneously are termed *fibrous cortical defects*. These appear like cortical "blisters" with very thin outer cortices. The larger lesions with more sclerotic, scalloped margination also occur eccentrically in metaphyses but are usually termed *nonossifying fibromas* or *fibroxanthomas*.

The benign cortical irregularity of the distal medial femur (cortical desmoid), with a predilection for children and adolescents, is a fibrous lesion located near the inser-

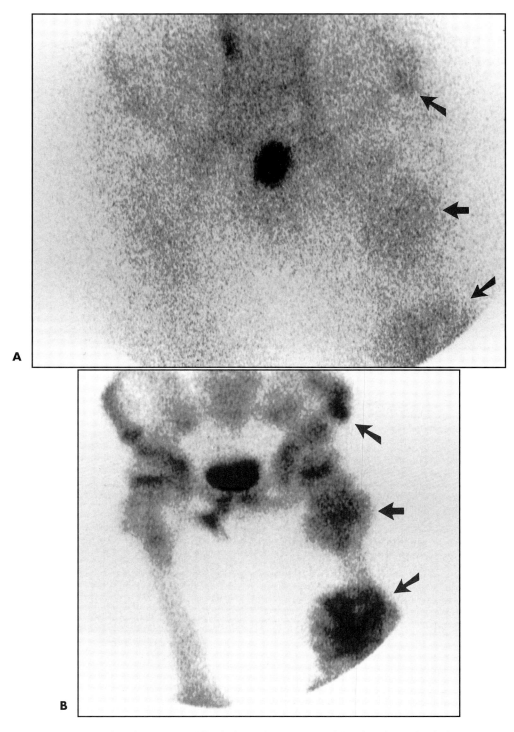

Fig. 16-18. Enchondromatosis (Ollier's disease) in a 7-year-old male. The multiple lesions throughout the skeleton exhibit the pattern shown in the pelvis and left femur on tissue-phase (**A**) and delayed bone (**B**) images. Uptake is increased but varies with the size and location of the lesion (*arrows*).

tion of the adductor magnus muscle.[320] Sometimes the periosteal reaction, cortical thickening, reactive bone formation, and bony fragments within the lesion are confused with malignancy (e.g., osteogenic sarcoma). The periosteal cortical thickening with microscopic evidence

of fibrous tissue proliferation and numerous osteoclasts can pathologically mimic malignancy if it is biopsied.

Normal to mildly increased focal uptake can occur on children's bone scans at the site of fibrous cortical defects or fibroxanthomas.[64] More marked increase in activity

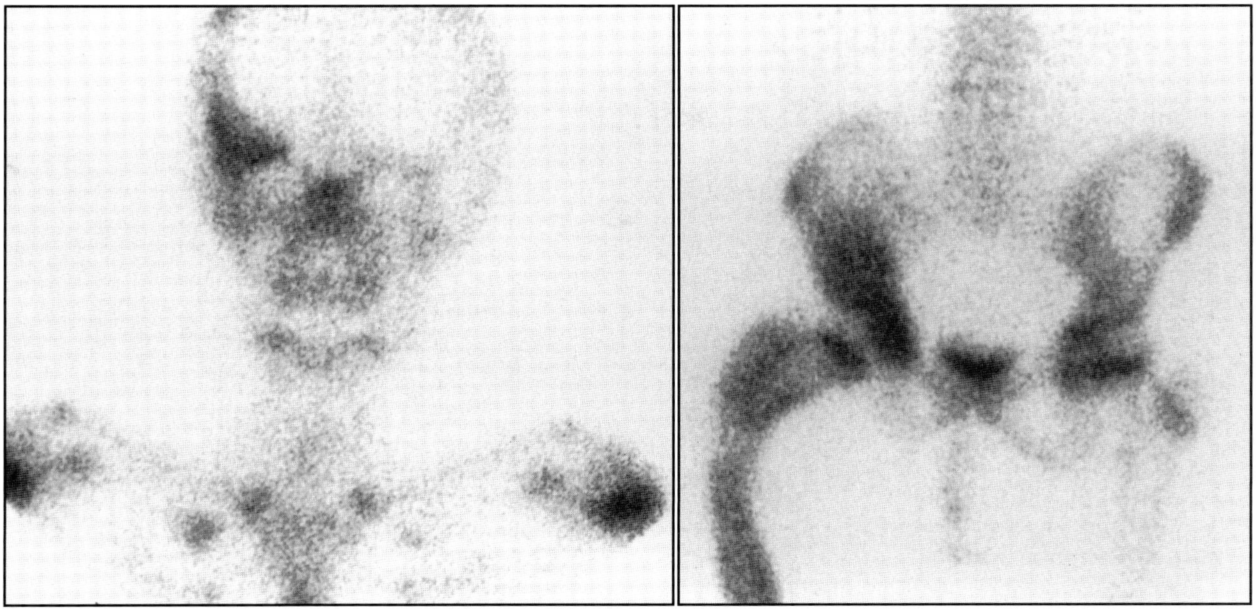

Fig. 16-19. Fibrous dysplasia in a 7-year-old female. Lesions show active tracer accumulation. Note that the skull (**A**), pelvic, and femoral (**B**) involvement is all on the right side of the body.

can be physiologic (conversion from nonossifying to ossifying fibroma) or posttraumatic (pathologic fracture). Detection of uncomplicated lesions depends on the size of the lesion, the resolution of the imaging equipment, and the relative osteogenic activity.[132] In the symptomatic individual whose radiograph causes concern for tumor, the bone scan differentiates the normal or minimally active benign cortical desmoid from the osteosarcoma with its avid activity.[64,379]

FIBROUS DYSPLASIA

Fibrous dysplasia is a benign, noninherited, and developmental or growth disorder in which normal bone is replaced by abnormal fibrous tissue containing small abnormally arranged bone trabeculae. Fibrous dysplasia occurs in polyostotic and monostotic forms; the radiographic and pathologic features of an individual monostotic and polystotic lesion are nearly identical in each form. Seventy-five percent to eighty percent of all patients with fibrous dysplasia have the monostotic form. Monostotic lesions occur most frequently in the femur, tibia, craniofacial bones, or ribs.[147] Long-bone lesions may be discovered because of deformity, pain secondary to incomplete fracture, or complete fracture. Fractures usually heal adequately.[153] The craniofacial form typically involves the maxilla or mandible but not the calvarium. The peak age of diagnosis of monostotic lesions is between 5 and 20 years.

Approximately 20% to 25% of patients with fibrous dysplasia have the polyostotic form. A few patients exhibit endocrine dysfunction, especially precocious puberty in girls (described by McCune and Albright). Other endocrine abnormalities that have been reported include precocious puberty in boys, hyperthyroidism, hyperparathyroidism, acromegaly, Cushing's disease, and diabetes mellitus.[170] Patients with polyostotic fibrous dysplasia become symptomatic at a median age of 8 years, and two thirds are symptomatic before the age of 10 years. The skeletal lesions primarily affect the lower extremities, and are often entirely or predominantly unilateral—that is, all the lesions are found on the same side of the body. The commonly involved bones are the femur, tibia, pelvis, metatarsals, fibula, or phalanges.

The radiographic appearance of fibrous dysplasia varies. It arises within the medullary cavity and replaces normal cancellous bone with a purely lytic or amorphous "ground-glass" appearance. The lesion is homogeneous and has no radiographically visible trabeculae. Fibrous dysplasia typically enlarges or expands the affected bone. In other cases focal nodules of cartilage in polyostotic fibrous dysplasia can produce foci of popcornlike calcification. Skeletal deformities are common, especially bowing of long bones, varus angulation or shepherd's crook deformity of the proximal femur, and abnormal tubulation of long bones without tapering from wider metaphysis to narrower diaphysis. Skull lesions affect primarily the base, causing thickening and sclerosis of sphenoid wings, sella, orbital roof, and the vertical portion of the frontal bone. Paranasal sinuses may be obliterated.

Bone scintigraphy is a sensitive imaging technique for detecting early lesions and identifying polyostotic involvement in fibrous dysplasia. Due to the increased vascularity of fibrous dysplasia lesions, there is active concentration of the bone-seeking radiopharmaceutical in both early and delayed phases (Fig. 16-19). In one report studying radiographically obvious lesions, a small percentage of cystic-type lesions (14%) and homogeneous ground-glass lesions (7%) exhibited no increase in radioisotope uptake.[226]

OSTEOFIBROUS DYSPLASIA (CAMPANACCI'S DISEASE) AND ADAMANTINOMA

Osteofibrous dysplasia, cortical fibrous dysplasia, or ossifying fibroma is a benign bone lesion that occurs most commonly in the tibia (92%). It is often confused with fibrous dysplasia. There is usually an associated tibial bowing in infants and young children with this lesion. The age at presentation ranges from birth to 20 years. Sixty percent of children are younger than 5 years of age.[49] Histologically the lesion consists of spicules of bone in a fibrous stroma, quite similar to fibrous dysplasia. The distinguishing features of osteofibrous dysplasia are zonal architecture, lamellar bone, and rimming of bone spicules by osteoblasts.

Adamantinoma or ameloblastoma can occur in association with either fibrous dysplasia or osteofibrous dysplasia.[267] Adamantinoma is an uncommon malignant tumor, but 14% occur in children. Scattered epithelioid islands typical of adamantinoma can be found in an area of osteofibrous dysplasia.[331] This is explained by the concept that adamantinoma is a pluripotential neoplasm with bimodal differentiation (epithelial and mesenchymal). The mesenchymal differentiation includes fibrous, fibrous dysplasia-like, and osteofibrous dysplasia-like stroma. These tumors have been termed differentiated adamantinomas. They are predominantly osteofibrous dysplasia in composition and are considered at the benign end of the spectrum of adamantinomas.[72]

The radiographic patterns are age related. Unilocular, expansile, and lytic lesions with well-defined sclerotic margins in the midtibia with anterior bowing are found in infancy. After 3 months of age, the osteolytic lesion usually is eccentric and multilocular. The medullary cavity is usually narrow and the overlying cortex is thinned. Most lesions stabilize and regress after puberty, and there is usually a conservative surgical approach. Bone scintigraphy in the few reported cases showed marked increase in radiotracer uptake.[193,227,349]

Giant Cell Tumor

Giant cell tumors comprise approximately 4% of all primary bone neoplasms.[216] A small percentage (1.7%) of giant cell tumors occur in children younger than 15 years of age.[334] These tumors are considered benign but may pursue a progressive and potentially malignant clinical course. This is characterized by recurrence, sarcomatous change, and development of metastases (both benign and malignant tumors). Giant cell tumors show a uniform distribution of osteoclast-like, multinucleated giant cells with a stroma of plump oval-to-spindle–shaped cells. The lesion has to be differentiated from many other giant cell–containing lesions, such as nonosteogenic fibroma, benign fibrous histiocytoma, aneurysmal bone cysts, chondroblastoma, chondromyxoid fibroma, brown tumor of hyperparathyroidism, giant cell reparative granuloma, and osteosarcoma with benign giant cells.[73]

Fifty percent of lesions are epiphyseal/metaphyseal in location, and reside in the long bones of the lower extremities. This predominantly lytic lesion is usually expansile and eccentrically placed in the larger long bones. Joint invasion should be considered when subarticular cortical bone is disrupted by the lesion or by pathologic fracture.

The giant cell tumor is an expansive, very vascular skeletal neoplasm that has been described to produce a fairly characteristic scintigraphic "doughnut" sign (64% of cases) on tissue-phase and delayed bone images.[127,380] The "doughnut" sign is produced by a thick collar of intense uptake of the radiotracer (accelerated osteoblastic activity of reactive bone) surrounding a relatively photopenic tumor mass. The "doughnut" pattern is not pathognomonic for giant cell tumor, but when it occurs eccentrically in the end of a long bone (distal femur, proximal tibia, and distal radius), the diagnosis of giant cell tumor must be seriously considered. This tumor often exhibits an extended pattern (similar to osteosarcoma), which can lead to overestimation of its true boundaries.[169] Adjunctive use of SPECT[195] or high-resolution magnification imaging may demonstrate the presence of the central photopenic defect in smaller tumors. The entire skeleton should be imaged with scintigraphy because giant cell tumors have a 10% incidence of metastases[215] and also can be multifocal. Bone scintigraphy is also helpful in detecting recurrences of tumor.[308]

Marrow Infiltrative Disease

EWING'S SARCOMA

Ewing's sarcoma, a primitive primary sarcoma of the bone, is the second most common malignant bone tumor of children and young adults. There is a slight male predominance. It arises most frequently in the femur and pelvic bones, followed by ribs and tibia. Ewing's sarcoma is a member of a heterogeneous group of lesions termed small round cell tumors (e.g., histiocytic lymphoma, neuroblastoma). The distribution corresponds to the red marrow distribution population, which varies with age as the body undergoes slow conversion of red to fatty marrow.[196] Flat bone involvement is more frequent in patients over 9 years of age with the more central red marrow distribution.

Plain radiography accurately predicts the histologic diagnosis in cases of Ewing's sarcoma. The tumor characteristically arises in a metaphyseal-diaphyseal location, and imparts a mottled, moth-eaten, poorly marginated appearance to the bone lesions. The tumor coming out of the medullary portion of the bone evokes multiple layers of periosteal reaction, which can appear spiculated ("hair-on-end") or lamellated ("onion-skinned"). Ewing's sarcoma in flat bones may show a lytic, sclerotic, or mixed radiographic appearance. There is generally an associated soft-tissue component.

Bone scintigraphy is used to determine the presence of additional lesions at presentation and at regular intervals during therapy.[26] Bone tracers do not localize to soft-tissue and lung metastases. There is a marked uptake of the bone-seeking agent on the tissue-phase and delayed images in the area of osseous involvement. Here the uptake is secondary to the vascularity of the tumor tissue and reactive bone, not osteoid formation by the tumor itself. The pattern of uptake tends to mimic osteomyelitis. The poorly defined, usually homogeneous uptake of the radiopharmaceutical in Ewing's sarcoma has been contrasted to a patchy pattern with osteosarcoma.[283] An unusual appearance secondary to compromised circulation in a very aggressive tumor is that of photopenic lesion. Similarly large tumor with compromised circulation can also produce a "cold" lesion.[45]

Osseous metastases will be detected in approximately 11% of patients at presentation; this is associated with a poor prognosis. The bone scan is important in initial tumor staging and is mandatory in patient follow-up after initial therapy. In one study 47% of patients were found to have osseous metastases within 6 months of diagnosis. Marked diminution of tracer uptake in the primary tumor occurs within 3 to 4 months after onset of radiation therapy.[266] Intense focal areas of uptake in the tumor site within 3 to 4 months after treatment may indicate tumor recurrence, infection, or pathologic fracture. On rare occasions a "flare" response or apparent worsening of the bone scan can occur within 6 months of commencing therapy. This takes place in the absence of increasing bone pain and represents an apparently "good" response to treatment with calcification in the soft tissues and shrinkage of the mass.[270] When an intense area of uptake persists at the tumor site for 3 to 4 months, the concern is for tumor recurrence.

Gallium-67 scintigraphy is very sensitive for this tumor but not very specific. Thallium-201 chloride, the myocardial perfusion agent, has been shown to be accurate in differentiating malignant from benign disease and in evaluating treatment of sarcomas. Ewing's sarcoma can be evaluated initially to confirm uptake and then reassessed following therapy. Some tumors are not as thallium-avid as the osteosarcomas. Imaging of axial lesions in the spine and pelvis is often difficult because of tracer excretion through the kidneys and bowel, and improved lesion detection occurs with SPECT.[282] Technetium-99m sestamibi, another myocardial potassium analog tracer, may supplant thallium-201 chloride because it has higher target-to-background ratios, yields better resolution, and has quicker imaging time (see Chapter 7). This is particularly applicable to the pediatric population.

LYMPHOMA AND LEUKEMIA

Lymphomas are the third most common neoplasm affecting the American pediatric population and the third most common primary malignant bone tumor (these were previously referred to as *reticulum cell sarcomas*). Primary lymphoma of bone may arise in any bone but approximately 50% arise in the long bones. Skeletal metastasis of both non-Hodgkin's and Hodgkin's lymphoma is well recognized and is much more common than primary lymphoma of bone. In metastatic non-Hodgkin's lymphoma, the most frequent osseous sites of involvement include the spine, sacrum, skull, and facial bones. The spine, predominantly thoracic and lumbar, and pelvis are the most frequent sites of bone involvement with Hodgkin's lymphoma. The incidence of metastatic bone disease is less than 20.5% in both types of lymphoma when considering initial and follow-up examinations.[60]

Leukemia, the most common childhood cancer, accounts for 35% of pediatric malignancies.[272] Acute lymphocytic leukemia (ALL) is the most common form of childhood leukemia and accounts for 80% to 85% of cases, with acute myeloid leukemia representing the remainder of the cases. The usual involvement of the skeletal system is by marrow infiltration. Osseous disease is seen in 47% of children at presentation and 70% to 90% during the course of the disease.[344] Systemic signs and symptoms include pallor, fatigue, and petechiae. These are a result of anemia and thrombocytopenia secondary to marrow infiltration. Leukopenia can occur 50% of the time. Bone pain is predominantly in the long bones and back.

In general on plain radiographs, lymphoma and leukemia produce similar changes in bone. Commonly recognized patterns of bone destruction include geographic, permeative, and moth-eaten forms.[306] Lytic, sclerotic, and mixed lesions as well as periosteal reaction may occur.

Bone scintigraphy is not reliable in the detection of all osseous disease in patients with lymphoma. Although the lesions usually manifest increased uptake, some sites in the axial skeleton are photopenic. Bone scintigraphy is not used to diagnose leukemia, but patients may be sent for a scan because of unexplained musculoskeletal complaints. In leukemia the bone scan can demonstrate osseous leukemic involvement with unifocal and multifocal abnormalities that predate radiographic changes (Fig. 16-20). Increased uptake of the bone tracer usually occurs in the metaphyses. Other patterns include diffuse uptake in the diaphyses and flat bones. Leukemic changes may mimic the symmetry seen with lesions of metastatic neuroblastoma.[118] Proliferation of the leukemic cells in the marrow spaces may interfere with blood supply and cause a photon-deficient pattern like that seen with infarction. In one series 80% of children manifested scintigraphic abnormalities at the time of their diagnosis. Positive radiographic correlation was found in only 52% of these cases.[59]

NEUROBLASTOMA

After ALL and brain tumors, the next most common malignancy in children is neuroblastoma. Accurate identification of bone and marrow metastases is extremely important in neuroblastoma, because therapy and prognosis relate directly to staging. Neuroblastomas originate from sympathetic neuroblasts of the neural crest. Two thirds of primary tumors are found in the upper abdomen. The skeletal system is the most frequent site of hematogenous metastases in all patients with neuroblastoma except infants, who more frequently show liver

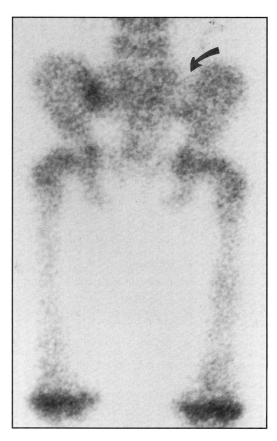

Fig. 16-20. Acute myelogenous leukemia. This 2-year-old male presented with a facial mass. Note the diffuse patchy pattern of uptake in this posterior image of the pelvis and femurs with photopenia (*arrow*) in the right sacroiliac joint.

involvement. The incidence of neuroblastoma is highest during the first 2 years of life.

Bone metastases from neuroblastoma are often metaphyseal and can be symmetric; however, asymmetric involvement is more common. Radiographically the lesions are patchy and lytic, with or without areas of sclerosis and periosteal reaction.[11] Bone scintigraphy is extremely sensitive in the detection of skeletal metastases in neuroblastoma. The scintigraphic skeletal survey is better (4% false-negative) than the radiologic skeletal survey (15% false-negative) for the detection of osseous spread. A false-negative examination is possible when the metastatic lesion is metaphyseal and contiguous to a very active growth plate.[188] Extreme care and time must be expended when performing bone scintigraphy in children with neuroblastoma. Magnification images (pinhole collimation) may be required to resolve equivocal abnormalities near the physes. Blurring of the growth plate is suspicious for metastatic involvement.[163] Although 70% of lesions show increased uptake, photopenic lesions occasionally occur.[65] With therapy, cold lesions revert to normal or develop increased activity.

Besides revealing skeletal metastases, the bone scan may also detect primary and secondary tumors[247] because of the tumor's uptake of the bone tracer. In an undiagnosed child presenting with bone pain, the bone scan may show a characteristic diagnostic pattern for neuroblastoma: tracer uptake in the metastatic bone lesions and the primary (soft-tissue) lesion simultaneously (Fig. 16-21). In one study 91% of primary tumors accumulated the radiopharmaceutical.[151] Uptake of the radiopharmaceutical is seen in tumors with and without macrocalcification or microcalcification. One report speculates that uptake of the bone-seeking tracer by a neuroblastoma might be related to the metabolic rate or activity rather than total amount of calcium within the tumor.[258] Twenty-eight percent of the extraosseous metastases of neuroblastoma were reported to concentrate the radiopharmaceutical.[247] Radioactivity can be observed in ascites, liver, lung, anterior mediastinum, and posterior mediastinum.

The specificity of detection of neuroblastoma lesions has been increased with the development of the tracer iodine-131-metaiodobenzylguanidine (I-131 MIBG), a physiologic analog of norepinephrine and guanethidine. It is highly accurate in the detection of neuroblastoma metastases, primary tumors, and posttreatment recurrence. In one series of intraabdominal lesions ranging from bean-to-fist size, I-131 MIBG was compared with gallium and bone scintigraphy. One hundred percent of lesions were detected on I-131 MIBG scanning, whereas only 57% and 50% of lesions were detected with gallium and bone tracer, respectively. Iodine-131 MIBG sensitivity seems to correlate with elevations of urinary vanillylmandelic acid (VMA), dopamine levels, and serum neuron-specific enolase levels. Normally or minimally elevated markers were seen in patients with negative scans.[149] Iodine-123 MIBG is not generally available but offers the advantage of higher counts, shorter imaging time, and better resolution. Metaphyseal lesions in children probably can be detected more confidently with I-131 MIBG because there is less interference from the activity in the growth plates. Diffuse symmetric involvement of the skeleton is not a diagnostic problem because of specificity of the radiopharmaceutical for tumor.[342] Indium-111 octreotide scintigraphy is a somatostatin analog that has very promising results in imaging tumors of neuroendocrine origin (paragangliomas, glomus tumors, tumors of neural crest origin).[202] Neuroblastoma cells are derived from neural crest cells, the precursors of the sympathetic neurons and adrenal chromaffin cells. High levels of somatostatin, a neuropeptide transmitter, are demonstrated in primary neuroblastoma tumors and this accounts for tumor incorporation of the labeled somatostatin analog.[292]

HISTIOCYTOSIS X

The reticuloendothelioses (e.g., histiocytosis X) are not truly neoplasms but are characterized by a varied and abnormal proliferation of histiocytes. The clinical and pathologic findings encompass isolated bone involvement (solitary or multifocal, eosinophilic granulomas), a relatively benign disseminated disease (Hand-Schüller-Christian disease), and a highly malignant disseminated disease form (Letterer-Siwe disease). Musculoskeletal

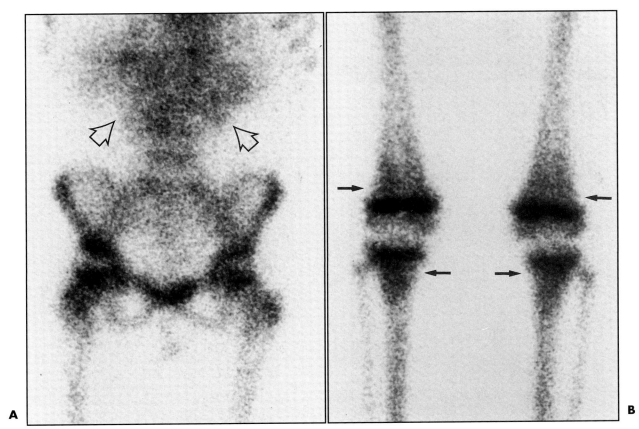

Fig. 16-21. Metastatic neuroblastoma in a 3-year-old female. There is uptake by the primary tumor (*open arrows*) and metastasis to the pelvis and right femur. (**A**) Metaphyseal involvement obscures the growth plates about the knees and can appear symmetric (**B**) (*arrows*).

manifestations occur 78% of the time. The occurrence rate in children younger than age 15 years is 1 in 350,000.[397] The etiology remains obscure.

There is a predilection for marrow involvement with the flat bones of the skull and pelvis being the most common sites. Other common sites include the metaphyseal-diaphyseal (rarely epiphyseal) regions of the ribs and femurs, and the bodies of the vertebrae (vertebrae plana). The radiographic characteristics (purely lytic, lytic with central nidus of bone, to lytic with sclerotic margination) vary within the patient because the lesions are in various stages of activity and healing. Characteristic "beveled" lesions result in the skull and ilium because of differential destruction of the inner and outer tables of the skull and the anterior and posterior surfaces of the ilium.

The radiographic skeletal survey and bone scan appear complementary in the detection of osseous lesions. Neither study by itself is able to identify all osseous foci.[200,332] The radiographic skeletal survey is reported to be superior to bone scintigraphy in the detection of most osseous lesions, but skeletal scintigraphy is more reliable for detection of recurrences on follow-up examinations.[69] Approximately 30% to 40% of lesions in histiocytosis are not detectable by bone scintigraphy. The ability of scintigraphy to identify an osseous lesion on bone scintigraphy depends on its location, size, symbiosis, or

induced osteoblastic reaction by the host bone. In patients with severe multifocal involvement, the likelihood of false-negative bone scan is greater.[388] Small areas of bone destruction are difficult to detect, particularly when located near a very active physis in the immature skeleton. Some lesions are quiescent and covered by superimposed normal bone activity, whereas others can elicit periosteal reaction. Most lesions evoke increased radiotracer accumulation on the scan (Fig. 16-22). Large, aggressive, lytic lesions may not allow a reactive bone response by the host skeleton and may therefore be cold or photopenic. Gallium scans have been variable in demonstrating activity in the soft-tissue and osseous lesions of histiocytosis.

GAUCHER'S DISEASE

Gaucher's disease represents an inborn error of lipid metabolism. The underlying defect is a deficiency in the activity of glucosyl ceramide β glucoxidase. The result is an accumulation of glucocerebroside in RE cells. An abundance of Gaucher's cells in the RE system results in hepatosplenomegaly, lymph node replacement, and marrow packing (expansion). The metaphyseal regions of the long bones, especially in the lower extremities, change their modeling as a result of marrow packing and develop the radiographic "Erlenmeyer flask" deformities.

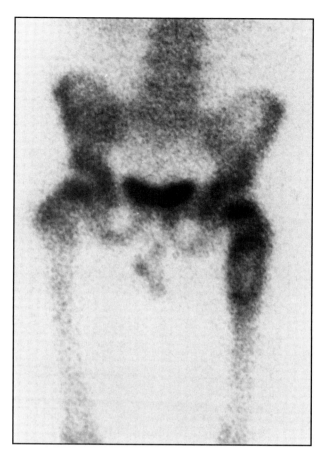

Fig. 16–22. Histiocytosis in a 3-year-old female. Disseminated disease exhibits a variety of scintigraphic patterns. Homogenously increased uptake is seen in the right ilium; the proximal left femur shows a "doughnut" lesion.

Packing also leads to encroachment of the intramedullary circulation; this ultimately can produce ischemia and osteonecrosis. Osteomyelitis is less common than "pseudoosteomyelitis."[21] In pseudoosteomyelitis, or bone crisis, there is localized pain, tenderness, erythema, and swelling. The patient's temperature may be elevated in conjunction with the erythrocyte sedimentation rate and the white blood cell count. Blood cultures and aspirates are sterile.

The problem of differentiating infarction from infection is similar to that in the sickle cell hemoglobinopathies when those patients present with fever and pain.[274] Bone scintigraphic findings in Gaucher's disease include widening of the metaphyses of the long bones and increased metaphyseal uptake.[55] Focal photopenia on marrow, bone, and gallium scintigraphy is a criterion for early infarction or pseudoosteomyelitis. In most cases of osteomyelitis, the bone scan is quite active. The difficulty arises when interpreting the scan of a patient in the non-acute setting after some bone healing and repopulation of the marrow have begun. The specificity for detecting infection has improved with the advent of the tagged white blood cell scanning.

SOFT-TISSUE TUMORS AND TUMORLIKE CONDITIONS

Extraosseous Tumors

The technetium phosphate complexes on rare occasions accumulate in benign soft-tissue tumor such as neurofibroma,[290] hemangioma,[242] hamartoma, lipoma,[56] desmoid,[214] or aggressive fibromatosis.[167] Localization of the radiophosphates in a soft-tissue tumor may be related to calcification within the tumor, local phosphate enzymes, increased blood flow, and/or alteration of capillary permeability. In a hemangioma, for example, there can be localization of tracer in the tumor because of sluggish, prolonged blood pooling. Desmoid tumor, on the other hand, is thought to exhibit chemiabsorption and with aggressive fibromatosis, involvement of the adjacent bone provokes accumulation. Soft-tissue sarcomas (e.g., rhabdomyosarcomas, leiomyosarcomas, fibrosarcomas) display activity because of their hypervascularity. In addition, tumors occasionally develop calcification secondary to hemorrhage or necrosis within the tumor mass itself; such areas with intact blood supply can exhibit tracer accumulation. Ninety-five percent accuracy is reported in detecting the involvement of local bone by soft-tissue sarcomas.[187] Gallium is an alternative agent also effective in detecting the location of soft-tissue sarcomas. The coincidental finding of extraosseous uptake of radiophosphate compounds by primary and secondary neural crest tumors is discussed in the section on neuroblastoma.

RHABDOMYOSARCOMA

Rhabdomyosarcoma is a malignant soft-tissue tumor of muscle origin. In children the most common sites, in descending order, are the head and neck, genitourinary tract, and extremities. Rhabdomyosarcoma, a relatively common childhood tumor, is exceeded in incidence only by tumors of the central nervous system, neuroblastoma, and Wilms' tumor. There are three histologic types of rhabdomyosarcoma identified: embryonal, alveolar, and pleomorphic. This discussion emphasizes changes in the extremities where tumors are usually the alveolar type. Sometimes a tumor contains calcification. If contiguous to bone, a tumor can erode the periosteum and cortex raising a question as to origin. Patients may present with skeletal metastases. Radiographs most commonly demonstrate metastases in the metaphyses of the extremities and in the spine; a destructive or diffusely permeative pattern without sclerotic margins is characteristic.[339]

Skeletal scintigraphy is useful for defining contiguous osseous involvement. There is some debate as to the bone scan's ability to identify skeletal metastases of rhabdomyosarcoma. Some metastases may elude detection because their aggressive osteolysis outstrips reactive response or because of a metaphyseal location adjacent to an active physis.[315] Calcification occurs in areas of hemorrhage or necrosis within the primary tumor.[35] Gallium can concentrate in nodal metastases as well as

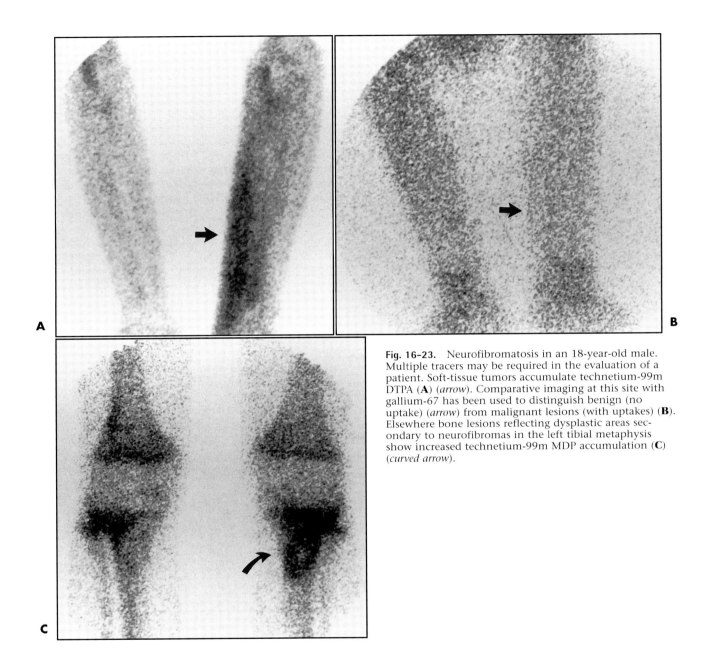

Fig. 16-23. Neurofibromatosis in an 18-year-old male. Multiple tracers may be required in the evaluation of a patient. Soft-tissue tumors accumulate technetium-99m DTPA (**A**) (*arrow*). Comparative imaging at this site with gallium-67 has been used to distinguish benign (no uptake) (*arrow*) from malignant lesions (with uptakes) (**B**). Elsewhere bone lesions reflecting dysplastic areas secondary to neurofibromas in the left tibial metaphysis show increased technetium-99m MDP accumulation (**C**) (*curved arrow*).

the primary tumor. Particularly in the head and neck and extremity locations, rhabdomyosarcoma is amenable to thallium-201 scintigraphy for assessment of multifocal extent and response to therapy.[88]

NEUROFIBROMATOSIS

Neurofibromatosis is a relatively common hereditary disorder (autosomal dominant with a variable penetrance) that can cause a dishistiogenesis of tissues predominantly of mesodermal and neuroectodermal origin. The phacomatosis produces neuroectodermal and mesodermal aberrations of the skin, nervous system, bones, and soft tissues. Nervous tissue overgrowth, seen primar-

ily as neurofibromas and schwannomas, may include any of the nerve tissue constituents. Rarely neurofibrosarcoma can occur. This mendelian dominant inherited disorder with variable genetic expression occurs mainly as NF-1, which affects 1 in 4000 persons. There is a 50% spontaneous mutation rate in neurofibromatosis.

The skeletal system is affected by overgrowth (focal gigantism), abnormally loose periosteum (subperiosteal hemorrhage and hematoma), underdevelopment (hypoplasia of the sphenoid bone with resultant exophthalmos, lambdoid sutural defects,[138] absent and hypoplastic pedicles[233]), osseous dysplasia (ribbon ribs, scalloped vertebrae[236]), sharp angle scoliosis, congenital pseudarthroses (predominantly in the tibia and fibula), multiple fibrous lesions of the lower extremities, and dysplastic protrusio acetabuli.[244] Pseudarthroses may radiographically appear as an hour-glass constriction (dysplastic), cystic (area of lysis), or sclerotic type (narrowed medullary canal). Overtubulation can lead to thin, elongated long bones. In elephantoid overgrowth of the extremities, the redundant soft tissues are usually composed combinations of hemangiomatous, lymphangiomatous, and neurofibromatous tissues. The underlying bone is usually elongated and has a wavy, irregular cortex. The periosteum in neurofibromatosis is abnormal, and subperiosteal hemorrhage can occur secondary to mesodermal dysplasia.[313] Focal gigantism is usually attributed to the increased blood flow from the contiguous soft-tissue involvement, but focal gigantism can occur in the absence of abnormal adjacent tissue.

Uptake of the bone agent in an extraosseous neurofibroma occasionally occurs.[290] This is explained by calcification and necrosis in the tumor. However, in another patient, uptake of the bone radiotracer in soft-tissue lesions of the back, buttocks, and thighs regions was explained by sluggish circulation.[159] The tracer localization was attributed to prolonged soft-tissue (blood pool) retention. The soft-tissue overgrowth accompanying neurofibromatosis can be evaluated by technetium-99m diethylenetriamine pentaacetic acid (DTPA) and gallium-67 citrate. Accumulation of technetium-99m DTPA (the commonly used renal scanning agent) has been reported in the soft-tissue tumors of neurofibromatosis.[245] Both plexiform and well-circumscribed focal lesions can be detected. The temporal scintigraphic pattern with neurofibroma is slight to moderate lesion activity in the first 30 minutes after radiopharmaceutical injection and moderate to marked uptake (i.e., progressive intensification) on further delayed imaging (Fig. 16-23, A). This technique, which can detect lesions as small as 1.5 cm, can be used to detect occult neurofibromas in equivocal cases or to survey the body for the location of internal sites. The whole-body survey has advantages of cross-sectional modalities that study smaller volumes. Examination of the paraspinal region lends itself to the use of SPECT, which is able to detect subtle differences in soft-tissue uptake. SPECT is helpful in detecting small lesions because multiplanar reconstruction removes superimposed activity. Preoperative imaging can guide the surgeon in placement of graft material with posterior fusion for kyphoscoliosis. Selecting areas devoid of plexiform neurofibromas helps to prevent bone resorption and ultimate failure of the fusion.

Pain is not a reliable sign of malignant degeneration in the tumors in neurofibromatosis. CT and MRI do not have infallible criteria for distinguishing benign and malignant differentiation in these tumors.[217] The pattern of technetium-99m DTPA accumulation in neurofibrosarcoma has not been determined. Preferential gallium accumulation by malignant tumors of neurofibromatosis has promise as a means for detecting malignant degeneration (Fig. 16-23, B). In one small series gallium uptake occurred in the malignant neoplasms and none of the benign lesions.[137]

Hemangiomas, Vascular Malformations, and Lymphangiomas

The classification of pediatric vascular lesions has recently changed with division into two major categories: hemangiomas and vascular malformations. In general, hemangiomas exhibit rapid growth during the neonatal period and then regress; their main vascular constituent is capillary. Almost all vascular malformations are also present at birth; however, these enlarge in proportion to the child's growth and do not involute. Most represent what were formerly considered cavernous or mixed hemangiomas. These lesions can occur anywhere in the musculoskeletal system: soft tissues, muscle, and sometimes in bone. Lymphangiomas are collections of dilated lymphatics and are classified according to size: capillary, cavernous, or multilocular (cystic hygroma). More than 50% of these lesions are present at birth. Histologically, lesions mixed patterns with angiomatous and lymphangiomatous characteristics at different sites.

Capillary hemangiomas in soft tissues may contain phleboliths (remnants of old, calcified thrombi), which are visible on radiographs. Vascular malformations appear as diffuse soft-tissue masses with loss of normal tissue planes. Cystic angiomatosis of bone (diffuse lymphangiomatosis and hemangiomatosis) is characterized by diffuse cystic lesions and is often associated with visceral involvement.[177] Multiple primary hemangiomas of bone are differentiated from the diffuse type by being localized to a few bones. Bony involvement in cystic angiomatosis includes most of the axial skeleton as well as the femur, humerus, tibia, radius, and fibula. Osseous changes are usually trophic with either increased or decreased bone size, bowing, osteoporosis, cortical thickening, erosions, and phleboliths. Skeletal angiomatosis with involvement of multiple bones is rare. Patients can have skeletal lesions entirely intraosseous or in association with soft-tissue involvement. Radiographically osseous vascular malformations have lytic areas surrounded by sclerosis. In the vertebrae these lesions usually produce a striated or streaked appearance in the vertebral bodies. The small bones of the feet and hands may also be affected.

Soft-tissue lymphangiomas produce a mass effect and usually do not have distinguishing radiographic features. Sometimes the intraosseous lymphangiomas are lytic, well defined, and surrounded by a sclerotic margin. Osseous lymphangiomatosis is rare and may be monostatic or disseminated. A diffuse form of lymphangiomatosis/hemangiomatosis occurs in an entity termed *Gorham disease* ("vanishing bone disease"). In this disease an absent or disappearing portion of the skeleton is associated with regional hemangiomas and/or lymphangiomas. Regeneration of the destroyed bone does not occur. There is a prevalence for involvement of the shoulder and pelvic girdle.

Vascular malformations of bone can display normal, increased, or decreased bone activity on delayed scintigraphic images.[231] The increased activity of skeletal angiomatosis may also be appreciated only on angiographic and blood pool phases of the study.[279] Soft-tissue vascular malformations with cavernous elements may be detected on bone scintigraphy. In this instance the blood pool activity is still in the lesion when delayed images are obtained. This pattern results from slow, sluggish circulation within the lesion, not because of adsorption by phleboliths or bone matrix.[242] Technetium-99m tagged red blood cells can also be used effectively to identify vascular abnormalities of cavernous type.[107] Normal activity is present initially, followed by gradually increasing accumulation of radioactivity in the soft-tissue mass on later images. In vanishing bone disease or Gorham disease, slightly increased activity (somewhat linear or streaky) is found in the soft tissues adjacent to the area of bone resorption. This pattern is visualized on both red blood cell scans and soft-tissue scans done with technetium-99m DTPA.[234] (See section on neurofibromas.) Lymph-

angiomas may be detected by lymphoscintigraphy (technetium-99m antimony trisulfide colloid or technetium-99m human serum albumin) if they communicate with the lymphatic system. Accumulation of the activity may be seen transiently on the early images.[385] Bone scintigraphy may demonstrate multifocal bone involvement (areas of increased uptake) in hemangiomatosis.[5] Multiple "doughnut" lesions have been described in hemangioendothelioma of bone.[264] (The differential diagnosis of "doughnut" lesions is discussed in the section on aneurysmal bone cysts.)

Congenital Limb Enlargement

Congenital limb enlargement (focal gigantism) can result from single or multiple aberrations in the vascular (Klippel-Trénaunay, Parkes-Weber), lymphatic (congeni-

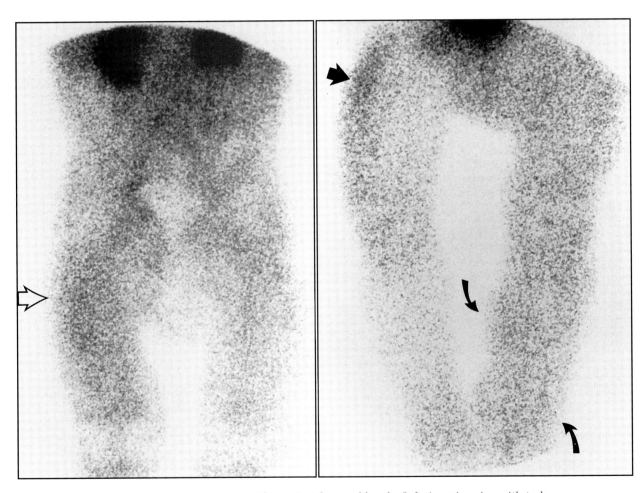

Fig. 16-24. Klippel-Trénaunay syndrome in a 2-year-old male. Soft-tissue imaging with technetium-99m DTPA shows early pooling in the mid right thigh (*open arrow*) and delayed pooling of activity in the left leg (*curved arrows*) and upper right thigh (*thick arrow*) secondary to variable capillary, interstitial, and venous abnormalities. (**A**) Immediate tissue phase. (**B**) Delayed phase (30 to 45 minutes). Patterns of uptake and washout depend on tissue composition of the particular lesion. (*From Mandell GA, Alexander MA, Harcke HT: A multiscintigraphic approach to imaging of lymphedema and other causes of the congenitally enlarged extremity. Semin Nucl Med 1993; 23:334; with permission.*)

tal lymphedema), neuroectodermal (neurofibromatosis), and fibrofatty (*Proteus* syndrome) tissues. Klippel-Trénaunay and some aspects of neurofibromatosis (von Recklinghausen's disease) are discussed here because of the associated musculoskeletal findings. The soft-tissue tumors of neurofibromatosis are discussed under the tumor section.

KLIPPEL-TRÉNAUNAY SYNDROME

Klippel-Trénaunay syndrome is a complex vascular anomaly with a spectrum of lymphatic (hypoplasia, aplasia, lymphangioma), capillary (capillary hemangiomas, port-wine nevi), and venous (varicose veins, venous hypoplasia, aplasia) components. The syndrome is referred to as an angioosteohypertrophy because of associated bony and soft-tissue hypertrophy. Limb hypertrophy results in increased length and circumference. Macrodactyly, syndactyly, and polydactyly also occur.

Bone scintigraphy demonstrates the enlarged deformed extremity and can reflect both the diffuse abnormal soft-tissue uptake and the enlarged osseous components.[350] Lymphoscintigraphy, soft-tissue studies with technetium-99m DTPA[252] (Fig. 16-24), and technetium-99m tagged red blood cell studies can further define the vascular nature of the capillary and cavernous vascular malformations, lymphangiomas, deficiencies of the veins and/or lymphatics, and the varicosities.[235]

LIPOMATOSIS

Fatty tissue lesions are associated with both focal and diffuse soft-tissue enlargements in children. The tumors may be isolated or part of a more encompassing syndrome. Large aggressive lesions can invade local musculature and provoke bony cortical thickening or deformities.[203] Congenital bone anomalies can be associated with deep lipomas. Such bone dysplasia can result in the form of localized overgrowth or deformity.

Lipoblastoma (circumscribed form) or lipoblastomatosis (diffuse form) are both characterized by proliferation of immature "embryonal" lipoblasts in myxoid stroma compartmentalized by fibrous septa. Eighty percent occur in children under the age of 3 years.[205]

Aggressive lipomatosis can produce separation and pressure changes to regional bones as well as overgrowth (macrodactyly or focal gigantism). Bone alteration (such as an enlarged pedicle, transverse process, or femoral neck) has been described with regional soft-tissue lipomas. An anomalous iliac or sacroiliac osseous appendage can occur with intramuscular lipoma, intraspinal lipoma, or lipomeningocele.

Bone-seeking tracers will localize in some lipomas because of their intrinsic dystrophic calcifications. Increased soft-tissue activity can be seen in uncalcified liposarcomas, probably on the basis of the hypervascularity of these lesions.[56] With soft-tissue scanning technique (technetium-99m DTPA) employing sequential (immediate and late) body imaging, fibrofatty lesions fail to accumulate radiotracer. This distinguishes them from neurofibromas and hemangiomas, which will show different patterns.

Myositis Ossificans Progressiva (Fibrodysplasia Ossificans Progressiva)

Myositis ossificans progressiva is usually sporadic in occurrence but may be inherited as an autosomal dominant disorder with variable penetrance. It is usually recognized in early childhood and is associated with a malformation of the great toe or thumb in 70% to 90% of patients.[322] Lesions can develop acutely and are associated with hemorrhagic edema followed by round cell infiltration and capillary proliferation. In the succeeding phase of the disease, there is an increase of collagenous fibrous tissue and degeneration of muscle fibers with evolution into osseous tissue.

Bone is formed in the fascia, aponeuroses, tendons, and/or muscles. Initially involvement is classically in the cervical area, back, or near the joint of a limb. Radiographically the calcification is in periarticular tissues together with gradual bony and fibrous ankylosis of involved joints. Cervical vertebrae are inhibited in their growth, and dislocation of the shoulder and hip joints results from fixation of the shafts of the long bones and continued growth of the proximal metaphyses. There is usually shortening of the proximal phalanx of the thumb, sometimes hypoplasia of the first metacarpal, and clinodactyly of the fifth digit. Metaphyseal flaring with spiking at the edges of the metaphyses in the long bones has recently been reported as a radiographic finding before growth plate fusion.[298]

The foci of ossification in fibrodysplasia ossificans are demonstrated by bone scintigraphy.[97] As with other forms of heterotopic bone formation, serial scans are used to monitor response to treatment and detect the occurrence of new lesions.[134]

Soft-Tissue Abnormalities

HEMATOMA

Subperiosteal hematomas in the neonate are related to calvarial birth trauma (cephalohematoma). In older children subperiosteal hematomas (seen most commonly in the lower extremities) occur secondary to insufficient osseous matrix (scurvy or osteogenesis imperfecta),[105] severe periosteal trauma (child abuse syndrome), or with neuromuscular deficiency (congenital insensitivity to pain or meningomyelocele). In neurofibromatosis the hematoma is seen in focal gigantism and is secondary to osseous dysplasia and loose periosteum.[198,240]

On the bone scan a "doughnut" appearance is produced by peripheral accumulation of the bone radiotracer in the area where microcalcification begins and there is absence of uptake centrally.[104] Changes on bone scan images antedate the radiographic appearance of ossification by several weeks. The intensity of the radiotracer activity is highest early in the process of osteogenesis, and as the heterotopic bone matures, uptake decreases and approaches normal. If scintigraphy is performed later in the process when centripetal calcification takes place, the photopenic center will disappear as conversion of the fibrous center to solid ossification occurs. Musculoskeletal "doughnuts" are not specific for hematoma and can be seen, for example, in giant cell tumors of bone, osteo-myelitis, and coccidiomycosis.

SUBCUTANEOUS FAT/RHABDOMYOLYSIS

Fat necrosis occurs in the neonate as a complication of sepsis, anoxia, hypotension, and other stresses. Clinically subcutaneous protuberances are palpable especially around the cheeks, shoulders, buttocks, and thighs. Fat breakdown leads to fatty acid crystal accumulation, fibroplastic proliferation, and the deposition of calcium salts. Radionuclide accumulation in soft tissue reflects these areas of calcification.[390]

Rhabdomyolysis (damaged muscle) can result in diffusely increased tissue uptake of bone-seeking radiotracer. This has been reported in muscles following extensive exercise or a seizure.[66,213] Focal rhabdomyolysis in children can be secondary to electrical burns, frostbite, meperidine (Demerol) or iron dextran injections,[38] and crush injuries.

CONGENITAL, INHERITED, AND/OR DEVELOPMENTAL ABNORMALITIES

Congenital Osseous Anomalies

The most noticeable congenital derangements of the skeleton visualized by bone scintigraphy are those associated with duplication (supernumerary) or underdevelopment (hypoplasia or aplasia). A classic redundancy of the skeleton is the occurrence of bifid ribs in the thoracic cage. The children with bifid ribs of the chest (usually the third or fourth levels) classically present because someone suddenly feels or notices a chest wall mass. Bone scintigraphy may have been ordered to rule out the presence of a chondroid or osseous neoplasm.

Deficiencies in chondrogenesis and osteogenesis express themselves as absence or reduction of tracer uptake on bone images. Pedicular hypoplasia or aplasia can manifest either as an area of decreased uptake on the ipsilateral side[371] or an area of relative increased uptake on the contralateral side, where a compensatory sclerosis and hypertrophy develops in the pedicle. Photopenia secondary to absent bone must be differentiated from a cold lesion where marrow is replaced by tumor, infarction, or infection. Similarly the contralateral area of increased radiotracer accumulation has a differential from fracture and neoplasm. Examples of absent or deficient uptake (relative photopenia) include undersegmentations of the spine (wedge vertebra and hemivertebra) (Fig. 16-25), myelodysplasia, cleidocranial dysostosis, sphenoid dysplasia, exstrophy of the bladder,[317] fenestrated sternum,[232] absent sternum,[246] absent or hypoplastic radius, fibular hemimelia (absent fibula), and clawfoot deformities. When discussing aberrant patterns of bone uptake that show no uptake where skeletal activity would be expected, one must also think of bone destruction or replacement by tumor or purulent materi-

al as well as lack of inherent osteogenesis (e.g., the fenestrated sternum). Correlative radiographic imaging usually resolves the differential diagnosis.

Congenital Urinary Tract Abnormalities

Approximately 50% of the injected technetium phosphate complexes are excreted by the kidneys, hence coexisting urinary tract abnormalities can be detected. These may be present as much as 15% of the time.[1,228] Irregularly enlarged but functioning kidneys are seen with polycystic kidney disease. Stasis of activity in a collecting system can occur transiently with an extrarenal-type pelvis and to a more pronounced degree in an enlarged dilated system associated with ureteropelvic obstruction, vesicoureteral reflux, or congenital megacalycosis. Congenital anomalies such as absent kidney, ectopic kidney (Fig. 16-26), horseshoe kidney,[99] thoracic kidney, and hypoplastic kidney are readily recognized.

Other detectable anomalies involve the ureter and bladder. An intravesical defect can be produced by a ureterocele. Constipation secondary to neurogenic deficiency or on a functional basis can cause extrinsic pressure on the bladder.[237] Very enlarged, atonic, neurogenic bladders secondary to a meningomyelocele or other neuromuscular-deficient states may have to be catheterized to drain the bladder to visualize the bony pelvis. Idiopathic megaureters or enlarged ureters secondary to reflux may also become apparent during bone imaging. Additional examples of urinary tract imaging during bone scanning are included in Chapters 17 and 18.

Inherited and/or Developmental Abnormalities

EPIPHYSEAL PLATES, APOPHYSEAL PLATES, AND ACCESSORY CENTERS

The scintigraphic appearance of the growth plate changes with age. In the infant and young child the physis is thicker and oval-shaped.[145] With maturation it becomes linear, and in adolescence the closing physis shows progressively decreasing activity. Growth plates close at different times in different parts of the skeleton. Skeletal maturation occurs earlier in girls than boys. The growth plates can be influenced by direct trauma (fractures), infection (meningococcemia), and hypervitaminosis (vitamin A intoxication) with premature closure of a portion of the physis. Chronic hyperemia accelerates regional growth plate closure. Indolent infectious, inflammatory (rheumatoid arthritis, chondrolysis), and tumor/tumorlike (osteoid osteoma, fibrous dysplasia) disease processes can be responsible for premature closure at a site. At all ages, normal physes of the knee have greater activity in the medial half than the lateral half of the femoral growth plate. The opposite finding occurs in the normal proximal tibial physis. Through childhood and adolescence the growth plates reduce in activity relative to the adjacent metaphysis.

Mechanical loading and stress factors influence scintigraphic uptake at the growth plate. When an extremity is immobilized for a prolonged period, activity in the

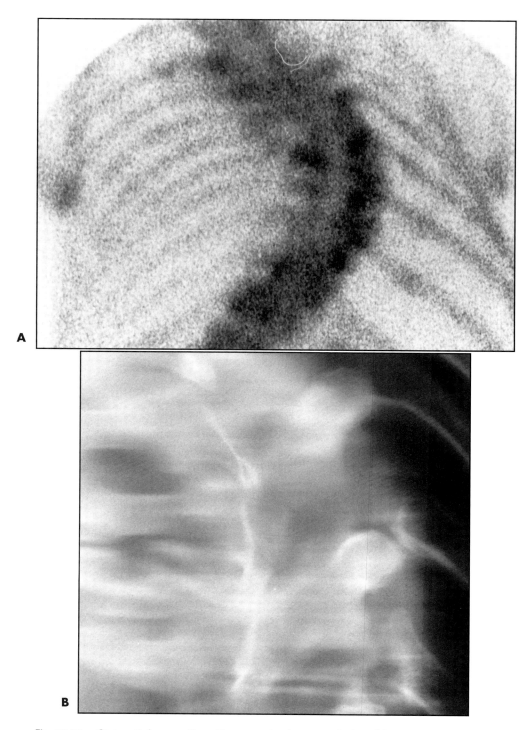

Fig. 16–25. Congenital anomalies of bone create aberrant scintigraphic patterns. Radiographic/scintigraphic correlation provides clarification in this 21-year-old male with congenital scoliosis secondary to thoracic fusion/segmentation abnormality. Posterior scan (**A**) and spine tomogram (**B**).

physis decreases in comparison with the contralateral mobile physis. Immobilization in a cast had been used as nonoperative therapy for SCFE. Angular deformities such as genu varum (bow legs) and genu valgum (knock knees) cause more of the body weight to be supported by the lat-

eral and medial portion of the plate, respectively. These portions of the growth plate become more active. Tibia vara, or Blount disease, is one condition that defies the rules and manifests increased uptake in the medial growth plates of the distal femur and proximal tibia.

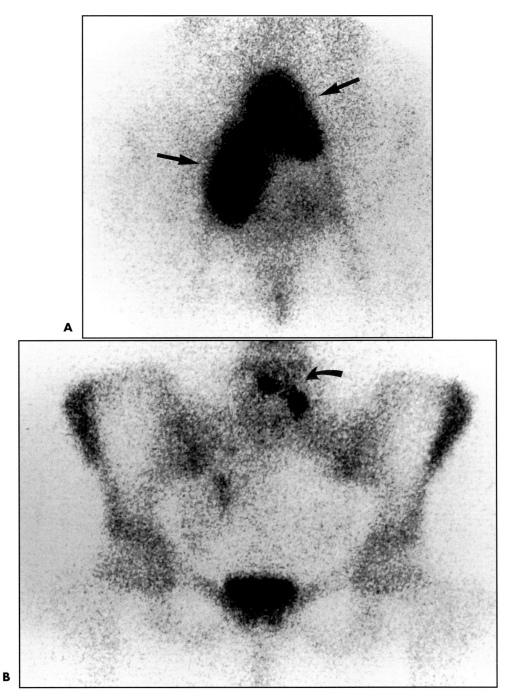

Fig. 16-26.   Fused pelvic kidneys appearing as lumbar spine uptake in a 16-year-old female. The tissue-phase activity (**A**), which shows the fused kidneys (*straight arrows*), is the key to explaining the focal "lesions" in the spine on the delay bone images (**B**) (*curved arrow*).

Bone scintigraphy can be used to diagnose conditions involving the growth plate that are not detectable by plain radiography. Increased physeal activity is seen acutely in Salter type I fractures[141] and SCFE.[346] Angular deformity can result from metaphyseal injury near (but not involving) the growth plate of a long bone. Valgus resulting from medial activity and varus from lateral

uptake near the physis are attributed to local acceleration of growth in a part of the plate.[146,399] Systemic conditions such as rickets and osteomalacia can result in generalized increase in growth plate uptake throughout the skeleton. Intentional surgical closure of a growth plate (epiphysiodesis) is performed in children who have progressive leg length discrepancy. The procedure can be done by a simple percutaneous technique with scintigraphy used to assess the success of the procedure. It takes approximately 4 months for surgical healings, at which time the blood pool and delayed images demonstrate decreased uptake in the plate if the surgery has been successful.

At different ages particular apophyses and accessory ossification centers appear (sometimes asymmetrically) in the juvenile and adolescent skeleton; this can be a source of confusion to those interpreting pediatric bone scintigrams. In the feet, for example, ossification centers that are fusing (i.e., the talus [os trigonum] or the tibia [os peroneum]) are detected because of the better resolution of modern gamma cameras. In symptomatic patients with an apparent os subfibulare, an avulsion fracture may be present; this may or may not be associated with laxity of the anterior talofibular ligament. Clearly, the avulsion fracture is not a normal variant, and bone scintigraphy therefore will demonstrate active uptake.[18] The accessory navicular is situated adjacent to the medial and posterior

margins of the navicular. It is present in 4% to 14% of the population.[207] In asymptomatic individuals the center usually fuses with the navicular. In symptomatic persons, usually adolescent females, the navicular bone remains unfused bilaterally and can be detected by scintigraphy as the lesion causing pain.[208] The os trigonum adjacent to the posterior margin of the talus is triangular and up to 15 mm in size; it is more commonly bilateral than unilateral. The posterior margin of the talus and the unfused ossification center are vulnerable to trauma, particularly in plantar flexion of the ankle. The os trigonum syndrome encompasses the symptomatic individuals. In the proper clinical scenario, the bone scan showing focal increased uptake is an integral part of the ostrigonum syndrome.[181] Sometimes accessory centers such as the bipartite patella can be associated with pain and tenderness, and in these instances increased activity is noted on bone scan.[296]

Apophyses related to posterior and transverse spinous processes sometimes occur, and on planar and SPECT

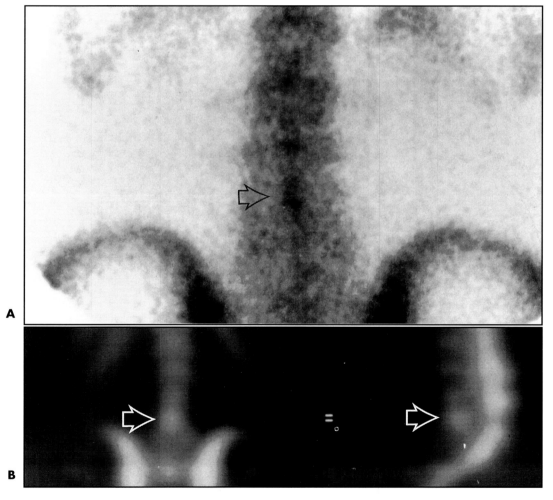

Fig. 16-27. An unfused posterior spinous process apophysis in a 16-year-old male was noted to cause increased uptake on planar (**A**) and SPECT images (**B**) (*arrows*).

images uptake at these sites can be confused with traumatic injuries[239] (Fig. 16-27). Secondary centers that usually ossify at puberty and fuse with the primary centers by age 25 years include the ring epiphyses, the superior articular processes, the transverse processes, the inferior articular processes, and the posterior spinous process. When fusion is actively occurring, the osteoblastic activity increases and previously unrecognized secondary centers become visible. Secondary centers are usually multiple and bilateral. The time of fusion can vary, and the persistent epiphysis can mimic fracture or neoplasm. Correlation of the scan with good-quality radiographs can prevent errors.

DYSPLASTIC PROXIMAL FEMORAL EPIPHYSIS (COMPLICATED VERSUS UNCOMPLICATED)

Bilateral developmental irregularities and pathologic deformities of the proximal femoral epiphyses occur in multiple epiphyseal dysplasia. These radiographic changes can be mistaken for bilateral idiopathic AVN (Legg-Perthes disease).[70] On the other hand, patients with multiple epiphyseal dysplasia can also develop AVN. Multiple epiphyseal dysplasia involves a heterogeneous population with a spectrum of mild to severe epiphyseal involvement.[4] Meyer described a type of dysplasia limited to the femoral head, almost exclusively occurring in boys less than 4 years of age and frequently with a family history of hip problems.[269] Forty-two percent of these patients had bilateral disease, and this probably is a manifestation of a very mild form of multiple epiphyseal dysplasia. The predominant genetic factor is autosomal dominance with complete penetrance but variable expression.

Radiographically multiple epiphyseal dysplasia is characterized by delayed appearance of the epiphyseal center (which is also often irregular and fragmented in appearance). When ossification of the proximal femoral epiphysis finally begins, usually at about 2 years of age, it progresses slowly and results in less than expected volume of mineralization for the patient's age. The epiphyses of the hips, shoulders, and ankles are most commonly involved. Serial radiographic examinations in frontal and lateral (frog-leg) projections are necessary for proper evaluation of patients with both uncomplicated or complicated multiple epiphyseal dysplasia. Sclerosis and fissuring are usually superimposed on the dysplastic epiphysis. When AVN occurs, it is usually unilateral and asymmetric. If the ischemic process is bilateral, it does not occur simultaneously in the two hips. Reversible epiphyseal sclerosis can sometimes be seen in association with renal osteodystrophy.[109] This phenomenon is probably similar to the osteosclerosis produced in the "rugger jersey" spine and would demonstrate increased uptake on bone scintigraphy.

When a patient with epiphyseal dysplasia lacks serial radiographic examinations, bone scintigraphy is helpful in differentiating the complicated form (dysplasia with AVN) from the uncomplicated form (dysplasia alone). High-resolution views of the hips (pinhole collimation) in anterior (neutral) and frog-leg (lateral) views must be compared with similar radiographic projections. In multiple epiphyseal dysplasia without AVN, the distribution of the tracer activity matches the ossification pattern on the radiograph. There is usually slightly increased activity in the dysplastic epiphysis relative to the femoral neck and a normal, nondysplastic epiphysis. A technical problem with interpretation arises when only a small amount of epiphyseal ossification is present, making it difficult to resolve epiphyseal activity from the adjacent activity of the physis. The early and intermediate phases of AVN are characterized by a scintigraphic and radiographic discordance or mismatch; no activity (photopenia) is present in areas where radiographic ossification is apparent.[249]

DEVELOPMENTAL DYSPLASIA OF THE HIP

Congenital dislocation and/or dysplasia of the hip is diagnosed in the infant by the combination of physical examination and ultrasonography. As part of the condition, the ossification of the femoral head may be delayed. During treatment the head is at risk for AVN. AVN of the femoral head does not occur in developmental dysplasia of the hip (DDH) unless treatment has been initiated. It can occur after all types of immobilization (pillow, harness, splint, cast) or surgical intervention.[128] Development of necrosis in the femoral head may be due to interference with the nutritional and matrix physiology of the epiphyseal and physeal germinal cartilage and bone cells. Failure of appearance of the femoral ossification center during the year after reduction or failure of growth of an established center over this same span are accepted as good evidence of AVN. Characteristic signs of neck broadening and flattening and sclerosis of the head may become evident later. A transient growth disturbance may be recognized radiographically by several granular foci rather than a single homogeneous center of ossification. Hip dislocations may be associated with other developmental disorders such as congenital coxa vara and proximal focal femoral deficiency.

Scintigraphic findings vary with the position of the femoral head and duration of the dislocation. Delayed calcification will be paralleled by delay in appearance and extent of bone radiopharmaceutical uptake at the location. AVN superimposed on dysplasia will be recognized by a photopenic femoral head. In long-standing dislocation deformity of the acetabulum, the physis and epiphysis are scintigraphically apparent.

PROTRUSIO ACETABULI

Acetabular protrusion (protrusio acetabuli) is the medial displacement of the inner wall of the acetabulum, accompanied by medial migration of the femoral head. The deformity may be unilateral or bilateral. The process most commonly arises in childhood but usually does not manifest clinically until late in the second decade and adulthood.

A transient form of acetabular protrusion can occur in normal children. These children have a relatively inward bulging of the medial acetabular wall that disappears by the end of puberty. The failure of correction of this normal developmental variation of acetabular configuration may result in protrusio acetabuli. Protrusio acetabuli is a feature of inflammatory processes such as rheumatoid arthritis, osteoarthritis, seronegative spondyloarthropathies, idiopathic chondrolysis, infection, and JRA. Matrix deficiency in osteomalacia or osteoporosis can lead to protrusio acetabuli. Metabolic or connective tissue deficiencies that produce this change in the acetabulum include hyperparathyroidism, hyperthyroidism, osteogenesis imperfecta, hypophosphatasia, mucopolysaccharidoses, and Marfan's syndrome.[20,387] Acetabular protrusion has been reported with skeletal dysplasia such as fibrous dysplasia, Turner's syndrome, and recently in neurofibromatosis.[244] It can also be secondary to a cellular infiltrative process such as histiocytosis in children and secondary to extrinsic radiation therapy.

On plain radiography a straight, true anteroposterior position of the pelvis is mandatory to accurately assess protrusio acetabuli. In growing prepubertal children it is not abnormal for the acetabular line (the curved line of the medial wall of the acetabulum) to be medial to the vertical to slightly oblique ilioischial line (the quadrilateral surface of the acetabulum).[186] Protrusio acetabuli definitely exists when the acetabular line is 3 mm or more medial to the ilioischial line in men and 6 mm or more in women. Narrowing of the joint space can be associated with idiopathic protrusio and concurrent chondrolysis, infection, rheumatoid arthritis, and ankylosing spondylitis.[89,90]

A nuclear medicine study is not used to diagnose protrusio but to detect synovial inflammatory conditions that lead to or aggravate the deformity. On anterior and posterior views of the pelvis, a convex medial bulge of activity may be seen at the site of protrusio into the pelvis. The cases with an increase in acetabular/joint line activity have been associated with rheumatoid arthritis and chondrolysis. Normal soft-tissue and bone uptake are appreciated on blood pool and delayed scintigrams, respectively, in the uncomplicated idiopathic variety of acetabular protrusion.

SCHEUERMANN'S DISEASE

Scheuermann's disease (juvenile kyphosis), a common cause of structural kyphosis of the thoracic spine, is a well-defined clinical entity involving wedging of three or more consecutive vertebrae. The criteria for diagnosis is anterior wedging of 5 or more degrees. The exact etiology of this condition is not known. The incidence is 0.4% to 8.0% of the general population.[223] There is a lumbar form of this thoracic disease, sometimes referred to as "atypical" or lumbar Scheuermann's disease; this form is usually painful. Radiographic features of the lumbar disease include involvement of one or more vertebrae (from T10 to L5) with radiographs showing "scooped" defects in the anterior end plate (herniated Schmorl nodes), end plate irregularities, and disk space narrowing.[28] There is an increased incidence of idiopathic scoliosis in atypical lumbar Scheuermann's disease (43% to 70%).[251] Adolescents with lumbar Scheuermann's disease tend to be more athletic and have a history suggesting increased axial stress to the spine. This condition is self-limiting and benign, and confusion with other pathologic entities of the spine and overtreatment should be avoided.

Bone scintigraphy is usually normal in patients with thoracic Scheuermann's disease.[394] Traditionally bone

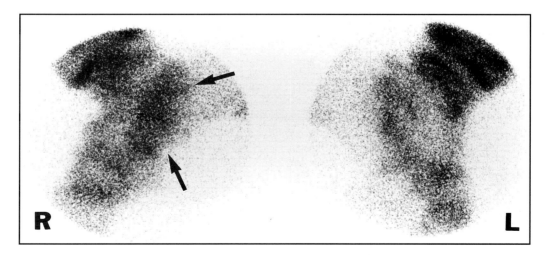

Fig. 16–28. Tarsal coalition (subtalar joint) in a 12-year-old male. Lateral magnification (pinhole) views over the medial aspect of the feet show increased tracer uptake on the right (*arrows*).

scanning has been used to exclude other etiologies for back pain, such as spondylolysis and diskitis. In the lumbar form of Scheuermann's disease, when one or two levels are involved, the clinical picture can be confused with infection or neoplastic disease. In these instances bone scintigraphy has been used. The bone scan findings in lumbar Scheuermann's disease consist of subtle increases in activity on planar scintigraphy and SPECT.[251] The mildly positive findings are less intense than the uptake seen in acute infections and traumatic events.

TARSAL COALITION

Abnormal fusion of two or more independent centers of the hindfoot is termed *tarsal coalition* (also called synostosis and fusion). The most frequent coalitions are between the talus and calcaneus and between the calcaneus and navicular bone.[357] With subtalar coalition the middle facet just behind the sustentaculum tali is the usual location, followed by the anterior, and then posterior facets.[309] Tarsal coalition is attributed to failure of normal segmentation during embryogenesis. Mesodermal union of the tarsal bones occurs in the following order of frequency: bony, fibrous, and cartilaginous. The ossified coalitions are the least mobile. Symptoms do not occur until the second decade, probably because of the flexibility of the early fibrous and cartilaginous stage of the bar. As a rule the talocalcaneal synostoses with the spastic flatfoot type of presentation are more symptomatic than the calcaneonavicular synostoses. The coexistence of calcaneonavicular and talocalcaneal coalitions occurs between 17% and 30% of the time.[211,357]

Standard anteroposterior and lateral weight-bearing radiographs are notoriously poor for revealing the presence of talocalcaneal synostoses. Routine radiography (including the oblique view) usually suffices to rule out calcaneonavicular, calcaneocuboid, and talonavicular coalitions. CT is usually quite effective in determining the location, extent, and nature of coalitions.[157,329]

Bone scintigraphy can be employed in cases with equivocal radiographic and CT changes.[80,122] Focal concentration of activity in the subtalar space is associated with coalition (Fig. 16-28). The active accumulation of radiotracer usually occurs in the bone adjacent to the articular surfaces where abnormal movement evokes stress reactions rather than at the precise location of the synostosis. However, during transformation of a nonosseous to an osseous bridge, increased accumulation of activity is found not only at the talocalcaneal articulations, but also at the point of the developing fusion. High-resolution pinhole images are helpful in diagnosing the equivocal nonosseous subtalar coalition.[243] SPECT can also be a helpful adjunct to magnification bone scintigraphy because it detects small focal accumulations of uptake in the subtalar region. Almost all coalitions of the middle facet can be diagnosed by combining scintigraphy and CT scans. With earlier detection of coalitions by advanced imaging techniques, extirpation of the cartilaginous and fibrous bars can be performed with limited resection; this is thought to minimize the occurrence of later degenerative changes.

Miscellaneous Proliferative Disorders of Osteogenesis

OSTEOPETROSIS

Osteopetrosis (Albers-Schönberg disease) is a diffuse sclerosing dysplasia related to osteoclastic dysfunction. It can occur in either a benign or a malignant form. The aggressive infantile form with diffuse sclerotic bone marrow space obliteration is characterized by anemia, thrombocytopenia, and an increased susceptibility to infection. In the skull the base is most severely affected.[305] The milder forms develop later, usually have a lesser percentage of marrow space obliteration, and are more compatible with survival to an older age. Mild forms of the disease most often have dominant inheritance, whereas severe forms usually have recessive inheritance.

The major clinical and skeletal manifestations of osteopetrosis can be explained by the fact that the resorption of endochondral cartilage is markedly diminished, while bone formation continues at a normal rate. The roentgenographic hallmark of all types of osteopetrosis is a generalized radiodensity (sclerosis) of the medullary portion of bone. Modeling defects are apparent in the metaphyseal regions with Erlenmeyer flask deformities. Bone-within-bone appearances are noted in the spine. Sclerosis is more prominent at the base of the skull.

Bone scintigraphy has demonstrated increased radiopharmaceutical uptake throughout the skeleton in malignant osteopetrosis. In the benign form of the disease, the frontal bones, facial bones, flared ends of long bones, distal ends of metacarpals, and proximal ends of phalanges show increased uptake interspersed with areas of normal activity. The diffuse, avid uptake in osteopetrosis can produce a "superscan" appearance with faint visualization of the kidneys. Focal exaggerated areas of even greater increase in uptake may indicate superimposed pathologic fracture or osteomyelitis.

OSTEOPOIKILOSIS, OSTEOPATHIA STRIATA, MELORHEOSTOSIS

Osteopoikilosis is a rare hereditary disorder with round or oval, usually asymptomatic, areas of dense bone in the long bones and pelvis. Densities range in size from a few millimeters to a few centimeters in diameter. The bone scan is usually normal in this process[389] but on rare occasions shows multiple foci of increased activity corresponding to the sclerotic foci of the roentgenograms.[280] Osteopathia striata is another rare, benign sclerotic dysplasia of bone that is characterized by production of longitudinal dense striations in the metaphyses of bones.[389] Bone scintigraphy does not exhibit any increased uptake.

Melorheostosis is a rare, non-hereditary disorder characterized by asymmetric symptomatic endosteal and periosteal thickening of cortical bone that generally occurs in a single extremity or single bone of an adolescent or young adult.[302] It may include the pelvis or scapula and sometimes can result in deformity and limitation of motion. The overlying skin may be similar in appearance to scleroderma. One proposed etiology is an insult to a segmental sensory spinal nerve. The flowing wax pattern of cortical thickening on radiography is considered pathognomonic of melorheostosis. The bone radiotracer accumulates avidly in the areas of increased, eccentric bone sclerosis.[85,178] The presence of increased blood flow and metabolic activity have been documented by the increased tracer uptake on the three phases of bone scintigraphy.[76] The crossing of joints with asymmetric involvement by increased activity may be specific for melorheostosis.[76,85]

BONE ISLAND

An enostosis is a focus of compact bone within the spongiosa, representing a developmental error: arrested resorption of mature bone during the process of endochondral ossification. A bone island is completely asymptomatic and recognized by its characteristic radiologic appearance. The importance of correctly recognizing this lesion is to avoid mistaking it for a sclerotic primary or metastatic tumor of bone.

The majority of bone islands do not exhibit increased uptake of radiotracer on skeletal scintigraphy. There are, however, reports of some histologically proven bone islands having increased radionuclide uptake on bone scan. The growth activity and size of the bone island have been linked with positive bone scan findings. Greenspan et al demonstrated histologically cold islands to consist of compact, or compact and trabecular, bone with little remodeling and very little cellular activity.[131] The hot islands contained substantial amounts of woven bone, blood vessels, and osteoblastic activity.

DIAPHYSEAL DYSPLASIA (ENGELMANN'S DISEASE AND RIBBING'S DISEASE)

Progressive diaphyseal dysplasia of the Engelmann variety is an autosomal dominant hereditary dysplasia involving the metaphyses and diaphyses of the long bones. The dysplasia of endomembranous ossification results in periosteal and endosteal proliferation of sclerotic bone and a broadening of the long bones. Sometimes the base of the skull is affected. Histologically there is a combination of bone resorption and formation. Ribbing's disease has less extensive skeletal involvement (tibiae and femora), usually occurs after puberty, and may have an autosomal recessive inheritance. Histologically, there is just bone formation.[341]

Areas of sclerosis on radiography usually accumulate the bone radiotracer, but maturation of the process can lead to quiescence and a normal appearance of the bone scan.[199,224] Corticosteroid therapy results in clinical improvement and reduction of diaphyseal uptake of the bone agent.[381] The scintigram also can anticipate the process with increased activity in areas that radiographically appear unremarkable. The bone scan pattern is similar to that in Engelmann's disease but exhibits milder involvement.

ERDHEIM–CHESTER DISEASE

Erdheim-Chester disease is a lipoidosis characterized by foamy histiocytic infiltration of the skeleton and other viscera. Diffuse sclerosis of the metaphyses and diaphyses of the long bones is characteristic on radiography.

On bone scintigraphy there is intense accumulation of the bone radiotracer in these areas.[321]

TUMORAL CALCINOSIS

Tumoral calcinosis is a rare disease characterized by large periarticular calcific masses. The onset of the disease is in childhood, sometimes familial,[33] and usually in black males. It can be idiopathic or secondary to sarcoidosis and is associated with hyperphosphatemia. The calcified conglomerates contain a white suspension of carbonate and calcium phosphonate crystals. There is a connective tissue capsule with a wall rich in mononuclear cells and alkaline phosphatase.

Bone imaging has shown increased radiopharmaceutical uptake corresponding closely in extent to palpable and radiographic evidence of soft-tissue calcification.[40,95] The intense uptake is probably related to the local active osteogenic process. In phosphate depletion therapy a reduction in the size of the mass and its intensity of radiotracer uptake can be noted.[12]

CALCINOSIS UNIVERSALIS/CALCINOSIS CIRCUMSCRIPTA

Intramuscular deposition of calcium phosphate (calcinosis universalis) can occur in inflammatory and collagen vascular disorders (scleroderma, polymyositis, pyomyositis, and dermatomyositis).[16,75,354] The localization of the bone tracer in the soft tissues can antedate radiographic appreciation of the calcification by 18 months on the average. Soft-tissue accumulation of the bone agent can occur in small calcified deposits in the cutaneous and subcutaneous regions adjacent to the extensor aspects of joints and fingertips (calcinosis circumscripta).

Periosteal Proliferations

IDIOPATHIC HYPERTROPHIC OSTEOARTHROPATHY

Hypertrophic osteoarthropathy results in symmetric periosteal production in association with clubbing of the fingers and painful extremities. Hypertrophic osteoarthropathy in patients in the first two decades of life occurs in asthma, cystic fibrosis, bronchiectasis, mediastinal disease (Hodgkin's disease, thyroid, and thymic tumors), cardiovascular disease (cyanotic congenital heart disease, bacterial endocarditis), and gastrointestinal disease (regional enteritis, ulcerative colitis, congenital biliary atresia, lymphoma). The etiology is not definitely known.

Bone scintigraphy reveals diffuse increased uptake in areas of skeletal involvement of the appendicular skeleton.[84,370] The process can be reversed with elimination of the inciting process such as tumor or infection, with normalization of radiographs and scintigrams and disappearance of symptoms.[197]

METABOLIC PERIOSTITIS

Layered periosteal new bone formation is a feature of prostaglandin therapy, healing rickets, scurvy, hypervitaminosis A and D, thyroid arachnopachy, and Caffey's disease. Prostaglandin E_1 intravenous injections are used in infants with ductal-dependent congenital heart disease to maintain ductal patency and prolong life until palliative or corrective surgery is feasible. Osseous complications of prostaglandin therapy include pseudo-widening of the cranial sutures, underossification of the calvarial bones, periostitis, and skin edema.[260] Periosteal reaction can occur as early as 9 days following the initiation of prostaglandin therapy. The distribution of prostaglandin-induced periostitis is usually symmetric and includes the long bones of the extremities, ribs, clavicles, and rarely the mandible.[314]

Findings of hypervitaminosis A include pronounced craniotabes and occipital edema, skin desquamation, fissuring of the lips, pains in the legs and forearms, neurologic disturbances, anorexia, and irritability and hepatosplenomegaly.[307] Hypercalcemia has been described with hypervitaminosis A. Radiographic findings in children over 6 months of age receiving anywhere from 75,000 to 500,000 units of vitamin A include cortical hyperostosis (diaphysitis) in decreasing order of frequency of the ulna, tibia, clavicle, metatarsals, fibula, and ribs. Tender swelling of the covering soft tissues can accompany the affected bones.[46] Other deformities include cup-shaped deformities and widened metaphyses in the long bones. High doses of vitamin A produce an enzymatic dissolution of the cartilaginous matrix by release of lysosomes from the chondrocytes. If the diagnosis is made early and the intake of vitamin A discontinued, usually the osseous changes are reversible. With continued hypervitaminosis, crippling deformities of the long bones with early partial or complete closure of the growth plates

occur even years after initial insult.

The periosteal proliferation of Caffey's disease typically presents during the first 5 months of life. It is frequently less symmetric than prostaglandin or vitamin A in the induced periostitis. The disease almost always involves the mandible and clavicle and is accompanied by the clinical findings of tenderness, swelling, and hyperirritability. A prostaglandin inhibitor, indomethacin, was used for 2-week therapy in some children with return to normal of elevated prostaglandin E serum levels and dramatic relief of symptoms.[158]

Bone scintigraphy will demonstrate increased radionuclide uptake in affected bones whether the site is symptomatic or asymptomatic.[273] The ulna, tibia, and metatarsals commonly have uptake in hypervitaminosis A (Fig. 16-29). The long bones, ribs, and clavicle have increased accumulation of the radionuclide in prostaglandin therapy. The mandible and clavicle are commonly involved in Caffey's disease but not usually implicated in hypervitaminosis A or prostaglandin therapy. Bone scintigraphy has been used to assess the activity of the growth plates secondary to the vitamin A poisoning.

Osteopenia Secondary to Metabolic Disorders

Osteopenia describes the skeleton with less than normal bone mass. The increased radiolucency (decreased density) of bones may result from a deficient connective tissue matrix (osteoporosis) or a disturbed calcium and phosphorus metabolism (osteomalacia).

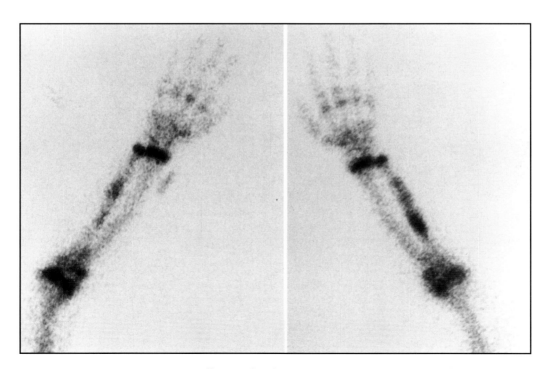

Fig. 16-29. Hypervitaminosis A effect on the ulnas in a 5-year-old male receiving high doses of retinoic acid in association with chemotherapy for neuroblastoma. The scan was performed as a routine survey for metastasis.

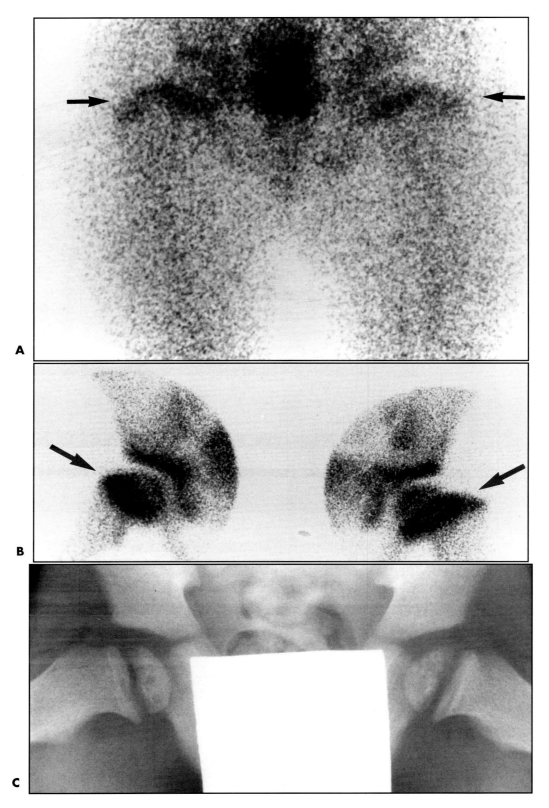

Fig. 16-30. Hypophosphatemic rickets in a 4-year-old female. Growth plate activity is increased for age on tissue-phase (**A**) and delayed (**B**) images (*arrows*). The radiograph shows metaphyseal changes reflecting healing rickets (**C**).

OSTEOPOROSIS (E.G., OSTEOGENESIS IMPERFECTA, JUVENILE OSTEOPOROSIS)

Osteogenesis imperfecta, idiopathic juvenile osteoporosis, long-term steroid therapy, Cushing's disease, and scurvy are disorders producing childhood osteoporosis. Osteogenesis imperfecta is discussed as a representative example of osteoporosis because of the particular applicability of bone scintigraphy to this disorder.

Osteogenesis imperfecta is an inherited disorder of connective tissue that affects the skeleton, ligaments, skin, sclerae, and dentin. There is abnormal maturation of collagen, and a primary defect in extracellular bone matrix. Periosteal bone formation is decreased. Osteoblastic activity is slow, and there is failure to replace fetal bone with normal lamellar bone, resulting in thin, delicate cortices. The number of osteoblasts and osteocytes increases in an attempt to compensate for their lack of efficiency. Blue sclerae result from brown choroid shining through the abnormally thin sclerae. The previous classification of a congenital form with high infant mortality and the tarda form with normal life expectancy has been abandoned. This disorder is now subclassified according to different modes of inheritance and specific biochemical defects in collagen.

In osteogenesis imperfecta, mineralization varies and some mild forms have essentially normal-looking density on plain radiographs. Gracile bones and diaphyseal bowing are the most common features of the milder forms. Short, thick limbs occur almost exclusively in the congenital form. Cystic changes in flared metaphyses is another expression of osteogenesis imperfecta; the metaphyses can be undermodeled or overmodeled. Fracture healing may be normal, or have increased callus or pseudarthrosis formation. Vertebrae can be wedge-shaped or biconcave. Intrasutural bones (wormian bones) are present in the lambdoid sutures and platybasia, with or without basilar impression, is possible.

Bone scintigraphy can be used to determine the presence and age of fractures. Recent fractures (within the last few months) show intense uptake of the radionuclide on both tissue and delayed images. In later stages of healing, the intensity of the radionuclide uptake on delayed images lessens and blood pool activity normalizes. In osteoporosis bone scans may show poor uptake of the radionuclide and increasing the time between injection and acquisition delayed images (3 to 4 hours) may be helpful. If a very acute fracture is suspected, it is desirable to wait 48 to 72 hours before performing bone scanning in patients with osteopenia.

OSTEOMALACIA

Osteomalacia encompasses several disorders in which there is a defect in, or failure of, bone mineralization. When osteomalacia occurs in children, it is known as rickets, and the effects include physeal manifestations of defective mineralization. Causes of osteomalacia in children include nutritional rickets, neonatal deficiency rickets, hypophosphatemic rickets, hyperparathyroidism, renal osteodystrophy, and X-linked hypophosphatemia (familial vitamin D–resistant rickets).

Neonatal deficiency rickets occurs in preterm infants with prolonged, complicated conditions resulting in inadequate nutrition. On chest radiographs of premature infants, fractures of ribs, vertebrae, and proximal long bones may raise the suspicion of rickets. Radiographic changes of rickets include widening of the growth plate, loss of density in the zone of provisional calcification, and irregularity and fraying of the metaphysis. Bowing of the bones into a genu varum or valgum deformity often occurs, depending on the age of the patient and on the degree of weight-bearing. In hypophosphatemic rickets, abnormalities of the peripheral skeleton are common. Looser zones (pseudofractures) occur in the ischial and pubic rami, ribs, scapulae, and the medial aspect of the femoral necks. These occur in areas of stress and probably represent minor insufficiency fractures.

A combination of multiple "hot spots" or pseudofractures in the axial skeleton and long bones suggests osteomalacia. Osteomalacia, with its rapid bone turnover, usually demonstrates prominent uptake in the mandible and calvarium, prominent costochondral junctions, faint kidney images, and increased uptake in the axial skeleton and long bones.[103] In vitamin D–resistant rickets there is usually markedly increased uptake of the growth plates that returns to normal with adequate therapy (Fig. 16-30). A generalized increase in uptake in the axial and peripheral skeleton with more prominent uptake in the metaphyseal regions of the long bones can occur in renal osteodystrophy. The bone scan appearance in neonatal rickets represents an exception. There is usually a generalized decrease in uptake throughout the skeleton. Focal regions of increased activity indicate associated insufficiency fractures.[330]

REFERENCES

1. Adams KJ, Shuler SE, Witherspoon LR, et al: A retrospective analysis of renal abnormalities detected on bone scan. *Clin Nucl Med* 1980; 5:1.
2. Ami TB, Treves ST, Tumeh S, et al: Stress fractures after surgery for osteosarcoma: A scintigraphic assessment. *Radiology* 1987; 163:157.
3. Amundsen TR, Siegel MJ, Siegel BA: Osteomyelitis and infarction in sickle cell hemoglobinopathies: Differentiation by combined technetium and gallium scintigraphy. *Radiology* 1984; 153:807.
4. Andersen PE, Schantz K, Bollerslev J, et al: Bilateral femoral head dysplasia and osteochondritis: Multiple epiphyseal dysplasia tarda, spondyloepiphyseal dysplasia tarda, and bilateral Legg-Perthes disease. *Acta Radiol* 1988; 29:705.
5. Anez LF, Gupta SM, Berger D, et al: Scintigraphic evaluation of multifocal hemangioendothelioma of bone. *J Nucl Med* 1993; 34:297.
6. Aprin H, Roseborough EJ, Hall JE: Chondrosarcoma in children and adolescents. *Clin Orthop* 1982; 166:226.
7. Armas RR, Goldsmith SJ: Gallium scintigraphy in bone infarction: Correlation with bone imaging. *Clin Nucl Med* 1984; 9:1.
8. Aronson J, Karvin K, Siebert J, et al: Efficiency of the bone scan for occult limping toddlers. *J Pediatr Orthop* 1992; 12:38.

9. Ash JM, Gilday DL: The futility of bone scanning in neonatal osteomyelitis: Concise communication. *J Nucl Med* 1980; 21:417.

10. Atkinson RN, Paterson DC, Morris LL, et al: Bone scintigraphy in diskitis and related disorders in children. *Aust N Z J Surg* 1978; 48:374.

11. Baker M, Siddiqui AR, Provisor A, et al: Radiographic and scintigraphic skeletal imaging in patients with neuroblastoma: Concise communication. *J Nucl Med* 1983; 24:467.

12. Balachandran S, Abbud Y, Prince MJ, et al: Tumoral calcinosis: Scintigraphic studies of an affected family. *Br J Radiol* 1980; 53:960.

13. Barker DJP, Hall AJ: The epidemiology of Perthes' disease. *Clin Orthop* 1983; 209:89.

14. Barron BJ, Robinson L, Huyden D, et al: Scintigraphic manifestations of "sternal cupping." *J Nucl Med* 1994; 35:1167.

15. Bellah RD, Summerville DA, Treves ST, et al: Low back pain in adolescent athletes: Detection of stress injury to the pars interarticularis with SPECT. *Radiology* 1991; 180:509.

16. Bellina CR, Bianchi R, Bombardieri S, et al: Quantitative evaluation of 99m-Tc pyrophosphate muscle uptake in patients with inflammatory and noninflammatory muscle disease. *J Nucl Med Allied Sci* 1978; 22:89.

17. Benashel H, Bok B, Cavailloles F, et al: Bone scintigraphy in Perthes disease. *J Pediatr Orthop* 1983; 3:302.

18. Berg EE: The symptomatic os subfibulare: Avulsion fracture of the fibula associated with recurrent instability of the ankle. *J Bone Joint Surg Am* 1991; 73A:1251.

19. Bernstein BH, Singsen BH, Kent JT, et al: Reflex neurovascular dystrophy in childhood. *J Pediatr* 1978; 93:211.

20. Bible MW, Pinals RS, Palmieri GMA, et al: Protrusio acetabuli in osteoporosis and osteomalacia. *Clin Exp Rheumatol* 1983; 1:323.

21. Bilchik TR, Heyman S: Skeletal scintigraphy of pseudo-osteomyelitis in Gaucher's disease. Two case reports and review of the literature. *Clin Nucl Med* 1992; 17:279.

22. Bishop JO, Oley TJ, Stephenson CT, et al: Slipped capital femoral epiphysis: A study of 50 cases in black children. *Clin Orthop* 1978; 135:93.

23. Bjorksten B, Gustavson KH, Erickson B, et al: Chronic recurrent multifocal osteomyelitis and pustulosis palmoplantaris. *J Pediatr* 1978; 93:227.

24. Blasier RD, Monson RC: Acquired spondylolysis after posterolateral spinal fusion. *J Pediatr Orthop* 1987; 7:215.

25. Bloem JL, Mulder JD: Chondroblastoma: A clinical and radiological study of 104 cases. *Skeletal Radiol* 1985; 14:1.

26. Bloem JL, Taminiau AHM, Euldrink F, et al: Radiologic staging of primary bone sarcoma: MR imaging, scintigraphy, angiography, and CT correlated with pathologic examination. *Radiology* 1988; 169:805.

27. Blumberg K, Patterson RJ: The toddler's cuboid fracture. *Radiology* 1991; 179:93.

28. Blumenthal SL, Roach J, Herring JA: Lumbar Scheuermann's: A clinical series and classification. *Spine* 1986; 12:929.

29. Bodner RJ, Heyman S, Drummond DS, et al: The use of single photon emission computed tomography (SPECT) in the diagnosis of low back pain in young adults. *Spine* 1988; 13:1155.

30. Borden S IV: Roentgen recognition of plastic bowing of the forearm in children. *AJR Am J Roentgenol* 1977; 125:524.

31. Borkow SE, Kleiger B: Spondylolisthesis in the newborn. A case report. *Clin Orthop* 1976; 117:23.

32. Borman RR, Johnson RA, Sherman FC: Gallium scintigraphy for diagnosis of septic arthritis and osteomyelitis in children. *J Pediatr Orthop* 1986; 6:317.

33. Bostrom B: Tumoral calcinosis in an infant. *Am J Dis Child* 1981; 135:245.

34. Bowen A: Plastic bowing of the clavicle in children. *J Bone Joint Surg Am* 1983; 65A:403.

35. Brasch RC, Kim OH, Kushner JH, et al: Ossification in soft tissue embryonal rhabdomyosarcoma. *Pediatr Radiol* 1981; 11:99.

36. Bressler EL, Conway JJ, Weiss SC: Neonatal osteomyelitis examined by bone scintigraphy. *Radiology* 1984; 152:685.

37. Bressler EL, Marn CS, Gore RM, et al: Evaluation of ectopic bone by CT. *AJR Am J Roentgenol* 1987; 148:931.

38. Brill DR: Radionuclide imaging of non-neoplastic soft-tissue disorders. *Semin Nucl Med* 1981; 11:277.

39. Brower AC: The osteochondroses. *Orthop Clin North Am* 1983; 14:99.

40. Brown ML, Thrall JH, Cooper Ra, et al: Radiography and scintigraphy in tumoral calcinosis. *Radiology* 1977; 124:757.

41. Brown SJ, Dadparvar S, Slizofski WJ, et al: Triple-phase bone image abnormalities in Lyme arthritis. *Clin Nucl Med* 1989; 14:730.

42. Brown T, Wilkinson RH: Chronic recurrent multifocal osteomyelitis. *Radiology* 1988; 166:493.

43. Brusschwein DA, Brown ML, McLeod RA: Gallium scintigraphy in the evaluation of disk space infections: Concise communication. *J Nucl Med* 1980; 21:925.

44. Busch MT, Morrissey RT: *Clin Orthop* 1987; 18:637.

45. Bushnell D, Shirazzi P, Khedkar N: Ewing's sarcoma seen as "cold" lesions on bone scans. *Clin Nucl Med* 1983; 8:173.

46. Caffey J: Chronic poisoning due to excess to vitamin A. Description of the clinical and roentgen manifestations in seven infants and young children. *AJR Am J Roentgenol* 1951; 12.

47. Caffey J: Traumatic cupping of the metaphysis of growing bones. *AJR Am J Roentgenol* 1970; 108:451.

48. Cahill BR, Borg BC: 99m-technetium phosphate compound joint scintigraphy in management of juvenile osteochondritis dissecans of the femoral condyles. *Am J Sports Med* 1983; 11:329.

49. Campanacci M, Laus M: Osteofibrous dysplasia of tibia and fibula. *J Bone Joint Surg Am* 1981; 63A:367.

50. Capanna R, DalMonte A, Gitelis S, et al: The natural history of unicameral bone cyst after steroid injection. *Clin Orthop* 1982; 166:204.

51. Capitanio MA, Kirkpatrick JA: Early roentgen observation in acute osteomyelitis. *AJR Am J Roentgenol* 1970; 108:488.

52. Caro PA, Borden S IV: Plastic bowing of the ribs in children. *Skeletal Radiol* 1988; 17:255.

53. Carty H, Maxted MB, Fielding JA, et al: Isotope scanning in the "irritable hip syndrome." *Skeletal Radiol* 1984; 11:32.

54. Cawley K, Dvorak A, Wilmot M: Normal anatomic variant: Scintigraphy of the ischiopubic synchondrosis. *J Nucl Med* 1983; 4:14.

55. Cheng TH, Holman BL: Radionuclide assessment of Gaucher's disease. *J Nucl Med* 1978; 19:1333.

56. Chew FS, Hudson TM: Radionuclide imaging of lipoma and liposarcoma. *Radiology* 1980; 136:741.

57. Chew JS, Hudson TM: Radionuclide bone scanning of osteosarcoma: Falsely extended uptake patterns. *AJR Am J Roentgenol* 1982; 139:49.

58. Chung SMK: The arterial supply of the developing proximal end of the human femur. *J Bone Joint Surg Am* 1976; 58A:961.

59. Clausen N, Gotze H, Pedersen A, et al: Skeletal scintigraphy and radiography at onset of acute lymphocytic leukemia in children. *Med Pediatr Oncol* 1983; 11:291.

60. Cohen MD, Siddiqui A, Weetman R, et al: Hodgkin disease and non-Hodgkin lymphomas in children: Utilization of radiological modalities. *Radiology* 1986; 158:499.

61. Committee on Drugs. Guidelines for monitoring and management of pediatric patients during and after sedation for diagnostic and therapeutic procedures. *Pediatrics* 1992; 89:1110.

62. Conway JJ: A scintigraphic classification of Legg-Calve-Perthes disease. *Semin Nucl Med* 1993; 13:274.

63. Conway JJ, Collins M, Tanz RR, et al: The role of bone scintigraphy in detecting child abuse. *Semin Nucl Med* 1993; 23:321.

64. Conway JJ, Gooneratne N, Simon G: Radionuclide evaluation of distal femoral metaphyseal irregularities which simulate neoplasm. *J Nucl Med* 1975; 16:521.

65. Cook AM, Waller S, Loken MR: Multiple "cold" areas demonstrated on bone scintigraphy in patient with neuroblastoma. *Clin Nucl Med* 1982; 7:21.

66. Cornelius EA: Nuclear medicine imaging in rhabdomyolysis. *Clin Nucl Med* 1982; 7:462.

67. Coventry MB, Ghormley RK, Kernohan JW: Intervertebral disk: Its microscopic anatomy and pathology. *J Bone Joint Surg Am* 1945; 27A:105.

68. Cristofaro RL, Appel MH, Gelb RI, et al: Musculoskeletal manifestations of Lyme disease in children. *J Pediatr Orthop* 1987; 7:527.

69. Crone-Munzebrock W, Brassow F: A comparison of radiographic and bone scan findings in histiocytosis X. *Skeletal Radiol* 1993; 9:170.

70. Crossnan JF, Wynn-Davies R, Fulford GE: Bilateral failure of the capital femoral epiphysis: bilateral Perthes disease, multiple epiphyseal dysplasia, pseudoachondroplasia, spondyloepiphyseal dysplasia congenita and tarda. *J Pediatr Orthop* 1983; 3:297.

71. Crowe JE, Swischuk LE: Acute bowing fractures of the forearm in children: a frequently missed injury. *AJR Am J Roentgenol* 1977; 128:981.

72. Czerniak B, Rojas-Corona RR, Dorfman HD: Morphologic diversity of long bone adamantinoma: The concept of differentiated (regressing) adamantinoma and its relationship to osteofibrous dysplasia. *Cancer* 1989; 64:2319.

73. Dahlin DC: Giant cell tumor: Highlights of 407 cases. 1984; 144:955.

74. Dahlin DC, McLeod RA: Aneurysmal bone cyst and other neoplastic conditions. *Skeletal Radiol* 1982; 8:243.

75. Datz FL, Lewis SE, Conrad MR, et al: Pyomyositis diagnosed by radionuclide imaging and ultrasonography. *South Med J* 1980; 73:649.

76. Davis DC, Skylawer R, Cole RL: Melorheostosis on three-phase bone scintigraphy. Case report. *Clin Nucl Med* 1992; 17:561.

77. DeCristofaro R, Biagini R, Boriani S, et al: Selective arterial immobilization in the treatment of aneurysmal bone cyst and angioma of bone. *Skeletal Radiol* 1992; 21:523.

78. Demangeat H, Constantinesco A, Brunot B, et al: Three-phase bone scanning in reflex sympathetic dystrophy of the hand. *J Nucl Med* 1988; 29:26.

79. Detmer DE: Chronic leg pain. *Am J Sports Med* 1980; 8:141.

80. Deutsch AL, Resnick D, Campbell G: Computed tomography and bone scintigraphy: In the evaluation of tarsal coalition. *Radiology* 1982; 144:137.

81. DiAngelis JA, Fisher RL, Ozonoff MB, et al: 99m Tc-polyphosphate bone imaging in Legg-Perthes' disease. *Radiology* 1975; 115:407.

82. Dich VQ, Nelson JD, Haltalin KC: Osteomyelitis in infants and children. *Am J Dis Child* 1989; 129:1153.

83. Dominguez R, Oh KS, Young LW, et al: Acute chondrolysis complicating Legg-Calvés-Perthes disease. *Skeletal Radiol* 1987; 16:377.

84. Donnelly B, Johnson PM: Detection of hypertrophic pulmonary osteoarthropathy by skeletal imaging with 99m-Tc-labeled diphosphonate. *Radiology* 1975; 114:389.

85. Drane WE: Detection of melorheostosis on bone scan. *Clin Nucl Med* 1986; 12:548.

86. Drane WE, Tipler BM: Heterotopic ossification (myositis ossificans) in acquired immune deficiency syndrome. Detection by gallium scintigraphy. *Clin Nucl Med* 1987; 12:308.

87. Dunbar JS, Owen HF, Nogrady MB, et al: Obscure tibial fracture of the infants—the toddler's fracture. *J Can Assoc Radiol* 1954; 15:136.

88. Durak H, Ugar O, Ozgur F: Giant rhabdomyosarcoma with necrosis visualized with Tl-201 chloride. *Clin Nucl Med* 1991; 16:947.

89. Dwosh IL, Resnick D, Becker MA: Hip involvement in ankylosing spondylitis. *Arthritis Rheum* 1976; 19:683.

90. Edelstein G, Murphy WA: Protrusio acetabuli: Radiographic appearance in arthritis and other conditions. *Arthritis Rheum* 1983; 26:1511.

91. El-Khoury GY, Mickelson MR: Chondrolysis following slipped capital femoral epiphysis. *Radiology* 1977; 1234:327.

92. Elliott S, Hutson A, Wastle ML: Bone scintigraphy in the assessment of spondylolysis in patients attending a sports injury clinic. *Clin Radiol* 1988; 39:269.

93. Ellison MJ, Isaac L, Smith WI, et al: Intraoperative scintigraphic localization of the nidus of osteoid osteoma. *Clin Nucl Med* 1984; 11:640.

94. Englaro EE, Gelfand MJ, Paltiel HJ: Bone scintigraphy in preschool children with lower extremity pain of unknown origin. *J Nucl Med* 1992; 33:351.

95. Eugenidis N, Locher JT: Tumor calcinosis imaged by bone scanning. *J Nucl Med* 1988; 18:34.

96. Even-Sapir E, Martin RH, Mitchell MJ, et al: Assessment of painful late effects of lumbar spinal fusion with SPECT. *J Nucl Med* 1994; 35:416.

97. Fang MA, Reinig JW, Hill SC, et al: Technetium-99m MDP demonstration of heterotopic ossification in fibrodysplasia ossificans progressiva. *Clin Nucl Med* 1986; 11:8.

98. Fernandez-Ulloa M, Vasavada PJ, Black RR: Detection of acute osteomyelitis with indium-111 labeled white blood cells in a patient with sickle cell disease. *Clin Nucl Med* 1989; 14:97.

99. Fink-Bennett D, Dworkin H: Incidental detection of a horseshoe kidney on radionuclide bone images. *Radiology* 1977; 123:392.

100. Fischer GW, Popich GA, Sullivan DE, et al: Discitis: A prospective diagnostic analysis. *Pediatrics* 1978; 62:543.

101. Fischer KC, Shapir S, Treves S: Visualization of the spleen with a bone-seeking radionuclide in a child with sickle cell anemia. *Radiology* 1977; 122:398.

102. Fisher RL: An epidemiological study of Legg-Perthes disease. *J Bone Joint Surg Am* 1972; 54A:769.

103. Fogelman I, McKillop JH, Cowden EA, et al: The role of bone scanning in osteomalacia. *J Nucl Med* 1978; 19:245.

104. Front D, Hardoff R: Doughnut phenomenon in bone scintigraphy. *Clin Nucl Med* 1978; 3:82.

105. Front D, Hardoff R, Levy T, et al: Bone scintigraphy in scurvy. *J Nucl Med* 1978; 19:916.

106. Front D, Israel O, Jerushalmi J, et al: Quantitative bone scintigraphy using SPECT. *J Nucl Med* 1989; 30:240.

107. Front D, Royal HD, Israel O: Scintigraphy of hepatic hemangiomas: The value of Tc-99m labeled red blood cells: Concise communication. *J Nucl Med* 1981; 22:684.

108. Gamble JR, Rinsky LA: Chronic recurrent multifocal osteomyelitis: A distinct clinical entity. *J Pediatr Orthop* 1986; 6:579.

109. Garver P, Resnick D, Niwayama G, et al: Epiphyseal sclerosis in renal osteodystrophy simulating osteonecrosis. *AJR Am J Roentgenol* 1981; 136:1239.

110. Gates GF: Scintigraphy of discitis. *Clin Nucl Med* 1977; 2:20.

111. Gelberman RH, Bauman TD, Menon J, et al: The vascularity of the lunate bone in Kienböck's disease. *J Hand Surg* 1980; 5:272.

112. Gelfand MJ, Silberstein EB: Radionuclide imaging: Use in diagnosis of osteomyelitis in children. *JAMA* 1977; 237:245.

113. Gelfand MJ, Strife JL, Graham EJ, et al: Bone scintigraphy in slipped capital femoral epiphysis. *Clin Nucl Med* 1983; 8:613.

114. Gerscovich EO, Greenspan A: Osteomyelitis of the clavicle: Clinical, radiologic and bacteriologic findings in ten patients. *Skeletal Radiol* 1994; 23:205.

115. Ghelman B, Thompson FM, Arnold WD: Intraoperative radioactive localization of an osteoid osteoma. *J Bone Joint Surg Am* 1981; 63A:826.

116. Giedion A, Kesztler R, Muggiasca F: The widened spectrum of multiple cartilaginous exostoses (MCE). *Pediatr Radiol* 1975; 3:93.

117. Gilday DL, Ash JM, Green MD: Child abuse: Its complete evaluation by one radiopharmaceutical (abstract). *J Nucl Med* 1980; 21:10.

118. Gilday DL, Ash JM, Reilly BJ: Radionuclide skeletal survey for pediatric neoplasms. *Radiology* 1977; 123:399.

119. Gille P, Nachin P, Aubert S, et al: Intraoperative radioactive localization of an osteoid osteoma: Four case reports. *J Pediatr Orthop* 1986; 6:596.

120. Giulano AE, Feig S, Eilber RF: Changing metastatic patterns of osteosarcoma. *Cancer* 1984; 54:2160.

121. Goldman AB, Becker MH, Braunstein P, et al: Bone scanning—osteogenic osteosarcoma. *AJR Am J Roentgenol* 1975; 124:83.

122. Goldman AB, Pavlov H, Schneider R: Radionuclide bone scanning in subtalar coalitions: Differentiations considerations. *AJR Am J Roentgenol* 1982; 138:427.

123. Goldman AB, Schneider R, Martel W: Acute chondrolysis complicating slipped-capital femoral epiphysis. *AJR Am J Roentgenol* 1978; 130:945.

124. Goldsmith D, Feldman N, Heyman S, et al: Nuclear imaging in childhood reflex neurovascular dystrophy (CRND). *Arthritis Rheum* 1986; 29(suppl 4): 92.

125. Goldstein H, McNeil BJ, Zufali E, et al: Changing indications for bone scintigraphy in patients with osteosarcoma. *Radiology* 1980; 135:177.

126. Golimbu C, Firozinia H, Rafii M, et al: Acute traumatic fibular bowing associated with tibial fracture. *Clin Orthop* 1982; 182:211.

127. Goodgold HM, Chen DCP, Majd M, et al: Scintigraphic features of giant cell tumor. *Clin Nucl Med* 1984; 9:526.

128. Gore DR: Iatrogenic avascular necrosis of the hip in young children: A review of six cases. *J Bone Joint Surg Am* 1974; 56A:493.

129. Green M, Nyhan WL, Fousek MD: Acute hematogenous osteomyelitis. *Pediatrics* 1956; 17:368.

130. Green NE, Beauchamp RD, Griffin PP: Primary subacute epiphyseal osteomyelitis. *J Bone Joint Surg Am* 1981; 63A:107.

131. Greenspan A, Steiner G, Knutzon R: Bone island (enostosis): Clinical significance and radiologic and pathologic correlation. *Skeletal Radiol* 1991; 20:85.

132. Greyson ND, Pang S: The variable appearance of nonosteogenic fibroma of bone. *Clin Nucl Med* 1981; 6:242.

133. Guze BH, Hawkings RA, Marcus CS: Technetium-99m white blood cell imaging: False-negative results in Salmonella osteomyelitis associated with sickle cell disease. *Clin Nucl Med* 1989; 14:104.

134. Guze BH, Scheibert H: The nuclear bone image and myositis ossificans progressiva. *Clin Nucl Med* 1989; 14:161.

135. Haase D, Martin R, Marrie T: Radionuclide imaging in pyogenic vertebral osteomyelitis. *Clin Nucl Med* 1980; 5:533.

136. Haase GM, Ortiz V, Sfaianakis GN, et al: The value of radionuclide bone scanning in the early recognition of deliberate child abuse. *J Trauma* 1980; 20:873.

137. Hammond JA, Driedger AA: Detection of malignant change in neurofibromatosis (von Recklinghausen's disease) by gallium-67 scanning. *Can Med Assoc J* 1978; 119:352.

138. Handa J, Koyama T, Shimizu Y, et al: Skull defect involving the lambdoid suture in neurofibromatosis. *Surg Neurol* 1975; 3:119.

139. Handmaker H, Giammona ST: Improved early diagnosis of acute inflammatory skeletal-articular disease in children: A two-radiopharmaceutical approach. *Pediatrics* 1984; 73:661.

140. Hannon KM, Wetta WJ: Failure of technetium bone scanning to detect pseudoarthroses in spinal fusion for scoliosis. *Clin Orthop* 1977; 123:42.

141. Harcke HT: Bone scintigraphy in children: Trauma. *Ann Radiol* 1983; 26:675.

142. Harcke HT: Bone imaging in infants and children: A review. *J Nucl Med* 1978; 19:324.

143. Harcke HT, Conway JJ, Tachdjian MO, et al: Scintigraphic localization of bone lesions during surgery. *Skeletal Radiol* 1985; 13:211.

144. Harcke HT, Larkin M, Clancy M: Evaluation of spinal fusions by bone scintigraphy (abstract). *J Nucl Med* 1980; 21:9.

145. Harcke HT, Mandell GA: Scintigraphic evaluation of the growth plate. *Semin Nucl Med* 1993; 23:266.

146. Harcke HT, Zapf SE, Mandell GA, et al: Angular deformity of the lower extremity: Evaluation with quantitative scintigraphy. *Radiology* 1987; 164:437.

147. Harris WH, Dudley HR, Barry RV: The natural history of fibrous dysplasia. *J Bone Joint Surg Am* 1962; 44A:207.

148. Hartmann JT, Gates DJ: Recovery from cartilage necrosis following slipped capital femoral epiphysis. *Clin Orthop* 1982; 165:99.

149. Hattner RS, Huberty JP, Engelstad BL, et al: Localization of m-iodo (131-I) benzylguanidine in neuroblastoma. *AJR Am J Roentgenol* 1984; 143:373.

150. Haueisen DC, Weiner DS, Weiner SD: The characterization of "transient synovitis of the hip" in children. *J Pediatr Orthop* 1986; 6:11.

151. Heisel MA, Miller JH, Reid BS, et al: Radionuclide scan in neuroblastoma. *Pediatrics* 1983; 71:206.

152. Helms CA, Hattner RS, Vogler JB: Osteoid osteoma: radionuclide diagnosis. *Radiology* 1984; 151:779.

153. Henry A: Monostotic fibrous dysplasia. *J Bone Joint Surg Br* 1969; 51B:300.

154. Herman JH, Herzig EB, Crissman JD, et al: Idiopathic chondrolysis—an immunopathological study. *J Rheumatol* 1980; 7:694.

155. Hernandez RJ, Conway JJ, Poznanski AK, et al: The role of computed tomography and radionuclide scintigraphy in the localization of osteomyelitis in flat bones. *J Pediatr Orthop* 1985; 5:151.

156. Herndon WA, Alexieva BT, Schwindt ML, et al: Nuclear imaging for musculoskeletal infections in children. *J Pediatr Orthop* 1985; 5:343.

157. Herzenber JE, Goldner JL, Martinez S, et al: Subtalar joint coalition: A clinical and anatomic study. *Foot Ankle* 1986; 6:273.

158. Heyman E, Laver J, Beer S: Prostaglandin synthetase inhibitor in Caffey's disease. *J Pediatr* 1982; 101:314.

159. Holbert RL, Lamki LM, Holbert JM: Uptake of bone scanning agent in neurofibromatosis. *Clin Nucl Med* 1987; 12:66.

160. Holder LE, Cole LA, Myerson MS: Reflex sympathetic dystrophy in the foot: Clinical and scintigraphic criteria. *Radiology* 1992; 184:531.

161. Holder LE, Michael RH: The specific scintigraphic pattern of "shin splints" in the lower leg: Concise communication. *J Nucl Med* 1984; 25:865.

162. Howard JB, Highenboten CL, Nelson JS: Residual effects of septic arthritis in infancy and childhood. *JAMA* 1978; 236:932.

163. Howman-Giles RB, Gilday DL, Ash JM: Radionuclide skeletal survey in neuroblastoma. *Radiology* 1979; 131:497.

164. Howman-Giles RB, Trochei M, Yeates K, et al: Partial growth plate closure: Apex view on bone scan. *J Pediatr Orthop* 1985; 5:109.

165. Howman-Giles RB, Uren R: Multifocal osteomyelitis in childhood. Review of radionuclide bone scan. *Clin Nucl Med* 1992; 17:274.

166. Hudson TM: Scintigraphy of aneurysmal bone cyst. *AJR Am J Roentgenol* 1984; 142:761.

167. Hudson TM, Bertoni F, Enneking WF: Scintigraphy of aggressive fibromatosis. *Skeletal Radiol* 1985; 13:26.

168. Hudson TM, Hawkins IF Jr: Radiologic evaluation of chondroblastoma. *Radiology* 1981; 139:1.

169. Hudson TM, Schiebler M, Springfield DS, et al: Radiology of giant cell tumors of bone: Computed tomography, arthro-tomography, and scintigraphy. *Skeletal Radiol* 1984; 11:85.

170. Hudson TM, Stiles RG, Monson DK: Fibrous lesions of bone. *Radiol Clin North Am* 1993; 31:279.

171. Hughes AW: Idiopathic chondrolysis of the hip: A case report and review of the literature. *Ann Rheum Dis* 1985; 44:268.

172. Humphrey A, Gilday DL, Brown RG: Bone scintigraphy in chondroblastoma. *Radiology* 1980; 137:497.

173. Ingram AJ, Clarke MS, Clark CS, et al: Chondrolysis complicating slipped capital femoral epiphysis. *Clin Orthop* 1982; 165:99.

174. Israeli A, Zwas ST, Horoszowski H, et al: Use of radionuclide method in preoperative and intraoperative diagnosis of osteoid osteoma of the spine: Case report. *Clin Orthop* 19XX; 175:192.

175. Jackson RL, Llaurado JG: Visualization by dynamic and static osseous scintigraphy of pelvic chondrosarcoma in multiple hereditary exostoses. *Clin Nucl Med* 1987; 12:113.

176. Jackson RP, Reckling FW, Mants FA: Osteoid osteoma and osteoblastoma. Similar histologic lesions with different natural histories. *Clin Orthop* 1977; 128:303.

177. Jacobs JE, Kimmelstiel P: Cystic angiomatosis of the skeletal system. *J Bone Joint Surg Am* 1953; 35A:403.

178. Janousek J, Preston DF, Martin NL, et al: Bone scan in melorheostosis. *J Nucl Med* 1979; 4:75.

179. Jarvis J, McIntyre W, Udjus K, et al: Osteomyelitis of the ischiopubic synchondrosis. *J Pediatr Orthop* 1985; 5:163.

180. Jaudes PK: Comparison of radiography and radionuclide bone scanning in the detection of child abuse. *Pediatrics* 1984; 73:166.

181. Johnson RP, Collier BD, Carrera GF: The os trigonum syndrome: Use of the bone scan in diagnosis. *J Trauma* 1984; 24:761.

182. Jones BS: Adolescent chondrolysis of the hip joint. *A Afr Med J* 1971; 45:196.

183. Jones DC, Cady RB: "Cold" bone scans in acute osteomyelitis. *J Bone Surg* 1981; 63B:376.

184. Jones MM, Moore WM, Brewer EJ, et al: Radionuclide bone/joint imaging in children with rheumatic complaints. *Skeletal Radiol* 1988; 17:1.

185. Jurik AG, Moller BN: Inflammatory hyperostosis and sclerosis of the clavicle. *Skeletal Radiol* 1986; 15:284.

186. Katz JF: Precise identification of radiographic acetabular landmarks. *Clin Orthop* 1979; 141:166.

187. Kaufman JH, Cedermark BJ, Parthasarthy KL, et al: The value of "67"-Ga scintigraphy in soft-tissue sarcoma and chondrosarcoma. *Radiology* 1977; 123:131.

188. Kaufman RA, Thrall JH, Keyes JW, et al: False-negative bone scans in neuroblastoma metastatic to the ends of long bones. *AJR Am J Roentgenol* 1978; 130:131.

189. Kay JJ, Winchester PH, Freiberger RH: Neonatal septic "dislocation" of the hip: True dislocation of pathological epiphyseal separation? *Radiology* 1975; 114:671.

190. Keret D, Kumar SJ: Unicameral bone cysts in the humerus and femur in the same child. *J Pediatr Orthop* 1987; 7:712.

191. Kerr R: Radiology of the seronegative spondyloarthropathies. *Clin Exp Rheum* 1987; 5(S1):101.

192. Kingston S: The role of technetium and gallium imaging in musculoskeletal disorders. *Clin Rheum Dis* 1983; 9:347.

193. Klein M, Becker MH, Genieser NB, et al: Case Report 161. *Skeletal Radiol* 1981; 6:307.

194. Kloiber R, Paulovsky W, Portner O, et al: Bone scintigraphy of the hip joint effusion in children. *AJR Am J Roentgenol* 1983; 140:995.

195. Krasnow AZ, Isitman AT, Collier BD, et al: Flow study and SPECT imaging for the diagnosis of giant cell tumor of bone. *Clin Nucl Med* 1988; 13:89.

196. Kricun ME: Red-yellow marrow conversion: Its effect on the location of some solitary bone lesions. *Skeletal Radiol* 1985; 14:10.

197. Kroon HM, Pauwels EKJ: Bone scintigraphy for the detection and follow-up of hypertrophic osteoarthropathy. *Diagn Imaging* 1982; 51:47.

198. Kullman L, Wouters HW: Neurofibromatosis, gigantism and subperiosteal hematoma. *J Bone Joint Surg Br* 1972; 54B:130.

199. Kumar B, Murphy WA, Siegel BA: Progressive diaphyseal dysplasia (Engelmann's disease): Scintigraphic-radiologic-clinical correlations. *Radiology* 1981; 140:87.

200. Kumar R, Balachandran S: Relative roles of radionuclide scanning and radiographic imaging in eosinophilic granuloma. *Clin Nucl Med* 1980; 12:538.

201. Kumar SJ, Harcke HT, MacEwen GD, et al: Osteoid osteoma of the proximal femur. New techniques in diagnosis and treatment. *J Pediatr Orthop* 1984; 4:669.

202. Kwekkeboom DJ, van Urk H, Bernard KHP, et al: Octreotide scintigraphy for the detection of paragangliomas. *J Nucl Med* 1993; 34:873.

203. Lachman RS, Finkelstein MD, Mehringer CM, et al: Congenital aggressive lipomatosis. *Skeletal Radiol* 1983; 9:248.

204. Lange RH, Lange TA, Rao BK: Correlative radiographic, scintigraphic, and histological evaluation of exostoses. *J Bone Joint Surg Am* 1984; 66A:1454.

205. Langloh JT, Reing CM, Chun BK, et al: Lipoblastomatosis. A case report. *J Bone Joint Surg Am* 1978; 60A:130.

206. Lantto EH, Kaukonen JP, Kukkola A, et al: Tc-99m HMPAO labeled leukocytes superior to bone scan in detection of osteomyelitis in children. *Clin Nucl Med* 1992; 17:7.

207. Lawson JP: Clinically significant radiologic anatomic variants of the skeleton. *AJR Am J Roentgenol* 1994; 163:249.

208. Lawson JP, Ogden JA, Sella E, et al: The painful accessory navicular. *Skeletal Radiol* 1984; 12:250.

209. Lawson JP, Steere AC: Lyme arthritis: radiologic findings. *Radiology* 1985; 154:37.

210. Laxer RM, Malleson PN, Morrison RT, et al: Technetium 99m-methylene diphosphonate bone scans in children with reflex neurovascular dystrophy. *J Pediatr* 1985; 106:437.

211. Lee MS, Harcke HT, Kumar SJ, et al: Subtalar joint coalition in children: New observations. *Radiology* 1989; 172:635.

212. Lemahjieu RA, Van Laere C, Verbruggen LA: Reflex sympathetic dystrophy: An underreported syndrome in children. *Eur J Pediatr* 1988; 147:47.

213. Lentle B, Percy JS, Rigal WM, et al: Localization of Tc-99m pyrophosphate in muscle after exercise. *J Nucl Med* 1978; 19:223.

214. Lessig HJ, Devenney JE: Localization of bone-seeking agent within a desmoid tumor. *Clin Nucl Med* 1979; 4:164.

215. Levin E, DeSmet AA, Neff JR: Role of radiologic imaging in management of planning of giant cell tumor of bone. *Skeletal Radiol* 1984; 12:79.

216. Levin E, DeSmet AA, Neff JR: Scintigraphic evaluation of giant cell tumor bone. *AJR Am J Roentgenol* 1984; 143:343.

217. Levine E, Huntrakoon M, Wetzel LH: Malignant nerve-sheath neoplasms in neurofibromatosis: Distinction from benign tumors by imaging techniques. *AJR Am J Roentgenol* 1987; 149:1059.

218. Lewis JS, Rosenfeld NS, Hoffer PB, et al: Acute osteomyelitis in children: Combined Tc-99m and Ga-67 imaging. *Radiology* 1986; 158:795.

219. Lewis RJ, Ketcham AS: Maffucci's syndrome: Functional and neoplastic significance. *J Bone Joint Surg Am* 1973; 55A:1465.

220. Lieberman CM, Hemingway DL: Scintigraphy of shin splints. *Clin Nucl Med* 1980; 5:31.

221. Lisbona R, Rosenthal L: Role of radionuclide imaging in osteoid osteoma. *AJR Am J Roentgenol* 1979; 132:77.

222. Lowe HG: Necrosis of articular cartilage after slipping of the capital femoral epiphysis. Report of six cases with recovery. *J Bone Joint Surg Br* 1970; 52B:108.

223. Lowe TG: Current concepts review: Scheuermann's disease. *J Bone Joint Surg Am* 1990; 72A:940.

224. Lundy MMK, Billingsley JL, Redwine MD, et al: Scintigraphic findings in progressive diaphyseal dysplasia. *J Nucl Med* 1982; 23:324.

225. Mabney JD, Fitch RD: Plastic deformation in pediatric fractures: Mechanism and treatment. *J Pediatr Orthop* 1989; 9:310.

226. Machida K, Makita K, Nishikawa J, et al: Scintigraphic manifestation of fibrous dysplasia. *Clin Nucl Med* 1986; 11:426.

227. Macintosh D, Xipell JM, Thomas DP: Ossifying fibroma of bone. Report of two cases. *Australas Radiol* 1986; 30:124.

228. Maher FT: Evaluation of renal and urinary tract anomalies noted on scintiscans: A retrospective study of 1711 radioisotope skeletal surveys performed in an 18-month period. *Mayo Clin Proc* 1975; 50:370.

229. Mahoney DH Jr, Shepherd DA, DePuey EG, et al: Childhood multifocal osteosarcoma: Diagnosis by 99m technetium bone scan. A case report. *Med Pediatr Oncol* 1979; 6:347.

230. Makhija MC: Bone scanning in aneurysmal bone cyst. *Clin Nucl Med* 1981; 6:500.

231. Makhija M, Boffill ER: Hemangioma, a rare cause of photopenic lesion on skeletal imaging. *Clin Nucl Med* 1986; 7:487.

232. Mandell GA: Mid-line circular photopenic defects of the sternum. *Br J Radiol* 1983; 56:761.

233. Mandell GA: The pedicle in neurofibromatosis. *AJR Am J Roentgenol* 1978; 130:675.

234. Mandell GA: Unpublished data.

235. Mandell GA, Alexander MA, Harcke HT: A multiscintigraphic approach to imaging of lymphedema and other causes of the congenitally enlarged extremity. *Semin Nucl Med* 1993; 23:334.

236. Mandell GA, Casselman EC: Vertebral scalloping in neurofibromatosis. *Radiology* 1978; 7:178.

237. Mandell GA, Harcke HT: Extrinsic causes of vesical filling defects. *Clin Nucl Med* 1987; 12:204.

238. Mandell GA, Harcke, HT: Scintigraphic manifestations of infraction of the second metatarsal (Freiberg's disease). *J Nucl Med* 1987; 28:249.

239. Mandell GA, Harcke HT: Scintigraphy of persistent vertebral transverse process epiphysis. *Clin Nucl Med* 1987; 12:359.

240. Mandell GA, Harcke HT: Subperiosteal hematoma: Another scintigraphic "doughnut." *Clin Nucl Med* 1986; 11:35.

241. Mandell GA, Harcke HT, Bowen JR, et al: Transient photopenia in the femoral head following arthrography. *Clin Nucl Med* 1989; 14:397.

242. Mandell GA, Harcke HT, Davis N: Accumulation of technetium-99m MDP in an intramuscular hemangioma. *Clin Nucl Med* 1986; 11:487.

243. Mandell GA, Harcke HT, Hugh J, et al: Detection of talocalcaneal coalitions by magnification bone scintigraphy. *J Nucl Med* 1990; 31,1797.

244. Mandell GA, Harcke HT, Scott CI Jr, et al: Protrusio acetabuli in neurofibromatosis: Nondysplastic and dysplastic forms. *Neurosurgery* 1992; 30:550.

245. Mandell GA, Herrick WC, Harcke HT, et al: Neurofibromas: Location by scanning with Tc-99m DTPA. Work in progress. *Radiology* 1985; 157:803.

246. Mandell GA, Heyman S: Absent sternum on bone scan. *Clin Nucl Med* 1983; 8:327.

247. Mandell GA, Heyman S: Extraosseous uptake of technetium-99m MDP in secondary deposits of neuroblastoma. *Clin Nucl Med* 1986; 11:337.

248. Mandell GA, Keret D, Harcke HT, et al: Chondrolysis: detection by bone scintigraphy. *J Pediatr Orthop* 1992; 12:80.

249. Mandell GA, Mackenzie WG, Scott CI Jr, et al: Identification of avascular necrosis in the dysplastic proximal femoral epiphysis. *Skeletal Radiol* 1989; 118:273.

250. Mandell GA, Meek RS: Infarctions of ilia in young patients. *Clin Nucl Med* 1993; 18:559.

251. Mandell GA, Morales RW, Harcke HT, et al: Bone scintigraphy in patients with atypical lumbar Scheuermann's disease. *J Pediatr Orthop* 1993; 13:622.

252. Mandell GA, Scott CI Jr., Harcke HT, et al: Scintigraphic differentiation of congenital soft-tissue extremity enlargement with Tc-99m DTPA. *Skeletal Radiol* 1989; 18:33.

253. Manson D, Wilmot DM, King S, Laxer RM: Physeal involvement in chronic recurrent multifocal osteomyelitis. *Pediatr Radiol* 1989; 20:76.

254. Marcove RC: Chondrosarcoma: Diagnosis and treatment. *Orthop Clin North Am* 1977; 8:811.

255. Martel W, Holt JF, Cassidy JT: Roentgenographic manifestations of juvenile rheumatoid arthritis. *AJR Am J Roentgenol* 1962; 88:400.

256. Martin NL, Prestgon DF, Robinson RG, et al: Osteoblastomas of the axial skeleton shown by skeletal scanning: Case report. *J Nucl Med* 1976; 17:187.

257. Martin W, Riddervold HO: Acute plastic bowing of the fibula. *Radiology* 1979; 131:639.

258. Martin-Simmerman P, Cohen MD, Siddiqui A, et al: Calcification and uptake of Tc-99m diphosphonates in neuroblastoma: Concise communication. *J Nucl Med* 1984; 25:656.

259. Matin P: The appearance of bone scan following fractures including intermediate and long-term studies. *J Nucl Med* 1979; 20:1227.

260. Matzinger MA, Briggs VA, Dunlap HJ, et al: Plain film and CT observations in prostaglandin-induced bone changes. *Pediatr Radiol* 1992; 22:264.

261. Maurer AH, Chen DC, Camargo EE, et al: Utility of three phase skeletal scintigraphy in suspected osteomyelitis: Concise communication. *J Nucl Med* 1981; 22:941.

262. McCullough RW, Gandsman EJ, Kitchman H, et al: Computerized blood-flow analysis in osteochondroses dissecans. *Clin Nucl Med* 1986; 11:511.

263. McKillop JH, Etcubanas E, Goris ML: The indications for and limitations of bone scintigraphy in osteogenic sarcoma. *Cancer* 1981; 48:1133.

264. McNamara D, Beauregard GC, Lemieux RJ: Scintigraphic "doughnut sign" on skeletal imaging due to hemangioendothelioma of bone. *J Nucl Med* 1993; 34:297.

265. McNeil BJ: Value of bone scanning in neoplastic disease. *Semin Nucl Med* 1984; 14:277.

266. McNeil BJ, Cassidy JR, Geiser CF, et al: Fluorine-18 bone scintigraphy in children with osteosarcoma or Ewing's sarcoma. *Radiology* 1973; 109:627.

267. Merkel SF: Ossifying fibroma of long bone. Its distinction from fibrous dysplasia and its association with adamantinoma of long bone. *Am J Clin Pathol* 1978; 69:91.

268. Mesgarzadeh M, Sapega AA, Bonakdarpour A, et al: Osteochondritis dissecans: Analysis of mechanical stability with radiography, scintigraphy, and MR imaging. *Radiology* 1987; 165:775.

269. Meyer J: Dysplasia epiphysealis capitis femoris: A clinical-radiological syndrome and its relationship to Legg-Calvés-Perthes disease. *Acta Orthop Scand* 1964; 34:183.

270. Meyer JR, Shulkin BL: Flare response in Ewing's sarcoma. *Clin Nucl Med* 1991; 16:807.

271. Michael RH, Holder LE: The soleus syndrome. A cause of medical tibial stress (shin-splints). *Am J Sport Med* 1985; 13:87.

272. Miller DR: Acute lymphoblastic leukemia. *Pediatr Clin North Am* 1980; 27:269.

273. Miller JH, Hayon II: Bone scintigraphy in hypervitaminosis A. *AJR Am J Roentgenol* 1985; 144:767.

274. Miller JH, Ortega JA, Heisel MA: Juvenile Gaucher disease simulating osteomyelitis. *AJR Am J Roentgenol* 1981; 137:880.

275. Miller JH, Osterkamp JA: Scintigraphy in acute plastic bowing of the forearm. *Radiology* 1982; 142:742.

276. Miller JH, Sanderson RA: Scintigraphy of toddler's fracture. *J Nucl Med* 1988; 29:2001.

277. Mills GQ, Marymount JH III, Murphy DA: Bone scan utilization in the differential diagnosis of exercise induced lower extremity pain. *Clin Orthop* 1980; 149:207.

278. Mok PM, Reilly BJ, Ash JM: Osteomyelitis in the neonate: Clinical aspects and the role of radiography and scintigraphy in the diagnosis and management. *Radiology* 1982; 145:677.

279. Moore WH, Dhenke RD: Radiotracer imaging in a case of diffuse skeletal hemangiomatosis. *Clin Nucl Med* 1981; 6:405.

280. Mungovan JA, Tung GA, Lambiase RE, et al: Tc-99m MDP uptake in osteopoikilosis. *Clin Nucl Med* 1994; 19:6.

281. Murray IPC: Photopenia in skeletal scintigraphy of suspected bone and joint infection. *Clin Nucl Med* 1982; 7:13.

282. Nadel HR: Thallium-201 for oncological imaging in children. *Semin Nucl Med* 1993; 23:243.

283. Nair N: Bone scanning in Ewing's sarcoma. *J Nucl Med* 1985; 26:349.

284. Namey TC, McIntyre J, Buse M, et al: Nucleographic studies of the axial spondyloarthritides: Quantitative sacroiliac scintigraphy in early HLA-B27 associated sacroiliitis. *Arthritis Rheum* 1977; 20:1058.

285. Nelson HT, Taylor A: Bone scanning in the diagnosis of osteomyelitis. *Eur J Nucl Med* 1980; 5:267.

286. Nickerson R, Brewer E, Person D: Early histologic and radionuclide changes in children with reflex sympathetic dystrophy syndrome (RSDS). *Arthritis Rheum* 1985; 20(suppl 4):72.

287. Nickerson RW, Person DA, Brewer EJ, et al: Value of scintigraphy and vasodilator medication in reflex neurovascular dystrophy (RND). *Pediatr Res* 1982; 16:166 (abstracted).

288. Nixon GW: Acute hematogenous osteomyelitis. *Pediatr Ann* 1976; 5:64.

289. Nixon GW: Hematogenous osteomyelitis of metaphyseal-equivalent locations. *AJR Am J Roentgenol* 1978; 130:123.

290. Nolan HG: Intense uptake of 99mTc-diphosphonate by an extraosseous neurofibroma. *J Nucl Med* 1974; 15:1207.

291. Nuovo MA, Norman A, Chumas J, et al: Myositis ossificans with atypical clinical, radiographic, or pathologic findings: A review of 23 cases. *Skeletal Radiol* 1992; 21:87.

292. O'Dorisio MS, Chen F, O'Dorisio TM, et al: Characterization of somatostatin receptors on human neuroblastoma tumors. *Cell Growth Differ* 1994; 5:108.

293. Oever van den M, Merrick MV, Scott JHS: Bone scintigraphy in symptomatic spondylolysis in the lumbar spine. *J Bone Joint Surg Br* 1987; 69B:453.

294. Ogden JA: Changing patterns of proximal femoral vascularity. *J Bone Joint Surg Am* 1974; 56A:941.

295. Ogden JA, Lister G: Pathology of neonatal osteomyelitis. *Pediatrics* 1975; 55:474.

296. Ogden JA, McCarthy SM, Joki P: The painful bipartite patella. *J Pediatr Orthop* 1982; 2:263.

297. Olgilve J, Sherman J: Spondylolysis in Scheuermann's disease. *Spine* 1986; 12:251.

298. O'Reilly M, Renton P: Metaphyseal deformities of fibrodysplasia ossificans progressiva. *Br J Radiol* 1993; 66:112.

299. Orava S, Jormakka E, Hulkko A: Stress fractures in young athletes. *Arch Orthop Trauma Surg* 1981; 98:271.

300. Orzel JA, Rudd TG, Nelp WB: Heterotopic bone formation: Clinical, laboratory, and imaging correlation. *J Nucl Med* 1985; 26:125.

301. Oudjhane K, Newman B, Oh KS, et al: Occult fracture in preschool children. *J Trauma* 1988; 28:858.

302. Pajarinen P, Alhava E, Tehnberg V: Melorheostosis: A case report with special reference to bone mineral density, bone circulation, and bone scan. *Ann Clin Gynaecol* 1978; 67:36.

303. Palestro CJ, Kim CK, Swyer AJ, et al: Radionuclide diagnosis of osteomyelitis: Indium-111 leukocyte and technetium-99m methylene diphosphonate bone scintigraphy. *J Nucl Med* 1991; 32:1861.

304. Park CH, Kapadia D, O'Hara AE: Three phase bone scan findings in stress fractures. *J Bone Joint Surg* 1977; 59:869.

305. Park HM, Lambertus J: Skeletal and reticuloendothelial imaging in osteopetrosis. *J Nucl Med* 1977; 18:1091.

306. Parker BR, Marglin S, Castellino RA: Skeletal manifestations of leukemia, Hodgkin disease and non-Hodgkin lymphoma. *Semin Roentgenol* 1980; 15:302.

307. Pease CN: Focal retardation and arrestment of growth of bones due to vitamin A intoxication. *JAMA* 1962; 182:980.

308. Peimer CA, Schuller AL, Mankin HJ: Multicentric giant-cell tumor of bone. *J Bone Joint Surg Am* 1980; 62A:652.

309. Peterson HA: Partial growth plate arrest and its treatment. *J Pediatr Orthop* 1984; 4:246.

310. Perlman MD, Wertheimer SJ: Tarsal coalition. *J Foot Surg* 1986; 25:58.

311. Petty RE, Malleson P: Spondyloarthropathies of childhood. *Pediatr Rheum* 1986; 33:1079.

312. Pickett WJ, Falstein EJ, Chacko A, et al: Comparison of radiographs and radionuclide skeletal surveys in battered children. *South Med J* 1983; 76:207.

313. Pitt M, Mosher JR, Edeiken J: Abnormal perisoteum in bone in neurofibromatosis. *Radiology* 1972; 103:143.

314. Poznanski AK, Fernbach SK, Berry TE: Bone changes from prostaglandin therapy. *Skeletal Radiol* 1985; 14:20.

315. Quddus FF, Espinola D, Kramer SS, et al: Comparison between x-ray and bone scan detection of bone metastases in patients with rhabdomyosarcoma. *Med Pediatr Oncol* 1983; 11:125.

316. Ramanna L, Waxman A, Binney G, et al: Thallium-201 scintigraphy in bone sarcoma: Comparison with gallium-67 and technetium-MDP in the evaluation of chemotherapeutic response. *J Nucl Med* 1990; 31:567.

317. Rao BK, Weir JG, Lieberman LM: Extrophy of the bladder: Diagnosis on a bone scan. *Clin Nucl Med* 1981; 6:552.

318. Ratcliffe JF: Anastomotic basis for the pathogenesis and radiologic feature of vertebral osteomyelitis and its differentiation from childhood diskitis. A microarteriographic investigation. *Acta Radiol Diag* 1985; 26:137.

319. Reilnus WR, Conway WF, Totty WG, et al: Carpal avascular necrosis: MR imaging. *Radiology* 1986; 160:689.

320. Resnick D, Greenway G: Distal femoral cortical defects, irregularities, and excavations. *Radiology* 1982; 142:345.

321. Resnick D, Greenway G, Genant H, et al: Erdheim-Chester disease. *Radiology* 1982; 142:289.

322. Rogers JG, Geho WB: Fibrodysplasia ossificans progressiva. *J Bone Joint Surg Am* 1979; 61A:909.

323. Rogers LF, Malave S, Jr, White H, et al: Plastic bowing, torus and greenstick supracondylar fractures of the humerus: Radiographic clues to obscure fractures of the elbow in children. *Radiology* 1978; 128:145.

324. Rolfe EB, Garvie NW, Khan MA, et al: Isotope bone imaging in suspected scaphoid trauma. *Br J Radiol* 1981; 54:762.

325. Rosenbaum DM, Blumhagen JD: Acute epiphyseal osteomyelitis in children. *Radiology* 1985; 156:68.

326. Rosenthal L, Hill RO, Chung S: Observation of the use of Tc-99m-phosphate imaging in peripheral bone trauma. *Radiology* 1978; 119:637.

327. Russell AS, Lentle BC, Percy JS: Investigation of sacroiliac disease: Comparative evaluation of radiological and radionuclide techniques. *J Rheumatol* 1975; 2:45.

328. Saltzman L, Lee VW, Grant P: Gallium uptake in myositis ossificans. Potential pitfalls in diagnosis. *Clin Nucl Med* 1987; 12:308.

329. Sarno RC, Carter BL, Semine MC: Computed tomography in tarsal coalition. *J Comput Assist Tomogr* 1984; 8:1155.

330. Saul PD, Lloyd DJ, Smith FW: The role of bone scanning in neonatal rickets. *Pediatr Radiol* 1983; 13:89.

331. Schahowicz F, Santini-Arayo E: Adamantinoma of the tibia masked by fibrous dysplasia. *Clin Orthop* 1989; 238:294.

332. Schaub T, Ash JM, Gilday DL: Radionuclide imaging in histiocytosis X. *Pediatr Radiol* 1987; 17:397.

333. Schauwecker DS: Osteomyelitis: Diagnosis with In-111 labeled leukocytes. *Radiology* 1989; 171:141.

334. Schuttle HE, Taconis WK: Giant cell tumor in children and adolescents. *Skeletal Radiol* 1993; 22:173.

335. Sebes JI: Diagnostic imaging of bone and joint abnormalities associated with sickle cell hemoglobinopathies. *AJR Am J Roentgenol* 1989; 152:1153.

336. Seitsalo S, Osterman K, Poussa ML: Scoliosis associated with lumbar spondylolisthesis. A clinical survey of 190 young patients. *Spine* 1988; 8:899.

337. Sever JW: Apophysitis of the os calcis. *New York Med J* 1912; 95:1025.

338. Shahriaree H, Harkness JW: A family with spondylolisthesis. *Radiology* 1970; 94:631.

339. Shapeero LG, Couanet D, Vanel D, et al: Bone metastases as the presenting manifestation of rhabdomyosarcoma in childhood. *Skeletal Radiol* 1993; 22:433.

340. Sherman FC, Wilkinson RH, Hall JE: Reactive sclerosis of a pedicle and spondylolysis in the lumbar spine. *J Bone Joint Surg Am* 1977; 59A:49.

341. Shier CK, Krasicky GA, Ellis BI, et al: Ribbing's disease: radiographic-scintigraphic correlation and comparative analysis with Engelmann's disease. *J Nucl Med* 1987; 28:244.

342. Shulkin BL, Shen SW, Sisson JC, et al: Iodine-131 MIBG scintigraphy of the extremities in metastatic pheochromocytoma and neuroblastoma. *Clin Nucl Med* 1988; 13:46.

343. Siddiqui AR, Ellis JH: "Cold spot" on bone scan site of primary osteosarcoma. *Eur J Nucl Med* 1982; 7:480.

344. Simmons CR, Harle TS, Singleton EB: The osseous manifestations of leukemia in children. *Radiol Clinics North Am* 1968; 6:115.

345. Slizofski WJ, Collier BD, Flately TJ, et al: Painful pseudarthrosis following lumbar spinal fusion: Detection by combined SPECT and planar bone scintigraphy. *Skeletal Radiol* 1987; 16:136.

346. Smergel EM, Harcke HT, Pizzutillo PD, et al: Use of bone scintigraphy in the management of slipped capital femoral epiphysis. *Clin Nucl Med* 1987; 12:39.

347. Smith FW, Gilday DL: Scintigraphic appearance of the osteoid osteoma. *Radiology* 1980; 137:191.

348. Smith FW, Gilday DL, Ash JM, et al: Unsuspected costovertebral fractures demonstrated by bone scanning in the child abuse syndrome. *Pediatr Radiol* 1980; 10:103.

349. Smith NM, Byard RW, Foster B, et al: Congenital ossifying fibroma (osteofibrous dysplasia) of the tibia—a case report. *Pediatr Radiol* 1991; 21:449.

350. Snow RD, Lecklitner ML: Musculoskeletal findings in Klippel-Trénaunay syndrome. *Clin Nucl Med* 1991; 16:928.

351. Spencer RP, Levison ED, Baldwin RD, et al: Diverse bone scan abnormalities in "shin splints." *J Nucl Med* 1979; 20:1271.

352. Stark JE, Glasier CM, Blasier RD, et al: Osteomyelitis in children with sickle cell disease: Early diagnosis with contrast-enhanced CT. *Radiology* 1991; 179:731.

353. Starshak RJ, Simons GW, Sty JR: Occult fracture of the calcaneus—another toddler's fracture. *Pediatr Radiol* 1984; 14:37.

354. Steinfeld JR, Thorne NA, Kennedy TF: Positive 99m-Tc-pyrophosphate bone scan in polymyositis. *Radiology* 1977; 122:168.

355. Stewart CA, Siegel ME, King D, et al: Radionuclide and radiographic demonstration of condensing osteitis of clavicle. *Clin Nucl Med* 1988; 13:177.

356. Stewart TD: The age incidence of neural arch defects in Alaska natives, considered from the standpoint of etiology. *J Bone Joint Surg Am* 1953; 35A:937.

357. Stormont DM, Peterson HA: The relative incidence of tarsal coalition. *Clin Orthop* 1983; 181:28.

358. Struhl S, Edelson C, Pritzker H, et al: Solitary (unicameral) bone cyst: The fallen fragment sign revisited. *Skeletal Radiol* 1989; 18:261.

359. Sty JR, Babbitt DP, Sheth K: Abnormal 99mTc methylene diphosphonate accumulation in the kidneys of children with sickle cell disease. *Clin Nucl Med* 1980; 5:445.

360. Sty J, Simons G: Intraoperative 99m technetium bone imaging in the treatment of benign osteoblastic tumors. *Clin Orthop* 1982; 165:223.

361. Sty JR, Starshak RJ: The role of bone scintigraphy in the evaluation of the suspected abused child. *Radiology* 1983; 146:369.

362. Swanson D, Blecker I, Gahbauer H, et al: Diagnosis of diskitis by SPECT technetium-99m MDP. A case report. *Clin Nucl Med* 1987; 12:210.

363. Swee RG, McLeod RA, Beabout JW, et al: Osteoid osteoma: Detection, diagnosis and localization. *Radiology* 1979; 130:117.

364. Sunberg SB, Savage JP, Foster BK: Technetium phosphate bone scan in diagnosis of septic arthritis in childhood. *J Pediatr Orthop* 1989; 9:579.

365. Sutherland AD, Savage JP, Paterson DC, et al: The nuclide bone scan in the diagnosis and management of Perthes disease. *J Bone Joint Surg Br* 1980; 62B:300.

366. Szer IS, Taylor E, Steere AC: The long-term course of Lyme arthritis in children. *N Engl J Med* 1991; 325:159.

367. Tanaka T, Rossier AB, Hassey RW, et al: Quantitative assessment of para-osteo-arthropathy and its maturation on serial radionuclide bone images. *Radiology* 1977; 123:217.

368. Taylor L, Newberger EH: Child abuse in the international year of the child. *New Engl J Med* 1979; 301:1205.

369. Teates CD, Brower AC: Bone scans in condensing osteitis of clavicle. *South Med J* 1978; 71:736.

370. Terry DW, Isitman AT, Holmes RA: Radionuclide bone images in hypertrophic pulmonary osteoarthropathy. *AJR Am J Roentgenol* 1975; 124:571.

371. Tessler F, Lander P, Lisbona R: Congenital absence of a pedicle with photon deficiency on a bone scan. *Clin Nucl Med* 1981; 6:498.

372. Thayer C, Rogers LF: Unicentric osteosarcoma of bone with subsequent skeletal metastases. *Skeletal Radiol* 1979; 4:148.

373. Thiessen P, Hoffman A, Linden A, et al: Magnetic resonance imaging, radiography, and bone scintigraphy in patients with sacroiliitis (abstract). *J Nucl Med* 1989; 30:842.

374. Thomas HM: Calcaneal fracture in childhood. *Br J Surg* 1969; 56:664.

375. Tibone J, Sakimura I, Nickel VL, et al: Heterotopic ossification around the hip in spinal cord injured patients. *J Bone Joint Surg Am* 1978; 60A:769.

376. Trueta J: The three types of acute hematogenous osteomyelitis. A clinical and vascular study. *J Bone Joint Surg Br* 1959; 41-B:671.

377. Ueno D, Rikimaru S, Kawashima Y, et al: Bone imaging of sternoclavicular hyperostosis in palmoplantar pustulosis. *Clin Nucl Med* 1986; 11:420.

378. Uno K, Matsui N, Nohira K, et al: Indium-111 leukocyte imaging in patients with rheumatoid arthritis. *J Nucl Med* 1986; 27:339.

379. Velchik MG, Heyman S, Makler St, et al: Bone scintigraph: Differentiating benign cortical irregularities of the distal femur from malignancy. *J Nucl Med* 1984; 25:72.

380. Veluvola P, Collier BD, Isitman AT, et al: Scintigraphic skeletal "doughnut" sign due to giant cell tumor of the fibula. *Clin Nucl Med* 1984; 99:631.

381. Verbruggen LA, Bossuyt A, Schreuer R, et al: Clinical and scintigraphic evaluation of corticosteroid treatment in a case of progressive diaphyseal dysplasia. *J Rheumatol* 1985; 12:809.

382. Vinchinsky EP, Labin BH: Sickle cell anemia and related hemoglobinopathies. *Pediatr Clin North Am* 1980; 27:429.

383. Vyas K, Eklem M, Seto H, et al: Quantitative scintigraphy of sacroiliac joints: Effects of age, gender, and laterality. *AJR Am J Roentgenol* 1981; 136:589.

384. Wahner HW: Radionuclides in the diagnosis of fracture healing. *J Nucl Med* 1978; 19:1356.

385. Wells RG, Ruskin JA, Sty JR: Lymphoscintigraphy. Lower extremity lymphangioma. *Clin Nucl Med* 1986; 11:523.

386. Wenger DR, Bobechko WP, Gilday DL: The spectrum of intervertebral disk space infection in children. *J Bone Joint Surg Am* 1978; 60A:100.

387. Wenger DR, Ditkoff TJ, Herring JA, et al: Protrusio acetabuli in Marfan's syndrome. *Clin Orthop* 1980; 147:134.

388. Westra SJ, Van Woerden H, Postma A, et al: *Eur J Nucl Med* 1983; 8:303.

389. Whyte MP, Murphy WA, Siegel BA: 99m Tc-pyrophosphate bone imaging in osteopoikilosis, osteopathia striata, and melorheostosis. *Radiology* 1981; 140:87.

390. Williams JL, Capitanio ML, Harcke HT: Bone scanning in neonatal fat necrosis. *J Nucl Med* 1978; 19:861.

391. Williamson SL, Williamson MR, Siebert JJ, et al: Indium 111 white blood cell scanning in the pediatric population. *Pediatr Radiol* 1986; 16:493.

392. Wiltse LL, Newman PH, Macnab I: Classification of spondylolysis and spondylolisthesis. *Clin Orthop* 1976; 117:23.

393. Wingstrand H, Egund N, Carlin NO, et al: Intracapsular pressure in transient synovitis of the hip. *Acta Orthop Scand* 1985; 56:204.

394. Winter WA, Versart BEEMJ, Verdegaal WP: Bone scintigraphy in patients with juvenile kyphosis. *Diagn Imaging* 1981; 50:186.

395. Wioland M, Bonnerot V: Diagnosis of partial and total physeal arrest by bone single-photon emission computed tomography. *J Nucl Med* 1993; 34:1410.

396. Woodhouse CF: Dynamic influence of vascular occlusion affecting the development of avascular necrosis of the femoral head. *Clin Orthop* 1964; 32:119.

397. Wroble RR, Weinstein SL: Histiocytosis X and scoliosis and osteolysis. *J Pediatr Orthop* 1988; 8:213.

398. Young MRA, Lowry JH, Ferguson WR: 99mTC-MDP bone scanning of injuries of the carpal scaphoid. *Injury* 1981; 19:14.

399. Zionts LE, Harcke HT, Brooks KM, et al: Posttraumatic tibia valga: A case demonstrating asymmetric activity at the proximal growth plate on technetium bone scan. *Pediatr Orthop* 1987; 7:458.

400. Zionts LE, Leffers D, Oberto MR, et al: Case report. Plastic bowing of the femur in neonates. *J Pediatr Orthop* 1984; 4:749.

401. Zwas ST, Elkanovitch R, Frank G: Interpretation and classification of bone scintigraphic findings in stress fractures. *J Nucl Med* 1987; 28:452.

IN THIS CHAPTER

CHAPTER 17

SOFT TISSUE UPTAKE OF BONE AGENTS

H. W. Gray

Arthur Z. Krasnow

For over 20 years bone scintigraphy has been the most commonly performed nuclear medicine procedure being applied to a wide range of diagnostic problems in clinical practice. The early polyphosphates provided excellent kidney and urinary tract images due to a prolonged renal excretion phase; it was soon recognized[112] that unsuspected renal and urinary tract pathology could be detected incidentally during bone scintigraphy. The newer diphosphonates with their faster soft-tissue clearance provide in addition an ideal vehicle for showing accumulation of bone-seeking agents in both neoplastic and nonneoplastic soft tissue. Initially thought to relate to macroscopic or microscopic tissue calcification,[144] soft-tissue uptake has been observed within such a plethora of pathologic entities that any simplistic concept of a uniform mechanism for soft-tissue deposition of technetium diphosphonates has become untenable.

Despite considerable research effort and critical clinical observation, our overall understanding of the underlying mechanisms of ^{99m}Tc-labeled phosphate uptake at a tissue or cellular level is still rudimentary. Unexpected soft-tissue uptake of ^{99m}Tc-MDP (methylene diphosphonate) can provide the inexperienced observer with a source of uncertainty and doubt. Conversely, the often serendipitous finding of soft-tissue uptake in a recogniz-able pattern greatly enhances the diagnostic value of the study. This chapter reviews the wide range of disease processes where recognition of nonskeletal soft-tissue uptake of ^{99m}Tc-MDP is of value in clinical practice. For more information on uptake of bone tracer by soft tissue, readers are directed to the many excellent articles and texts available.* Emphasis in this chapter has been placed first on the diagnosis that can be made by chance from the bone scan, and second on the use of bone imaging for detection of specific conditions known to reliably accumulate bone imaging agents. No distinction has been made between the various ^{99m}Tc-labeled phosphates because of the evidence that they behave qualitatively in a similar manner.[25]

PATHOPHYSIOLOGY

The underlying mechanisms for uptake of bone-seeking agents in many soft tissues remain uncertain, although clinical experience and experimental evidence have provided some insights. Only in heterotopic new

*References 19, 29, 39, 100, 105, 125, 141.

bone formation (e.g., myositis ossificans) is the mechanism similar to that for the skeleton.[25,49,80,127] Several theories to account for soft-tissue uptake of ^{99m}Tc-phosphates have been proposed. It is now clear that in most individual cases, multiple factors are probably involved.

A common mechanism for soft-tissue localization of bone-seeking radiopharmaceuticals relates to the altered tracer handling dynamics consequent on an expansion of the interstitial fluid compartment. The slower washout of tracer from a pleural effusion or ascitic collection provides a "pure" example of this mechanism. Other exemplars such as infection, inflammation, or tumor probably reflect not only increased interstitial volume but increased blood flow and vascularity. Increased blood flow to a vascular organ or tissue would permit more tissue contact with ^{99m}Tc-phosphate and, certainly this effect can be recognized in the syndrome of reflex sympathetic dystrophy.[24] On the other hand, Chew et al[29] found no evidence of hypervascularity in soft tissue sarcomas which accumulated bone tracer. It would appear possible therefore that altered sympathetic tone and the opening of local vascular plexuses is more important than neovascularization.

Soft-tissue calcification has long been recognized as an important causal factor in the soft-tissue uptake of ^{99m}Tc-phosphates.[49,144] This mechanism is thought to be operative in dystrophic calcification from whatever cause, since most tissue calcium is in the form of hydroxyapatite.[52] The calcium phosphate molar ratio, crystalline surface area, and presence of other metallic ions may also influence the amount of diphosphonate absorption[48] and may explain the absence of ^{99m}Tc-phosphate uptake in some tumors despite recognizable calcification on the radiograph.[51,97]

Metastatic calcification occurs in renal failure when the solubility product for calcium and phosphate is exceeded and hydroxyapatite crystals precipitate in the soft-tissue interstitial space.[121] McLaughlin[102] and Rosenthall et al[124] confirmed the affinity of ^{99m}Tc-phosphate for calcium precipitates by correlating diffuse lung uptake of tracer in hypercalcemic patients with the pathologic identification of calcium deposition in the alveolar septa. Watson et al[169] showed resolution of the lung uptake on correction of the hypercalcemia. Conger and Alfrey[34] demonstrated in vitro that ^{99m}Tc-phosphates form a strong chemical bond to hydroxyapatite crystals and a weak bond to the amorphous salt (Whitlockite) found in the lungs of uremic patients.[35] It is likely that the higher magnesium content of Whitlockite significantly diminishes the bone tracer binding and explains the lack of sensitivity of bone tracers for detecting metastatic lung calcification in dialysis patients.[4]

The abnormal intracellular flux of ionic calcium seen after ischemic or other damage to cell membrane integrity has been clearly shown to be a preliminary factor in the increased uptake of ^{99m}Tc-phosphates by ischemic or dying cells.[168] The intracellular solubility product for calcium and phosphate may be exceeded with precipitation of calcium salts around mitochondria, which have nucle-

ating properties.[136,137] ^{99m}Tc-pyrophosphate localizes to intracellular calcium as amorphous calcium phosphate and crystalline hydroxyapatite but also to calcium complexed to myofibrils and other macromolecules in the myoplasm.[20,40]

There is evidence that transchelation of ^{99m}Tc may occur where there is a high local tissue concentration of calcium or iron to facilitate dissociation of ^{99m}Tc from the phosphate ligand and may lead to its deposition at the reaction site.[103] This mechanism would be operative for uptake in infarction or in tissues with a high iron content like iron injection sites[23,163] or the spleen in hemolysis.[106] McRae also suggested ionic iron may catalyze the formation of a new ^{99m}Tc-ligand with a tissue distribution different from ^{99m}Tc-phosphate. This may explain the high renal uptake of ^{99m}Tc when bone imaging is performed in systemic iron overload.[31] Binding of ^{99m}Tc-phosphate to receptor sites on tissue enzymes, such as acid phosphatase, has been suggested to account for breast uptake in normals and cancer patients.[131,180] Little hard evidence is available to substantiate this attractive theory.

Collagen can nucleate the growth of hydroxyapatite crystals.[55] Rosenthall and Kay[126] have argued that ^{99m}Tc-phosphates may have a greater affinity for immature collagen than for the crystal surface of bone. This theory is supported by the localization of bone-seeking agents in healing surgical scars[116] and in fibrothorax.[119]

BONE SCAN APPEARANCES

Incidental Findings

As the bone scan is invariably obtained for skeletal assessment, the detection of soft-tissue abnormalities provides a valuable bonus and is serendipity in action. The unexpected finding relates most often to the kidney and the urinary tract because of the high photon density achieved within this organ system during radiopharmaceutical excretion. Less commonly, new information is gained that delineates unsuspected benign or malignant tumors, areas of unsuspected infarction, or unforeseen effects or complications from known disease processes. The prevalence of renal abnormalities on unselected bone scans is approximately 15%.[1,95,112,148] Peller et al[114] reported that of 1000 consecutive patients referred for investigation of known or suspected neoplasia, 8% had localized soft-tissue abnormalities on bone scans referable to primary or secondary sites of involvement.

KIDNEY AND URINARY TRACT

Unlike the early ^{99m}Tc-phosphates with their high renal excretion,[32] current agents like MDP have a much higher skeletal uptake. Consequently the renal excretion is lower and the incidental renal images at 4 hours are of poor quality. However, by contrasting digitized lumbar views or by overexposing the analog lumbar view to "burn out" the spine, one can obtain acceptable kidney images. Other workers have routinely imaged the kidneys at 5 minutes after injection to ensure adequate high count-density views of kidney,[28] but it is unclear whether this extra time and effort is worthwhile. Occasionally the diagnostic value may be enhanced by extra views in the lateral or oblique position for kidney or the caudal (squat) position for bladder.[57]

The most specific signs of renal disease on bone imaging can be broadly classified as renal asymmetry, mass lesions, urinary or renal tract dilatation, or abnormalities of uptake, size, or displacement. Less valuable signs are bilateral decreased renal uptake and focal areas of increased uptake.

RENAL ASYMMETRY. Clearcut renal asymmetry is a sensitive and specific sign of renal disease[148,167] and may

be noted in up to 10% of routine bone scans.[66] Minor asymmetry is of less value, and despite acquisition of other views, the abnormal kidney may be difficult to pinpoint. Some cases are simply caused by horizontal orientation of one kidney.[105]

There are three broad patterns of asymmetry. In the first pattern a unilateral nonfunctioning kidney is accompanied by a normal or hypertrophied contralateral kidney. This may occur in congenital absence, severe chronic pyelonephritis, following nephrectomy, or in idiopathic nonfunction.[1,95,167] In the second pattern a unilateral shrunken kidney may result from chronic pyelonephritis, radiation nephritis,[148] idiopathic small kidney, chronic hydronephrosis without urinary stasis[1,167] or renal artery stenosis.[105] This pattern can be

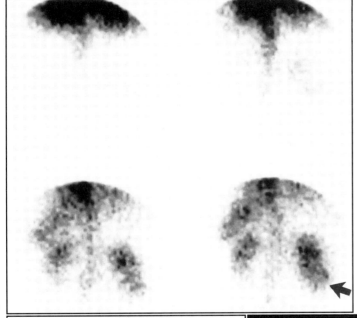

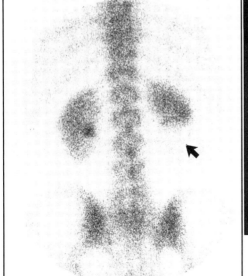

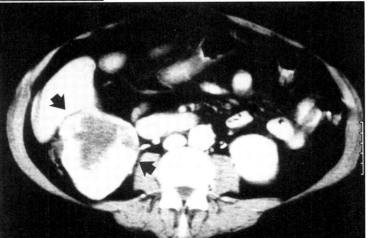

Fig. 17-1. Renal abnormality. In this patient with renal cell carcinoma there is normal blood flow—**A**, posterior image—but absent delayed tracer uptake (**B**) to the mass in the lower pole of the right kidney (*arrow*). **C**, CT scan at the level of the renal mass (*arrows*).

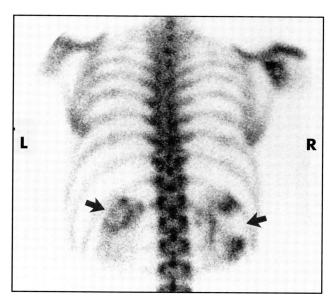

Fig. 17-2. Renal abnormality. Multiple photon-deficient areas in both kidneys due to lung carcinoma metastases (*arrows*).

simulated by the presence of a renal mass at either pole, which is not directly visualized.[11] The third pattern of unilateral enlargement with a normal contralateral kidney has been reported in hydronephrosis[167] and in the presence of renal cell carcinoma[105] or Wilms' tumor.[43] It is also possible to see unilateral kidney enlargement in catastrophic vascular disease such as renal vein thrombosis, severe renal artery stenosis, and acute renal infarction.[84,86,148] Excessive uptake in a neuroblastoma can mimic a large kidney as can abnormal uptake in stomach.

MASS LESIONS. The mass lesion represented by a focal photon-deficient area is an uncommon but reliable indicator of renal disease. In a pediatric series Sty et al[148] reported that Wilms' tumor was the most common neoplasm. Solitary cysts, polycystic disease, and renal abscess were all uncommon in their experience. In an adult population primary renal cell carcinoma (Fig. 17-1) and single or multiple renal cysts are equally common, whereas metastatic disease (Fig. 17-2) and renal abscess are uncommon.[1,95,167]

It is clear that many small lesions will be missed despite the acquisition of good-quality images. In the series of Biello et al,[11] 10 of 20 mass lesions detected by intravenous urography (IVU) were missed on bone imaging providing a sensitivity of 50% and specificity of 100%. There is no evidence that renal flow studies[54] or a 2-minute blood pool image[28] improve the rate of detection.

OBSTRUCTIVE UROPATHY. The appearance of increased tracer accumulation within a dilated renal pelvis and ureter is the most common soft-tissue abnormality on bone imaging. Compared with the IVU as the gold standard, bone agents were found to have a sensitivity of 73% and specificity of 100% for detection of ureteropyelocaliectasis.[11] Although bilateral abnormalities on bone scanning were 100% concordant with the IVU, unilater-

al abnormalities on scanning were found in 50% of cases with bilateral disease, bone imaging detecting the most severely affected side. By itself, increased accumulation of tracer in the renal pelvis alone was found to be an unreliable and insensitive (11%) indicator of true pelviureteric junction obstruction. IVU is usually normal or reveals an extrarenal pelvis or duplex calyceal system in such cases. Maher[95] found prostatic carcinoma to be the most frequent cause of urinary obstruction seen on bone imaging, with secondary carcinoma in the pelvis a less common cause.

In pediatric practice Sty et al[148] confirmed that dilatation and increased uptake in the ureter, pelvis, and intrarenal collecting system was definitive in documenting an obstructive uropathy. Enlargement or contraction of the kidneys seemed to depend on the degree and duration of the obstruction, which was reported with congenital defects, calculi and blood clot, lymph node enlargement, pelvic and retroperitoneal masses, and following surgery.

ABNORMAL KIDNEY UPTAKE, SIZE, AND POSITION. The miscellaneous renal abnormalities associated with increased tracer accumulation, increased kidney size, and abnormality of position are rarely found on bone imaging in adults. Koizumi et al[81] defined "hot kidneys" as kidneys showing diffusely increased uptake in the posterior projection greater than that of the lumbar spine (Fig. 17-3). They found that 13 of 2056 patients (0.63%) fulfilled this criteria. All were men with a diagnosis of liver cirrhosis, lymphoreticular or other tumor, sideroblastic anemia, or diabetes mellitus. Anticancer chemotherapy or iron overload appeared to be common factors. Intense renal uptake of bone agents was first described by Lutrin et al[93] in children treated with cyclosporin, vincristine, and doxorubicin within the previous 7 days. Trackler and Chinn[160] reported similar findings after the administration of amphotericin B and proposed tubular or interstitial damage with microcalcification as a likely mechanism. Iron overload following repeated blood transfusion or hemochromatosis has been noted to alter the biodistribution of bone agents with uptake at iron injection sites[23,163] and intense concentration in kidney.[31,113] Transchelation of ^{99m}Tc with synthesis of a renal rather than a bone-seeking agent has been proposed.[103] Diffuse increase in kidney uptake has also been reported early after kidney irradiation[92,177] and in thalassemia major,[161] nephrocalcinosis,[17] urinary obstruction at an early phase,[148] hypercalcemia,[22] myoglobinuria,[151] and in children[149] or adults[13] with sickle cell disease.

Bilateral renal enlargement is uncommon in adults[167] but has been reported in thalassemia major[161] and myeloma.[1] Sty et al[148] considered bilateral renal enlargement to be the most common abnormality in children and reported it not only in urologic conditions but also leukemia, lymphoma, hyperuricemic nephropathy, and renal toxicity from chemotherapy.

A unilateral pelvic kidney is the congenital abnormality most likely to be encountered.[1] Recognition is essential as it may mimic lumbosacral disease. Polycystic and horseshoe kidneys[45] are rare.

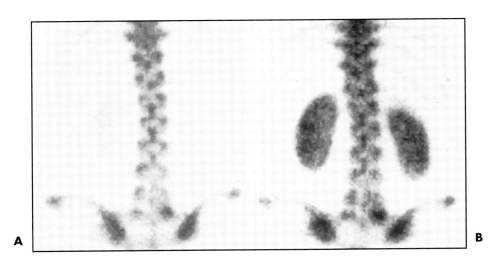

Fig. 17-3. Renal abnormality. Renal uptake before (**A**) and 10 days after (**B**) receiving cyclophosphamide and doxorubicin chemotherapy. The diffuse increase in renal activity is thought to be related to drug toxicity. *(From Gray HW: Soft tissue uptake of bone agents, in Fogelman I (ed): Bone Scanning in Clinical Practice, Springer Verlag, Berlin, 1987; with permission.)*

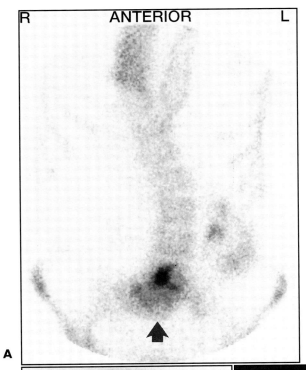

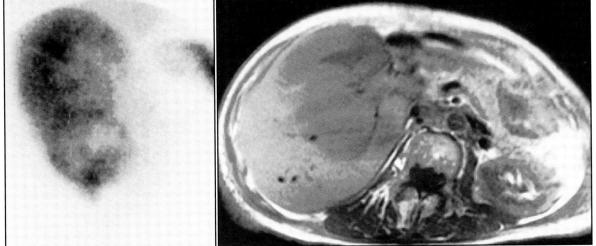

Fig. 17-4. Renal abnormality. **A**, Abnormal activity in the midline of the lower pelvis (*arrow*) is actually the right kidney being displaced by an enlarged liver (from lymphoma metastasis). Tc-99m sulfur colloid (**B**) and MRI (**C**) display the massive size of the liver.

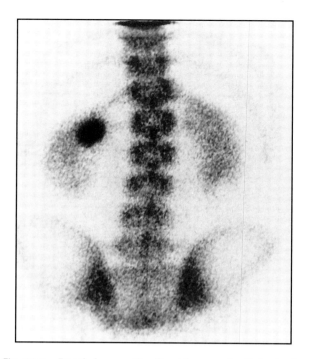

Fig. 17-5. Renal abnormality. Focal increased activity in the left upper pole due to urinary stasis in an area of caliectasis. *(From Gray HW: Soft tissue uptake of bone agents, in Fogelman I (ed): Bone Scanning in Clinical Practice, Springer Verlag, Berlin, 1987; with permission.)*

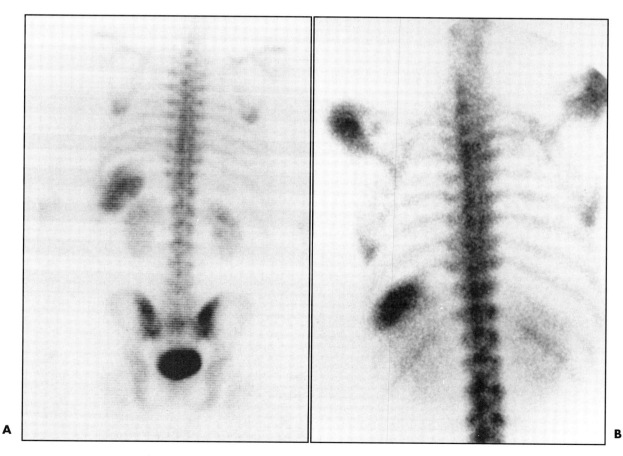

Fig. 17-6. Splenic uptake. Splenic uptake of Tc-99m MDP in two patients. Patient (**A**) had widely metastatic choriocarcinoma but no good explanation for the splenic activity. Patient (**B**) had sickle cell disease.

Renal displacement is a rarity[167] (Fig. 17-4). Inferior displacement by a retroperitoneal mass[105] or neuroblastoma[70,139] has been reported.

Abnormal tracer accumulation may be seen incidentally in the intraperitoneal[105] or retroperitoneal space[41,87] as a complication of renal surgery. The appearance is dramatic and unlikely to cause confusion.

ABSENT OR FAINT RENAL UPTAKE. A low count-density within the kidneys during bone scanning is an unreliable sign of renal disease.[167] It was first reported in Paget's disease[138] but is most common in metastatic disease[155] and is secondary to rapid and enhanced uptake of radiopharmaceutical by the abnormal bone. Not surprisingly, similar "superscan" appearances occur in renal osteodystrophy, primary hyperparathyroidism, and hyperthyroidism.[47,91] Adams et al[1] found this pattern in 34 of 215 scans (16%) with abnormal renal images, and in no patient was renal disease confirmed. He commented that although extensive bone involvement by tumor was the most common factor in adults, intense epiphyseal concentration, cellulitis, and neuroblastoma were the usual factors in children. Differentiation of the superscan appearance caused by bone disease from other causes has been reported with a bone-to-soft-tissue index[36] and with an 8-minute lumbar vertebral uptake.[77] Clearly it is unwise to make an inference regarding kidney function without further specific investigation in patients with faint or absent kidney images.

FOCAL UPTAKE IN KIDNEY. Focal areas of increased tracer accumulation in kidney are most often due to stasis within the collecting system (Fig. 17-5) and rarely indicate renal disease.[61,167] Winter[175] cautioned against the adoption of supine imaging, which favors postural pooling and reported that postambulation or delayed views usually confirm the diagnosis.

Rarely a lesion of the twelfth rib may simulate a renal lesion[105] or stasis in an upper calyx a rib lesion.[173] Focal uptake has also been reported in a primary renal tumor[145] and in secondary renal tumors.[53] Focal uptake in the renal bed simulating a normal kidney has been observed in recurrent renal carcinoma[110] and in neuroblastoma.[70]

In summary, valuable new information on kidney structure and function can be obtained during bone scanning in at least 15% of patients. Renal asymmetry is the most common abnormality with mass lesions and

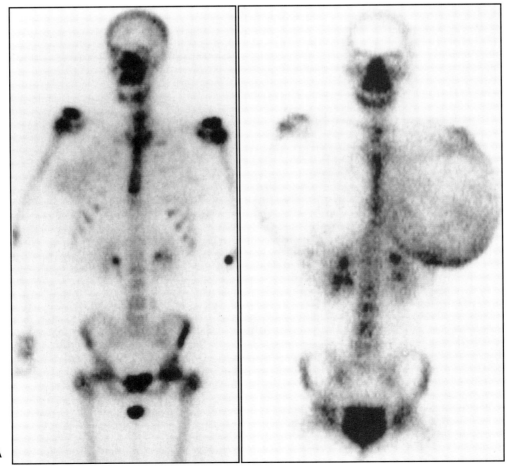

Fig. 17-7. Breast uptake. **A,** Focal increased activity in a right breast carcinoma. **B,** Diffuse uptake in the left breast in a patient with inflammatory breast carcinoma.

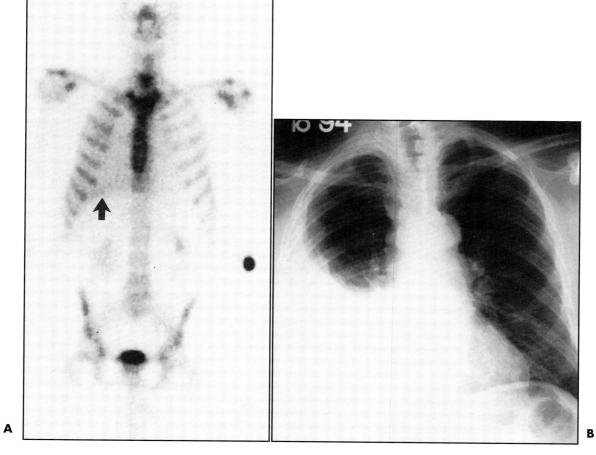

Fig. 17-8. Chest uptake. Diffuse uptake in a patient with a malignant pleural effusion from adenocarcinoma of the lung (*arrow*). **A**, Anterior planar image. **B**, Chest x-ray.

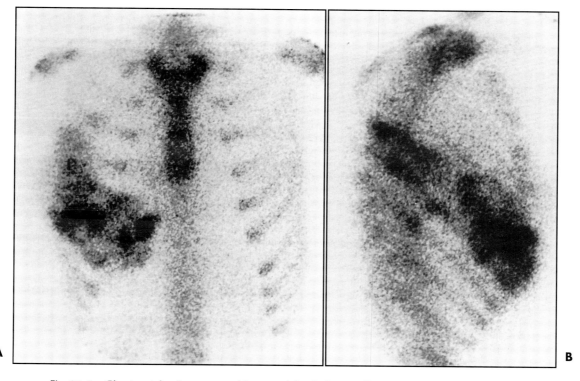

Fig. 17-9. Chest uptake. Large area of increased focal chest wall activity in an anaplastic sarcoma with osteogenic features. **A**, Anterior view. **B**, Right lateral view. *(From Gray HW: Soft tissue uptake of bone agents, in Fogelman I (ed): Bone Scanning in Clinical Practice, Springer Verlag, Berlin, 1987; with permission.)*

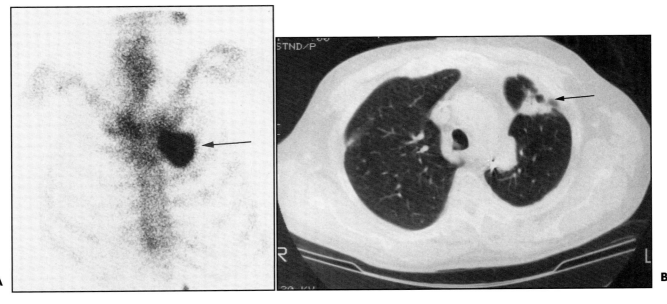

Fig. 17-10. Chest uptake. Focal increased uptake in a parenchymal lung metastasis from osteogenic sarcoma (*arrows*). **A**, Anterior planar image. **B**, CT scan.

obstructive uropathy the most specific. Overall experience indicates that a renal abnormality on bone scanning is unlikely to be a false-positive result and requires further investigation. However, normal renal images do not exclude a renal abnormality.

SPLEEN

Unsuspected splenic visualization during bone imaging usually results from homozygous or heterozygous sickle cell disease.[58,64,143] Accumulation may be faint or striking (Fig. 17-6) and is related to the presence of splenic infarction, anoxia, and/or a high local tissue concentration of iron. Rarely uptake can indicate secondary carcinoma of spleen.[50]

Care is required to distinguish spleen from uptake in stomach, ribs, lung, or a laterally displaced kidney. Adrenal deposition may cause uncertainty, but it is rare and usually bilateral with a more medial position.

Other rare causes of splenic uptake include lymphoma or leukemia,[106,176] metastatic carcinoma,[38] trauma,[153] and glucose-6-phosphate dehydrogenase deficiency.[89]

BREAST

Breast uptake of bone agents is often seen incidentally. Unfortunately the finding is nonspecific and has been reported in the normal breast as well as in those harboring benign or malignant disease (Fig. 17-7).[10,21,101,133]

The mechanism of uptake is uncertain but may be related to high tissue calcium levels[141] or to binding with receptor sites of acid phosphatase.[131] Bone formation in the breast is rare.[33]

In the largest series Holmes et al[69] showed that 95% of benign lesions including fibroadenomas, mammary dysplasia, and cystic mastitis had bilateral uptake, whereas 25% of malignant lesions showed a similar pattern.

Those workers concluded that only unilateral breast uptake merited further investigation unless the uptake was seen in the contralateral breast following mastectomy. In this latter situation malignancy was rarely found. As further caveats Bledin et al[15] reported that nonmammary uptake in the ribs on the mastectomy side was seen in 75% of patients and should not be confused with a pathologic process, whereas Thrall et al[158] reported uptake in a pathologic rib fracture simulating unilateral breast uptake.

CHEST

Excluding uptake in breast, unilateral uptake over the chest during bone scanning is usually an incidental finding in malignant pleural effusions (Fig. 17-8). Siegal et al[140] found bone radiopharmaceutical in the noncellular phase of the effusion, and other workers have confirmed the specificity for malignant rather than benign disease processes.[5,85] The effusion can appear as diffuse uptake over the lower chest in erect views, which becomes homogeneous over the hemithorax in supine position. When the effusion is loculated, it may appear as intense and well-circumscribed uptake. Less commonly, uptake in a hemithorax can result from a tumor of the chest wall (Fig. 17-9), from lung and pleural uptake in bronchogenic carcinoma, from radiotherapy to chest,[166] or from radiation pneumonitis.[130] Metastatic disease of lung (Fig. 17-10) is readily identifiable by the more focal nature of the uptake.[62,79] Rarely, idiopathic pulmonary ossification results in focal uptake of bone agents.[44]

BRAIN

Localization of bone agents in brain is most commonly seen in cerebral infarction[90] (Fig. 17-11). Less commonly, uptake may be noted in primary and metastatic

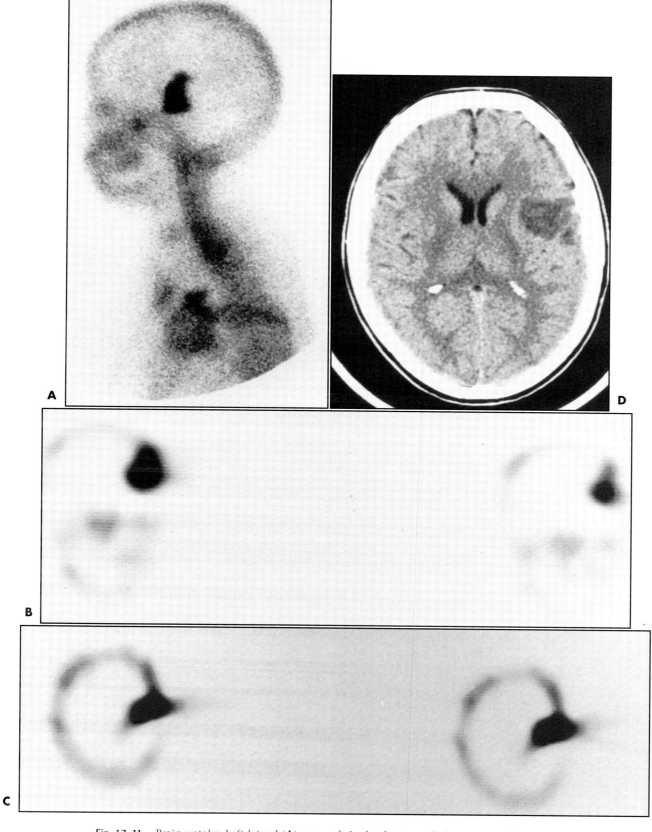

Fig. 17–11.   Brain uptake. Left lateral (**A**), coronal single photon emission computed tomography (SPECT) (**B**), and transaxial SPECT (**C**) images show focal increased activity in brain parenchyma due to a recent cerebral vascular accident. **D**, CT scan.

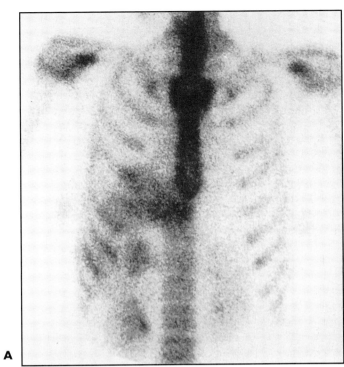
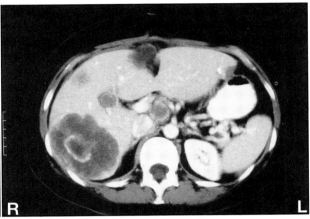

Fig. 17-12. Abdominal uptake. Multiple focal areas of increased activity in the liver due to necrosis in colon carcinoma metastases. **A**, Planar anterior image. **B**, CT scan.

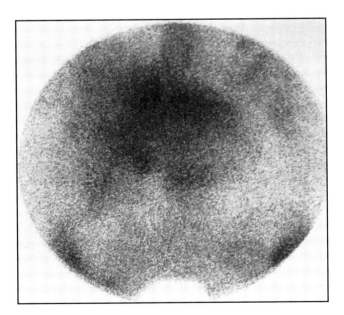

Fig. 17-13. Abdominal uptake. Diffuse right upper quadrant activity in the liver of a patient with amyloidosis. *(From Krasnow AZ et al: Nuclear medicine evaluation of amyloidosis, in* Nuclear Medicine Annual 1992, *Raven Press, New York, 1992; with permission.)*

carcinoma, chronic subdural hematoma, arteriovenous malformation, and various inflammatory lesions.[59,99] Additional views may be necessary to exclude uptake in the calvaria.

Uptake in brain occurs only when there is disorganization of the blood-brain barrier. Because uptake of bone agents in cerebral infarction usually exceeds that of pertechnetate,[59,170] the mechanism is likely to be related in part to the calcium content of the cerebral infarct.

ABDOMEN

Incidental detection of hepatic metastases on bone scanning (Fig. 17-12) is a relatively common occurrence.[71] The primary tumor is usually found in colon,[51,60] lung,[107,118] esophagus,[171] breast,[9] or prostate.[65] Unless the metastases are calcified,[159] the mechanism for uptake remains unclear. Wilson et al[174] found no association between localization of bone agent and the presence of necrosis, calcification, or recent change in size of the secondary deposit. The differential diagnosis of unexpected right upper quadrant localization includes artifactual uptake, rib metastases, malignant pleural effusion,[140] inflammatory carcinoma of breast,[27] and hepatic necrosis.[94] Diffuse liver uptake can be seen when there is amyloid deposition (Fig. 17-13). A generalized diffuse increase in uptake over the abdomen usually indicates malignant ascites (Fig. 17-14). Multiple focal areas of increased

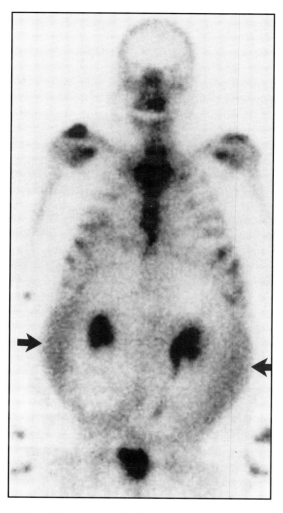

Fig. 17-14. Abdominal uptake. Increased activity in both lateral aspects of the abdomen (*arrows*) due to malignant ascites from lymphoma.

activity in the abdomen can be seen in periotoneal carcinomatosis (Fig. 17-15).

MISCELLANEOUS

UNSUSPECTED PRIMARY. It is unusual for a primary tumor to emerge during bone imaging for known secondary disease. Jackman et al[72] reported the detection of a renal cell carcinoma while investigating a photon-rich secondary deposit in upper humerus.

METASTATIC CALCIFICATION. The diagnosis of metastatic calcification on clinical grounds is difficult; accordingly the condition is often unrecognized.[30,68] It is often discovered by chance[121] when hypercalcemic patients are screened for metastases by bone scanning. Diffuse uptake of tracer is seen in lung first of all and in more severe cases may also be noted in heart, liver, stomach, and kidney. This results from soft-tissue microcalcification, which can occur in chronic renal failure (Fig. 17-16), hyperparathyroidism, milk-alkali syndrome, hypervitaminosis D, bone metastases, myeloma, and lymphoma.[6,124,132,146,178] Reimaging with bone agents may be used to evaluate the success[169] or otherwise[67] of appropriate treatment.

AMYLOIDOSIS. In amyloidosis the glycoprotein amyloid P component binds to pleated protein fibrils in a calcium-dependent way. Consequently normal tissue is destroyed and organ function disturbed. After a biopsy diagnosis, bone imaging can be used to determine the extent of disease (Fig. 17-17).[73,179] Although insensitive, diffuse hepatic or cardiac uptake point to amyloid infiltration. This diagnosis is likely if diffuse hepatic and/or soft-tissue uptake of bone-seeking agents is present with normal muscle enzymes.[83,164]

LOWER LIMB UPTAKE. An unusual increase in tracer accumulation is occasionally seen unilaterally in lower extremities during routine bone imaging. The pattern may result from lymphedema secondary to lymphatic obstruction, circulation stasis caused by pelvic obstruction or deep vein thrombosis, or cellulitis resulting from trauma, infection, or radiation (Fig. 17-18).[96] This should

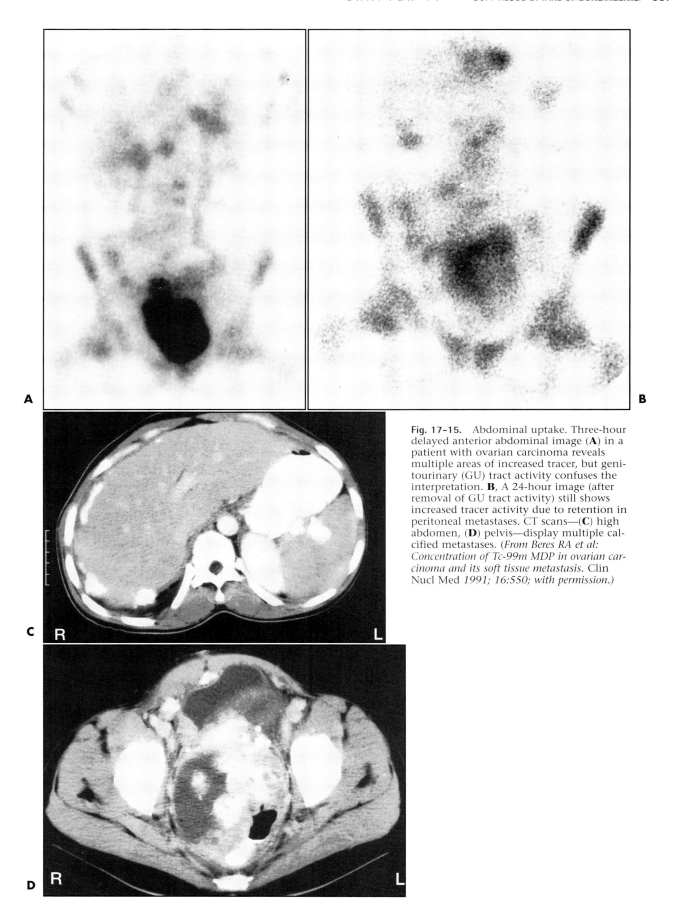

Fig. 17-15. Abdominal uptake. Three-hour delayed anterior abdominal image (**A**) in a patient with ovarian carcinoma reveals multiple areas of increased tracer, but genitourinary (GU) tract activity confuses the interpretation. **B**, A 24-hour image (after removal of GU tract activity) still shows increased tracer activity due to retention in peritoneal metastases. CT scans—(**C**) high abdomen, (**D**) pelvis—display multiple calcified metastases. (*From Beres RA et al: Concentration of Tc-99m MDP in ovarian carcinoma and its soft tissue metastasis.* Clin Nucl Med *1991; 16:550; with permission.*)

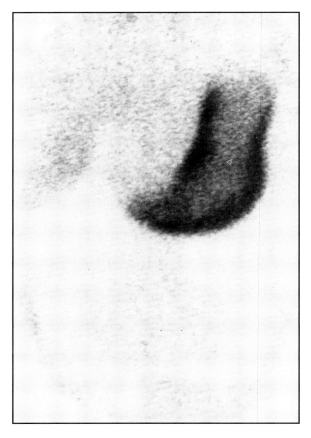

Fig. 17-16. Metastatic calcification. Increased stomach and soft-tissue activity due to hypercalcemia caused by breast carcinoma and renal failure.

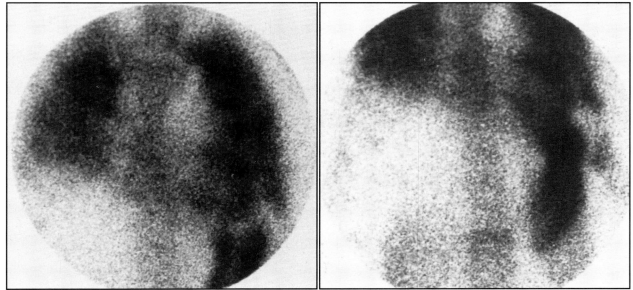

Fig. 17-17. Amyloidosis. Anterior chest (**A**) and anterior abdomen (**B**) images reveal increased tracer in the lungs, heart, and gastrointestinal (GI) tract from amyloid deposition. *(From Krasnow AZ et al: Nuclear medicine evaluation of amyloidosis, in Nuclear Medicine Annual 1992, Raven Press, New York, 1992; with permission.)*

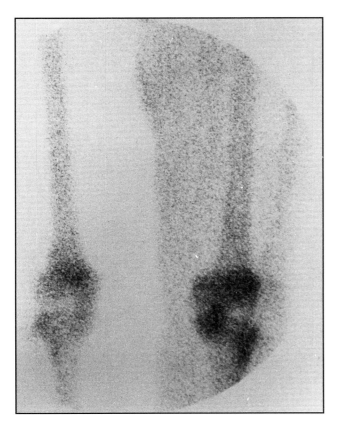

Fig. 17–18. Lower extremity uptake. Diffuse soft-tissue tracer deposition in the entire left lower extremity due to lymphedema (from liposarcoma).

be distinguishable from the syndrome of reflex sympathetic dystrophy.[82]

Although increased bone tracer uptake around the hip or knee joint invariably points to degenerative joint disease, it must be remembered that rarely such appearances can indicate soft-tissue uptake in synovium associated with synovial chondromatosis (Fig. 17-19). In the early stages of this condition, a rim of increased ^{99m}Tc-MDP can be seen along the femoral head, resembling degenerative joint disease, but x-rays of the joint are often normal.[39,181]

Diagnostic Applications

^{99m}Tc-phosphates have been used to provide important diagnostic information on conditions known to reliably accumulate bone agents in soft tissue. Common applications include the search for tissue damage or infarction, the assessment of heterotopic ossification, and the screening for soft-tissue calcification. Less commonly, bone agents have been used for staging of soft-tissue tumors.

MYOCARDIAL INFARCTION

The technique of ^{99m}Tc pyrophosphate imaging for myocardial infarction[16] has been widely applied[12] but is now seldom used. Focal uptake in myocardium is nonspecific and was seen in unstable angina,[172] ventricular aneurysm,[2] calcified heart valves,[74] and myocardial contusion.[56] Diffuse uptake in myocardium has been reported in alcoholic myopathy,[2] amyloid heart (Fig. 17-20),[18] cardiac toxicity induced by adriamycin,[150] severe hypercalcemia,[6,8] and after cardioversion.[111] Diffuse uptake may also be noted in the elderly and is of uncertain significance.[76] Increased activity more peripherally in the heart can be seen in malignant pericardial effusions (Fig. 17-21).

RHABDOMYOLYSIS. Calcium can be detected radiographically in severe muscle damage.[3] The mechanism for uptake of ^{99m}Tc-phosphates in skeletal muscle is therefore analogous to that in heart muscle. Significant muscle uptake of bone agents has been reported in trauma,[141] ischemia,[46] idiopathic and alcohol-related rhabdomyolysis,[14,142] and after severe exercise,[122] where it can differentiate between joint and muscle injury, bone infarction, or stress fracture.[98] Imaging for a diagnosis of rhabdomyolysis, Cornelius[37] found bone agents superior to other modalities, being more sensitive than radiography and more specific than ultrasound. Increased uptake in muscle has also been described in patients with polymyositis (Fig. 17-22). Additional details on muscle injury are discussed in Chapter 13. One must distinguish the curvilinear tracer uptake in calcified femoral arteries from muscle uptake in thigh.

MISCELLANEOUS. In pediatric practice ^{99m}Tc-phosphates have been used for detection of necrotizing enterocolitis of the newborn[135] and for bowel infarction.[108]

Lyons et al[94] and Echeuarria et al[42] have independently reported intense concentration of bone tracer in severe centrilobular necrosis of liver. It is not clear whether such uptake indicates reversible or irreversible disease. Vascular activity can be present when there is excessive thrombosis (Fig. 17-23).

HETEROTOPIC NEW BONE FORMATION

The formation of bone outside the skeleton is unusual but readily detected on bone scanning (Fig. 17-24). In muscle, myositis ossificans occurs rarely as a congenital disorder but most commonly after direct muscle trauma,[154] in patients with paraplegia,[156] or following hip surgery.[128] Bone imaging is more sensitive than radiography in detecting ectopic bone formation and if used serially can indicate the optimum time for excision.[104] Ectopic bone formation around the hip in paraplegia can mimic deep vein thrombosis. Imaging is particularly valuable in identifying the nature of this complication.[109,117]

SOFT–TISSUE CALCIFICATION

Deposition of calcium phosphate in soft tissue (calcinosis) occurs in scleroderma and dermatomyositis. Sfakianakis et al[134] have shown that calcinosis universalis is common in the sceleroderma and dermatomyositis of childhood and that bone tracers localize to the calcified lesion 18 months on average before they are seen radiographically. Uptake of bone agents also occurs in calci-

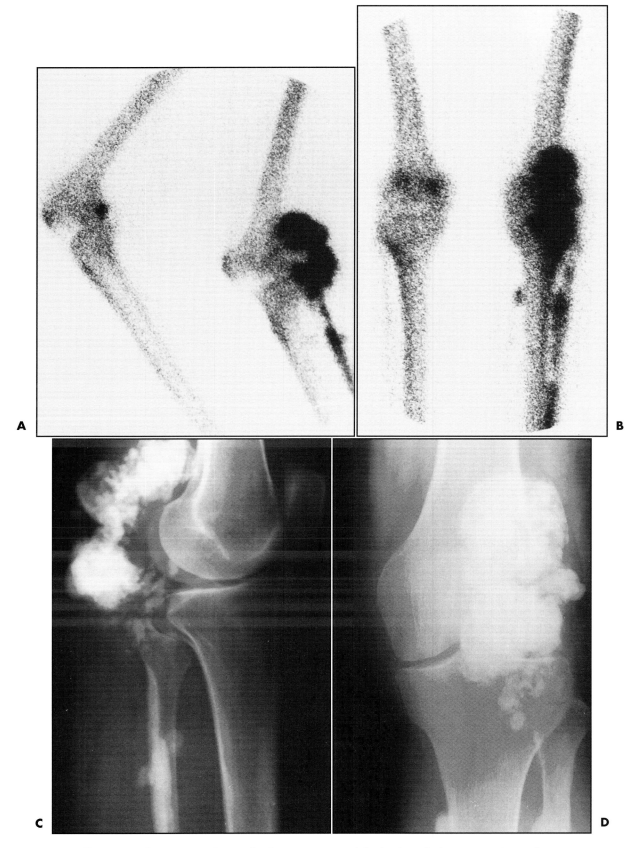

Fig. 17–19. Lower extremity uptake. Intense tracer activity in the soft tissues posterior to the left knee extends down the calf in a patient with synovial chondromatosis. **A**, Left lateral view. **B**, Anterior view. Lateral (**C**) and anterior (**D**) x-rays of the left knee show extensive calcification.

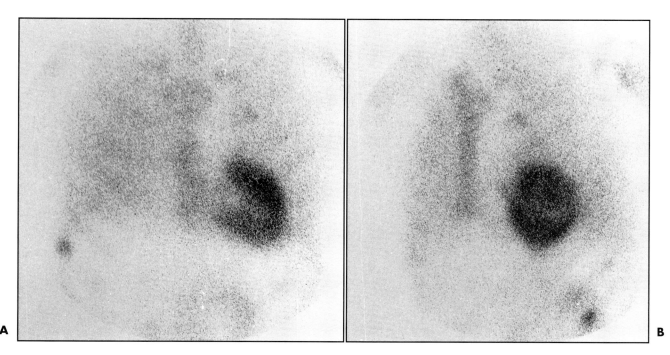

Fig. 17-20. Heart uptake. Intense diffuse myocardial muscle uptake in a patient with amyloidosis. **A**, Anterior view. **B**, Left anterior oblique view.

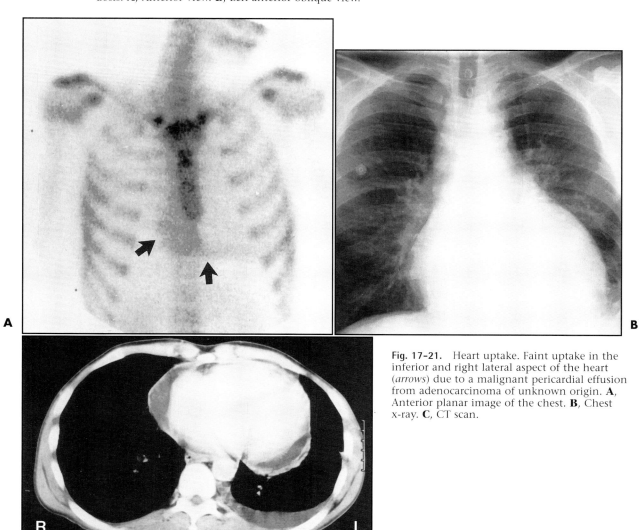

Fig. 17-21. Heart uptake. Faint uptake in the inferior and right lateral aspect of the heart (*arrows*) due to a malignant pericardial effusion from adenocarcinoma of unknown origin. **A**, Anterior planar image of the chest. **B**, Chest x-ray. **C**, CT scan.

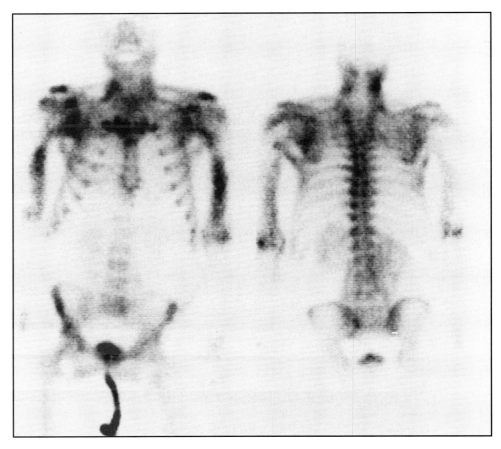

Fig. 17-22. Muscle uptake. Increased activity in the muscles of the neck, shoulders, upper extremities, and lower spine due to polymyositis from lung carcinoma; the bone scan activity returned to normal after tumor resection.

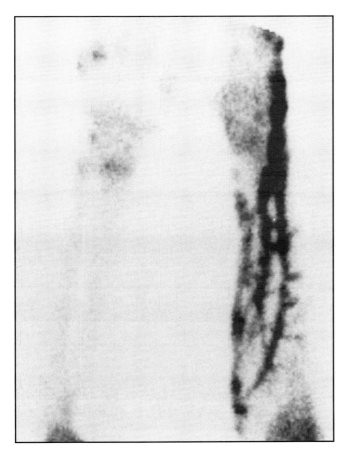

Fig. 17-23. Vascular uptake. Three-hour delayed image of the upper extremities shows activity in the venous vessels of the left arm because of thrombosis of an arteriovenous (AV) fistula (used for renal dialysis).

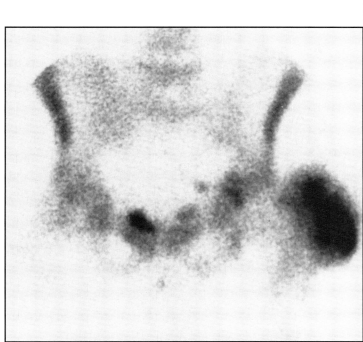

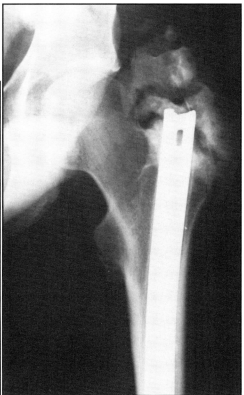

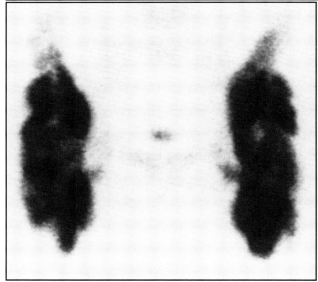

Fig. 17-24. Heterotopic ossification (HO). There is increased tracer above the left greater trochanter in one patient due to previous instrumentation (**A** and **B**). Intense activity around both hips of another patient with quadraplegia indicates very active disease (**C**).

nosis circumscripta, where small calcified deposits appear in the cutaneous and subcutaneous tissue over the extensor aspects of joints and fingertips. Scintigraphy may have an additional role in detecting calcinosis tumoralis, the localized but extensive calcification around joints, and also in determining the effectiveness of diet or steroid therapy.[88] Focal uptake can occur after electrical cardioversion (Fig. 17-25).

STAGING OF SOFT-TISSUE TUMORS

Most malignant and many benign tumors of soft tissue accumulate ^{99m}Tc-phosphate (Fig. 17-26).[29,63,78] Uptake is usually greater in malignant than in benign tumors, but there is considerable overlap. Absence of uptake is strong evidence for a benign lesion. Preoperative staging with bone imaging agents evaluates the relationship of the primary tumor to the adjacent bone.

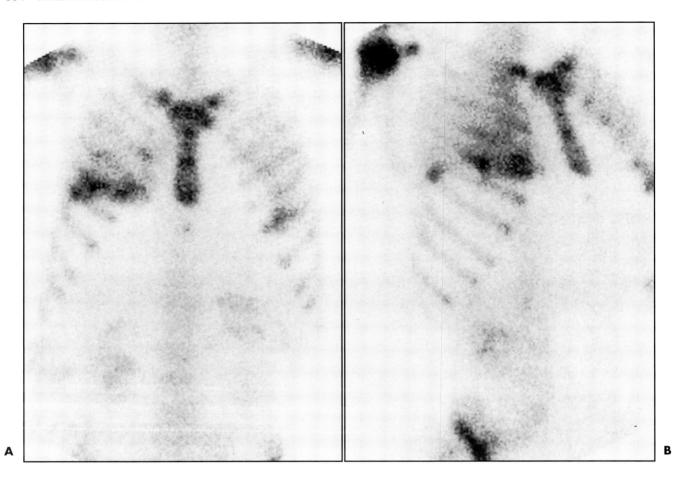

Fig. 17-25. Skin uptake. Increased tracer activity at the site of electrical cardioversion. **A**, Anterior view. **B**, RAO of the chest.

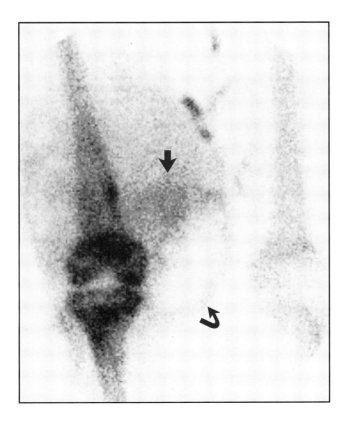

Fig. 17-26. Soft-tissue tumor. Liposarcoma in the right thigh shows areas of increased activity, possibly from tumor necrosis (*straight arrow*), and decreased activity, from cystic regions (*curved arrow*). There is only a small area of increased activity in cortical bone.

Increased tracer uptake in bone adjacent to a soft-tissue sarcoma indicates bone involvement by the tumor itself or by the reactive mesenchymal tissue around it. Such involvement may also be present when uptake in the soft-tissue lesion is contiguous with the bone and cannot be separated even on appropriate multiple scan views.

Bone scintigraphy to determine the extent of an osteosarcoma and its bone metastases may be of value for detection of nonpulmonary soft-tissue metastases (Fig. 17-10).[157] The sensitivity for scintigraphic detection of pulmonary metastases is only 21%, however,[165] with computed tomography (CT) and magnetic resonance imaging (MRI) providing the major contribution to diagnosis.

Bone imaging indicates the position and extent of a neuroblastoma in up to 90% of cases,[115] documents the presence of bone metastases,[147] and alerts the clinician to displacement or obstruction of a kidney.[70] Distant metastases in soft tissue may be detected,[123,152,162] but CT has better spatial resolution and is the investigation of choice.[7]

Primary and secondary medullary carcinoma of thyroid may accumulate bone agents[120] because of the tendency for the tumors to calcify. In the series of Johnson et al,[75] 4 out of 34 patients with medullary carcinoma of thyroid had soft-tissue metastases in liver, cervical nodes, and mediastinum detected by bone imaging. Two of these patients had soft-tissue metastases without bone involvement.

REFERENCES

1. Adams KJ, Shuler SE, Witherspoon LR, Neely HR: A retrospective analysis of renal abnormalities detected in bone scans. *Clin Nucl Med* 1980; 5:1.
2. Ahmad M, Dubiel JP, Verdon TA, et al: Technetium-99m stannous pyrophosphate myocardial imaging in patients with and without left ventricular aneurysm. *Circulation* 1976; 58:833.
3. Akmal M, Goldstein DA, Telfer N, et al: Resolution of muscle calcification in rhabdomyolysis and acute renal failure. *Ann Intern Med* 1978; 89:928.
4. Alfrey AC, Solomons CC, Ciricillo J, Miller NL: Extraosseous calcification: Evidence for abnormal pyrophosphate metabolism in uraemia. *J Clin Invest* 1976; 57:692.
5. Aprile C, Bernardo G, Carena M, et al: Accumulation of ^{99m}Tc-Sn-pyrophosphate in pleural effusions. *Eur J Nucl Med* 1978; 3:219.
6. Arbona GL, Antonmattei S, Tetalman MR, Scheu JD: Tc-99m-diphosphonate distribution in a patient with hypercalcaemia and metastatic calcification. *Clin Nucl Med* 1980; 5:422.
7. Armstrong EA, Harwood-Nash DCF, Ritz CR, et al: CT of neuroblastomas and ganglioneuromas in children. *AJR Am J Roentgenol* 1982; 139:571.
8. Atkins HL, Oster ZH: Myocardial uptake of a bone tracer associated with hypercalcaemia. *Clin Nucl Med* 1984; 9:613.
9. Baumert JE, Lantieri RL, Horning S, McDougall IR: Liver metastases of breast carcinoma detected on ^{99m}Tc-methylene diphosphonate bone scan. *AJR Am J Roentgenol* 1980; 134:389.
10. Berg GR, Kalisher L, Osmond JD, et al: ^{99m}Tc-diphosphonate concentration in primary breast carcinoma. *Radiology* 1973; 109:393.
11. Biello DR, Coleman RE, Stanley RJ: Correlation of renal images on bone scan and intravenous pyelogram. *Am J Roentgenol Radium Ther Nucl Med* 1976; 127:633.
12. Bingham JB, McKusick KA, Strauss HW: Cardiovascular nuclear medicine, in Maisey MN, Britton KE, Gilday DL (eds): *Clinical Nuclear Medicine*, Chapman and Hall, London, 1983, p 1.
13. Binnur K, Firat G, Sukran T, Metin E: Tc-99m HMDP uptake by the kidney in sickle cell disease. *Clin Nucl Med* 1992; 17:236.
14. Blair RJ, Schroeder ET, McAfee JG, Duxbury CE: Skeletal muscle uptake of bone seeking agents in both traumatic and non-traumatic rhabdomyolysis with acute renal failure. *J Nucl Med* 1975; 16:515.
15. Bledin AG, Kim EE, Haynie TP: Bone scintigraphic findings related to unilateral mastectomy. *Eur J Nucl Med* 1982; 7:500.
16. Bonte FJ, Parkey RW, Graham KD, et al: A new method for radionuclide imaging of myocardial infarcts. *Radiology* 1974; 110:473.
17. Bossuyt A, Verbeelen D, Jonckheer MH, et al: Usefulness of ^{99m}Tc-methylene diphosphonate scintigraphy in nephrocalcinosis. *Clin Nucl Med* 1979; 4:333.
18. Braun SD, Lisbona R, Novales-Diaz JA, Sniderman A: Myocardial uptake of ^{99m}Tc-phosphate tracer in amyloidosis. *Clin Nucl Med* 1979; 4:244.
19. Brill DR: Radionuclide imaging of non-neoplastic soft tissue disorders. *Semin Nucl Med* 1981; 11:277.
20. Buja LM, Tofe AJ, Kulkarni PV, et al: Sites and mechanisms of localisation of technetium-99m phosphorus radiopharmaceuticals in acute myocardial infarcts and other tissues. *J Clin Invest* 1977; 60:724.
21. Burnett KR, Lyons KP, Theron Brown W: Uptake of osteotropic radionuclides in the breast. *Semin Nucl Med* 1984; 14:48.
22. Buxton-Thomas MS, Wraight EP: High renal activity on bone scintigrams: A sign of hypercalcaemia. *Br J Radiol* 1983; 56:911.
23. Byun HH, Rodman SG, Chung KE: Soft tissue concentration of ^{99m}Tc-phosphates associated with injections of iron dextran complex. *J Nucl Med* 1976; 17:374.
24. Carlson DH, Simon H, Wegner W: Bone scanning and diagnosis of reflex sympathetic dystrophy secondary to herniated lumbar discs. *Neurology* 1977; 27:791.
25. Charkes ND: Mechanisms of skeletal tracer uptake. *J Nucl Med* 1979; 20:794.
26. Chaudhuri TK: Liver uptake of ^{99m}Tc-diphosphonate. *Radiology* 1976; 119:485.
27. Chaudhuri TK, Chaudhuri TK, Gulesserian HP, et al: Extraosseous noncalcified soft tissue uptake of ^{99m}Tc-polyphosphate. *J Nucl Med* 1974; 15:1054.
28. Chaynes ZW, Strashun AM: Improved renal screening on bone scans. *Clin Nucl Med* 1980; 5:94.
29. Chew FS, Hudson TM, Enneking WF: Radionuclide imaging of soft tissue neoplasms. *Semin Nucl Med* 1981; 11:266.
30. Chhabria PB, Stankey RM, Pinksy ST: Extraskeletal uptake of ^{99m}Tc-Sn-pyrophosphate in hypercalcaemia associated with carcinoma of the urinary bladder. *Clin Nucl Med* 1977; 2:87.
31. Choy D, Murray IPC, Hoschi R: The effect of iron on biodistribution of bone scanning agents in humans. *Radiology* 1981; 140:197.

32. Citrin DL, Bessent RG, McGinley E, Gordon D: Dynamic studies with ^{99m}Tc-HEDP in normal subjects and in patients with bone tumours. *J Nucl Med* 1975; 16:886.

33. Cole-Beuglet C, Kirk ME, Selovan R, et al: Bone within the breast. *Radiology* 1976; 119:643.

34. Conger JD, Alfrey AC: Scanning for pulmonary calcification. *Ann Intern Med* 1976; 84:224.

35. Conger JD, Hammond WS, Alfrey AC, et al: Pulmonary calcification in chronic dialysis patients: Clinical and pathological studies. *Ann Intern Med* 1975; 83:330.

36. Constable AR, Cranage RW: Pitfalls of absent or faint kidney sign on bone scan. *J Nucl Med* 1981; 22:658.

37. Cornelius EA: Nuclear medicine imaging in rhabdomyolysis. *Clin Nucl Med* 1982; 7:462.

38. Costello P, Gramm HF, Steinberg D: Simultaneous occurrence of functional asplenia and splenic accumulation of diphosphonate in metastatic breast carcinoma. *J Nucl Med* 1977; 18:1237.

39. Datz FL: *Gamuts in Nuclear Medicine*, Appleton and Lange, Norwalk, Conn., 1987, p 97.

40. Dewanjee MK, Kahn PC: Mechanism of localisation of ^{99m}Tc-labelled pyrophosphate and tetracycline in infarcted myocardium. *J Nucl Med* 1976; 17:639.

41. Dhawan V, Sziklas JJ, Spencer RP, Gordon IJ: Surgically related extravasation of urine detected on bone scan. *Clin Nucl Med* 1977; 2:411.

42. Echeuarria RA, Bonanno C, Davis DK: Uptake of ^{99m}Tc-pyrophosphate in liver necrosis. *Clin Nucl Med* 1977; 9:322.

43. Edeling CJ: ^{99m}Tc-methylene diphosphonate uptake in a primary Wilms' tumour. *Eur J Nucl Med* 1983; 8:30.

44. Felson B, Schwartz J, Lukin RR, Hawkins HH: Idiopathic pulmonary ossification. *Radiology* 1984; 153:303.

45. Fink-Bennet D, Dworkin H: Incidental detection of a horseshoe kidney on radionuclide bone images. *Radiology* 1977; 123:392.

46. Floyd JL, Prather JL: ^{99m}Tc-EHDP uptake in ischemic muscle. *Clin Nucl Med* 1977; 2:281.

47. Fogelman I, McKillop JH, Boyle IT, Greig WR: Absent kidney sign associated with symmetrical and uniformly increased uptake of radiopharmaceutical by the skeleton. *Eur J Nucl Med* 1977; 2:257.

48. Francis MD, Ferguson DL, Tofe AJ, et al: Comparative evaluation of three diphosphonates: In vitro absorption (C-14 labelled) and in vivo osteogenic uptake (Tc-99m complexed). *J Nucl Med* 1980; 21:1185.

49. Francis MD, Russell RGG, Fleisch H: Diphosphonates inhibit formation of calcium phosphate crystals in vitro and pathological calcification in vivo. *Science* 1969; 165:1264.

50. Fujimoto H, Murakami K, Nosaka K, Arimizu N: Splenic metastases of hepatocellular carcinoma: Accumulation of Tc-99m HDP. *Clin Nucl Med* 1992; 17:99.

51. Garcia AC, Yeh SDJ, Benua SCD, Benua RS: Accumulation of bone seeking radionuclides in liver metastases from colon carcinoma. *Clin Nucl Med* 1977; 2:265.

52. Gatter RA, McCartney DJ: Pathological tissue calcifications in man. *Arch Pathol* 1967; 84:346.

53. Gerhold JP, Klingensmith WC, Loeffel SC: Focal uptake of Tc-99m-MDP in renal metastases from squamous cell carcinoma of the lung. *Clin Nucl Med* 1980; 5:522.

54. Glass EC, DeNardo GL, Hines HH: Immediate renal imaging and renography with ^{99m}Tc-methylene diphosphonate to assess renal blood flow, excretory function and anatomy. *Radiology* 1980; 135:187.

55. Glimcher MJ, Krane SM: The organisation and structure of bone and the mechanism of calcification, in Ramachandron GN (ed): *Treatise on Collagen,* Academic, New York, 1968, p 137.

56. Go RT, Doty DB, Chiu CL, Christie JH: A new method of diagnosing myocardial contusion in a man by radionuclide imaging. *Radiology* 1975; 116:107.

57. Goldfarb CR, Ongseng F, Kuhn M, Metzger T: Non-skeletal accumulation of bone seeking agents: Pelvis. *Semin Nucl Med* 1988; 18:159.

58. Goy W, Crowe WJ: Splenic accumulation of ^{99m}Tc-diphosphonate in a patient with sickle cell disease: Case report. *J Nucl Med* 1976; 17:108.

59. Grames GM, Jansen C, Carlsen EN, Davidson TR: The abnormal bone scan in intracranial lesions. *Radiology* 1975; 115:129.

60. Guiberteau MJ, Potsaid MS, McKusick KA: Accumulation of ^{99m}Tc diphosphonate in four patients with hepatic neoplasm: Case reports. *J Nucl Med* 1976; 17:1060.

61. Harbert JC, Vieras F, Boyd CM: Focal renal activity on bone scans. *J Nucl Med* 1976; 17:426.

62. Hardy JG, Anderson GS, Newble GM: Uptake of ^{99m}Tc-pyrophosphate by metastatic extragenital seminoma. *J Nucl Med* 1976; 17:1105.

63. Harwood SJ, Wang TY, Camblin JG, Carroll RG: Internal focal uptake of technetium-99m diphosphonate in a soft tissue mass. *Semin Nucl Med* 1991; 21:335.

64. Harwood SJ: Splenic visualisation using ^{99m}Tc-methylene diphosphonate in a patient with sickle cell disease. *Clin Nucl Med* 1978; 3:308.

65. Haseman MK: Accumulation of a bone imaging agent in liver metastases from prostatic carcinoma. *Clin Nucl Med* 1983; 8:488.

66. Hattner RS, Miller SW, Schimmel D: Significance of renal asymmetry in bone scans: Experience of 795 cases. *J Nucl Med* 1975; 16:161.

67. Herry JY, Chevet D, Moisan A, et al: Pulmonary uptake of Tc-99m labelled methylene diphosphonate in a patient with a parathyroid adenoma. *J Nucl Med* 1981; 22:888.

68. Holmes RA: Diffuse interstitial pulmonary calcification. *JAMA* 1974; 230:1018.

69. Holmes RA, Manoli RS, Isitman AT: Tc-99m labelled phosphates as an indicator of breast pathology. *J Nucl Med* 1975; 16:536.

70. Howman-Giles RB, Gilday DL, Ash JM: Radionuclide skeletal survey in neuroblastoma. *Radiology* 1979; 131:497.

71. Ibis E, Krasnow AZ, Isitman AT, et al:. Liver uptake of technetium-99m-labelled phosphate compounds: An updated gamut. *Semin Nucl Med* 1992; 22:202.

72. Jackman SJ, Maher FT, Hattery RR: Detection of renal cell carcinoma with ^{99m}Tc polyphosphate imaging of bone. *Mayo Clin Proc* 1974; 49:297.

73. Janssen S, Piers DA, Rijswijk MH, et al: Soft tissue uptake of ^{99m}Tc-diphosphonate and ^{99m}Tc-pyrophosphate in amyloidosis. *Eur J Nucl Med* 1990; 16:663.

74. Jengo JA, Mena I, Joe SH, Criley JM: The significance of calcific valvular heart disease in Tc-99m pyrophosphate myocardial infarction scanning: Radiographic scintigraphic and pathological correlation. *J Nucl Med* 1977; 18:776.

75. Johnson DG, Colman RE, McCook TA, et al: Bone and liver images in medullary carcinoma of the thyroid gland: Concise communication. *J Nucl Med* 1984; 25:419.

76. Jones A, Keeling D: Benign myocardial uptake of hydroxy methylene diphosphonate. *Nucl Med Commun* 1994; 15:21.

77. Kajubi SK, Chayes ZW: Superscan prediction—another benefit of early renal views in bone scans. *J Nucl Med* 1985; 26:428.

78. Kida T, Hoshi K, Hoshino R, et al:. Tc-99m methyl-enediphosphonate (Tc-99m MDP) and Ga-67 concentration in soft tissue malignant fibrous histiocytoma (MFH): Case report. *Ann Nucl Med* 1993; 7:57.

79. Kim EE, Domstad PA, Choy YC, DeLand FH: Accumulation of Tc-99m phosphate complexes in metastatic lesions from colon and lung carcinoma. *Eur J Nucl Med* 1980; 5:299.

80. King WR, Francis MD, Michael WR: Effect of disodium ethane-1-hydroxy-1, 1-diphosphonate on bone formation. *Clin Orthop* 1971; 78:251.

81. Koizumi K, Tonami N, Hisada K: Diffusely increased Tc-99m MDP uptake in both kidneys. *Clin Nucl Med* 1981; 6:362.

82. Kozin F, Soin JS, Ryan LM, et al: Bone scintigraphy in the reflex sympathetic dystrophy syndrome. *Radiology* 1979; 138:437.

83. Kula FW, Engel WK, Line BR: Scanning for soft tissue amyloid. *Lancet* 1977; I:92.

84. Lamki LM, Wyatt JK: Renal vein thrombosis as a cause of excess renal accumulation of bone seeking agents. *Clin Nucl Med* 1983; 8:267.

85. Lamki L, Cohen P, Driedger A: Malignant pleural effusion and Tc-99m MDP accumulation. *Clin Nucl Med* 1982; 7:331.

86. Lantieri RL, Lin MS, Martin W, Goodwin DA: Increased renal accumulation of Tc-99m MDP in renal artery stenosis. *Clin Nucl Med* 1980; 5:305.

87. Lecklitner ML, Tauxe WN: Bone scintigraphy and post operative ureteropelvic urine extravasation. *Eur J Nucl Med* 1983; 8:346.

88. Leicht E, Berberich R, Lauffenburger T, Haas HG: Tumoral calcinosis: Accumulation of bone seeking tracers in the calcium deposits. *Eur J Nucl Med* 1979; 4:419.

89. Lieberman CM, Hemingway DL: Splenic visualisation in a patient with glucose-6-phosphate dehydrogenase deficiency. *Clin Nucl Med* 1979; 4:405.

90. Low RD, Hicks RJ, Gill G, Arkles LB: Tc-99m MDP uptake in a cerebral infarct. *Clin Nucl Med* 1992; 17:968.

91. Lunia SL, Heravi M, Goel V, et al: Pitfalls of absent or faint kidney sign on bone scan. *J Nucl Med* 1980; 21:894.

92. Lutrin CL, Goris ML: Pyrophosphate retention by previously irradiated renal tissue. *Radiology* 1979; 133:207.

93. Lutrin CL, McDougall IR, Goris ML: Intense concentration of technetium-99m-pyrophosphate in the kidneys of children treated with chemotherapeutic drugs for malignant disease. *Radiology* 1978; 128:165.

94. Lyons KP, Kuperus J, Green HW: Localisation of Tc-99m pyrophosphate in the liver due to massive liver necrosis: Case report. *J Nucl Med* 1977; 18:550.

95. Maher FT: Evaluation of renal and urinary tract abnormalities noted on scintiscans. *Mayo Clin Proc* 1975; 50:370.

96. Manoli RS, Soin JS: Unilateral increased radioactivity in the lower extremities of routine 99mTc pyrophosphate bone imaging. *Clin Nucl Med* 1978; 3:374.

97. Martin-Simmerman P, Cohen MD, Siddiqui A, et al: Calcification and uptake of Tc-99m diphosphonates in neuroblastomas: Concise communication. *J Nucl Med* 1984; 25:656.

98. Matin P, Lang G, Carretta R, Simon G: Scintigraphic evaluation of muscle damage following extreme exercise: Concise communication. *J Nucl Med* 1983; 24:308.

99. Matsui K, Yamada H, Chiba K, Iio M: Visualisation of soft tissue malignancies by using 99mTc polyphosphate, pyrophosphate and diphosphonate (99mTc-P). *J Nucl Med* 1973; 14:632.

100. McAfee JG, Silberstein EB: Non-osseous uptake, in Silberstein EB, McAfee JG (eds): *Differential Diagnosis in Nuclear Medicine*, McGraw Hill, New York, 1984, p 300.

101. McDougall IR, Pistenma DA: Concentration of 99mTc diphosphonate in breast tissue. *Radiology* 1974; 112:655.

102. McLaughlin AF: Uptake of 99mTc bone scanning agent by lungs with metastatic calcification. *J Nucl Med* 1975; 16:322.

103. McRae J, Hambright P, Valk P, Bearden AJ: Chemistry of 99mTc tracers. (ii) In vitro conversion of tagged HEDP and pyrophosphate (bone seekers) into gluconate (renal agent). Effects of Ca and Fe (2) on in vivo distribution. *J Nucl Med* 1976; 17:208.

104. Muheim G, Donath A, Rossier AB: Serial scintigrams in the course of ectopic bone formation in paraplegic patients. *Am J Roentgenol Radium Ther Nucl Med* 1973; 118:865.

105. Neely HR, Witherspoon LR, Shuler SE: Genitourinary findings incidental to bone imaging, in Silberstein EB (ed): *Bone Scintigraphy*, Futura, Mount Kisko, New York, 1984, p 370.

106. Nisbet AP, Maisey MN: Splenic accumulation of technetium 99m methylene diphosphonate. *Br J Radiol* 1982; 55:454.

107. Oren VO, Uszler JM: Liver metastases of oat cell carcinoma of lung detected on 99mTc-diphosphonate bone scan. *Clin Nucl Med* 1978; 3:355.

108. Ortiz VN, Sfakianakis GN, Haase GM, et al: The value of radionuclide scanning in early diagnosis of intestinal infarction. *J Pediatr Sur* 1978; 13:616.

109. Orzel JA, Rudd TG, Nelp WB: Heterotopic bone formation (myositis ossificans) and lower extremity swelling mimicking deep venous disease. *J Nucl Med* 1984; 25:1105.

110. Ozarda AT, Haynie TP, Gutierrez CR: Recurrent renal cell carcinoma following nephrectomy mimicking a normal kidney on bone scan. *Eur J Nucl Med* 1983; 8:148.

111. Palestro CJ, Steele MK, Kim CK, Goldsmith SJ: Myocardial uptake of Tc-99m MDP following cardioversion. *Clin Nucl Med* 1991; 16:273.

112. Park CH, Glassman LM, Thompson NL, Mata JS: Reliability of renal imaging obtained incidentally in 99mTc polyphosphate bone scanning. *J Nucl Med* 1973; 14:534.

113. Parker JA, Jones AG, Davis MA, et al: Reduced uptake of bone seeking radiopharmaceuticals related to iron excess. *Clin Nucl Med* 1976; 1:267.

114. Peller PJ, Ho VB, Kransdore MJ: Extraosseous Tc-99m MDP uptake: A patho-physiologic approach. *Radiographics* 1993; 13:715.

115. Podrasky AE, Stard DD, Hattner RS, et al: Radionuclide bone scanning in neuroblastoma: Skeletal metastases and primary tumour localisation with 99mTc-MDP. *AJR Am J Roentgenol* 1983; 141:469.

116. Poulose KP, Reba RC, Eckelman WC, Goodyear M: Extraosseous localisation of 99mTc pyrophosphate. *Br J Radiol* 1975; 48:724.

117. Prakash V, Lin MS, Perkash I: Detection of heterotopic calcification with 99mTc pyrophosphate in spinal cord injury patients. *Clin Nucl Med* 1978; 3:167.

118. Que L, Wiseman J, Hales IB: Small cell carcinoma of the lung: Primary site and hepatic metastases both detected on Tc-99m pyrophosphate bone scan. *Clin Nucl Med* 1980; 62:60.

119. Ravin CE, Hoyt TS, De Blanc H: Concentration of 99m-technetium polyphosphate in fibrothorax following pneumonectomy. *Radiology* 1977; 122:405.

120. Reuter E, Bethge N, Matthes M, Koppenhagen K: 99mTc-phosphonates for imaging of amyloid in C-cell carcinoma. *Eur J Nucl Med* 1983; 8:398.

121. Richards AG: Metastatic calcification and bone scanning. *J Nucl Med* 1975; 16:1087.

122. Rivera-Luna H, Spiegler EJ: Incidental rectus abdominis muscle visualisation during bone scanning. *Clin Nucl Med* 1991; 16:523.

123. Rosenfield N, Treves S: Osseous and extraosseous uptake of fluorine-18 and technetium-99m polyphosphates in children with neuroblastoma. *Radiology* 1974; 111:127.

124. Rosenthal DI, Chandler HL, Azizi F, Schneider PB: Uptake of bone imaging agents by diffuse pulmonary metastatic calcification. *Am J Roentgenol Radium Ther Nucl Med* 1977; 129:871.

125. Rosenthall L: Extraskeletal localisation of radiophosphate, in Rosenthall L, Lisbona R (eds): *Skeletal Imaging*. Prentice-Hall, London, 1984, p 261.

126. Rosenthall L, Kaye M: Technetium 99m pyrophosphate kinetics and imaging in metabolic bone disease. *J Nucl Med* 1975; 16:33.

127. Rossier AB, Bussat PH, Infant F, et al: Current facts on para-osteo-arthropathy (POA). *Paraplegia* 1973; 2:35.

128. Russell RGG, Kanis JA: Ectopic calcification and ossification, in Nordin BEC (ed): Metabolic Bone and Stone Disease, Churchill Livingston, Edinburgh, 1984, p 344.

129. Saha GB, Herzberg DL, Boyd CM: Unusual in vivo distribution of 99mTc-diphosphonate. *Clin Nucl Med* 1977; 2:303.

130. Sarreck R, Sham R, Alexander LL, Cortez EP: Increased 99mTc-pyrophosphate uptake with radiation pneumonitis. *Clin Nucl Med* 1979; 4:403.

131. Schmitt GH, Holmes RA, Isitman AI, Hensley Lewis JD: A proposed mechanism for 99mTc-labelled polyphosphate and diphosphonate uptake by human breast tissue. *Radiology* 1974; 112:733.

132. Seid K, Lin D, Flowers WM: Intense myocardial uptake of Tc-99m MDP in a case of hypercalcaemia. *Clin Nucl Med* 1981; 6:565.

133. Serafini AN, Raskin MM, Zard LC, Watson DD: Radionuclide breast scanning in carcinoma of the breast. *J Nucl Med* 1974; 15:1149.

134. Sfakianakis GN, Damoulaki-Sfakianaki E, Bass JC, et al: Tc-99m polyphosphate scanning in calcinosis universalis of dermatomyositis. *J Nucl Med* 1975; 16:568.

135. Sfakianakis GN, Ortiz VN, Haase GM, Boles ET: Tc-99m diphosphonate abdominal imaging in necrotising enterocolitis. *J Nucl Med* 1978; 19:691.

136. Shen AC, Jennings RB: Myocardial calcium and magnesium in acute ischaemic injury. *Am J Pathol* 1972; 67:417.

137. Shen AC, Jennings RB: Kinetics of calcium accumulation in acute myocardial ischaemic injury. *Am J Pathol* 1972; 67:441.

138. Shirazi PH, Ryan WG, Fordham EW: Bone scanning in evaluation of Paget's disease of bone. *Crit Rev Clin Radiol Nucl Med* 1974; 5:523.

139. Siddiqui AR, Cohen M, Moran DP: Enhanced differential diagnosis of abdominal masses using inferior vena cava, renal and bone imaging with single foot injection of Tc-99m methylene diphosphonate (MDP) in children. *J Nucl Med* 1982; 23:P7.

140. Siegel ME, Walker WJ, Campbell JL: Accumulation of 99mTc-diphosphonate in malignant pleural effusions: Detection and verification. *J Nucl Med* 1975; 16:883.

141. Silberstein EB: Nonosseous localisation of bone seeking radiopharmaceuticals, in Silberstein EB (ed): *Bone Scintigraphy*, Futura, Mount Kisco, New York, 1984, p 347.

142. Silberstein EB, Bove KE: Visualisation of alcohol induced rhabdomyolysis: A correlative radiotracer, histochemical, and electron microscopic study. *J Nucl Med* 1979; 20:127.

143. Silberstein EB, Delong S, Cline J: Tc-99m diphosphonate and sulphur colloid uptake by the spleen in sickle disease: Interrelationship and clinical correlates: Concise communication. *J Nucl Med* 1984; 25:1300.

144. Silberstein EB, Francis MD, Tofe AJ, Slough CL: Distribution of 99mTc-Sn diphosphonate and free 99mTc-pertechnetate in selected hard and soft tissues. *J Nucl Med* 1975; 16:58.

145. Singh BN, Ryerson TW, Kesala BA, Mehta SP: 99mTc-diphosphonate uptake in renal cell carcinoma. *Clin Nucl Med* 1977; 2:95.

146. Stone CK, Sisson JC: What causes uptake of technetium 99m methylene diphosphonate by tumours? A case where the tumour appeared to secrete a hypercalcaemia-causing substance. *J Nucl Med* 1985; 26:250.

147. Sty JR, Babbitt DP, Casper JT, Boedecker RA: 99mTc-methylene diphosphonate imaging in neural crest tumours. *Clin Nucl Med* 1979; 4:12.

148. Sty JR, Babbit DP, Kun L: Atlas of 99mTc-methylene diphosphonate renal images in paediatric oncology. *Clin Nucl Med* 1979; 4:122.

149. Sty JR, Babbitt DP, Sheth K: Abnormal Tc-99m methylene diphosphonate accumulation in the kidneys of children with sickle cell disease. *Clin Nucl Med* 1980; 5:445.

150. Sty JR, Garrett R: Abnormal myocardial image with 99mTc pyrophosphate in a child on chemotherapy. *Clin Nucl Med* 1977; 2:65.

151. Sty JR, Starshak RJ: Abnormal Tc-99m MDP renal images associated with myoglobinuria. *Clin Nucl Med* 1982; 7:476.

152. Sty JR, Starshak RJ, Casper JT: Extraosseous accumulation of Tc-99m MDP: Metastatic intracranial neuroblastoma. *Clin Nucl Med* 1983; 8:26.

153. Sty JR, Starshak RJ, Hubbard A: Accumulation of Tc-99m MDP in the spleen of a battered child. *Clin Nucl Med* 1982; 7:292.

154. Suzuki Y, Hisada K, Takeda M: Demonstration of myositis ossificans by 99mTc pyrophosphate bone scanning. *Radiology* 1974; 111:663.

155. Sy WM, Patel D, Faunce H: Significance of absent or faint kidney sign on bone scan. *J Nucl Med* 1975; 16:454.

156. Tanaka T, Rossier AB, Hussey RW, et al: Quantitative assessment of para-osteo-arthropathy and its maturation on serial radionuclide bone images. *Radiology* 1977; 123:217.

157. Teates CD, Brower AC, Williamson BRJ: Osteosarcoma extraosseous metastases demonstrated on bone scans and radiographs. *Clin Nucl Med* 1977; 2:298.

158. Thrall JH, Ghaed N, Geslien GE, et al: Pitfalls in Tc-99m polyphosphate skeletal imaging. *Am J Roentgenol Radium Ther Nucl Med* 1974; 121:739.

159. Tokuue K, Furuse M: Usefulness of the [99mTc]-MDP scan in the detection of calcified liver metastases. *Nucl Med* 1990; 29:231.

160. Trackler RT, Chinn RYW: Amphotericin B therapy. A cause of increased renal uptake of Tc-99m MDP. *Clin Nucl Med* 1982; 7:293.

161. Valdez VA, Bonnin JM, Martini T, Herrera NE: Abnormal liver and bone scans in a case of metastatic neuroblastoma. *Clin Nucl Med* 1978; 3:337.

162. Valdez VA, Jacobstein JG: Visualisation of a malignant pericardial effusion with Tc-99m EHDP. *Clin Nucl Med* 1980; 5:210.

163. Van Antwerp JD, Hall JN, O'Mara RE, Schuyler VH: Bone scan abnormality produced by interaction of Tc-99m diphosphonate with iron dextran (Imferon). *J Nucl Med* 1975; 16:577.

164. Van Antwerp JD, O'Mara RE, Pitt MJ, Walsh S: Technetium 99m diphosphonate accumulation in amyloid. *J Nucl Med* 1975; 16:238.

165. Vanel D, Henry-Amar M, Lumbroso J, et al: Pulmonary evaluation of patients with osteosarcoma: Roles of standard radiography, tomography, CT, scintigraphy and tomoscintigraphy. *AJR Am J Roentgenol* 1984; 143:519.

166. Vieras F: Radiation induced skeletal and soft tissue bone scan changes. *Clin Nucl Med* 1977; 2:93.

167. Vieras F, Boyd CM: Diagnostic value of renal imaging incidental to bone scintigraphy with [99mTc]-phosphate compounds. *J Nucl Med* 1975; 16:1109.

168. Wahner HW, Dewanjee MK: Drug induced modulation of Tc-99m pyrophosphate tissue distribution: What is involved? *J Nucl Med* 1981; 22:555.

169. Watson NW, Cowan RJ, Maynard CD, Richards F: Resolution of metastatic calcification revealed by bone scanning: Case report. *J Nucl Med* 1977; 18:890.

170. Wenzel WW, Heasty RG: Uptake of [99mTc]-stannous polyphosphate in an area of cerebral infarction. *J Nucl Med* 1974; 15:207.

171. Wilkinson RH, Gaede JT: Concentration of Tc-99m methylene diphosphonate in hepatic metastases from squamous cell carcinoma. *J Nucl Med* 1979; 20:303.

172. Willerson JT, Parkey RW, Bonte FJ, et al: Technetium stannous pyrophosphate myocardial scintigrams in patients with chest pain of varying aetiology. *Circulation* 1975; 51:1046.

173. Williamson BRS, Teates CD, Bray ST, et al: Renal excretion simulating bone disease on bone scans—a technique for solving the problem. *Clin Nucl Med* 1979; 4:200.

174. Wilson MA, Liss LF, Studey C: Calcification of hepatic metastases. *J Nucl Med* 1983; 24:P85.

175. Winter PF: Focal renal activity in bone scans. *J Nucl Med* 1976; 17:429.

176. Winter PF: Splenic accumulation of [99mTc] diphosphonate. *J Nucl Med* 1976; 17:850.

177. Wistow BW, McAfee JG, Sagerman RH, et al: Renal uptake of Tc-99m methylene diphosphonate after radiation therapy. *J Nucl Med* 1979; 20:32.

178. Wynchank S: [99mTc] methylene diphosphonate lung uptake in mixed small and large cell lymphoma. *Eur J Nucl Med* 1982; 7:47.

179. Yood RA, Skinner M, Cohen AS, Lee VW: Soft tissue uptake of bone seeking radionuclide in amyloidosis. *J Rheumatol* 1981; 8:760.

180. Zimmer AM, Isitman AT, Holmes RA: Enzyme inhibition of diphosphonate: A proposed mechanism of tissue uptake. *J Nucl Med* 1975; 16:352.

181. Zwas ST, Friedman B, Nervbay T: Scintigraphic presentation of hip joint synovial chondromatosis. *Eur J Nucl Med* 1988; 14:411.

CHAPTER 18

DECEPTIONS IN NUCLEAR MEDICINE IMAGING OF BONE

Arthur Z. Krasnow

Robert S. Hellman

Ali T. Isitman

B. David Collier, Jr.

David W. Palmer

Kutlan Ozker

James R. Swinghammer

"Smooth runs the water where the brook is deep."
"The fox barks not when he would steal the lamb."

William Shakespeare

Abnormalities that appear on imaging studies may not always represent disease. Such dilemmas should be anticipated whenever mechanical equipment is used and human interaction is required. These problems occur often in nuclear medicine studies with several books, articles, and posters presenting some of the more common artifacts encountered.* The variety of imaging artifacts has increased over the years as technology has become more sophisticated. Some of the artifacts that occurred in the past were eliminated by modern instrumentation; however, other new abnormalities were created. With the

*References 48, 49, 56, 57, 59, 64, 99, 109, 122, 132, 133.

increase in study acquisition parameters including the use of newer radionuclides, interventional drugs, and novel procedures, the potential is great for the development of even more deceptive abnormalities.

Most authors have termed these types of imaging abnormalities as *artifacts*. We prefer to use a broader classification that includes conditions that lead to both incorrect abnormal (false-positive) and incorrect normal (false-negative) interpretations. This latter situation occurs when a true lesion is obscured by another condition. Thus the patient who is taking a medication that interferes with the localization of a radiopharmaceutical may display a scan appearance that is not necessarily artifactual but rather shows an altered distribution. This in turn masks any true anomalies (Fig. 18-1). In this chapter the terms *deception* and *artifact* will be used interchangeably. A number of pathologic conditions in nonskeletal

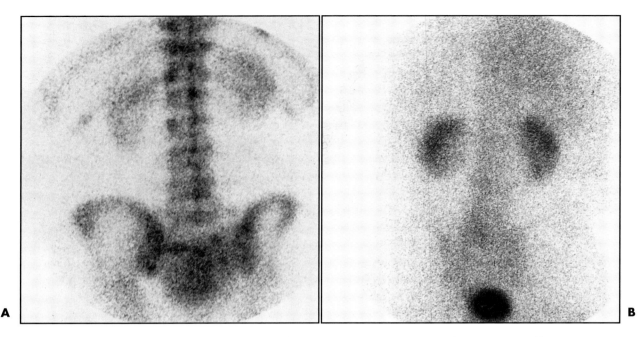

Fig. 18-1. Drug interference. **A**, Normal bone scan activity (posterior lumbar spine). **B**, Diffuse soft-tissue and kidney activity with little bone uptake is seen in the same patient while taking etidronate. *(From Krasnow AZ, Collier BD, Isitman AT, et al: False negative bone imaging due to etidronate disodium therapy.* Clin Nucl Med *1988; 13:264; with permission.)*

structures will accumulate bone-seeking radiopharmaceuticals, often simulating bone disease. These situations are discussed in Chapter 2.

We initially describe some of the general characteristics that are often present in deceptions that occur on bone scans as well as our approach to recognize them. We then discuss specific groups of abnormalities and show examples. Finally, we present some guidelines to reduce the occurrence of these aberrations.

RECOGNIZING BONE SCAN DECEPTIONS

The most important technique for detection of an image deception is for the interpreter to maintain a high index of suspicion. A study should be approached like a detective solving a crime. A nuclear medicine physician should be familiar with common deceptions and their variable appearance on a bone scan. However, caution is advised since pathologic conditions may have a similar appearance to that of a known artifact. Examples of this previously reported include a metastasis to the humerus at the deltoid muscle insertion site[71] and an osteosarcoma of the lower extremity appearing like urine contamination.[55]

The best way to review a bone scan is to evaluate it in an organized fashion. Assess each phase of the examination and each body region individually for any defects without concentrating solely on areas that are obviously abnormal. Artifacts and deceptions will often appear in multiple regions. Only by reviewing all the nuclear med-

icine films available can this pattern be recognized. Lesions that are present on planar images should also be seen on single photon emission computed tomography (SPECT) images, and intense abnormalities on SPECT images can usually be seen on planar images (Fig. 18-2). In addition, lesions seen on one set of SPECT images should also be seen on at least one and often all orthogonal (transverse, coronal, and sagittal) images since the same digital data are being sectioned in a different plane. An abnormality should be looked at and decided if it conforms exactly to what would be anticipated from the pathologic conditions in the differential diagnosis. Artifacts will often show a slightly different pattern with abnormal activity outside the expected regions. Is there a pattern present that would suggest free pertechnetate (Fig. 18-3) or interference from a patient's medications? Does the abnormality change over time as might happen from activity in the genitourinary tract?

There should be a higher index of suspicion for the presence of an artifact whenever an alteration in the standard operating procedure of a laboratory occurs. Changes in equipment, computer software, study protocols, dose procurement, and technology staff can all lead to unfamiliarity and the development of new deceptions in bone scan imaging.

Many artifacts have an obvious and classic appearance, whereas others may be subtle and more difficult to determine. There are several general characteristics that if present should lead the physician to highly suspect an artifact. A scan abnormality that has a very proportional geometric shape or is distributed symmetrically may be a clue that an artifact is present. A true pathologic lesion

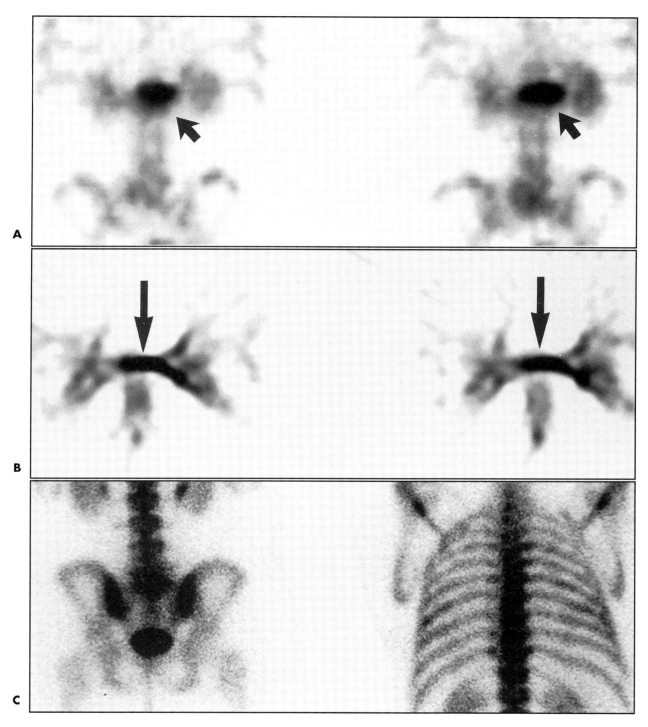

Fig. 18-2. Unconfirmed abnormality. Intense linear area of increased activity anterior to the vertebrae on coronal (**A**) and transaxial (**B**) SPECT images (*arrows*) is not seen on high intensity posterior planar images (**C**). This artifact occurred because of the transient appearance of excessive activity in the renal pelvis (change in tracer distribution artifact).

would not manifest as distinct as a circle, which is the appearance seen with an attenuation artifact from a cardiac pacemaker. Another clue is the presence of a very smooth, distinct border between an abnormality and the adjacent normal tissue. Pathologic conditions do not

usually occur in a precise fashion (Fig. 18-4). Finally, one needs to determine whether a lesion conforms to a known anatomic distribution. Artifacts will often cross outside these natural borders (Fig. 18-5).

Patient clinical information can help the reviewer

Fig. 18-3. Free pertechnetate. **A**, Increased activity is seen in the GI tract (*arrow*; anterior abdominal image). **B**, Complete lack of bone uptake indicates that this patient was injected with Tc-99m pertechnetate instead of Tc-99m MDP (anterior whole-body image).

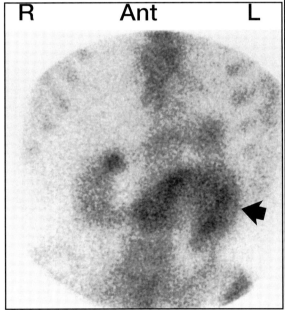

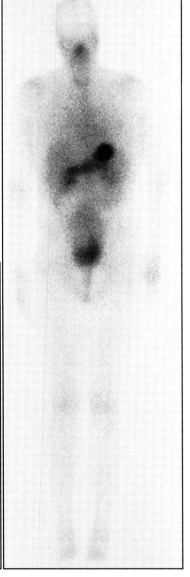

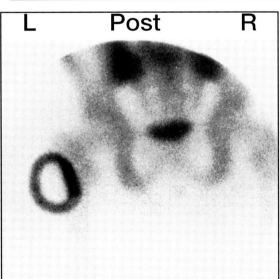

Fig. 18-4. Artifact clues. (1) Sharp borders, (2) spheric shape, and (3) extension beyond anatomic borders; this patient placed a contaminated straight urine catheter in his back pocket (posterior pelvic image).

avoid false interpretations. Box 18-1 lists the type of information that should be obtained. Review of the patient's x-rays and old bone scans might show discrepancies or findings that could explain an abnormality. The presence of osteophytes in the hip on x-ray could indicate why there is increased activity along the outer borders of the femoral head with less activity in the center, thereby simulating avascular necrosis (see Chapter 4, Fig. 4-10).

One of the most important pieces of information to ascertain is how a study was obtained. Problems with the radiopharmaceutical, the patient, and the acquisition may have transpired, leading to a false abnormality. Only by talking to the technologist who performed the study and determining any deviations from the normal technique can many of these deceptive findings be discovered.

By reviewing other bone scans and imaging studies performed the same day, an explanation for an artifact may be uncovered. Abnormalities occurring on all studies performed on the same imaging instrument would signify that the camera, or its electronics, are responsible. Alternately a series of flawed studies performed with the same radiopharmaceutical drawn from the same vial would indicate this agent as the culprit.

Finally, evaluation of the acquired images as a cine on the computer or a computer-generated image of the data[42] may alert the physician as to whether movement of the patient, camera, or table occurred. Cinegraphic review of SPECT images can provide information about

---

BOX 18-1. Patient Evaluation Questions

Patient History
- Reason for performing the study
- Age
- Medical diagnoses
- Medications
- Last menstrual cycle
- Previous surgeries (including dates)
- Recent procedures (including intramuscular injections)
- Recent studies (x-rays, nuclear examinations)
- Radiation therapy

Physical Examination
- Patient size and body habitus
- Surgical scars
- IV lines
- Other tubes
- Pacemaker, prosthetic bra, other external devices
- External drainage devices
- Arteriovenous fistula

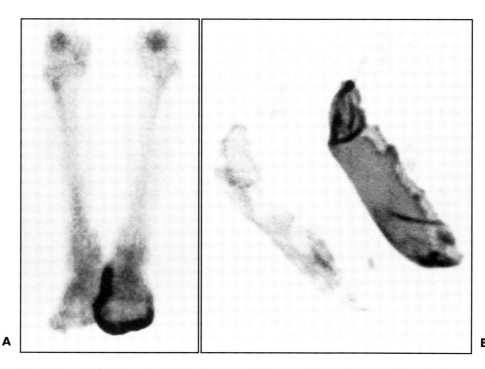

Fig. 18-5. Artifact clue. **A,** Activity is seen outside normal bone structures (anterior lower extremity image). **B,** Nearly all the activity is observed in the patient's contaminated sock when it is imaged by itself.

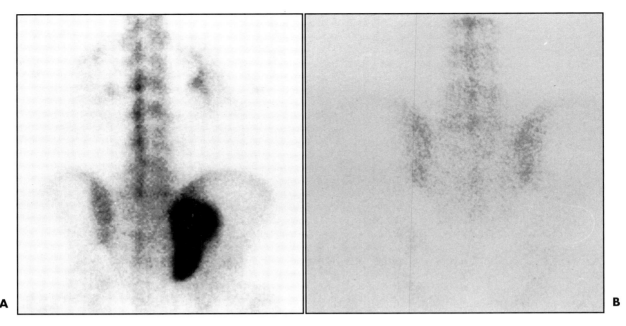

Fig. 18-6. Helpful maneuver. **A**, Right posterior oblique image of the spine and pelvis show intense abnormal activity in the right sacroiliac joint region. **B**, Twenty-four hour image reveals that the activity was radioactive urine in an asymmetrically placed distended bladder.

BOX 18-2. Maneuvers to Expose Deceptions

- Obtain multiple views of the abnormal region (caudal cranial view, vertex view, SPECT)
- Move the patient and or the camera
- Remove clothing, empty pockets
- Change collimator if defective
- Cleanse the skin
- Obtain 24-hour image to remove bladder activity
- Have patient stand, walk, urinate to remove urinary tract activity
- Use a second agent (Tc-99m sulfur colloid to ascertain bone marrow sites; Tc-99m DTPA to outline the genitourinary system)
- Move urine drainage bag or intravenous line
- Review images on the computer at various intensities (if digitally acquired)

BOX 18-3. General Organization Scheme of Deceptions in Bone Imaging

- Normal Variant
- Iatrogenic error: procedural
- Radiopharmaceutical error
- Equipment induced abnormality
- Setup error
- Injection error
- Imaging error
- Processing/filming error
- Patient-induced error

the depth of an abnormality, revealing its anatomic relationship to bone and kidneys.

A number of different maneuvers have been used to expose artifacts. Such procedures as removing a patient's clothes or obtaining different camera views are described in Box 18-2 (Fig. 18-6).

CATEGORIZING BONE SCAN DECEPTIONS

Each phase of the bone scan examination is susceptible to developing artifacts or deceptive images. Flow studies, planar images, and SPECT images can all reveal distinct types of deceptions because of their different acquisition techniques. SPECT images, because of more sophisticated procedural requirements, can display artifacts not seen on planar bone images. Each phase of the examination from patient preparation to the filming of the final product is subject to error. Box 18-3 lists our basic scheme for organizing bone scan artifacts and deceptions based on etiology. Table 18-1 elaborates on this categorization scheme and more specifically denotes abnormalities described in the nuclear medicine literature. Some of the references cited discuss general SPECT artifacts (not bone specific), but can occur in skeletal scintigraphy.

The normal variant category includes all scan abnormalities that occur because of the diversity in patient anatomy and physiology. A number of skeletal areas can

Text continued on p. 416.

TABLE 18-1
Gamut for Deceptions in Bone Imaging*

NORMAL VARIANT	Applicable Technique	Scan Appearance	Image in Text	References
MISTAKEN IDENTITY FOR PATHOLOGY				
Muscle insertion site: stippled ribs, deltoid insertion,				
patellar tendon insertion	Planar	Increased focal activity		46, 47
Prominent C2	Planar, SPECT	Increased focal activity		13
Prominent lumbar spinous process(es)	Planar, SPECT	Increased focal activity		93
Prominent sacral tubercle	Planar, SPECT	Increased focal activity		14
SI joint activity mistaken for posterior element disease	SPECT	—		
Tibia/fibula activity at articulation site	Planar, SPECT	—		
Lordosis of the spine	SPECT	Increased vertebral activity		
Increased vertebral activity above the diaphragm	SPECT	Increased vertebral activity	Fig. 18-7	
Delayed closure of the growth plate	Planar	Increased focal activity		87
Ischiopubic synchondrosis	Planar	Increased focal activity		29
Parietal thinning	Planar	Decreased focal skull activity		108
Spleen mimicking the kidney	Flow	—		
Shallow acetabulum	Planar	Decreased focal femoral head activity		66
Absent bone marrow in femoral head	Bone marrow imaging	Decreased focal femoral head activity		120
VARIATION IN SIZE, SHAPE, POSITION				
Abnormal kidney position	Flow, planar, SPECT	Kidney may appear small		1
Bone marrow packing (after prosthesis placement)	Bone marrow imaging	Increased focal activity at the tip of the prosthesis	Fig. 18-18	34
EXCRETION INTO A NORMAL ORGAN				
Bladder: asymmetry, diverticulum	Planar	Increased focal activity	Fig. 18-6, Fig. 18-8	117,119
Ureter	Planar	Increased focal activity (may be linear)	Fig. 18-8	53,54,135
Kidney: transplant, horseshoe	Planar	Increased focal activity	Fig. 18-8	58,128
NORMAL PHYSIOLOGY VARIATIONS				
Menstruation: uterine blush	Flow	Increased focal flow		85,112
Erection: penile blood flow	Flow	Increased focal flow	Fig. 18-10	

Continued

TABLE 18–1
Gamut for Deceptions in Bone Imaging, cont'd

	Applicable Technique	Scan Appearance	Image in Text	References
NORMAL VARIANT, cont'd				
NORMAL PHYSIOLOGY VARIATIONS, cont'd				
Food attenuation	Planar	Decreased focal activity		33
Hormones: lactation	Planar	Increased diffuse breast activity		81,94
Changing tracer distribution	SPECT	Increased activity (streaks)	Fig. 18-2, Fig. 18-9	15***(#),61***, 109,78,95***
DELAY WASHOUT				
Blood vessel	Planar	Increased focal activity		89
IATROGENIC ERROR: PROCEDURAL				
SURGICAL CHANGE OF ANATOMY				
Urinary tract diversion	Planar, SPECT	Intense increased focal activity in abdomen, GI tract		9,40,58,88,132
Mastectomy	Planar	Increased diffuse activity in the ribs		
Breast prosthesis	Planar	Decreased diffuse activity in the ribs		133
Breast prosthesis	Planar around the prosthesis	Increased focal ring of activity		73,109
Activity in a surgical scar	Planar	Increased focal linear activity		103,116,122
RADIOPHARMACEUTICAL ERROR				
FREE PERTECHNETATE		Increased diffuse soft-tissue activity; increased stomach, GI tract, salivary gland activity	Fig. 18-3	134
O$_2$ in vial	Planar			56,99,138**
Prolonged storage	Planar			38,137
Inadequate stannous ion	Planar			12****,79****, 138**
Order of agent mixing	Planar			138**
Unspecified etiology	Planar			35,48,49, 52,59,122
COLLOID FORMATION				
Aluminum	Planar	Increased diffuse liver activity; decreased bone activity		24**,25,56,72**, 99,141**

	Modality	Finding	Figure	References
Water in kit	Planar			56
Unspecified etiology	Planar			105
EXCESSIVE ALKALINE PH	Planar	Increased liver, gallbladder, GI tract activity		2,24**,28,115

EQUIPMENT-INDUCED ABNORMALITY

CAMERA

	Modality	Finding	Figure	References
Center of rotation	SPECT	Distorted anatomy; increased ring activity		64***(#),109
Crystal abnormality	Planar	Increased or decreased focal area of activity	Fig. 18-11	109
PM tube defect	Planar	Absent focal activity at PM tube site		48,49,56##
Tipped gantry	SPECT	Poor-quality images		

COLLIMATOR

	Modality	Finding	Figure	References
Dent/defect	Planar	Decreased focal activity		
Foreign body	Planar, SPECT	Decreased focal activity		
Center of rotation	SPECT	Distorted anatomy	Fig. 18-11	22***(#),44#, 140***(#)
Holes not parallel	SPECT	Poor-quality images		

SET UP ERROR

	Modality	Finding	Figure	References
WRONG AGENT	Planar	Depends on agent injected		
WRONG COLLIMATOR	Planar, SPECT	Increased diffuse soft-tissue activity	Fig. 18-12	56
IMAGES OBTAINED TOO SOON	Planar	Increased diffuse soft-tissue activity; decreased diffuse bone activity (age dependent)		104

INJECTION ERROR

WRONG SPACE

	Modality	Finding	Figure	References
Arterial	Flow	Increased soft-tissue activity distal to the injection site	Fig. 18-13	3,109
Dose infiltration	Planar	Increased diffuse soft-tissue activity; lymph node visualization; bandage activity	Fig. 18-13	23,48,49,70***(##), 122,132, 21**(##),39,97, 114****(##),16, 100,129,131*****

POOR BOLUS

	Modality	Finding	Figure	References
	Flow	Decreased flow activity		

TECHNIQUE

	Modality	Finding	Figure	References
Into existing line	Planar	Increased focal activity (linear)	Fig. 18-13	48,99,109
Tourniquet use	Flow	Increased flow to injected extremity	Fig. 18-13	37,82
Clumping of the agent	Planar	Increased focal uptake in lungs (multiple)		121

Continued

TABLE 18-1
Gamut for Deceptions in Bone Imaging, cont'd

	Applicable Technique	Scan Appearance	Image in Text	References
IMAGING ERROR				
CAMERA TOO FAR FROM PATIENT (SPECT: TOO LARGE A RADIUS OF ROTATION)	Planar, SPECT	Poor-quality images	Fig. 18-12	56
PATIENT POSITIONING ERROR				
Tilt	Flow, planar, SPECT	Asymmetric bone structures		30***(#)
In and out of FOV	SPECT	Bone structure cutoff; increased streaking activity		64***(#),109
Extravasation from injection site overlying a bone site	Planar	Increased focal activity		99
TABLE MOTION	Planar, SPECT	Distorted anatomy		109
ACQUISITION				
Incomplete angle sampling	SPECT	Focal rings of increased activity	Fig. 18-14	11***(#), 60***,64***(#)
180-degree rotation	SPECT	Areas of increased and decreased activity	Fig. 18-14	10***(#)
Use of wrong matrix	Planar, SPECT	Poor-quality images		
Wrong energy peak	Planar, SPECT	Increased diffuse soft-tissue activity	Fig. 18-12	99,109
Low counts	SPECT	Poor-quality images (mottled areas)	Fig. 18-12	64***(#),109
Nonlevel camera head (longitudinal and transaxial)	SPECT	Poor-quality images		64***(#)
SPECTRAL OVERLAP (DUAL AGENT STUDY)	Planar	Increased activity from the second agent	Fig. 18-15	45
PIXEL OVERFLOW	SPECT	Absent focal activity next to an area of increased activity	Fig. 18-14	19*****,60***
PROCESSING/FILMING ERROR				
PHOTOGRAPHIC INTENSITY	Flow, planar, SPECT	Increased or decreased activity		
DOUBLE EXPOSURE	Planar	Multiple superimposed bones	Fig. 18-16	133
FILTER/SMOOTHING ERROR	SPECT	Poor-quality images	Fig. 18-16	64***(#),109
MIRRORED IMAGES	Flow, planar, SPECT	Reversed image		
UNIFORMITY ERROR	SPECT	Increased or decreased ring of activity		64***(#),109
WRONG LABEL	Flow, planar, SPECT	Wrong patient identified		
ASYMMETRICAL SECTIONING	SPECT	Asymmetrical bones		
ZIPPER EFFECT (HISTORICAL)	Planar	Absent focal activity (linear)		51

	Type of study	Finding	Figure	References
DUST IN THE PROCESSOR	Flow, planar, SPECT	Absent focal activity		
PATIENT-INDUCED ERROR				
TWO SEPARATE STUDIES				
Tc-99m MDP/I-131 (preceding)	Planar	Increased focal activity at non-bone sites	Fig. 18-17	48,64,109,132 64***(#),109
CONTAMINATION				
Urine: catheter, phimosis, spill	Planar, SPECT	Increased focal activity on skin	Fig. 18-4, Fig. 18-5, Fig. 18-17	48,49,55,56, 62,122,132
Sweat	Planar	Increased focal activity on skin		4
Blood (bandage, tampon)	Planar	Increased focal activity on skin		27,92,124
PATIENT MOTION	Flow, planar, SPECT	Poor quality images		49,109
ATTENUATION				
Intrinsic: penile prosthesis, surgical sponge, barium, orthopedic hardware, pacemaker, fat	Flow, planar, SPECT	Absent focal activity	Fig. 18-17	18,48,74,83, 106,133,139
Extrinsic: earrings, coins, medallions, belt buckles	Flow, planar	Absent focal activity	Fig. 18-17	49,56,63,122,132
OTHER DISEASE				
Age	Planar	Increased diffuse soft-tissue activity; decreased diffuse bone activity		136
Hypercalcemia	Planar	Absent kidney activity due to forced diuresis		76
Calcification of a vessel	Planar	Increased focal activity		122
DJD mimicking avascular necrosis of the femoral head	Planar, SPECT	Increased focal activity; decreased central activity		
Renal failure on dialysis: mimicking a superscan	Planar	Increased diffuse bone activity; absent kidneys	Fig. 18-17	
Hemochromatosis	Planar	Decreased diffuse bone activity; increased diffuse kidney activity		26,98
ARTHROGRAPHY	Planar	Decreased focal femoral head activity		86
SMALL ANGLE PHOTON SCATTER (FROM NEARBY INTENSE ACTIVITY)	Planar	Increased focal activity		56,102
DRUG INDUCED				
Local injection: iron	Planar	Increased focal soft-tissue activity		90,127
Local injection: calcium	Planar	Increased focal soft-tissue activity		8,75
Local injection: calcium (subcutaneous heparin)	Planar	Increased focal soft-tissue activity (usually multiple)		5,41,101*****

Continued

TABLE 18-1
Gamut for Deceptions in Bone Imaging, cont'd

	Applicable Technique	Scan Appearance	Image in Text	References
PATIENT-INDUCED ERROR, cont'd				
DRUG INDUCED, cont'd				
Local injection: chemotherapy	Planar	Increased diffuse soft-tissue activity in distal extremity		118
Systemic: iron	Planar	Decreased diffuse bone activity; increased diffuse soft-tissue activity; increased diffuse kidney activity		20,26,50,98,126
Systemic: transfusion	Planar	Decreased diffuse bone activity; increased diffuse soft-tissue activity; increased diffuse kidney activity		17,26,77,86,125
Systemic: iron colloid	Planar	Increased diffuse liver activity		43
Systemic: indomethacin	Planar	Decreased diffuse bone activity		96**
Systemic: aluminum	Planar	Decreased diffuse bone activity; increased diffuse soft-tissue activity		48,49
Systemic: gynecomastia-causing drugs	Planar	Increased diffuse breast activity		107,111
Systemic: steroids	Planar	Decreased diffuse bone activity		6**
Systemic: etidronate	Planar	Decreased diffuse bone activity; increased diffuse soft-tissue activity	Fig. 18-1	36,69,80, 110,130**
Systemic: gentamicin	Planar	Increased diffuse kidney activity		91**
Systemic: chemotherapy (methotrexate, vincristine)	Planar	Increased diffuse kidney activity; increased diffuse skull activity		32,77,84,91**
Systemic: contrast	Planar	Increased diffuse kidney and liver activity		31

*   GI, gastrointestinal; SI, sacroiliac; DJD, degenerative joint disease; PM, photomultiplier; FOV, field of view.
**   Animal study.
***   Phantom study.
**** Nonimaging study.
***** Animal and human study.
****** Phantom and human study.
#   Nonbone SPECT study.
Nonbone (other) study.

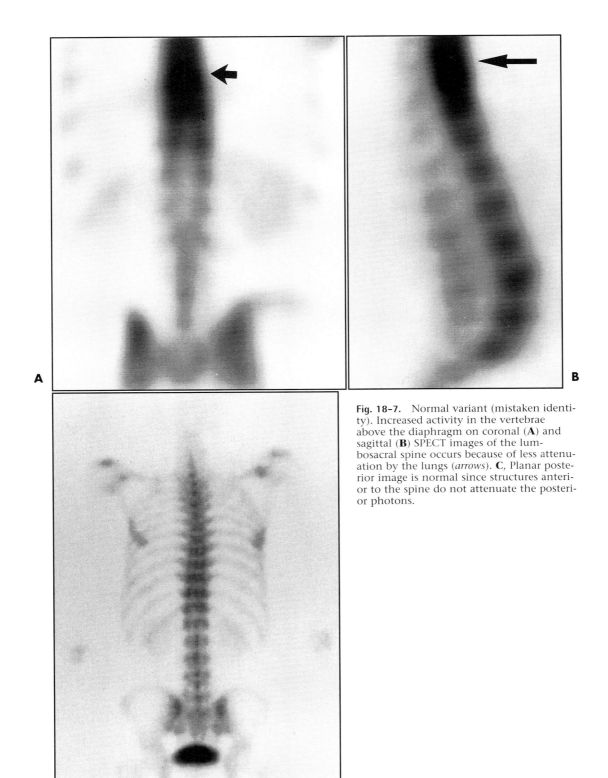

Fig. 18-7. Normal variant (mistaken identity). Increased activity in the vertebrae above the diaphragm on coronal (**A**) and sagittal (**B**) SPECT images of the lumbosacral spine occurs because of less attenuation by the lungs (*arrows*). **C**, Planar posterior image is normal since structures anterior to the spine do not attenuate the posterior photons.

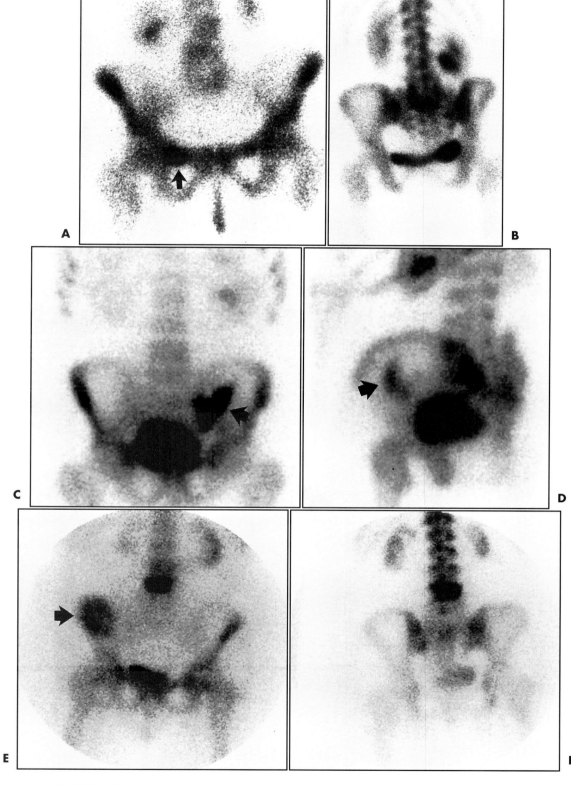

Fig. 18-8. Normal variants (genitourinary structures). **A**, Focal area of increased activity in the right superior pubic rami on the anterior pelvis image (*arrow*) is shown to be radioactive urine in the bladder on the posterior image (**B**). **C**, Increased activity in the left pelvis (*arrow*) is confirmed to be in the distal ureter on the left posterior oblique projection (**D**). **E**, Renal transplant overlying the right iliac crest (*arrow*) can easily be mistaken for a bone metastasis in this patient with known metastatic spread from breast cancer. **F**, The posterior pelvic image demonstrates that it is not in bone.

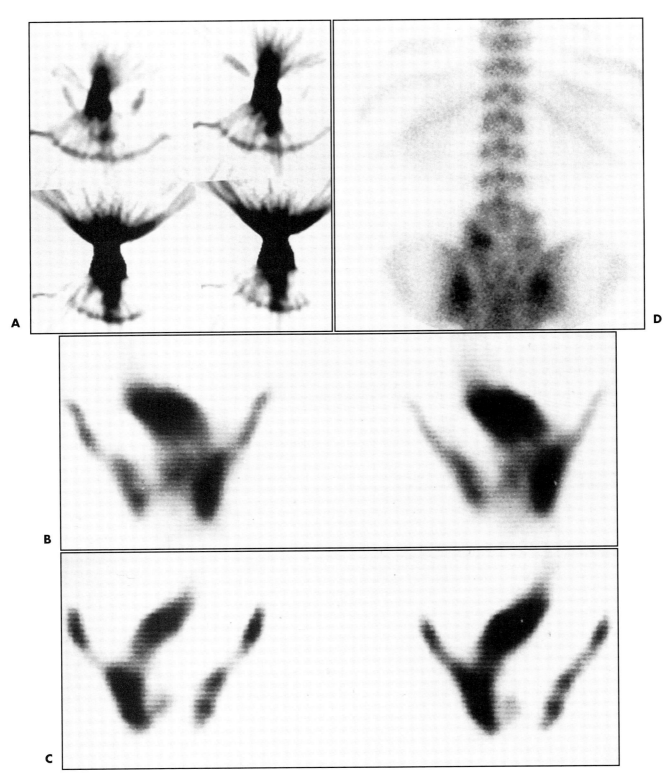

Fig. 18-9. Normal variants (normal physiology variation). **A**, A change in tracer distribution during the 20 to 30-minute SPECT study acquisition will cause streaking of the radioactivity as can be seen when imaging the pelvis (from the variable amount of radioactive urine in the bladder). **B** and **C**, Increased activity in opposite sacroiliac joints is seen when this patient was imaged on two different occasions, with the posterior planar image demonstrating normal activity in both joints (**D**). *(**B** and **C** from Krasnow AZ: Bone SPECT 1992: Clinical perspective and review, in Nuclear Medicine Annual 1992, Raven Press, New York, 1992, p 21; with permission.)*

appear more prominent in certain patients. These areas include those of muscle insertion, locations where adjacent bones are subject to different attenuation (Fig. 18-7), and regions where excessive curvature places one site closer to the camera. Changing a patient's positioning such as flexing their neck when imaging the cervical spine may be helpful.[13] Excretion into the genitourinary system can have an extremely variable appearance. Bladder and ureter activity can both simulate pelvic pathology (Fig. 18-8). Postvoid, caudal cranial, and 24-hour images may be helpful in proving that these scan abnormalities represent radioactive urine. Occasionally even a renal transplant may be mistaken for a pelvic mass (Fig. 18-8). Changing tracer deposition over time can have a profound effect on bone SPECT images (Fig. 18-9). This is most often seen when imaging the pelvis because of the constant change in the amount of radioactive urine in the bladder throughout the 20 to 30-minute acquisition. This artifact appears as streaks of increased activity that can overlap bone structures and hide or create abnormalities that mimic pathology. Increased activity in other nonbone structures can also cause deceptions, such as visualization of the penis (Fig. 18-10) or uterus on a blood flow study.

Iatrogenic errors and procedure abnormalities are those deceptions that occur because of surgical change of a patient's anatomy, often causing bone scan asymmetries. Removal of a breast will cause the ribs on that side of the chest to appear more intense because of less attenuation by overlying soft tissue. Surgical wounds will accumulate bone-seeking radiopharmaceuticals, especially when electrocautery is used,[103] with this activity becoming less apparent over time.[116] Urinary diversion procedures along with external drainage devices, can result in radioactive urine appearing in a number of unexpected places including the gastrointestinal tract.

Radiopharmaceutical errors include those where the radiochemical stability of the administered agent changes either before or after injection. A number of different situations can cause increased free pertechnetate, which will manifest as activity in the stomach and intestines. Thyroid activity is usually not seen because of the lack of organification and the 3-hour delay before imaging. The presence of unbound reduced, and hydrolyzed technetium, as well as aluminum from the molybdenum/technetium generator causes the formation of a colloidal suspension. This is removed by the reticuloendothelial system (RES) cells producing liver and spleen activity.

Equipment-induced abnormalities arise from technical problems with the instrumentation (Fig. 18-11). These can be due to the camera itself or to the collimator. They can sometimes be discovered by reviewing the daily quality control flood images. On SPECT examination, when there is excessive error in the center of rotation that is not corrected (with data from the specific collimator used), distorted images will appear.

Three classifications of abnormalities occur during the time of the exam performance: these are errors during the (1) setup, (2) the injection of the radiopharmaceuti-

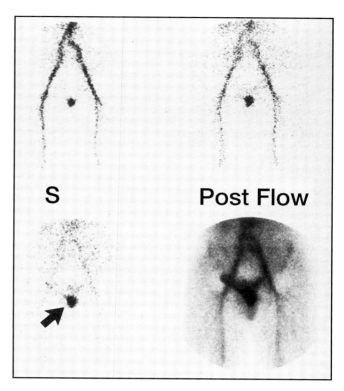

Fig. 18-10. Normal variant (normal physiology variation). Focal area of increased blood flow and hyperemia in the pelvis is due to a penile erection (*arrow*; anterior pelvic flow study).

cal, and (3) the actual acquisition period. Use of the wrong collimator or wrong agent will lead to poor-quality images that can hide pathologic findings (Fig. 18-12).

Injection errors occur quite frequently (Fig. 18-13). Subcutaneous injections generate increased background activity on planar images and can cause activity to accumulate in distal lymph nodes. An arterial injection will produce increased flow and uptake in the entire distal extremity (soft tissue and bone). A tourniquet left in place during injection will also create a dramatic flow discrepancy compared with the opposite extremity. Activity remaining in intravenous (IV) tubing may be mistaken for pathology if it overlies a bony structure.

Imaging errors can develop from positioning the camera either too far away from the patient or in an asymmetrical fashion. Other problems include using the wrong energy peak and acquiring a study for too short a time period (Fig. 18-12). Although 180-degree SPECT acquisitions of the spine provide quality diagnostic images,[123] such limited studies create deceptions when studying larger bones that are not asymmetrically placed in the body such as the skull and pelvis; 180-degree SPECT studies of these organs will show increased activity in those areas that were closest to the collimator during its limited arc (Fig. 18-14). If an insufficient number of acquisition stops are used on a SPECT examination, angular sampling errors are seen (Fig. 18-14). When performing a dual acquisition study with Tc-99m MDP and In-111 white blood cells (WBCs) for detection of

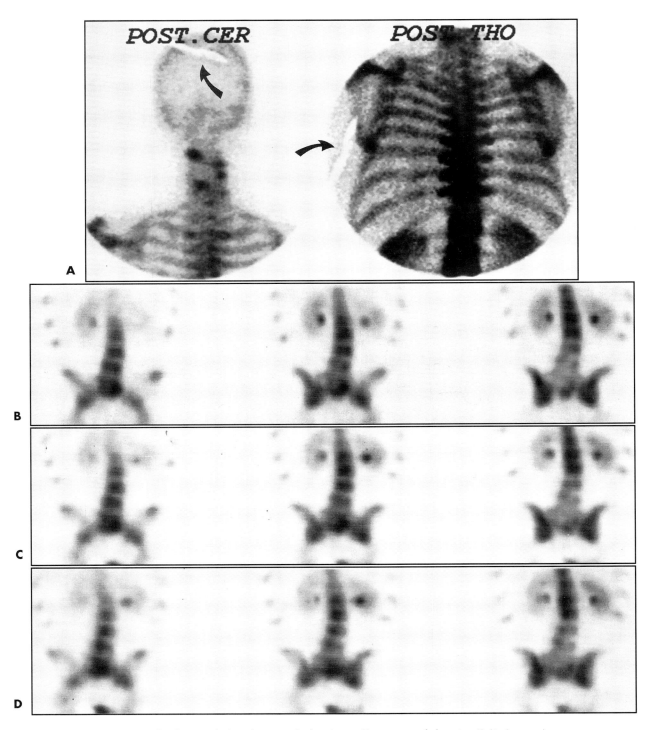

Fig. 18-11. Equipment induced errors. **A,** An almost linear area of absent activity is seen in different positions when using a camera with a cracked crystal (*arrows*). As the center of rotation gets worse, more image distortion occurs. Lumbosacral spine coronal SPECT images: (**B**) no error, (**C**) 6-mm deviation, (**D**) 9-mm deviation.

Continued.

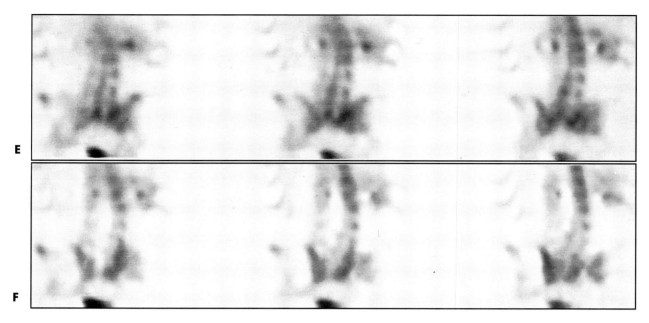

Fig. 18-11, cont'd. Equipment induced errors. Lumbosacral spine coronal SPECT images: (**E**) 18-mm deviation, (**F**) 32-mm deviation.

osteomyelitis, images obtained using the In-111 photopeaks will contain some Tc-99m photons due to pulse pileup. This can create the false impression of osteomyelitis (Fig. 18-15). SPECT images may suffer from pixel overload in which excessive activity causes adjacent photon-deficient zones (Fig. 18-14). This occurs more frequently when the acquisition is performed in byte mode rather than word mode on the computer.

Processing and filming errors are those that occur following image acquisition (Fig. 18-16). Care must be taken not to create the illusion of an abnormality by computer manipulation. Oversmoothing and undersmoothing of SPECT data can hide lesions, and photography can cause an abnormality to appear more or less significant than it actually is. Exposing a film more than once may lead to unusual images.

Finally, patient-induced errors occur because of intrinsic problems within the patients themselves (Fig. 18-17). This category includes photon deficient defects caused by attenuating substances such as orthopedic hardware, barium, and external metal objects. Radioactive urine, blood, and sweat can be transferred to any body region and appear at multiple sites. Such activity might also be present on the patient's clothing or on the imaging instrument. When the activity is on the camera or collimator, SPECT images will be severely affected. An area of intense tracer activity (e.g., extravasation at an injection

---

BOX 18-4. Nonpathologic Causes of Decreased Bone Lesion Detection

Poor Bone Uptake of the Agent
- Drug interference
- Subcutaneous injection
- Wrong agent used
- Imaged too soon after injection
- Large amounts of adipose tissue
- Poor agent preparation: free pertechnetate
- Prolonged storage of prepared dose
- Elderly patient

Lesion Size, Location, Activity
- Small lesions
- Lesions close to zones of normal increased activity (e.g., sacroiliac joints, growth plates)
- Deep central lesions

Technical
- Patient motion
- Wrong imaging technique (collimator, energy window, matrix size)
- Camera too far from patient
- Low count acquisition
- Filming technique
- Processing/filtering technique

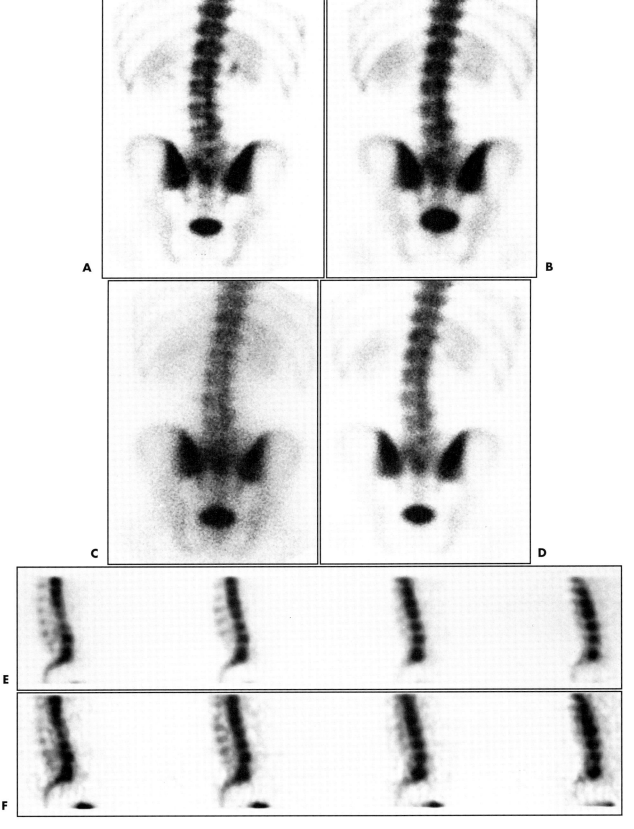

Fig. 18-12. Setup and imaging errors. A number of errors in study setup and acquisition can lead to suboptimal images. **A**, Normal posterior lumbosacral spine image; (**B**) the same patient is imaged using the LEAP collimator, (**C**) using the cobalt energy window, and (**D**) with the camera 12 in. away from the patient. In (**E**) a lumbosacral spine SPECT study was obtained in the standard fashion at 25 seconds per frame, and in (**F**) a second study on the same patient at 10 seconds per frame shows significant image degradation.

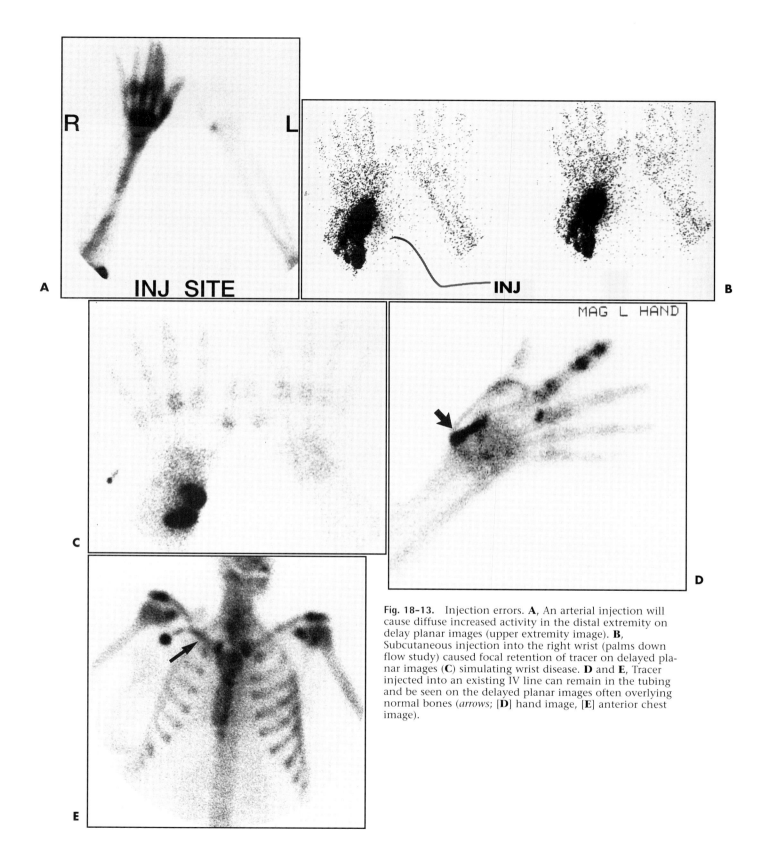

Fig. 18-13.   Injection errors. **A,** An arterial injection will cause diffuse increased activity in the distal extremity on delay planar images (upper extremity image). **B,** Subcutaneous injection into the right wrist (palms down flow study) caused focal retention of tracer on delayed planar images (**C**) simulating wrist disease. **D** and **E,** Tracer injected into an existing IV line can remain in the tubing and be seen on the delayed planar images often overlying normal bones (*arrows*; [**D**] hand image, [**E**] anterior chest image).

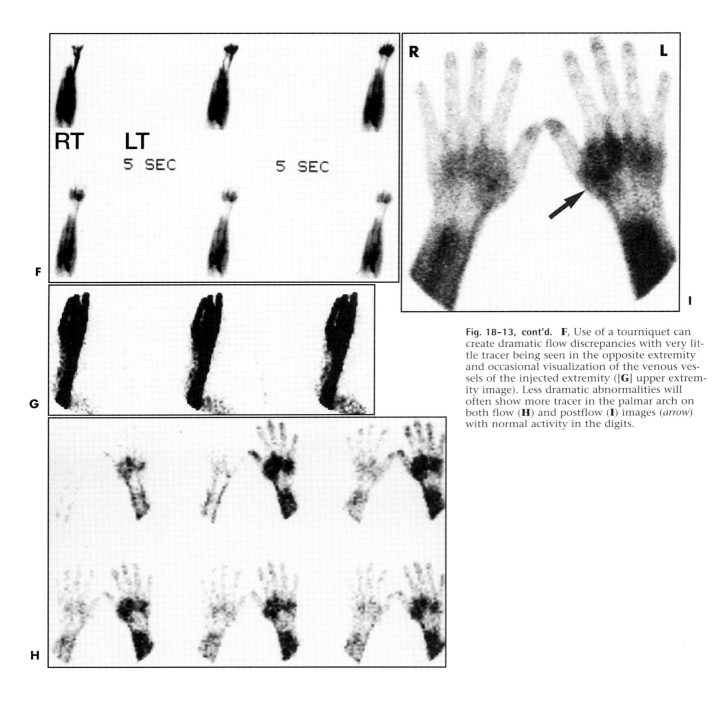

Fig. 18-13, cont'd. F, Use of a tourniquet can create dramatic flow discrepancies with very little tracer being seen in the opposite extremity and occasional visualization of the venous vessels of the injected extremity ([**G**] upper extremity image). Less dramatic abnormalities will often show more tracer in the palmar arch on both flow (**H**) and postflow (**I**) images (*arrow*) with normal activity in the digits.

site or bladder activity) can cause nearby bones to appear artifactually "hot." This is due to significant non-rejectable small angle scatter of photons from the bone onto the detector and hence the image. Patient motion will have a devastating effect on image quality and may be difficult to diagnose (see Chapter 4, Fig. 4-3). Other medical problems can affect bone scan images. A renal failure patient producing a superscan because dialysis removed all the background activity is one example. Several review papers discuss the interactions between patient medications and radiopharmaceuticals used in bone scanning and other nuclear medicine proce-

dures.[65,67,68] Local injection of iron and calcium can cause focal accumulation of tracer, while the presence of high serum iron levels from transfusions, systemic iron injections, and hemochromatosis will cause diffuse increased soft-tissue activity and low bone uptake.

Deceptions can also occur during bone marrow imaging. A clear knowledge of the normal distribution of these marrow-seeking agents is essential before interpreting abnormalities. Forty-five percent of normal people do not have femoral head activity on a bone marrow study. Therefore it is difficult to use this examination to diagnose avascular necrosis.[120] Increased bone marrow activ-

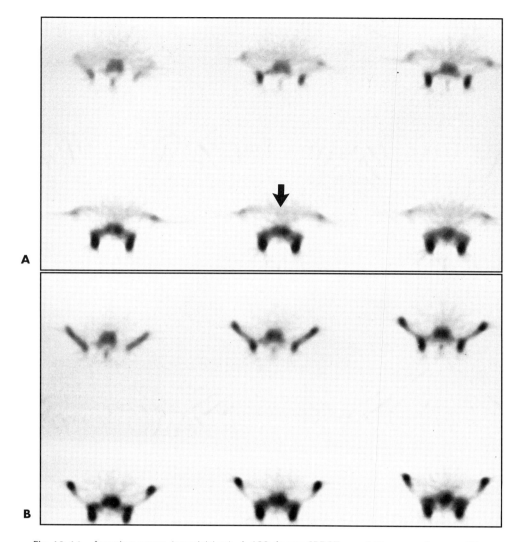

Fig. 18–14.   Imaging errors (acquisition). **A** 180-degree SPECT acquisitions produce quality images of the organs closest to the camera; when only the posterior 180-degree acquisition data were processed, there was good characterization of the spine but poor resolution of the anterior pelvis (*arrow*) compared with images generated from the full 360-degree study (**B**).

ity can be seen in the femur distal to a prosthesis (marrow packing). This may be confusing when evaluating for a prosthesis infection because labeled WBCs will also accumulate at this site of displaced marrow[34] (Fig. 18-18).

As in all nuclear medicine studies, there will be a subpopulation of patients who will have normal bone studies despite the presence of significant disease. Box 18-4 is a sublist of Table 18-1, which describes causes for decreased bone lesion detection due to conditions other than pathology.

REDUCING BONE SCAN DECEPTIONS

Many deceptions occur because of confusion about how the study is to be performed. Each nuclear medicine department should develop standard study protocols that are well documented and readily available for technologist use. The number of variations to this basic protocol for specific circumstances should be limited. Whenever a new procedure is introduced, time should be spent discussing it with the technologists and ensuring

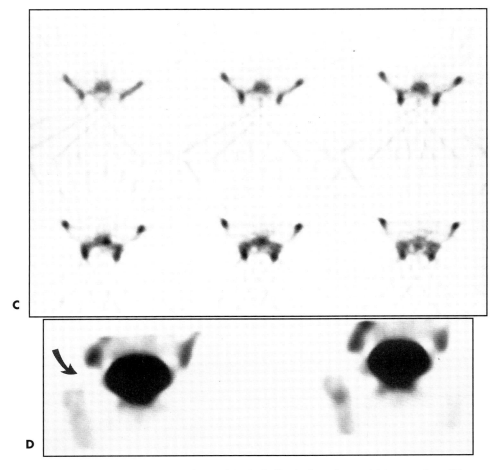

Fig. 18-14, cont'd.   Imaging errors (acquisition). **C,** Limited angle acquisitions such as 32 projections over 360-degrees will cause image streaking. **D,** Excessive activity (as can be seen in the bladder) can cause pixel overload on SPECT imaging with adjacent areas of photon deficiency (*arrow;* coronal SPECT images of the pelvis). (**D** *from Krasnow AZ et al: Bone SPECT 1992: Clinical perspective and review, in* Nuclear Medicine Annual 1992, *Raven Press, New York 1992, p 21; with permission.)*

that they understand how and why it is to be performed a particular way. Once a procedure protocol is established, few changes should be made. Technologists should be encouraged not to take any shortcuts and to alert the physician about any unusual occurrences.

Any change in department routine can lead to the occurrence of an image deception (new equipment, software, method of dose preparation and the use of inexperienced personnel). In these situations changes in study protocol may be necessary. In addition, proper training of new technologists is essential.

Strict adherence to routine quality control measures is imperative. When bone SPECT examinations are being performed, additional quality control measures are necessary (see Chapter 4, Box 4-5). Some authors have suggested supplementary testing procedures to specifically detect collimator abnormalities, particularly in those being used for SPECT imaging.[22,44,140] Abnormalities in these measures may alert the physician early that an artifact can be expected.

Bone scan examinations should be performed in appropriate clinical situations. The phases to be obtained (flow, planar, SPECT) will depend on the information desired. Planar images alone may be the most appropriate examination when imaging certain bony structures such as the cervical spine. The addition of a SPECT examination in this situation can create abnormalities that may confuse study interpretation (Fig. 18-19).

Careful preparation, handling, and storage of radiopharmaceuticals is essential. A number of situations can

Text continued on p. 430.

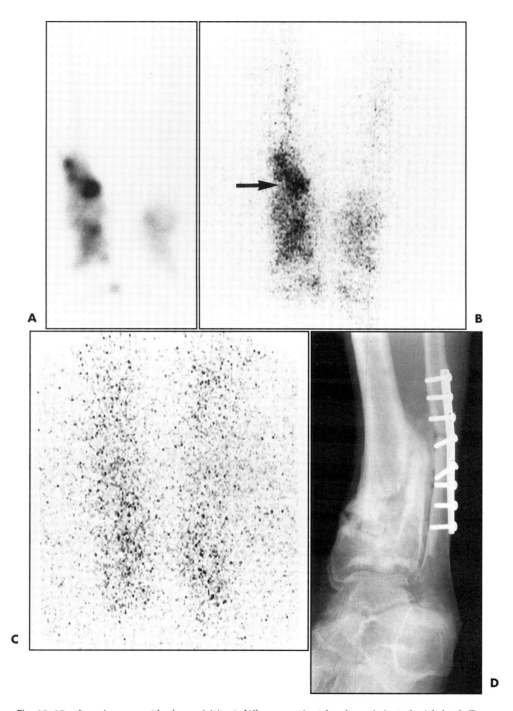

Fig. 18-15. Imaging error (dual acquisition). When a patient has been injected with both Tc-99m MDP and In-111 WBCs to diagnose osteomyelitis, areas of increased bone tracer uptake (**A**) will cause some photons to register in the higher In-111 window ([**B**] *arrow*). **C**, In-111 WBC images acquired before bone agent injection are more indicative of infection/inflammation. **D**, X-ray shows tibial fracture and orthopedic hardware explaining the increased bone scan activity.

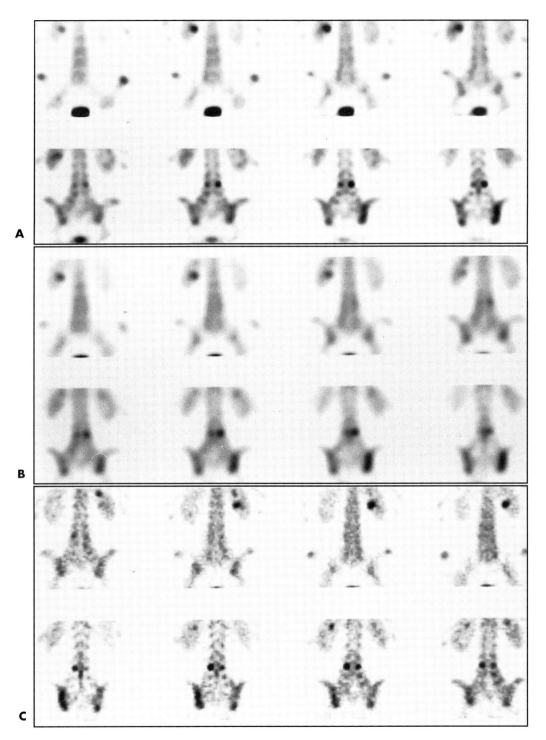

Fig. 18-16.   Processing/filming errors. **A**, Normal SPECT study; (**B**) oversmoothing, (**C**) undersmoothing (lumbosacral spine images).

Continued.

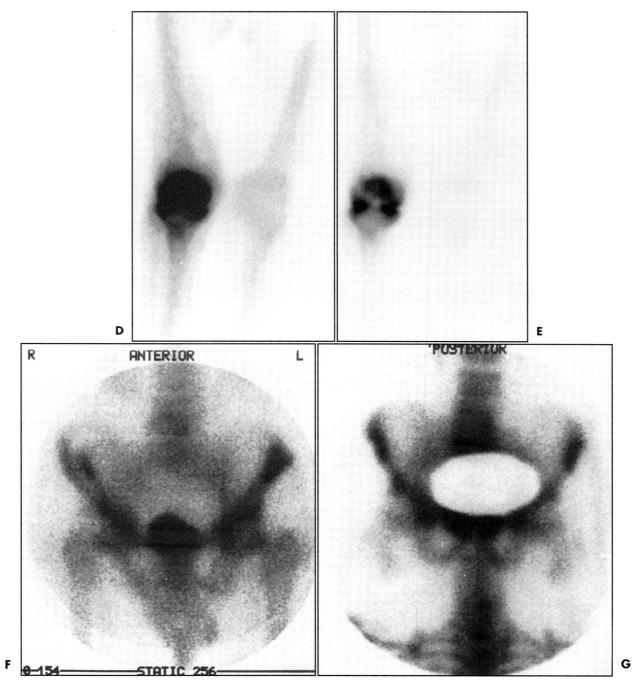

Fig. 18-16, cont'd. Processing/filming errors. **D,** Photographic intensity can create the appearance of a larger lesion: "darker images" make the abnormality appear to go deep into the femur and tibia when it is actually only in the bones adjacent to the joint (**E**). Double exposing a film can create subtle abnormalities (**F**) or very bizarre images (**G**).

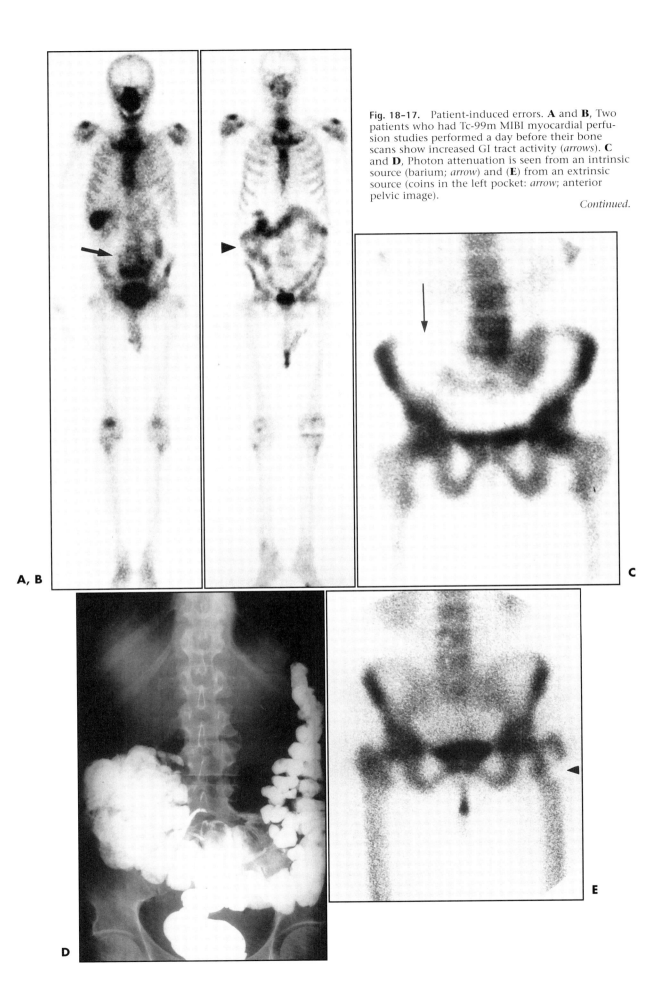

Fig. 18–17. Patient-induced errors. **A** and **B**, Two patients who had Tc-99m MIBI myocardial perfusion studies performed a day before their bone scans show increased GI tract activity (*arrows*). **C** and **D**, Photon attenuation is seen from an intrinsic source (barium; *arrow*) and (**E**) from an extrinsic source (coins in the left pocket: *arrow*; anterior pelvic image).

Continued.

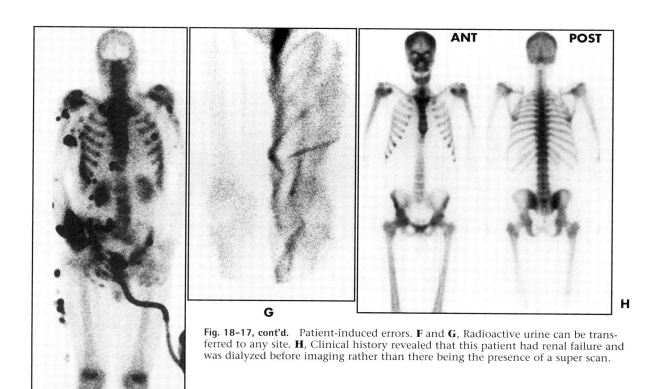

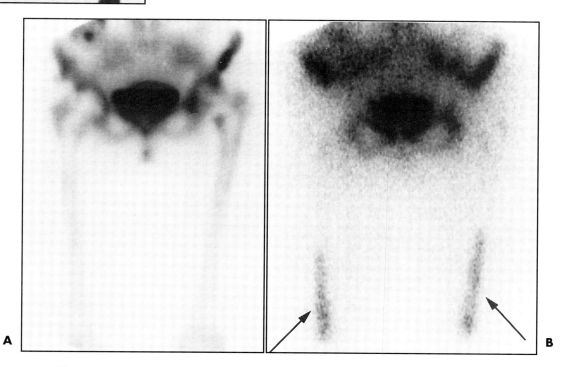

Fig. 18–17, cont'd. Patient-induced errors. **F** and **G**, Radioactive urine can be transferred to any site. **H**, Clinical history revealed that this patient had renal failure and was dialyzed before imaging rather than there being the presence of a super scan.

Fig. 18-18. Bone marrow/In-111 WBC abnormality. **A**, Bone scan image of the pelvis reveals bilateral photon-deficient areas indicating femoral prostheses. **B**, In-111 WBC imaging of this region shows increased WBC accumulation in the femurs distal to the tip of the prosthesis (*arrows*), suggesting osteomyelitis but instead is due to bone marrow packing from the surgical procedure (anterior pelvis and lower extremity images).

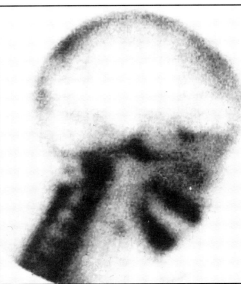

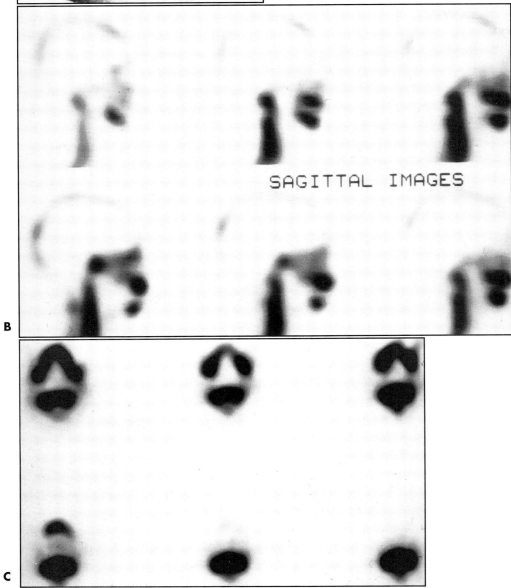

Fig. 18-19.   Unnecessary study. **A**, Planar right lateral image of the cervical spine shows a normal distribution of tracer activity. Sagittal (**B**) and transaxial (**C**) SPECT images, however, show intense activity in all of the cervical vertebrae. The addition of the SPECT examination can cause more confusion, leading to a false pathologic diagnosis.

lead to poor tagging efficiency including the presence of oxygen, the addition of an insufficient amount of stannous ion, and the long term storage of prepared doses at room temperature. Generator eluates should be routinely checked for the presence of aluminum breakthrough.

There are several guidelines to follow when preparing the patient for the imaging process. Only careful attention will avoid the injection of the wrong agent or the use of the wrong collimator. Each department should design safeguards to prevent these types of errors. Removal of metal objects and other attenuating materials from the patient's clothing before imaging is routine practice in most nuclear medicine departments. Also having the patient void before imaging can remove confusing genitourinary activity. Symmetric placement of bony structures as well as keeping the camera as close as possible to the patient will provide better diagnostic quality images. The injection site should be kept from overlapping other bone regions. Before starting a SPECT study, make sure the camera head is level and that the structure being imaged remains in the field of view throughout the acquisition. In general, SPECT images are count poor so that in order to improve resolution an attempt should be made to optimize the counting statistics. This includes injecting the maximum amount of activity and acquiring images for as long as feasible.

Constant attention and encouragment for the patient during an acquisition will reduce patient movement, thus decreasing image degradation. Motion can also be reduced by ensuring patient comfort with pillows and the liberal use of tape to secure body parts in a desired position.

When injecting a radiopharmaceutical, several precautions should be followed. A good IV access site should be secured. Injection into an existing IV is to be discouraged, although residual activity in the tubing does not occur frequently from the injection of many radiopharmaceuticals.[113] When a tourniquet is needed, avoid using a blood pressure cuff and wait at least 5 minutes after its removal before injecting the tracer.[37,82] Do not withdraw blood into the syringe since aggregates can form that will produce focal areas of increased activity in the lungs.[121]

Finally, a number of new computer software packages have been developed to compensate for some of the problems that occur in SPECT imaging including patient motion,[42] attenuation,[7] and bladder filling (the last causes a tracer distribution artifact on pelvis examinations).[15,61,78,95]

CONCLUSION

Numerous bone scan deceptions and artifacts have been described. Many more new abnormalities will appear in the future as instrumentation and imaging protocols become more sophisticated. Diligence is required to recognize and correct deceptions due to the equipment, the patient, and the performance of the study.

REFERENCES

1. Adams KJ, Shuler SE, Witherspoon LR, Neely HR: A retrospective analysis of renal abnormalities detected on bone scans. *Clin Nucl Med* 1980; 5:1.
2. Aldridge RE: Case of the quarter. *J Nucl Med Technol* 1976; 4:89.
3. Andrews GA, Theocheung JL, Andrews E, Tyler KR: Unintentional intra-arterial injection of a bone imaging agent. *Clin Nucl Med* 1980; 5:499.
4. Ajmani SK, Lerner SR, Pircher FJ: Bone scan artifact caused by hyperhidrosis: Case report. *J Nucl Med* 1977; 18:801.
5. Amico S, Lucas P, Liehn JC, Valeyre J: Unusual site of extraosseous uptake of Tc-99m HMDP due to subcutaneous heparin injections. *Eur J Nucl Med* 1989; 15:670.
6. Alazraki N, Scott S, Manaster BJ, et al: Effect of glucocorticoids on sensitivity of Tc-99m phosphate bone imaging for detection of trauma (abstract). *J Nucl Med* 1987; 28:606.
7. Bailey DL, Hutton BF, Walker PJ: Improved SPECT using simultaneous emission and transmission tomography. *J Nucl Med* 1987; 28:844.
8. Balsam D, Goldfarb CR, Stringer B, Farruggia S: Bone scintigraphy for neonatal osteomyelitis: Simulation by extravasation of intravenous calcium. *Radiology* 1980; 135:185.
9. Barakos JA, Colletti PM, Siegel ME, et al: Koch continent ileal urinary reservoir: Anatomy and potential pitfalls of radionuclide imaging. *Clin Nucl Med* 1987; 12:744.
10. Bice AN, Clausen M, Loncaric S, Wagner HN: Comparison of transaxial resolution in 180 degrees and 360 degrees SPECT with a rotating scintillation camera. *Eur J Nucl Med* 1987; 13:7.
11. Bieszk JA, Hawman EG: Evaluation of SPECT angular sampling effects: Continuous versus step and shoot acquisition. *J Nucl Med* 1987; 28:1308.
12. Billinghurst MW, Rempel S, Westendorf BA: Radiation decomposition of technetium-99m radiopharmaceuticals. *J Nucl Med* 1979; 20:138.
13. Black RR, Fernandez-Ulloa M: Anatomic and position-induced increased radiopharmaceutical uptake in the cervical spine on bone imaging. *Clin Nucl Med* 1988; 13:483.
14. Blei L, Cano RA, Jones AE, Johnston GS: The sacral tubercle—a cause for hot spots on bone scan. *Clin Nucl Med* 1978; 3:351.
15. Bok BD, Bice AN, Clausen M, et al: Artifacts in camera based single photon emission tomography due to time activity variation. *Eur J Nucl Med* 1987; 13:439.
16. Boxen I: Inadvertant lymphoscintigraphy? *Clin Nucl Med* 1985; 10:25.
17. Brill DR: Radionuclide imaging of non-neoplastic soft-tissue disorders. *Semin Nucl Med* 1981; 11:277.
18. Buchner BR, Joo KG, Baeumler GR: The case of the disappearing bladder. *Clin Nucl Med* 1984; 9:598.
19. Bunker SR, Handmaker H, Torre DM, Schmidt WP: Pixel overflow artifacts in SPECT evaluation of the skeleton. *Radiology* 1990; 174:229.
20. Byum HH, Rodman SG, Chung KE: Soft tissue concentration of Tc-99m phosphates associated with injections of iron dextran complex. *J Nucl Med* 1976; 17:374.
21. Castronova FP, McKusick KA, Strauss HW: The infiltrated radiopharmaceutical injection: Dosimetric considerations. *Eur J Nucl Med* 1988; 14:93.

22. Cerqueira MD, Matsuoka D, Ritchie JL, Harp GD: Influence of collimators on SPECT center of rotation measurements: Artifact generation and acceptance testing. *J Nucl Med* 1988; 29:1393.

23. Chatterton BE, Vannitamby M, Cook DJ: Lymph node visualization: An unusual artifact in the Tc-99m pyrophospate bone scan. *Eur J Nucl Med* 1980; 5:187.

24. Chaudhuri TK: The effect of aluminum and pH on altered body distribution of Tc-99m EHDP. *Int J Nucl Med Biol* 1976; 3:37.

25. Chaudhuri TK: Liver uptake of Tc-99m diphosphonate. *Radiology* 1976; 119:485.

26. Choy D, Murray IPC, Hoschl R: The effect of iron on the biodistribution of bone scanning agents in humans. *Radiology* 1981; 140:197.

27. Coates GG, Gass MA, Sicuro PL, Eisenberg B: The "breast pocket" sign: A clue to the possibility of spurious radionuclide uptake: A case report. *J Nucl Med Technol* 1994; 22:211.

28. Conway JJ, Weiss SC, Khentigan A, et al: Gallbladder and bowel localization of bone imaging radiopharmaceuticals (abstract). *J Nucl Med* 1979; 20:622.

29. Cowley KA, Dvorak AD, Wilmot MD: Normal anatomic variant: Scintigraphy of the ischiopubic synchondrosis. *J Nucl Med* 1983; 24:14.

30. Cradduck TD, Teresinska A: Head tilt and its effect on resolution orthogonal to transverse slices in SPECT (abstract). *J Nucl Med* 1986; 27:960.

31. Crawford JA, Gumerman LW: Alteration of body distribution of Tc-99m pyrophosphate by radiographic contrast material. *Clin Nucl Med* 1978; 3:305.

32. Creutzig H, Dach W: The "sickle sign" in bone scintigraphy. *Eur J Nucl Med* 1981; 6:99.

33. Croft B, Teates CD: "Lunch syndrome" a bone scanning artifact: Case report. *Clin Nucl Med* 1978; 3:137.

34. Cunningham DA: Abnormal bone marrow distribution following unsuccessful hip replacement: A potential confusion on white cell scanning. *Eur J Nucl Med* 1991; 18:67.

35. d'Avignon MB, Baum S: Increased jaw radioactivity on bone imaging. *Semin Nucl Med* 1982; 12:219.

36. DeMeo JH, Baliseiro J, Cole TJ: Etidronate sodium therapy—a cause of poor skeletal radiopharmaceutical uptake. *Semin Nucl Med* 1991; 21:332.

37. Desai A, Intenzo C: The tourniquet effect. *J Nucl Med* 1984; 25:697.

38. Dhawan V, Yeh SDJ: Labelling efficiency and stomach concentration in methylene diphosphonate bone imaging. *J Nucl Med* 1979; 20:791.

39. Dogan AS, Rezai K: Incidental lymph node visualization on bone scan due to subcutaneous infiltration of Tc-99m MDP: A potential false-positive. *Clin Nucl Med* 1993; 18:208.

40. DuCret RP, Boudreau RJ, Maguire FP, Althaus SJ: Sigmoid augmentation artifact in skeletal imaging. *Clin Nucl Med* 1988; 13:375.

41. Duong RB, Volarich DT, Fernandez-Ulloa M, Vasavada PJ: Tc-99m MDP bone scan artifact: Abdominal soft tissue uptake secondary to subcutaneous heparin injection. *Clin Nucl Med* 1984; 9:47.

42. Eisner RL, Noever T, Nowak D, et al: Use of cross correlation function to detect patient motion during SPECT imaging. *J Nucl Med* 1987; 28:97.

43. Eshima M, Shiozaki H, Ishino Y, Nakata H: Diffuse liver uptake of Tc-99m phosphate compound associated with intravenous injection of iron colloid solution. *Clin Nucl Med* 1993; 18:348.

44. Farrell TJ, Cradduck TD, Chamberlain RA: The effect of collimation on the center of rotation in SPECT (letter). *J Nucl Med* 1984; 25:632.

45. Fernandez-Ulloa M, Hughes JA, Krugh KB, Chin D: Bone imaging in infections: Artifacts from spectral overlap between a Tc-99m tracer and In-111 leukocytes. *J Nucl Med* 1983; 24:589.

46. Fink-Bennett D, Johnson J: Stippled ribs: A potential pitfall in bone scan interpretation. *J Nucl Med* 1986; 27:216.

47. Fink-Bennett D, Vicuna-Rios J: The deltoid tuberosity—a potential pitfall (the delta sign) in bone scan interpretation: Concise communication. *J Nucl Med* 1980; 21:211.

48. Fogelman I, Collier BD: *An Atlas of Planar and SPECT Bone Scans*, Martin Dunitz, London, 1989.

49. Fogelman I, Maisey M: *An Atlas of Clinical Nuclear Medicine*, Martin Dunitz, London, 1988.

50. Forauer AR, Grossman SJ, Joyce JM: Altered biodistribution of Tc-99m HMDP on bone scintigraphy from recent intravenous iron therapy. *Clin Nucl Med* 1994; 19:817.

51. Freitas JE, Dworkin HJ, Dees SM, Ponto R: Phantom feet on digital radionuclide images and other scary computer takes. *J Nucl Med* 1989; 30:1559.

52. Front D, Hardoff R, Mashour N: Stomach artifact in bone scintigraphy (letter). *J Nucl Med* 1978; 19:974.

53. Garty A, Siplovich L, Moguilner J: Pitfalls in the diagnosis of neuroblastoma by Tc-99m MDP scintigraphy: A case report. *Eur J Nucl Med* 1984; 9:564.

54. Garty I, Tanyman M, Reiner S: Accumulation of technetium-99m-MDP in distended ureter: A potential error in diagnosing osteoblastic bone activity. *Clin Nucl Med* 1985; 10:667.

55. Gelman R, Alexander MS, Sorandes TP: Extraosseous metastasis masquerading as urine contamination on bone scans. *J Nucl Med Technol* 1991; 19:87.

56. Gentili A, Miron SD, Adler LP: Review of some common artifacts in nuclear medicine. *Clin Nucl Med* 1994; 19:138.

57. Gentili A, Miron SD, Adler LP, Bellon EM: Artifacts in nuclear medicine (abstract). *J Nucl Med* 1992; 33:1068.

58. Gentili A, Miron SD, Adler LP: Incidental detection of urinary tract abnormalities with skeletal scintigraphy. *Radiographics* 1991; 11:571.

59. Gentilli A, Miron SD, Bellon EM: Nonosseous accumulation of bone seeking radiopharmaceuticals. *Radiographics* 1990; 10:871.

60. Gillen GJ, Gilmore B, Elliot AT: An investigation of the magnitude and causes of count loss artifacts in SPECT imaging. *J Nucl Med* 1991; 32:1771.

61. Gillen GJ, McKillop JH, Hilditch TE, et al: Digital filtering of the bladder in SPECT bone studies of the pelvis. *J Nucl Med* 1988; 29:1587.

62. Glassman AB, Selby JB: Another bone imaging agent false-positive: Phimosis. *Clin Nucl Med* 1980; 5:34.

63. Gupta SM, Panduranga A, Buckley M, et al: Significance of photon deficient areas in radionuclide bone scans. *J Nucl Med Technol* 1980; 8:208.

64. Harkness BA, Rogers WL, Clinthorne NH, Keyes JW: SPECT: Quality control procedures and artifact identification. *J Nucl Med Technol* 1983; 11:55.

65. Hesslewood S, Emmeline L: Drug interactions with radiopharmaceuticals. *Eur J Nucl Med* 1994; 21:348.

66. Higgens WL: Symmetric photon deficiency in the femoral heads on bone imaging: A normal variant (letter). *J Nucl Med* 1988; 29:266.

67. Hladik WB, Nigg KK, Rhodes BA: Drug induced changes in the biological distribution of radiopharmaceuticals. *Semin Nucl Med* 1982; 12:184.

68. Hladik WB, Saha GB, Study KT: *Essentials of Nuclear Science*. Williams and Wilkins, Baltimore, 1987.

69. Hommeyer SH, Varney DM, Eary JF: Skeletal nonvisualization in a bone scan secondary to intravenous etidronate therapy. *J Nucl Med* 1992; 33:748.

70. Hoop B: The infiltrated radiopharmaceutical injection: Risk consideration. *J Nucl Med* 1991; 32:890.

71. Hunter JV, Fogelman I: "Delta sign" in bone scan interpretation—a cautionary note. *J Nucl Med* 1987; 28:1229.

72. Jaresko GS, Zimmer AM, Pavel DG, Spies SM: The effect of circulating aluminum on the biodistribution of Tc-99m-Sn-diphosphonate in rats. *J Nucl Med Technol* 1980; 8:160.

73. Jayabalan V, Berry S: Accumulation of Tc-99m-pyrophosphate in breast prosthesis. *Clin Nucl Med* 1977; 2:452.

74. Karelitz JR, Richards JB: Pseudophotopenic defect due to barium in the colon. *Clin Nucl Med* 1978; 3:414.

75. Karimeddini MK, Spencer RP: Bone agent and radiogallium deposition around infiltrated calcium gluconate. *Clin Nucl Med* 1993; 18:797.

76. Karimeddini MK, Spencer RP: Forced diuresis: A cause of "absent" renal uptake of bone imaging agent. *Clin Nucl Med* 1987; 12:407.

77. Koizumi K, Tonami N, Hisada K: Diffusely increased Tc-99m MDP uptake in both kidneys. *Clin Nucl Med* 1981; 6:362.

78. Kouris K, Al-Ghussain NM, Higazi E, et al: Correction and evaluation of the bladder artifact in hip SPECT. *Eur J Nucl Med* 1989; 15:492 (abstract).

79. Kowalsky RJ, Dalton DR: Technical problems associated with the production of Tc-99m tin (II) pyrophosphate kits. *Am J Hosp Pharm* 1981; 38:1722.

80. Krasnow AZ, Collier BD, Isitman AT, et al: False negative bone imaging due to etidronate disodium therapy. *Clin Nucl Med* 1988; 13:264.

81. Landgarten S: Uptake of Tc-99m pyrophosphate by the lactating breast (letter). *J Nucl Med* 1977; 18:943.

82. Lecklitner ML, Douglas KP: Increased extremity uptake on three phase bone scans caused by peripherally induced ischemia prior to injection. *J Nucl Med* 1987; 28:108.

83. Lieberman C, Hemingway DL: Photopenic defect due to penis prosthesis. *Clin Nucl Med* 1979; 4:481.

84. Lutrin CL, McDougall IR, Goris ML: Intense concentration of Tc-99m pyrophosphate in the kidneys of children treated with chemotherapeutic drugs for malignancy. *Radiology* 1978; 128:165.

85. Mandell GA, Harcke T, Sharkey C, Brooks K: Uterine blush in multiphase bone imaging. *J Nucl Med* 1986; 27:51.

86. Mandell GA, Harke HT, Bower JR, Sharkey CA: Transient photopenia of the femoral head following arthrography. *Clin Nucl Med* 1989; 14:397.

87. Mandell GA, Heyman S: Dorsal defect of the patella on radionuclide bone scan. *Clin Nucl Med* 1983; 8:380.

88. Mariani G, Levorato D, Tuoni M, Giannotti P: Incidental imaging of the large bowel in patients with uretero-sigmoidostomy during bone scintigraphy with Tc-99m. *J Nucl Med Allied Sci* 1978; 22:153.

89. Massie JD, Mullens R: Tc-99m MDP uptake in lower extremity: An interesting artifact. *Clin Nucl Med* 1983; 8:447.

90. Mazzola AL, Barker MH, Belliveau RE: Accumulation of Tc-99m diphosphonate at sites of intramuscular iron therapy: case report. *J Nucl Med Technol* 1976; 4:133.

91. McAfee JG, Singh A, Roskopf M, et al: Experimental drug-induced changes in renal function and biodistribution of Tc-99m MDP. *Investigative Radiology* 1983; 18:470.

92. Murray IPC, Bass S: A false-positive artifact in the investigation of osteitis pubis. *Clin Nucl Med* 1991; 16:597.

93. Murray IPC, Frater CJ: Prominence of the C2 vertebrae on SPECT: A normal variant. *Clin Nucl Med* 1994; 19:855.

94. O'Connell MEA, Sutton H: Excretion of radioactivity in breast milk following Tc-99m-Sn polyphosphate. *Br J Radiol* 1976; 49:377.

95. O'Connor MK, Kelly BJ: Evaluation of techniques for the elimination of "hot" bladder artifacts in SPECT of the pelvis. *J Nucl Med* 1990; 31:1872.

96. Otsuka N, Ito Y, Nagai K, et al: Effects of prostaglandin on experimental bone malignancy and on scintigrams of bone and marrow. *J Nucl Med* 1981; 22:433.

97. Park HM, Hunt-Reimann A, Appledorn CR, Siddiqui A: A comet-tail imaging artifact due to a "hot" point source and faulty electronics. *Clin Nucl Med* 1993; 18:341.

98. Parker JA, Jones AG, Davis MA, et al: Reduced uptake of bone seeking radiopharmaceuticals related to iron excess. *Clin Nucl Med* 1976; 1:267.

99. Peller PJ, Ho VB, Kransdorf MJ: Extraosseous Tc-99m MDP uptake: A pathophysiological approach. *Radiographics* 1993; 13:715.

100. Penney HF, Styles CB: Fortuitous lymph node visualization after interstitial injection of Tc-99m MDP. *Clin Nucl Med* 1982; 7:84.

101. Planchon CA, Donadieu AM, Perez R, Cousins JL: Calcium heparinate induced extraosseous uptake in bone scanning. *Eur J Nucl Med* 1983; 8:113.

102. Popilock RM, Kim SM, Park CH: False-positive bone scan due to skin fold artifact: Case report. *J Nucl Med Technol* 1987; 15:11.

103. Postelnek DL, Chandeysson PL: Internal mammary artery artifact on bone scan of post-CABG patient. *Clin Nucl Med* 1993; 18:1092.

104. Potsaid MS, Guiberteau MJ, McKusick KA: Quality of bone scans compared with time between dose and scan. *J Nucl Med* 1977; 18:787.

105. Poulose KP, Reba RC, Eckelman WC, Goodyear M: Extraosseous localization of Tc-99m-Sn pyrophosphate. *Br J Radiology* 1975; 48:724.

106. Prakash V: Image of Harrington rods on a Tc-99m pyrophosphate scan. *Clin Nucl Med* 1979; 4:384.

107. Ramsingh P, Pujara S, Logic JR: Tc-99m pyrophosphate uptake in drug induced gynecomastia. *Clin Nucl Med* 1977; 2:206.

108. Rao BK, Lieberman LM: Parietal thinning: A cause of photopenia on bone scan. *Clin Nucl Med* 1980; 5:313.

109. Ryo UY, Alavi A, Collier BD, et al: *Atlas of Nuclear Medicine Artifacts and Variants*, Yearbook Medical Publishers, Chicago, 1990.

110. Sandler ED, Parisi MT, Hattner RS: Duration of etidronate effect demonstrated by serial bone scintigraphy. *J Nucl Med* 1991; 32:1782.

111. Schmitt GH, Holmes RA, Isitman AT, et al: A proposed mechanism for Tc-99m labelled polyphosphate and diphosphonate uptake by human breast tissue. *Radiology* 1974; 112:733.

112. Segall GM, Gurevich N: Uterine blush in multiphase imaging (letter). *J Nucl Med* 1986; 27:1500.

113. Segall GW, Gurevich N, McDougall IR: Adherence of radio-pharmaceuticals and labelled cells to intravenous tubing. *Clin Nucl Med* 1986; 11:830.

114. Shapiro B, Pillay M, Cox PH: Dosimetric consequences of interstitial extravasation following IV administration of a radiopharmaceutical. *Eur J Nucl Med* 1987; 12:522.

115. Sherkow L, Ryo UY, Fabich D, et al: Visualization of the liver, gallbladder and intestine on bone scintigraphy. *Clin Nucl Med* 1984; 9:440.

116. Shih W, Deland F, Domstad PA, Dillon ML: Unusual persistence of Tc-99m MDP uptake in the incisional scar after thoracotomy. *Clin Nucl Med* 1984; 9:596.

117. Silberstein EB, Volarich DO: Bladder diverticula masquerading as pubic metastasis. *Clin Nucl Med* 1982; 7:229.

118. Sorkin SJ, Horii SC, Passalagua A, Braunstein P: Augmented activity on bone scan following local chemoperfusion. *Clin Nucl Med* 1977; 2:451.

119. Spencer RP, Karimeddini MK: Photon scatter from asymmetric bladder activity. *Clin Nucl Med* 1986; 11:222.

120. Spencer RP, Lee YS, Sziklas JJ, et al: Failure of uptake of radiocolloid by the femoral heads—a diagnostic problem: Concise communication. *J Nucl Med* 1983; 24:116.

121. Tatum JL, Burke TS, Hirsch JI, Fratkin MJ: Artifactual focal accumulation of Tc-99m bone imaging tracer in the chest: Technicial note (bone imaging artifact). *Clin Nucl Med* 1985; 10:16.

122. Thrall JH, Ghaed N, Geslien GE, et al: Pitfalls in Tc-99m polyphosphate skeletal imaging. *Am J Roentgenol* 1974; 121:739.

123. Tondeur M, Ham H: 360 degrees or 180 degrees for bone SPECT of the spine. *Nucl Med Commun* 1994; 15:279.

124. Turton DB, Silverman ED: Tampon artifact in bone scintigraphy. *Clin Nucl Med* 1994; 19:1103.

125. Valdez VA, Jacobstein JG: Decreased bone uptake of Tc-99m polyphosphate in thalasemia major. *J Nucl Med* 1980; 21:47.

126. Van Antwerp JD, Hall JN, O'Mara RE: Soft tissue concentration of Tc-99m phosphates associated with injections of iron dextran complex (letter). *J Nucl Med* 1977; 18:855.

127. Van Antwerp JD, Hall JN, O'Mara RE, Hills SV: Bone scan abnormality produced by interaction of Tc-99m diphosphonate with iron dextran. *J Nucl Med* 1975; 16:577 (abstract).

128. Veluvolu P, Collier BD, Isitman AT, et al: False-positive planar bone images due to horseshoe kidney: Evaluation with blood pool image and SPECT. *Clin Nucl Med* 1985; 10:292.

129. Vieras F: Serendipitus lymph node visualization during bone imaging. *Clin Nucl Med* 1986; 11:434.

130. Wa HI, Hill P: Effects of acute administration of ethane hydroxydiphosphonate (EHDP) on skeletal scintigraphy with technetium-99m methylene. *Br J Radiology* 1981; 54:592.

131. Wallis JW, Fisher S, Wahl RL: Tc-99m MDP uptake by lymph nodes following tracer infiltration: Clinical and laboratory evaluation. *Nucl Med Commun* 1987; 8:357.

132. Weiss S, Conway JJ: Bone imaging artifacts. *J Nucl Med Technol* 1977; 5:17.

133. Wells LD, Bernier DR: *Radionuclide Imaging Artifacts*, Yearbook Medical Publishers, Chicago, 1980.

134. Williams JG: Pertechnetate and the stomach—a continuing controversy. *J Nucl Med* 1983; 24:633.

135. Williamson BRJ, Teates CD, Bray ST, et al: Renal excretion simulating bone disease on bone scans—a technique for solving this problem. *Clin Nucl Med* 1979; 4:200.

136. Wilson MA: The effect of age on the quality of bone scans using Tc-99m pyrophosphate. *Am J Roentgenol* 1981; 139:703.

137. Wilson MA, Pollack MJ: Gastric visualization and image quality in radionuclide bone scanning: Concise communication. *J Nucl Med* 1981; 22:518.

138. Yano Y, McRae J, VanDyke CD, Anger HO: Technetium-99m-labeled stannous ethane-1-hydroxy-1-disphosphonate: A new bone scanning agent. *J Nucl Med* 1973; 14:73.

139. Yeo EE, Low J: Intra-abdominal retained surgical sponges presenting as a photopenic mass on scintigraphy. *Clin Nucl Med* 1991; 16:543.

140. Yoshizumi TT, Suneja SK, Teal JS, et al: Defective parallel-hole collimator encountered in SPECT: A suggested approach to avoid potential problems (letter). *J Nucl Med* 1990; 31:1892.

141. Zimmer AM, Pavel DG: Experimental investigations of the possible cause of liver appearance during bone scanning. *Radiology* 1978; 126:813.

CHAPTER 19

PET BONE IMAGING

Randall A. Hawkins

Carl K. Hoh

Evaluation of the skeletal system with scintigraphy comprises a major part of the practice of nuclear medicine. As discussed in other chapters in this book, gamma camera bone-scanning methods continue to play a very significant role in managing diseases of the skeletal system. In addition to gamma camera bone-scanning methods, imaging the skeletal system with positron emission tomography (PET) is another approach to bone metabolic evaluations. Although PET studies of the musculoskeletal system have been relatively limited, initial studies indicate that the quantitative precision and image resolution of PET make it an attractive modality both for selected clinical and investigative applications in bone.

The positron-emitting radiopharmaceuticals [F-18]fluoride ion—a tracer of bone metabolic activity as mapped by [F-18]fluoride ion uptake in the hydroxyapatite crystal—and the glucose analog 2-[F-18]fluoro-2-deoxy-D-glu-

cose (FDG) have both been employed for evaluation of the skeletal system.[11,22,24,25] In fact, [F-18]fluoride ion was at one time the standard bone scanning agent,* but it was replaced for routine clinical use in the 1970s by Tc-99m labeled bone-seeking radiopharmaceuticals, because of the more optimal physical characteristics of Tc-99m for gamma camera systems.

Gamma camera bone-scanning methods will remain the standard nuclear medicine approach for skeletal evaluations for the foreseeable future because of their widespread availability and cost effectiveness. PET skeletal imaging, because of its better quantitative precision and, for most systems, better resolution,[41] is promising both as an investigative tool for better characterizing bone metabolism and as a potentially useful clinical problem-solving tool when standard bone scanning, coupled with plain radiographs, does not fully answer the clinical question. PET becomes a potentially cost-effective alternative to other tomographic imaging methods such as computed tomography (CT) and magnetic resonance imaging (MRI) in situations where it produces biologic information not attainable with other methods.

NOTE: This chapter is modified and extracted with permission from Hawkins RA, Hoh CK, Phelps ME: PET imaging of the skeletal system, in Sandler MP, Coleman RE, Wackers FJ TH., Patton JA, Gottschalk A, Hoffer PB (eds): *Diagnostic Nuclear Medicine*, ed 3, Williams and Wilkins, Baltimore, 1996.

*References 2, 12, 19, 32, 42, 48.

POSITRON EMISSION TOMOGRAPHY RADIOPHARMACEUTICALS AND METHODS

Blau et al[2] were the first to perform bone imaging with [F-18]fluoride ion. Following that initial work, [F-18]fluoride ion became the standard nuclear medicine bone-scanning agent.[12,19,32,42,48]

There is a large body of literature on the metabolism and pharmakokinetics of fluoride because of its role in the prevention of dental caries and also because of its potential as a therapeutic agent for osteoporosis.[33] In vitro studies have demonstrated that fluoride ion exchanges with the hydroxyl ion in the bone mineral hydroxyapatite crystal $[Ca_{10}(PO_4)_6(OH)_2]$ to form fluoroapatite: $Ca_{10}(PO_4)_6(F)_2$.[18] Although pharmacologic doses of fluoride affect bone cells and bone crystals,[33] the goal of PET bone imaging with [F-18]fluoride ion is to map the relative distribution and magnitude of bone uptake of tracer doses of this agent.

The first-pass extraction fraction of [F-18]fluoride ion through bone is high.[45,49] Based on an assumption of a 100% initial extraction of [F-18]fluoride through bone, Reeve et al[38] developed a method to estimate skeletal blood flow in humans based on measuring the rate of plasma clearance following intravenous injection of the agent [F-18]fluoride ion (i.e., without imaging).[50] Wooton et al[50] found a positive correlation between decreases in skeletal blood flow and decreases in the level of alkaline phosphatase in patients with Paget's disease treated with calcitonin with Reeve's method.

Charkes et al[3,4,5] were the first to develop an in vivo pharmakokinetic model of [F-18]fluoride ion distribution using compartmental modeling techniques and animal tissue sampling data. Although many excellent studies dealing with in vivo pharmakokinetics have been performed with plasma and tissue sampling methods alone,[29] PET and other imaging techniques produce direct tissue (image) measurements as a function of time. Coupled with plasma measurements of radionuclide concentrations as a function of time, tracer kinetic models, applied with PET imaging data, produce numeric estimates of a variety of physiologic and biochemical processes.[41]

The glucose analog 2-[F-18]fluoro-2-deoxy-D-glucose (FDG) is also a useful radiopharmaceutical for PET bone imaging. FDG, like glucose, is transported across capillary membranes via a carrier-mediated transport process, in the direction of a concentration gradient (facilitated diffusion). Both FDG and glucose are then phosphorylated by hexokinase, but because the phosphorylation product FDG-6-PO_4 cannot be metabolized further through the glycolytic cycle,[14] it accumulates in cells, unlike glucose-6-PO_4, which undergoes further metabolism through the Krebs cycle. Sokoloff et al[40] developed a mathematical model relating the net transport of C-14 deoxyglucose (DG) and accumulation of DG-6-PO_4 in tissue to glucose transport and metabolism based on Michaelis Menten kinetics. The original Sokoloff DG method, developed in rats for autoradiography, was extended to humans using PET and FDG by Reivich, Phelps, and colleagues.[26,36,39] Details of the FDG model, including assumptions and limitations of the method, are included in the literature.[21,23,26,36,39]

Although the mechanism of [F-18]fluoride ion uptake in bone, previously described, is different than the biochemical mechanisms underlying FDG transport and phosphorylation, both processes have in common a tissue phase distributed between two kinetically discrete compartments. For FDG these compartments are (1) free FDG and (2) "metabolically trapped" FDG-6-PO_4. For [F-18]fluoride ion these compartments are (1) "unbound" and (2) hydroxyapatite crystal–related "bound" [F-18]fluoride ion. Based on this similarity in tissue distribution kinetics, Hawkins et al[20] employed the well-known three-compartment model used in the FDG model to evaluate the kinetics of [F-18]fluoride ion uptake in bone with PET. PET kinetic studies with [F-18]fluoride ion produce numeric estimates for the forward (k) and reverse (k_2) rate constants for [F-18]fluoride ion transport into and out of bone, as well as for the forward rate constant k_3 for binding of [F-18]fluoride ion into the bound compartment in bone.

METHODS FOR POSITRON EMISSION TOMOGRAPHY BONE IMAGING

With both [F-18]fluoride ion and FDG, there are several potential approaches for acquiring PET bone images, including the following:

1. Standard transaxial attenuation corrected images at a preselected time after injection of [F-18]fluoride ion or FDG
2. Serial transaxial attenuation corrected images beginning simultaneously with injection of [F-18]fluoride ion or FDG (kinetic studies)
3. Whole-body images

Most PET systems contain rings of detectors, analogous to CT scanners in design.[41] The axial field of view of such devices is defined by the number of detector rings, and by the axial field of view of each ring, as well as by the acquisition and image reconstruction strategy employed. Some PET systems use two-dimensional detector systems similar to gamma camera designs.

PET emission data may be corrected for tissue attenuation with a transmission scan method using a Ga-68/Ge-68 transmission source. Because a strength of PET, as opposed to single photon emission computed tomography (SPECT), is the more accurate retrieval of voxel count density based on more accurate attenuation correction methods,[7] both approaches 1 and 2 are preferred if a truly quantitative, kinetic, study is desired.

A relative limitation of approaches 1 and 2, however, is the limited axial field of view of the scanner. The situation is very much analogous to SPECT. Although SPECT bone imaging is a very useful method for generating more anatomically precise cross-sectional bone scan images than planar gamma camera methods, SPECT is not convenient for total skeletal surveys, because the acquisition time for serial SPECT image sets that would include the whole body would be inconveniently long. Because obvious potential applications of [F-18]fluoride ion and FDG PET bone imaging include whole-body surveys for malignancies, Dahlbom et al[7] developed a whole-body PET imaging method that produces a tomographic and nontomographic (projection) image set of the whole body. The method is based on sequential acquisitions of standard transaxial PET image data sets at discrete locations in the body, followed by acquisitions at other body locations until the entire body (or more limited regions of interest) have been included in the data set. Standard transaxial images are reconstructed with filtered backprojection methods, and coronal and sagittal tomographic images are extracted from the stack of transaxial images via a sorting operation. Additionally, two-dimensional "projection" images, analogous to two-dimensional raw data sets with SPECT, are generated by appropriate sampling and sorting of the raw sinographic data. The end result is a whole-body image set consisting of transaxial, coronal, and sagittal tomographic images, together with two-dimensional projection images at various angles around the body.

There are two fundamental limitations to the whole-body PET method as it is usually currently employed. (1) The individual transaxial data sets are usually acquired for relatively short intervals (e.g., approximately 2 to 4 minutes) to permit acquisition of the whole-body data set in a reasonable time period (e.g., about 60 minutes). This results in transaxial image quality inferior to what would be generated with longer acquisitions (e.g., 10 to 30 minutes) over given body locations. (2) Whole-body PET images are usually acquired without attenuation correction, because standard transaxial transmission scanning at each bed position to generate an attenuation correction matrix would prohibitively lengthen the total time of the study. For this reason, whole-body skeletal PET images are primarily useful as qualitative maps of the whole-body distribution of [F-18]fluoride ion, FDG, or other compounds. However, in appropriate clinical contexts, such qualitative whole-body image sets can be very useful in mapping disease extent.

Refinements of the whole-body PET method that should increase both its quantitative precisions and clinical utility include development of practical attenuation correction approaches,[30] and application of alternative reconstruction methods such as the three-dimensional (3D) method.[6] The 3D reconstruction method makes it possible to use a much higher fraction of coincident events in the image reconstruction process, essentially by including coincident events between detector planes, as well as within individual or directly adjacent detector planes. This has the effect of significantly increasing the count rate efficiency of the PET system, with a potential result of decrease in acquisition time by up to a factor of 4 or more. Initial studies with simultaneous emission/transmission imaging indicate that it is feasible to devel-

op attenuation corrected whole-body PET image sets with quantitative precision rivaling standard sequential emission/transmission imaging methods.[30]

CLINICAL EXAMPLES OF POSITRON EMISSION TOMOGRAPHY BONE IMAGING

Normal Patterns

Figure 19-1 includes examples of [F-18]fluoride ion images acquired with the whole-body PET method. Selected two-dimensional projection as well as transaxial, coronal, and sagittal images are included. Note that the relative body distribution of [F-18]fluoride ion is very similar to the distribution of Tc-99m MDP (methylene diphosphonate) compounds, as expected, based on the biodistribution and metabolism of [F-18]fluoride ion.

Although the impact of the lack of attenuation correction on whole-body [F-18]fluoride ion images is evident from Fig. 19-1, it tends to be less apparent on selected tomographic images compared with FDG whole-body images for two reasons: (1) the bone/tissue contrast of [F-18]fluoride ion is high, and the relative uptake of [F-18]fluoride ion in bone, adjusted for bone size and partial volume effects, is relatively uniform, and (2) many bony structures are relatively near the body surface.

Additionally, because a single whole-body PET study can produce a large number of tomographic and projection images, it is very helpful to view such images on a workstation equipped with appropriate volume viewing software. Such display options are available on a variety of nuclear medicine workstations and, with the standardization of image file formats into DICOM3 and other standard file formats, display and viewing of such data sets on workstations designed for general imaging environments as part of larger PACS (picture archiving communication systems) will become progressively easier and more routine.

Another advantage of workstation viewing strategies for whole-body PET [F-18]fluoride ion and FDG bone studies is the ease of appropriate contrast adjustment (windowing) of images. Although FDG uptake in normal bone is low, normal bone marrow uptake produces a visible signal on appropriately windowed FDG images. This will be most evident in hematopoietically active marrow spaces, such as the vertebral bodies and proximal femoral shafts (Fig. 19-2).

Pathologic Conditions

PET bone imaging with [F-18]fluoride ion produces the expected findings of increased tracer uptake in the range of pathologic conditions known to also cause increased uptake of Tc-99m MDP and related compounds: neoplastic, inflammatory, traumatic, and other processes known to result in an acceleration of osteoblastic activity and bone blood flow.

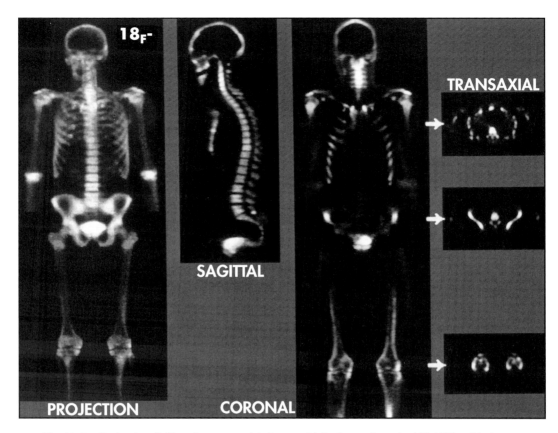

Fig. 19-1. Projection (*left*) and tomographic images (*right three columns*) of [F-18]fluoride ion distribution in a normal volunteer, illustrate the range of tomographic display options available with this technique. The right-hand column of images includes three transaxial images at the approximate levels of the midthoracic spine, pelvis, and knees, respectively. Single coronal (*second from right*) and sagittal (*second from left*) tomographic image sections are also included. Note the excellent delineation of the vertebral bodies and spinous processes, the tibial plateaus, and other bone structures. *(From Hawkins RA, Hoh C, Glaspy J, et al: The role of positron emission tomography in oncology and other whole-body applications. Semin Nucl Med 1992; 22:268; with permission.)*

In a series of 19 patients, with a range of malignant and benign skeletal conditions, Hoh et al[24] found that the tomographic (transaxial, coronal, and sagittal) [F-18]fluoride ion images had a 13% higher sensitivity for lesion detection than did the projection image set. Given that a fundamental advantage of any form of tomography is higher in-plane contrast,[41] this result is not surprising. Although projection images help the observer appreciate 3D relations, individual lesions may be visible only on the tomographic image set.

Because accelerated osteoblastic activity and bone blood flow are sensitive, but nonspecific, indicators of pathology, it is logical to expect that images of a different process, such as tissue glucose utilization mapped with FDG, should produce a different view of bone pathology. A feature shared by many aggressive neoplasms is an acceleration of their glycolytic rates.[47] Because bone (cortical and trabecular) has relatively low glucose utilization rates, compared with tissues such as the brain, heart, and striated muscle, whole-body PET FDG images in patients with skeletal primary or metastatic neoplasms frequently illustrate dramatic focal abnormalities that have very

high contrast compared with the background normal bone FDG uptake pattern. The [F-18]fluoride ion and FDG images in a patient with metastatic renal cell carcinoma (Fig. 19-2), illustrate this effect.

Review articles on whole-body PET imaging are available.[22,34,43] Several investigators have demonstrated that PET FDG imaging is useful for detecting and characterizing various types of primary and metastatic disease. A fundamental potential utility of the method is differentiating benign from malignant causes of increased uptake on "osteoblastic" bone scans, either PET [F-18]fluoride ion or gamma camera MDP studies. Although increased FDG uptake in bone is not pathognomic for cancer (inflammatory processes may also produce increased FDG uptake), and subcutaneous injections of FDG may result in significantly increased uptake in normal lymph nodes,[16,46] it is likely that the specificity of FDG will be higher than MDP or [F-18]fluoride ion for bone cancer detection. In a study of 25 patients with various types of musculoskeletal disorders, Adler et al[1] found that by quantifying FDG uptake in lesions, they could more accurately differentiate benign from malignant processes.

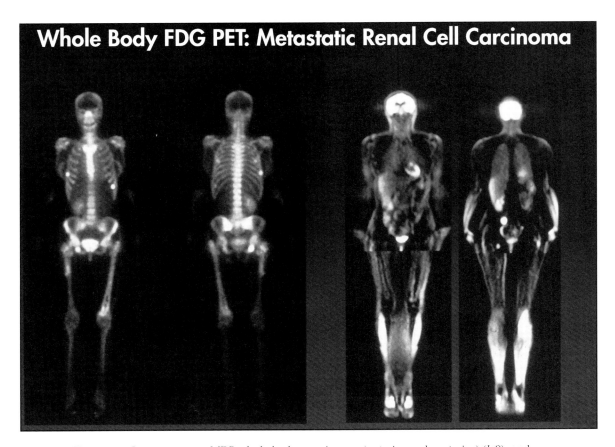

Whole Body FDG PET: Metastatic Renal Cell Carcinoma

Fig. 19-2. Gamma camera MDP whole-body scan images (anterior and posterior) (*left*), and two coronal whole-body PET FDG images (*right*) in a patient with metastatic renal cell carcinoma. The patient has previously undergone a right nephrectomy. On the PET FDG image on the right, note the increased uptake of FDG corresponding to increased uptake of MDP in the inferior pubic ramus on the right. The increased FDG uptake in bone, which normally has very low FDG uptake, is very consistent with metastatic disease. Rib lesions noted on MDP bone scan are not in the selected image planes on the PET FDG study. The patient had an intramedullary rod placed in the left femur. Note the displacement of the physiologic uptake of FDG in the hematopoietically active marrow space in the left femur compared with the normal FDG marrow pattern in the right femur. The cortical metastasis in the right proximal femur evident on the bone scan is anterior to the plane of the FDG images. There is physiologic uptake of FDG in the brain, heart, and soft tissues.

Kern et al,[28] in an earlier preliminary study, also found a good correspondence between FDG uptake and grade of malignancy in human musculoskeletal tumors.

This different mechanism of FDG and [F-18]fluoride ion uptake also can produce "uncoupling" of [F-18]fluoride ion and FDG uptake[1] in primary or metastatic bone tumors successfully responding to treatment, in which a persistent osteoblastic response, resulting in increased uptake on a PET [F-18]fluoride ion or gamma camera MDP bone scan, may indicate ongoing normal bone repair once the tumor, characterized by increased FDG uptake, has become suppressed. FDG imaging could be useful in differentiating the step-up in bone uptake of MDP or [F-18]fluoride ion that can occur during successful treatment, which should be associated with decreased FDG uptake, as opposed to tumor progression, which should be associated with increased FDG uptake.

QUANTITATIVE POSITRON EMISSION TOMOGRAPHY SKELETAL STUDIES

Quantitative applications of PET bone imaging to date have been relatively limited. The most likely potential application of quantitative PET FDG imaging in bone is disease characterization (e.g., differentiating benign from malignant conditions based on FDG uptake) and treatment monitoring, as discussed in previous reviews.[21,22] Additionally, quantitative PET FDG kinetic studies can be helpful in monitoring bone or marrow metabolic changes produced by pharmacologic agents, such as the effects of bone marrow stimulating growth factors (granulocyte-macrophage colony-stimulating factor [GM-CSF]) on hematopoietically active marrow uptake of FDG.[51] GM-CSF is one of a family of glycoprotein cytokines that stimulates bone marrow production of granu-

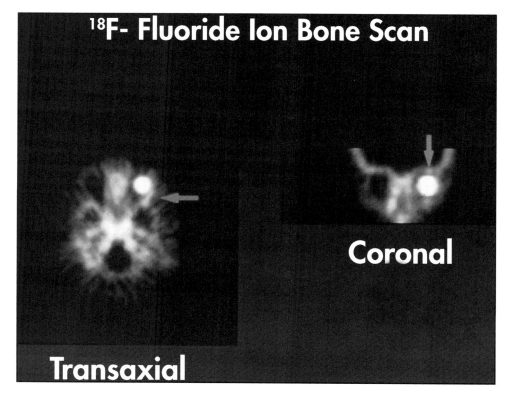

Fig. 19-3. [F-18]fluoride ion transaxial and coronal images through the skull in a patient with a left orbital hydroxyapatite, and a glass eye implant. There is uptake of [F-18]fluoride ion around the glass eye, and uptake of [F-18]fluoride ion in the implant equal to surrounding bony structures. Note the very good delineation of the orbital anatomy on the two image planes.

locytes and macrophages and is of significant therapeutic importance in some cancer patients with suppressed bone marrow.[8,15] Yao et al[51] found that bone marrow FDG uptake (glucose metabolic rate) increased by up to threefold during 3 to 10 days of GM-CSF therapy and progressively declined following therapy.

Quantitative PET studies with [F-18]fluoride ion are also potentially useful for evaluating bone metabolic disorders. Although single photon emitters such as Tc-99m MDP have been previously used to evaluate skeletal changes produced by hyperparathyroidism,[9,10,13,27] such methods have not been widely utilized. New-generation SPECT systems, equipped with transmission sources for attenuation correction, very well may result in renewed interest in the use of single photon bone-seeking tracers for quantitative bone metabolic studies.

Using a kinetic PET acquisition sequence with [F-18]fluoride ion, and the three-compartment kinetic model previously described, Messa et al[31] evaluated the utility of quantitative PET [F-18]fluoride ion kinetic studies in evaluation of patients with one form of metabolic bone disease: renal osteodystrophy. Using kinetically determined estimates of net [F-18]fluoride ion transport—K (in units of ml/min/ml of tissue), defined as $k_1 \cdot k_3/(k_2 + k_3)$—[20,31] they measured [F-18]fluoride ion uptake in normal volunteers, in eight patients with renal osteodystrophy, and compared the results to bone biopsy indicators of bone metabolic activity acquired from the renal osteodystrophy group.

Bone histomorphometry is a well-characterized tissue biopsy technique in which a variety of indices of bone mass, growth, and mineralization are measured quantitatively from biopsy samples. With oral tetracycline labeling, bone growth can be accurately measured with appropriate biopsy specimens.[17,35,37] Messa et al found a very good correlation between the PET index (K value) of bone metabolic activity obtained with dynamic [F-18]fluoride ion imaging and the histomorphometric index of bone formation rate. There was also a good correlation with K and serum alkaline phosphatase and parathyroid hormone levels (r > 0.8 in each case). Although this initial series needs validation in larger groups of patients, it illustrates the potential of quantitative PET bone imaging to better define metabolic characteristics of bone, some of which, such as bone formation rate, may otherwise be available only in direct tissue assay techniques.

CONCLUSIONS

Imaging the skeletal system with positron-emitting radiopharmaceuticals ([F-18]fluoride ion) was the first type of nuclear medicine bone scanning. The excellent resolution and quantitative precision of modern PET systems makes skeletal imaging with PET an attractive additional dimension to gamma camera skeletal scintigraphy in both clinical and investigative settings where the additional resolution and quantitative precision of PET produce information not available with standard nuclear medicine methods. Because modern gamma camera systems, including SPECT devices, produce very high quality bone images with Tc-99m methylene diphosphonate and related compounds, the most likely initial clinical application of PET bone imaging will be FDG studies to identify skeletal malignancies, and to differentiate benign from malignant causes of positive bone scans. PET bone studies with [F-18]fluoride ion produce numeric maps of fluoride ion transport to and binding in bone, in addition to very high quality bone scans (Fig. 19-3). The development of coincidence detection methods and specially designed collimators for gamma camera systems capable of imaging 511-keV annihilation photons produced by positron emitters is also making it possible to perform FDG skeletal studies with gamma camera systems. Although the sensitivity and resolution of gamma camera systems is much lower than PET systems for positron-emitting compounds, additional clinical studies should help define the relative roles and limitations of both SPECT and PET methods in this setting. Given the fundamental importance and utility of bone metabolism mapped by bone-seeking and other radiopharmaceuticals, qualitative and quantitative bone metabolic studies with radiopharmaceuticals promise to remain a very significant part of the practice of nuclear medicine.

REFERENCES

1. Adler LP, Blair HF, Makley JT: Noninvasive grading of musculoskeletal tumors using PET. *J Nucl Med* 1991; 32:1508.
2. Blau M, Nagler W, Bender MA: Fluorine-18: A new isotope for bone scanning. *J Nucl Med* 1962; 3:332.
3. Charkes ND, Brookes M, Makler PT. Studies of skeletal tracer kinetics. II. Evaluation of a five-compartment model of [18F]fluoride kinetics in rats. *J Nucl Med* 1979; 121:1150.
4. Charkes ND, Makler PT Jr, Phillips C: Studies of skeletal tracer kinetics. I. Digital computer solution of a five-compartment model of [18F]fluoride kinetics in humans. *J Nucl Med* 1978; 19:1301.
5. Charkes ND. Skeletal blood flow: Implications of bone-scan interpretation. *J Nucl Med* 1980; 21:91.
6. Cherry SR, Dahlbom M, Hoffman EJ: High sensitivity, total body PET scanning using 3-D data acquisition and reconstruction. *IEEE Trans Nucl Sci* 1992; 39:1088.
7. Dahlbom M, Hoffman EJ, Hoh CK, et al: Evaluation of a positron emission tomography scanner for whole body imaging. *J Nucl Med* 1992; 33:1191.
8. Demetri GD, Antman KH: Granulocyte-macrophage colony-stimulating factor (GM-CSF): Preclinical and clinical investigations. *Semin Oncol* 1992; 19:362.
9. Fogelman I, Bessent RG, Beastall G, et al: Estimation of skeletal involvement in primary hyperparathyroidism. *Ann Intern Med* 1980; 92:65.
10. Fogelman I, Bessent RG, Turner JG, et al: The use of whole-body retention of Tc-99m-diphosphonate in the diagnosis of metabolic bone disease. *J Nucl Med* 1978; 19:270.
11. Fowler JS, Wolf AP: Positron emitter-labeled compounds: Priorities and problems, in: Phelps M, Mazziotta J, Schelbert H(eds): *Positron Emission Tomography and Autoradiography: Principles and Applications for the Brain and Heart*, Raven, New York, 1986, p 391.
12. French RJ, McCready VR: The use of 18F for bone scanning. *Br J Radiol* 1967; 40:655.
13. Front D, Israel O, Jerushalmi J, et al: Quantitative bone scintigraphy using SPECT. *J Nucl Med* 1989; 30:240.
14. Gallagher BM, Fowler JS, Gutterson NI, et al: Metabolic trapping as a principle of radiopharmaceutical design: Some factors responsible for the biodistribution of [18F]2-deoxyglucose. *J Nucl Med* 1980; 19:1154.
15. Gasson JC: Molecular physiology of granulocyte-macrophage colony stimulating factor. *Blood* 1991; 7:1131.
16. Gold RH, Hawkins RA, Katz RD: Imaging osteomyelitis—From plain films to MRI: A pictorial essay. *AJR Am J Roentgenol* 1991; 157:365.
17. Goodman WG, Coburn JW, Slatopolsky E, Saluski IB: Renal osteodystrophy in adults and children, in Favus MJ (ed): *Primer on the Bone Metabolic Diseases and Disorders of Mineral Metabolism*, ed 1, American Society of Bone and Mineral Research, Kelseyville, Calif., 1990, p 200.
18. Grynpas MD: Fluoride effects on bone crystals. *J Bone Miner Res* 1990; 5(suppl 1):S169.
19. Harmer CL, Burns JE, Sams A, Spittle M: The value of fluorine-18 for scanning bone tumors. *Clin Radiol* 1969; 20:204.
20. Hawkins RA, Choi Y, Huang SC, et al: Evaluation of the skeletal kinetics of fluorine-18-fluoride ion with PET. *J Nucl Med* 1992; 33:633.
21. Hawkins RA, Choi Y, Huang SC, et al: Quantitating tumor glucose metabolism with FDG and PET. *J Nucl Med* 1992; 33:339.
22. Hawkins RA, Hoh C, Glaspy J, et al: The role of positron emission tomography in oncology and other whole-body applications. *Semin Nucl Med* 1992; 22:268.
23. Hawkins RA, Phelps ME, Huang SC: Effects of temporal sampling, glucose metabolic rate and disruptions of the blood brain barrier (BBB) on the FDG model with and without a vascular compartment: Studies in human brain tumors with PET. *J Cereb Blood Flow Metab* 1986; 6:170.
24. Hoh CK, Hawkins RA, Dahlbom M, et al: Whole body skeletal imaging with [18F]fluoride ion and PET. *J Comput Assist Tomogr* 1993; 17:34.
25. Hoh CK, Hawkins RA, Glaspy JA, et al: Cancer detection with whole-body PET using 2-[18F]fluoro-2-deoxy-D-glucose. *J Comput Assist Tomogr* 1993; 17:582.
26. Huang SC, Phelps ME, Hoffman EJ, et al: Noninvasive determination of local cerebral metabolic rate of glucose in man. *Am J Physiol* 1980; 238:E69.
27. Israel O, Front D, Hardoff R, et al: In vivo SPECT quantitation of bone metabolism in hyperparathyroidism. *J Nucl Med* 1991; 32:1157.
28. Kern KA, Brunetti A, Norton JA, et al: Metabolic imaging of human extremity musculoskeletal tumors by PET. *J Nucl Med* 1988; 29:181.
29. Lassen NA, Perl W: *Tracer Kinetic Methods in Medical Physiology*, Raven, New York, 1979.
30. Meikle SR, Bailey DL, Hutton BF, Jones WF: Optimisation of simultaneous emission and transmission measurements in PET, in *Proceedings IEEE Medical Imaging Conference*, 1993; p 1642.

31. Messa C, Goodman WG, Hoh CK, et al: Bone metabolic activity measured with positron emission tomography and [18F]fluoride ion in renal osteodystrophy: Correlation with bone histomorphometry. *J Clin Endocrinol Metab* 1993; 77:949.

32. Moon NF, Dworkin HJ, LaFluer PD: The clinical use of sodium fluoride F-18 in bone photoscanning. *JAMA* 1968; 204:974.

33. Murray TM, Singer FR (eds): *J Bone Miner Res* 1990; 5(suppl 1).

34. Ott RJ: The applications of positron emission tomography to oncology (editorial). *Br J Cancer* 1991; 63:343.

35. Parfitt AM, Drezner MK, Glorieux FH, et al: Bone histomorphometry: Standardization of nomenclature, symbols and units: Report of the ASBMR histomorphometry nomenclature committee. *J Bone Miner Res* 1987; 2:595.

36. Phelps ME, Huang SC, Hoffman EJ, et al: Tomographic measurements of local cerebral glucose metabolic rate in humans with (F-18)-2-fluoro-2-deoxy-D-glucose: Validation of method. *Ann Neurol* 1979; 6:371.

37. Recker RR: Bone biopsy and histomorphometry in clinical practice, in Favus MJ (ed): *Primer on the Bone Metabolic Diseases and Disorders of Mineral Metabolism*, ed 1, American Society of Bone and Mineral Research, Kelseyville, Calif., 1990, p. 101.

38. Reeve J, Arlot M, Wooton R, et al: Skeletal blood flow, iliac histomorphometry, and strontium kinetics in osteoporosis: A relationship between blood flow and corrected apposition rate. *J Clin Endocrinol Metab* 1988; 66:1124.

39. Reivich M, Kuhl D, Wolf A, et al: The [18F]fluorodeoxyglucose method for the measurement of local cerebral glucose utilization in man. *Circ Res* 1979; 44:127.

40. Sokoloff L, Reivich M, Kennedy C, et al: The [14C]deoxyglucose method for the measurement of local cerebral glucose utilization: Theory, procedure, and normal values in the conscious and anesthetized albino rat. *J Neurochem* 1977; 28:897.

41. Sorenson JA, Phelps ME (eds): *Physics in Nuclear Medicine*, ed 2, Grune & Stratton, Orlando, Fla., 1987.

42. Spencer R, Herbert R, Rish MW, Little WA: Bone scanning with 85Sr, 87mSr and 18F: Physical and radiopharmaceutical considerations and clinical experience in 50 cases. *Br J Radiol* 1967; 40:641.

43. Strauss LG, Conti PS: The applications of PET in clinical oncology. *J Nucl Med* 1991; 32:623.

44. Tse N, Hoh C, Hawkins R, et al: Positron emission tomography diagnosis of pulmonary metastases in osteogenic sarcoma. *Am J Clin Oncol* 1994; 17:22.

45. Van Dyke D, Anger HO, Yano Y, Bozzini C: Bone blood flow shown with 18F and the positron camera. *Am J Physiol* 1965; 209:65.

46. Wahl RL, Kaminski MS, Ethier SP, et al: The potential of 2-deoxy-2[18F]fluoro-D-glucose (FDG) for the detection of tumor involvement in lymph nodes. *J Nucl Med* 1990; 31:1831.

47. Warburg O: On the origin of cancer cells. *Science* 1956; 123:309.

48. Weber DA, Keyes JW Jr, Landman S, Wilson GA: Comparison of Tc-99m polyphosphate and F-18 for bone imaging. *Am J Roentgenol Radium Ther Nucl Med* 1974; 121:184.

49. Wooton R, Dore C: The single-passage extraction of 18F in rabbit bone. *Clin Phys Physiol Meas* 1986; 7:333.

50. Wooton R, Reeve J, Spellacy E, Tellez-Yudilevich M: Skeletal blood flow in Paget's disease of bone and its response to calcitonin therapy. *Clin Sci Molec Med* 1978; 54:69.

51. Yao WJ, Hoh CK, Hawkins RA, et al: Quantitative PET imaging of bone marrow glucose metabolic response to hematopoietic cytokins. *J Nucl Med* 1995; 36:794.

CHAPTER 20

BONE MINERAL ANALYSIS

Glen M. Blake

Ignac Fogelman

The past decade has seen the rapid evolution of new radiologic techniques for quantifying skeletal integrity.[31,76] More than any other method, however, the introduction of dual x-ray absorptiometry (DXA)[15,42,51,75,80] has been responsible for the recent rapid growth in clinical applications of bone densitometry.[81] Compared with the earlier technique of dual photon absorptiometry (DPA) based on a Gd-153 radionuclide source, DXA has advantages of high precision, short scanning times, low radiation dose, and stable calibration in the clinical environment.[5,48,59,63,72]

Perhaps the most important application of DXA has been its widespread use in prospective clinical trials of new therapies for osteoporosis.[28,59] Because of the well-established relation between bone mineral density (BMD) and fracture risk,* the demonstration of a statistically significant difference in the BMD changes of subjects on active drug and placebo is a primary objective of most trials of new treatments for osteoporosis. For such studies DXA provides a sensitive and specific method of measuring the BMD changes at selected sites in the skeleton. A second common use of DXA is for identifying perimenopausal and postmenopausal women with low bone

density who can be advised to take estrogen or other preventive therapies. Such patients may require follow-up scans after 2 or 3 years to monitor their response.

Whether monitoring subjects in clinical trials or patients taking established therapies, it is important that bone densitometry measurements are performed at sites where response can be reliably measured after a short interval. For many applications the lumbar spine has proved the ideal site because of the metabolically active trabecular bone in the vertebral bodies.[38] A DXA scan measures BMD (units: g/cm^2), defined as the integral mass of bone mineral per unit projected area. However, in the conventional posteroanterior (PA) scan of the spine (Fig. 20-1) this includes contributions from cortical bone and the spinous processes as well as the trabecular bone of the vertebral body. Further disadvantages of the PA scan include its susceptibility to spinal degenerative changes and aortic calcification (Fig. 20-2). The alternative technique of quantitative computed tomography (QCT)[11,12] permits direct measurement of the mineralization of trabecular bone in the lumbar spine (Fig. 20-3). QCT measures true physical density (units: g/cm^3) rather than the areal density of DXA. However, despite this, DXA remains the more widely used technique on the grounds of cost, precision, and radiation burden.[40,60]

*References 4, 16, 17, 26, 36, 82.

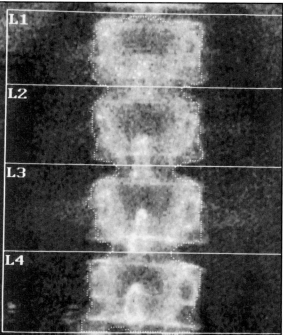

Fig. 20-1. A posteroanterior (PA) projection DXA scan of the lumbar spine in a postmenopausal patient (**A**) with results of bone mineral density (BMD) measurements (**B**). Areal BMD expressed in units of grams of hydroxyapatite per square centimeter of projected area is measured for the individual vertebrae L1 to L4 and is then averaged over their total area.

Region	Area (cm²)	BMC (grams)	BMD (g/cm²)
L1	12.85	10.01	0.779
L2	13.90	11.38	0.819
L3	14.81	11.52	0.778
L4	14.88	12.71	0.854
Total	56.44	45.61	0.808

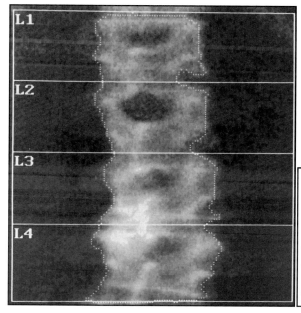

Fig. 20-2. Lumbar spine DXA scan of a patient with degenerative changes in L3 and L4 (**A**) showing the influence of such changes on the BMD results (**B**). BMD values are lower in L1 and L2 than for the patient in Fig. 20-1 but higher in L3 and L4 due to the degenerative changes.

Region	Area (cm²)	BMC (grams)	BMD (g/cm²)
L1	11.61	7.59	0.654
L2	12.47	7.86	0.630
L3	13.37	11.32	0.847
L4	15.46	13.83	0.894
Total	52.90	40.60	0.768

For many bone densitometry applications there is continuing interest in measurements of the peripheral skeleton. Such instrumentation is cheaper, takes up less space than a DXA scanner, and may give clinical data that are just as useful. X-ray absorptiometry of the forearm and ultrasound measurements of the calcaneus are the principal choices. The replacement of the I-125 radionuclide source used in single photon absorptiometry (SPA) by an x-ray tube has given rise to a technique referred to as single x-ray absorptiometry (SXA).[25,43] Like DXA, SXA measures the areal bone density. Thus a mea-

surement of the ultradistal region of the wrist sums contributions from both cortical and trabecular bone. An alternative new technology for forearm studies has been the development of small, dedicated computed tomography (CT) scanners to image the wrist (Fig. 20-4). This technique, referred to as peripheral QCT (pQCT),[9,47] measures the volumetric bone density of trabecular and cortical bone separately. Finally, improvements in technology have led to a revival of the technique of radiographic absorptiometry[14] in which the hand is x-rayed with a small calibration wedge (Fig. 20-5). Such a tech-

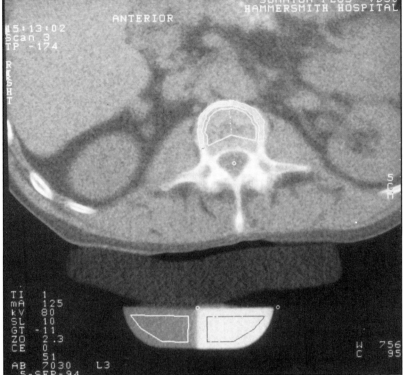

Fig. 20–3. A QCT scan of a lumbar vertebra. Volumetric BMD expressed in units of grams of hydroxyapatite per cubic centimeter can be measured separately in the trabecular bone and cortical shell of the vertebral body. The phantom below the patient serves to calibrate BMD in terms of the Hounsfield units of the CT image.

nique is inexpensive and widely accessible, although it requires careful quality control if it is to give useful data.

Another new peripheral technique, quantitative ultrasound (QUS) measurement of the calcaneus, is also now widely available (Fig. 20-6). Bone ultrasound systems use frequencies in the range of 200 to 600 kHz and measure broadband ultrasonic attenuation (BUA)[1,35,44,52,64] and the velocity of sound (VOS)[54] in the heel. The calcaneus is chosen for measurement because it is an easily accessible site of trabecular bone. An attraction of the peripheral x-ray systems is that studies over many years have demonstrated the ability of photon absorptiometry to predict fractures.[26,82] To date only one prospective study has related BUA measurements to fracture risk.[62] Further studies of fracture prediction are needed before QUS becomes an accepted technique.

At the present time DXA is the most widely used technique for bone densitometry studies. In part this is due to the good precision and stable calibration. Another factor is the continuing importance of measurements of the lumbar spine. However, there are also a wide variety of additional applications now available. These include BMD measurements of the proximal femur, distal forearm, and total body together with specialist applications such as body composition and vertebral morphometry.

As a result, the past 5 years have seen the rapid expansion of both research and routine clinical studies based on DXA.[81]

DXA TECHNOLOGY

Physical Principles of DXA

The fundamental principle behind DXA is the measurement of the transmission through the body of x-rays of two different photon energies. This enables the areal densities of two different tissues (conventionally bone and soft tissue) to be inferred. The physical principles are best illustrated with the DPA equation.[6,72] In the following equations primed variables denote the low-energy beam and unprimed variables the high-energy beam. The transmission of radiation through the body is given by

$$\text{Low energy: } I' = I_0' \exp[-(\mu_S' M_S + \mu_B' M_B)] \quad \textbf{(1a)}$$

$$\text{High energy: } I = I_0 \exp[-(\mu_S M_S + \mu_B M_B)] \quad \textbf{(1b)}$$

where μ is the mass attenuation coefficient, M is the areal density, and subscripts B and S denote bone and soft-tis-

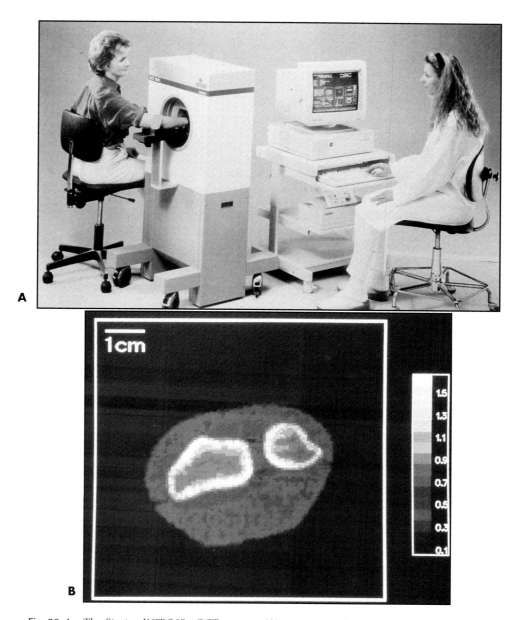

Fig. 20-4. The Stratec XCT-960 pQCT scanner (**A**) measures volumetric BMD in the distal forearm. Bone density is measured separately for trabecular and cortical bone in the distal radius (**B**). (*Courtesy of Stratec Medizintechnik, Germany.*)

sue, respectively. Equations 1a and 1b are simplified by writing J in place of the logarithmic transmission factor $-\ln(I/I_0)$, giving:

$$J' = \mu'_S M_S + \mu'_B M_B \qquad \textbf{(2a)}$$

$$J = \mu_S M_S + \mu_B M_B \qquad \textbf{(2b)}$$

Elimination of M_S gives the DPA equation:

$$M_B = \frac{J' - kJ}{\mu'_B - k\mu_B} \qquad \textbf{(3a)}$$

where

$$k = \frac{\mu'_S}{\mu_S} \qquad \textbf{(3b)}$$

In the earlier technology of DPA, the radionuclide source Gd-153 was chosen because its two photon emissions at 44 and 103 keV were close to the ideal energies for in vivo measurement of the lumbar spine.[76] At pho-

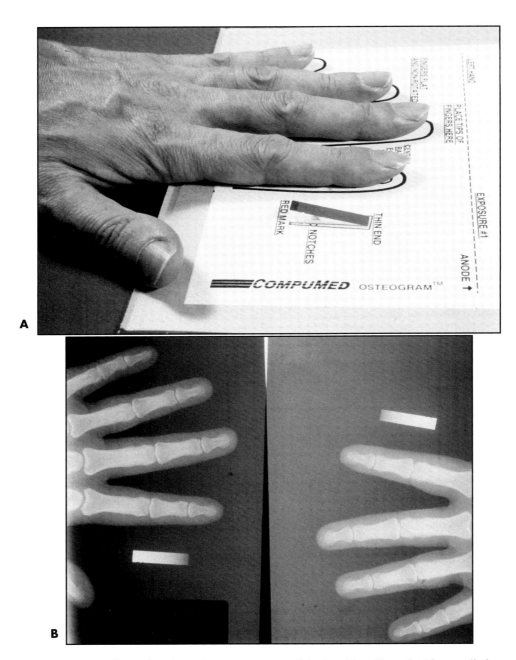

Fig. 20-5. In radiographic absorptiometry an x-ray of the hand is calibrated with a small aluminum wedge (**A**). The resulting film (**B**) can be digitized to measure BMD in the phalanges.

ton energies above 100 keV, there is little difference in the mass attenuation coefficients of bone and soft tissue, and transmission measurements reflect essentially the total mass of tissue in the beam. Photon energies around 40 keV are ideal for the low-energy beam because there is good contrast between bone and soft tissue without excessive attenuation to limit the signal reaching the detector.

The Radiation Source

The replacement of the Gd-153 radionuclide source with a x-ray tube improved the performance of DPA by combining high photon flux with the small focal spot size at the anode of the x-ray tube. The availability of an intense, narrow beam of radiation improved scanning time and image definition and led to a concomitant improvement in precision.

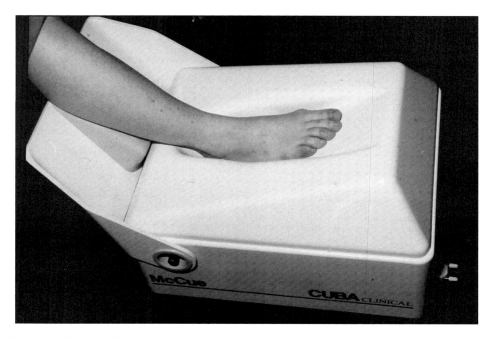

Fig. 20-6. Ultrasound systems measure broadband ultrasonic attenuation (BUA) and the velocity of sound (VOS) in bone in the frequency range of 200 to 600 kHz. The calcaneus is the usual measurement site. In the McCue CUBA Clinical system seen here, the transducers are coupled to the patient's heel with silicone rubber pads and gel.

However, the use of an x-ray tube as the radiation source requires the solution of several significant technical problems. As is evident from Equation 1, a highly stable source is essential. Image noise must be limited by photon statistics and not by instabilities in the x-ray generator. Because x-ray tubes produce polyenergetic spectra rather than the discrete line emissions of a radionuclide, the effects of beam hardening are a potential source of error.[6,72] In beam hardening lower-energy photons are preferentially removed from the radiation beam compared with higher-energy photons, leading to a progressive shift in spectral distribution to higher effective photon energies with increasing body thickness. As a result, the attenuation coefficients for bone and soft tissue in the DPA equation change with body thickness, and so vary from patient to patient and from site to site within the body.

Commercial DXA Systems

Manufacturers selling DXA equipment include Hologic (Waltham, Mass.), Lunar (Madison, Wisc.) and Norland (Fort Atkinson, Wisc.). The Lunar and Norland scanners use the K-absorption edge of a rare earth filter to split the polyenergetic x-ray beam into high- and low-energy components (Fig. 20-7) that mimic the emissions from Gd-153. Because the two components have inherently narrow spectral distributions, the problems associated with beam hardening are minimized. The Lunar DPX systems[51,81] have a cerium filter and use pulse height analysis at the detector to discriminate between high- and low-energy photons. A potential limitation of the latter is that at high count rates the dynamic range is restricted by the need to accurately correct for dead time in the electronics. The Norland systems[81] use a samarium filter and separate high- and low-energy detectors. Dynamic range is extended by a system for switching filters with different thicknesses of samarium into the beam.

In the Hologic QDR scanners[81] the dual energy x-ray beam is generated by switching the HV generator between 70 and 140 kVp during alternate half cycles of the mains supply. A rotating wheel (Fig. 20-8) containing bone and soft-tissue equivalent filters measures the attenuation coefficients in the DPA equation and calibrates the scan image pixel by pixel, correcting for the effects of beam hardening.[6,75] Pulse height analysis is not required, giving the instrument an inherently wide dynamic range.

Fan-Beam DXA

The first generation of DXA scanners used a pencil beam coupled to a single detector in the scanning arm. An important development in DXA technology was the introduction of scanners[61,73] with a fan beam coupled to a linear array of detectors (Fig. 20-9). Fan-beam studies are acquired by the scanning arm performing a single sweep across the patient instead of the two dimensional raster scan required by pencil-beam geometry. As a result, scan times are significantly shortened. A number of studies have demonstrated the equivalence of pencil- and fan-beam BMD measurements.[7,20,21,24,32] However, due to the fan beam geometry, measurements of projected

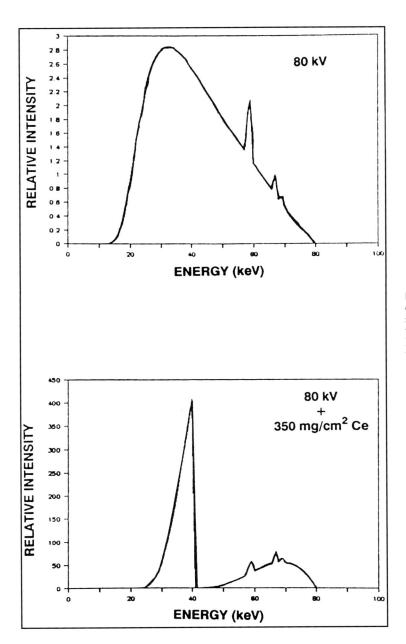

Fig. 20-7. The K-edge filtration technique produces a dual energy x-ray beam by filtering the continuous spectrum x-rays produced by an 80-kV generator (*top*) with a filter made from a rare earth metal (*bottom*). In Lunar DPX scanners a cerium filter with a K-absorption edge of 42 keV is used.

area and bone mineral content (BMC) are sensitive to the height of the measurement site above the scanning table.[7,20,21]

The first fan-beam system introduced, the Hologic QDR-2000, has a 32 detector array.[81] DXA scans of the spine or hip can be performed in either 45 or 90 seconds, depending on the image resolution required. The fastest mode is the 5-second "turbo" scan,[10] which functions primarily as a scout scan and is a useful aid to achieving exact and reproducible positioning of the patient. A high patient throughput, around twice that for first-generation DXA systems, is the major advantage of the QDR-2000.

In recent years commercial rivalry between manufacturers has provided an important spur to new technical developments. The most recent advance has been the introduction of a new generation of DXA scanners that produce images with much improved definition (Fig. 20-10). The Lunar Expert, a fan-beam system with 288 detectors, performs spine and hip scans in only 15 seconds. The conventional arrangement with the x-ray tube under the scanning table and the detector arm above is reversed to minimize geometric distortion from the fan beam. The improved resolution allows easier identification of vertebral structure together with the artifacts due to degenerative disease that are a significant limitation in conventional DXA. A new Hologic model, the QDR-4500 Acclaim (Fig. 20-11), introduces improvements in hardware and software that ease patient handling and further enhance image quality. A major motivation behind the

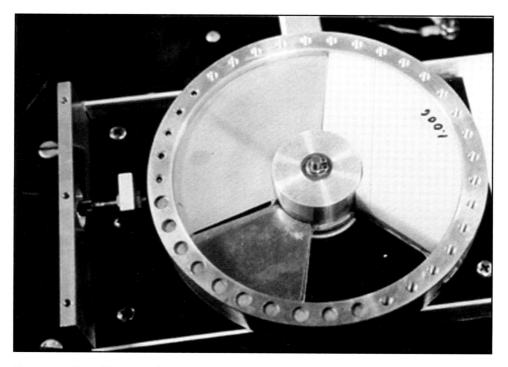

Fig. 20-8.   The calibration wheel used as the internal reference standard in Hologic scanners. The segments in the wheel include bone and soft-tissue equivalent filters together with an empty air sector. Each of these three segments has separate high- and low-energy x-ray sectors with and without an additional brass filter. In the wheel shown here, the BMD of the bone filter is 1.006 g/cm^2.

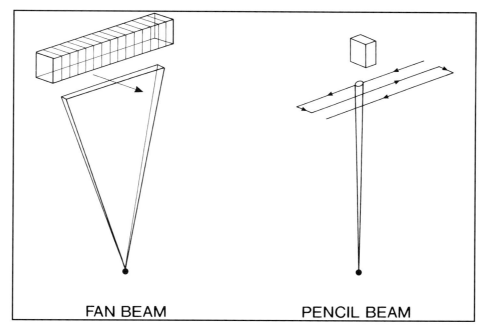

FAN BEAM   PENCIL BEAM

Fig. 20-9.   Comparison of x-ray beam and detector geometry for a pencil-beam configuration with a single detector (*right*) and a fan-beam configuration with a multidetector array (*left*).

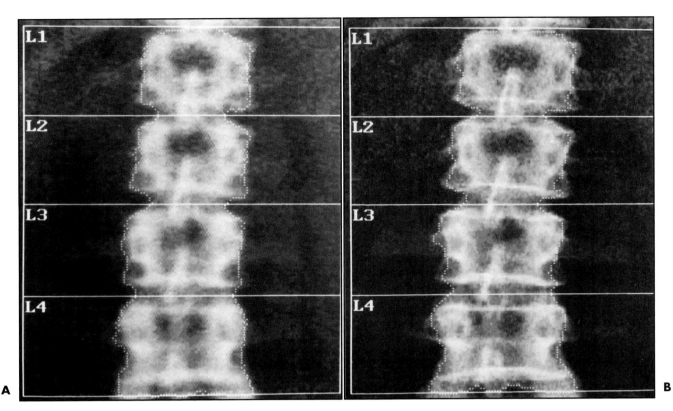

Fig. 20-10. Comparison of PA lumbar spine scans in the same subject produced by a first-generation QDR-1000 system (**A**) and a third-generation QDR-2000*plus* (**B**).

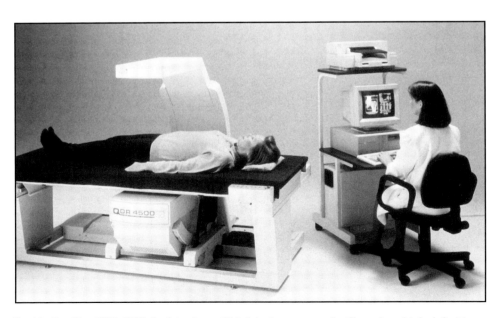

Fig. 20-11. The QDR-4500 Acclaim has a 216 detector array and will produce high-definition spine and hip images with scan times of 30 seconds. (*Courtesy of Itologic Inc., Waltham, Mass.*)

development of both the Expert and the Acclaim systems is a DXA scanner capable of producing vertebral morphometry studies with high resolution and short scan times.

DXA APPLICATIONS

Anteroposterior Lumbar Spine and Hip

The scanning software developed for first-generation DXA systems provided for clinical studies using PA projection scans of the lumbar spine (Fig. 20-1) and proximal femur. It is usual to examine BMD in the hip in three regions: the femoral neck, the greater trochanter, and Ward's triangle (Fig. 20-12). The latter measures the earliest site of postmenopausal bone loss in the proximal femur and is of interest because in principle it gives the best measure of trabecular bone in the hip. In practice, however, use of the Ward's triangle region is limited by the poor precision of measurements at this site, and the femoral neck is the region usually used.

For the majority of clinical studies, DXA scans of the PA spine and hip provide sufficient information. However, developments in DXA have made available new scanning modes and specialized applications that supplement the conventional spine and hip studies.

Distal Forearm

Studies of the radius are performed by placing the nondominant forearm on the scanning table and scanning the distal half from the midradius to the wrist (Fig. 20-13). Unlike SPA or SXA studies, DXA scans of the forearm can be performed in air and do not require the use of a water bath. Bone density measurements are made at

two principal sites.[46,66,83] The first of these, the ultradistal region, is a rectangular strip 1.5 cm wide immediately adjacent to the endplates of the radius and ulna (Fig. 20-13). This site is chosen because it is the area in the forearm with the highest percentage of trabecular bone. The second measurement site is the one-third region, a 2-cm wide strip centered over cortical bone at a point one-third the distance between the ulna styloid and the olecranon. BMD results at these sites are given for radius and ulnar either separately or combined.

DXA forearm scans provide BMD data equivalent to SPA and SXA scans.[25,46,83] Although forearm scans may be used to assess fracture risk or response to treatment, it is conventional, when possible, to perform such measurements at the spine and hip, since these are the principal fracture sites. Thus the principal applications of forearm DXA appear to be an adjunct to scanning of the spine and hip and a convenient site for monitoring cortical bone.

Total–Body Studies

Total-body DXA is of interest because of the comprehensive view it affords of changes across the whole skeleton (Fig. 20-14). Whole-body scans measure BMC and average BMD in the total skeleton together with subregions that include the skull, arms, ribs, thoracic and lumbar spine, pelvis, and legs.[33]

An interesting new application made possible by total-body DXA is body composition studies.[33,71] In those areas of a whole-body scan where the x-ray beam does not intersect bone, it is possible to use the attenuation at the two photon energies to measure separately the masses of fat and lean tissue. Over bone, however, only BMD and total (fat and lean) soft-tissue mass can be measured. Extrapolation of measurements of percentage body fat in soft tissue over adjacent bone means that a whole-body

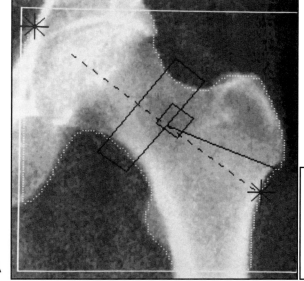

Fig. 20-12. A DXA scan of the proximal femur (**A**). The hip analysis software generates BMD measurements (**B**) in the femoral neck (*oblong box*), Ward's triangle (*small square box*), and the greater trochanter (*above solid diagonal line*).

Region	Area (cm²)	BMC (grams)	BMD (g/cm²)
Neck	5.01	3.14	0.626
Troch	10.84	6.36	0.587
Ward's	1.10	0.47	0.424
Total	36.82	29.58	0.804

A   B

DXA scan can provide estimates of total body fat and lean mass as well as BMC.

A wide variety of methods have been developed to measure body fat including hydrodensitometry, neutron activation analysis, total body potassium, total body water, and skinfold measurements. Each of these has individual limitations in its assumptions, calibration, and accuracy—complicating the assessment of the place of DXA in body composition studies. Body composition by DXA has evolved rapidly with a succession of software revisions that have refined accuracy. The present status has been reviewed by Nord and Payne.[56,57,58] With its high precision, low radiation dose to the patient, and general accuracy DXA is likely to become one of the principal methods of assessing body fat.

Prosthetic Implants

Another specialized application under evaluation is the study of the integrity of hip prostheses. In such patients scanning of the hip is complicated by the high x-ray attenuation of the metal implant. Software can now identify and reject the prothesis and automatically place regions of interest (ROIs) around the periprosthetic bone.[65] Studies are under way to determine whether serial DXA scanning after hip replacement can identify mechanical loosening and the durability of implants[77] and so aid improvements in the design of future implants.

Lateral Lumbar Spine

The rapid turnover of the metabolically active trabecular bone in the vertebral bodies makes the spine the optimum site for monitoring changes in bone mineralization.[38] DXA scans of the lumbar spine using the later-

al instead of the PA projection isolate the vertebral bodies from the posterior elements and better approximate the objective of measuring trabecular bone free of artifacts (Fig. 20-15).

Initial lateral DXA studies were performed using the decubitus method in which subjects lie on their side.[45,50,70,78] The first reports gave precisions with a coefficient of variation (CV) of 2% to 3%; however, later studies gave a CV of 5% to 6%.[8] The poor precision of the decubitus scan is partly the result of the difficulty in reproducing subjects' positions on follow-up scans, which leads to variation in the thickness and composition of the soft-tissue baseline. An important development in lateral studies has been the introduction of the new generation of fan-beam systems like the QDR-2000 equipped with a rotating scanning arm. This enables the lateral scan to be performed with the patient in the supine position and overcomes some of the difficulties associated with the decubitus scan. In supine lateral DXA, PA and lateral scans are acquired in pairs. After completion of the PA scan, the C-arm is rotated through 90 degrees and a lateral study performed without the patient moving. Information from both PA and lateral projections are combined to correct the errors due to variable soft-tissue baseline on the lateral scan using a technique referred to as baseline compensation.[8] Use of the supine position and baseline compensation algorithm has improved the short-term precision of vertebral body BMD measurements to 1%,[8,73] and the technique may have a use in clinical trials.

Vertebral Morphometry

Recent prospective clinical trials of new treatments for osteoporosis have given increased emphasis to the primary objective of such studies of demonstrating that thera-

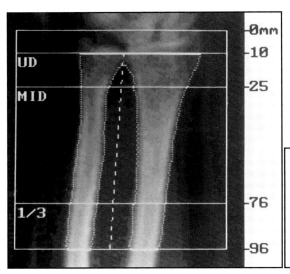

A

Fig. 20-13. A DXA scan of the distal forearm (**A**). BMD measurements (**B**) are made in the radius and ulna in the ultradistal (UD) and one-third radius (1/3) regions as well as a midregion between these two.

Region	Area (cm²)	BMC (grams)	BMD (g/cm²)
Ultradistal	6.38	2.09	0.327
Mid	12.53	6.04	0.482
One-Third	4.73	2.76	0.583
Total	23.64	10.88	0.460

B

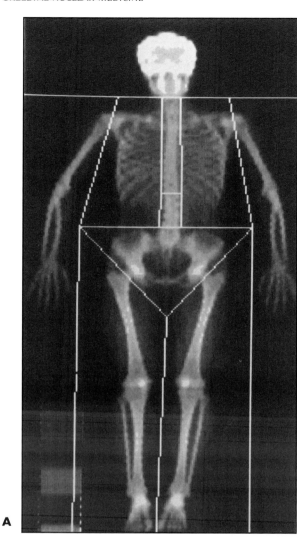

Fig. 20-14. A DXA scan of the total skeleton (**A**). As well as measuring bone mineral content (BMC) and bone mineral density (BMD) over the whole body, results are given separately for 10 subregions in the skeleton (**B**). From the same scan the body composition software will also estimate total-body and subregional fat and lean tissue masses.

Region	Area (cm²)	BMC (grams)	BMD (g/cm²)
L Arm	175.6	144.6	0.823
R Arm	189.7	150.4	0.793
L Ribs	148.6	104.0	0.700
R Ribs	138.1	95.0	0.688
T Spine	141.4	142.8	1.010
L Spine	50.3	61.1	1.213
Pelvis	231.6	286.5	1.237
L Leg	360.5	444.4	1.233
R Leg	367.3	459.1	1.250
Head	255.7	640.8	2.506
Total	2058.8	2528.6	1.228

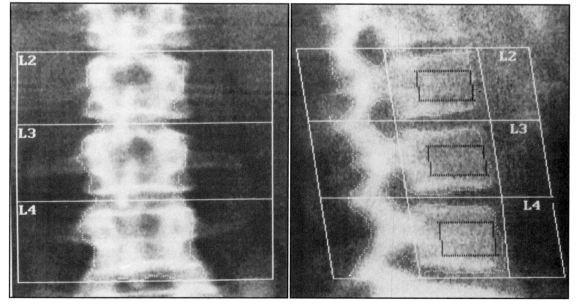

Fig. 20-15. Paired PA/lateral DXA scans of the lumbar spine showing the analysis for L2-L4. The PA scan is acquired first (*left*) and then the scanning arm rotated through 90 degrees to acquire the lateral scan (*right*). Vertebral body BMD is measured on the lateral scan anterior to the vertical line intersecting the neural arches, while midvertebral BMD is measured inside the black regions of interest within each vertebral body.

pies are successful in reducing the incidence of fragility fractures. Spinal crush fractures are important sequelae of osteoporosis, and it is usual to monitor the incidence of new vertebral deformities by performing serial morphometric measurements of vertebral body height on lateral radiographs of the lumbar and thoracic spine.[3,18,27,53]

The latest fan-beam DXA systems, the Hologic Acclaim and the Lunar Expert, are designed to perform fast, high-resolution lateral scans of the lumbar and thoracic spine (L4-T4) acquired with the patient in the supine position (Fig. 20-16). A major advantage of DXA systems for vertebral morphometry is the elimination of the geometric distortion associated with lateral radiographs that arises from the x-ray cone beam and can cause errors due to variable projection and magnification.[74] A further significant advantage is the much lower radiation dose to the patient from DXA compared with radiographs.[49] Initial studies of DXA vertebral morphometry have shown good agreement with radiographic studies after allowing for the elimination of the magnification error (Fig. 20-17). If DXA can be shown to give adequate image quality for reliably identifying vertebral deformities (Fig. 20-18), morphometry would be a major rationale for its use in future clinical trials and for monitoring patients with established spinal osteoporosis.

PRECISION

Precision errors are defined to characterize the reproducibility of a diagnostic technique. Accuracy errors, on the other hand, reflect the degree to which measured results deviate from true values. Despite the obvious importance of validating the accuracy of bone densitometry techniques, only a few studies of DPA or DXA have addressed this issue.[19,23,30,35,79] However, despite the general lack of accuracy data for studies of patients receiving treatment for osteoporosis, precision is usually the more important factor since it is essential to be able to reliably measure changes after a short time interval. The measurement of precision is therefore always an important element in the evaluation of new equipment and scanning applications.

Short-Term Precision

Most studies of equipment or new techniques include a measurement of short-term precision.* This involves performing a number of repeated measurements on a representative set of individuals to characterize the repro-

*References 8, 33, 43, 45, 51, 64, 73, 80.

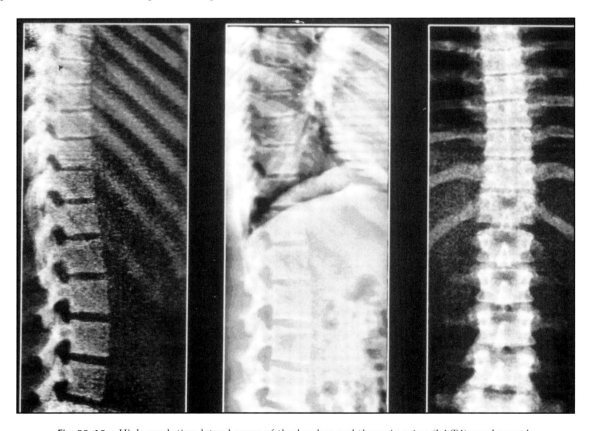

Fig. 20-16. High-resolution lateral scans of the lumbar and thoracic spine (L4-T4) can be used for morphometric x-ray absorptiometry (MXA) studies of vertebral deformities. These images were produced on a Hologic QDR-4500 system. An initial PA scan of the spine (*right*) generates a centerline in the middle of the spine that is tracked during the lateral scan to eliminate magnification errors. Both dual energy (*left*) and single energy (*center*) lateral images are available for analysis.

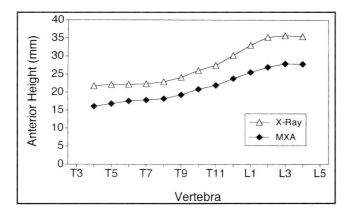

Fig. 20-17. Mean anterior vertebral heights (L4-T4) measured by MXA scanning in 150 postmenopausal women are compared with normative data from radiographic vertebral morphometry studies published by Black et al.[3] The x-ray measurements show a magnification error of approximately 20%.

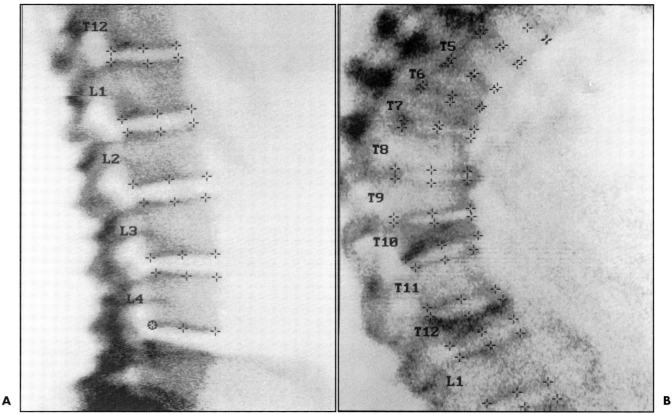

Fig. 20-18. MXA studies in a healthy postmenopausal woman without any vertebral deformities (**A**) and an osteoporotic woman with multiple vertebral crush fractures (**B**).

ducibility of the technique. Generally, short-term precision errors are assessed from measurements performed either on the same day or extending over a period of no more than 2 weeks. Since true changes in BMD may confound measurements made over a longer period, the assessment of short- and long-term precision requires different treatment of the data.

Short-term precision is evaluated by taking the mean and variance of two or more repeated measurements on each subject. The individual means and variances for all the subjects are then averaged and the root mean square standard deviation (RMS SD) calculated.[8] For many purposes the absolute error expressed by the RMS SD is the most satisfactory definition of short term precision. However, it is a popular convention to express precision data as the CV by dividing the SD by the mean for all subjects and expressing the result as a percentage:

$$CV = \frac{RMS\ SD(x)}{x} \times 100\% \qquad (4)$$

The reason why many authors prefer to use CV rather than SD to express precision data is probably because the significance of a result given as a CV is more readily comprehended. Thus the CV for a DXA measurement of PA

TABLE 20-1
Comparative Measurements of Precision

	DXA Spine BMD (g/cm²)	DXA Hip BMD (g/cm²)	Ultrasound BUA (dB/MHz)	Ultrasound VOS (m/sec)
Range of values (osteoporotic–normal)	0.65-1.05	0.55-0.90	45-80	1525-1600
Precision (SD)	0.010	0.018	3.2	16
Precision (CV)	1.0%	2.0%	4.0%	1.0%
Standardized coefficient of variation (SCV)	2.5%	5.0%	9.0%	20%

Data adapted from Herd RJM, Blake GM, Ramalingam T, et al: Measurements of postmenopausal bone loss with a new contact ultrasound system. *Calcif Tissue Int* 1993; 53:153; and Miller CG, Herd RJM, Ramalingam T, et al: Ultrasonic velocity measurements through the calcaneus: Which velocity should be measured? *Osteoporosis Int* 1993; 3:31.

spine BMD and a QUS measurement of ultrasonic velocity in the heel are both 1%.[8,54] Expressed as the RMS SD, however, the figures would be 0.01 g/cm² and 16 m/second, respectively (Table 20-1).

Not often appreciated are the large statistical errors inherent in many precision studies. If m repeated measurements are made on each of n subjects, there will be a total of $n \times m$ measurements. However, since it was necessary to calculate the mean BMD of each subject, there were only $n \times (m - 1)$ independent measurements from which to evaluate precision. This number—the degrees of freedom (df)—determines the statistical weight of the study. The error in the precision measurement cannot be smaller than the component arising from the finite data set available, which can be estimated from the chi-squared distribution[8] (Fig. 20-19). In practice, real differences in precision between subjects will make the errors in precision studies even larger.

Long-Term Precision

The assessment of the long-term reproducibility of a technique is complicated by the fact that the variations in the data will reflect true changes in bone mineral as well as imprecision in the measurements. Use of the SD to express the long-term precision would therefore result in an overestimate of the true precision errors of the technique.

In many subjects the plot of bone density against time approximates closely to a linear change (Fig. 20-20, *A*). A parameter that quantifies the sources of variability over and above the true linear change is the standard error of estimate (SEE) obtained from linear regression analysis of the data. However, the SEE will still include any variability due to nonlinear changes in bone density and therefore may not be appropriate in subjects who have recently commenced or discontinued treatment for osteoporosis (Fig. 20-20, *B*). As with short-term precision, results

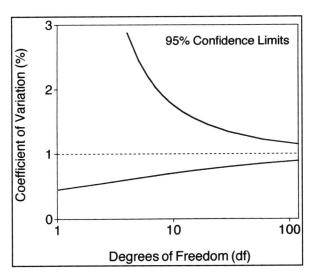

Fig. 20-19. Statistical errors in precision studies cannot be smaller than the component arising from the finite data set available which can be derived from the chi-squared distribution.[8] In this figure the 95% confidence limits are plotted as a function of the number of degrees of freedom (df) for a measured coefficient of variation (CV) of 1%. For a study with m measurements performed on each of n subjects: df = $n \times (m - 1)$.

from different individuals are combined to find the RMS average SEE. In a manner analogous to short-term precision, the long-term precision may be expressed as the CV by dividing the RMS SEE by the mean for all subjects and expressing the result as a percentage:

$$CV = \frac{RMS\ SEE(x)}{x} \times 100\% \qquad (5)$$

Long-term precision is a more realistic parameter for assessing the significance of changes measured in longitudinal studies than short-term precision. Even when the

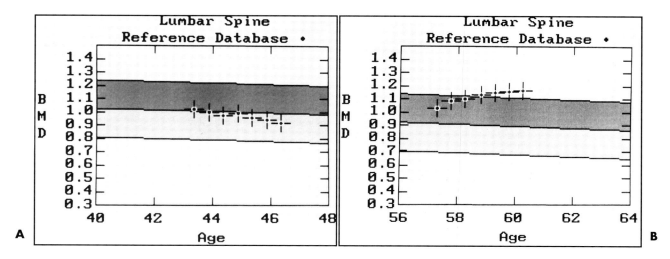

Fig. 20-20. In untreated subjects a plot of BMD against time approximates to a linear change (**A**). Long-term precision can be estimated from the standard error of estimate derived from a linear regression fit to the data. However, subjects who have recently started or stopped treatment show nonlinear changes (**B**) and cannot be used to derive figures for long-term precision.

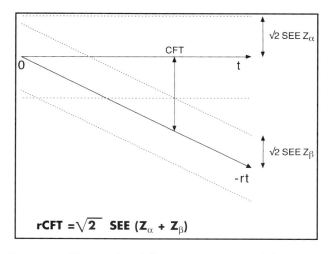

$$\textbf{rCFT} = \sqrt{2}\ \ \textbf{SEE}\ (\textbf{Z}_\alpha + \textbf{Z}_\beta)$$

Fig. 20-21. Characteristic follow-up time (CFT) is defined as the minimum time required to determine from a baseline and a single follow-up scan whether a subject's BMD is either falling at the expected rate r or is constant within specified type 1 (Z_α) and type 2 (Z_β) error limits. SEE is the long-term precision error measured by the standard error of the estimate. A factor of $\sqrt{2}$ is included to allow for the error in the difference between the baseline and follow-up scans.

underlying changes in bone mineral are truly linear, long-term precision would be expected to exceed short-term precision due to small drifts in instrumental calibration, variations in patient positioning, and changes in soft-tissue composition. Typically, in many studies long-term precision is around twice the short-term precision.

Standardized Coefficient of Variation

Short- or long-term precision data expressed by the CV are frequently used as a measure of the clinical performance of instrumentation. A limitation of using CV

for this purpose is the normalization of the precision error by the bone density parameter (Equations 4 and 5). This overlooks the significance of the size of the likely changes in bone density in limiting the sensitivity of equipment for measuring clinical response to treatment. To avoid this problem, Miller et al[54] proposed using the standardized coefficient of variation (SCV), defined as the RMS SD divided by a measure of the clinical range of the parameter:

$$SCV = \frac{RMS\ SD(x)}{range\ x} \times 100\% \qquad (6)$$

A convenient definition of the range is the difference in the values of the parameter between normal premenopausal women with peak bone mass and osteoporotic women (Table 20-1). In the example just given, although DXA PA spine BMD and QUS VOS both have a CV of 1%, when expressed as the SCV the precisions are 2.5% and 20%, respectively (Table 20-1). Miller et al argued that SCV is likely to be a more reliable measure than CV for evaluating the clinical utility of a technique.[54]

Characteristic Follow–Up Time

Glüer et al[29] have proposed the use of the characteristic follow-up time (CFT) as a measure of the sensitivity of a bone densitometry technique to monitor longitudinal change. CFT uses the follow-up time required for different techniques to measure statistically significant changes in BMD, with similar levels of confidence to compare the clinical utility of the techniques. Suppose a patient has a baseline BMD study. Let r be the expected annual rate of loss were the patient not receiving therapy (Fig. 20-21). After a period of t years a further scan is performed. The expected change in BMD at the time of the second scan is rt. Let SEE be the long-term precision error as measured by linear regression analysis. A 1 SD difference between the follow-up and baseline scans will be $\sqrt{2}$ SEE. The statistical significance of the expected change in BMD will be

$$Z_\alpha + Z_\beta = \frac{rt}{\sqrt{2}\ \text{SEE}} \qquad (7)$$

where α is the confidence level for a type 1 error and β the power for a type 2 error. The CFT is defined as the time to determine with 90% confidence ($Z_\alpha = 1.28$) and 80% power ($Z_\beta = 0.84$)[29] whether the patient is responding to treatment (i.e., BMD is stable) or not (i.e., BMD is falling at the expected rate). Substituting in Equation 7 gives

$$\text{CFT} = 3 \times \frac{\text{SEE}}{r} \qquad (8)$$

CFT is the time required to classify patients as either stable with no significant change of bone or losing bone at the rate r with the specified confidence and power. A shorter CFT represents a better sensitivity for monitoring the response to treatment in individual patients. Like SCV, CFT offers a more objective method than the CV for evaluating the clinical performance of instrumentation.

CLINICAL STUDIES OF BONE DENSITY

What is Normal?

One of the difficulties of interpreting the results of bone densitometry is that there is little consensus on how BMD measurements should be presented. To be clinically useful, BMD results for individual patients must be related to similar values obtained from a healthy reference population. The reference population is usually described in terms of the mean BMD and the population SD matched for age, sex, and race. A convenient method of displaying the results for an individual patient is to use a diagram in which the reference population is shown as the mean ± 2 SD (Fig. 20-22). Provided the reference data are accurate and appropriate, 95% of normal subjects will lie within the ±2 SD limits. The advantage of the plot shown in Fig. 20-22 is that the interpretation of the measured BMD relative to the reference range is immediately apparent.

THE Z-SCORE

The information given visually in Fig. 20-22 can also be expressed numerically by using Z-scores. The Z-score is defined by the following equation:

$$\text{Z-score} = \frac{\text{measured BMD} - \text{age-matched mean BMD}}{\text{population standard deviation}} \qquad (9)$$

and expresses by how many SDs a subject differs from the mean value for an age-, sex-, and race-matched reference population. Thus a subject lying on the central curve in Fig. 20-22 has a Z-score of zero, whereas subjects on the upper and lower curves have Z-scores of +2 and −2,

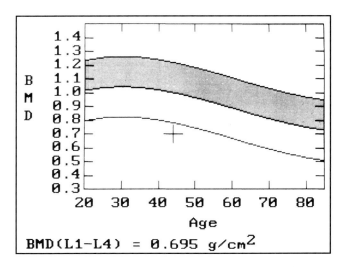

BMD(L1-L4) = 0.695 g/cm²

Fig. 20-22. PA lumbar spine BMD for a perimenopausal patient plotted with the normal reference curves. The middle curve shows the mean BMD in normal subjects ($Z = 0$), while the upper and lower curves show the ±2 standard deviation limits ($Z = \pm2$). This patient was recommended to commence estrogen replacement therapy.

respectively. An advantage of the Z-score is that although different manufacturers' instruments may have different normal ranges for BMD due to differences in technology, edge detection algorithms, and calibration, Z-score results should be identical provided that comparable reference populations are used.

A potential limitation of using Z-scores derived from age-dependent reference data like that shown in Fig. 20-22 is that the smooth variation of mean BMD and SD with age makes no allowance for whether a subject is premenopausal, perimenopausal or postmenopausal or the number of years since the menopause. In middle age these may be more relevant factors than chronologic age in the interpretation of BMD results. There is an argument therefore for plotting results for premenopausal and postmenopausal women separately and interpreting values for postmenopausal women as a function of years after the menopause.[67]

THE T-SCORE

The T-score is similar to the Z-score except that the mean and SD of the young adult age group (20 to 35 years) is used as the reference range, regardless of the age of the patient whose BMD is being interpreted. T-scores compare a given subject with the sex- and race-adjusted expected maximum BMD achieved in life. The T-score is defined by the following equation:

$$\text{T-score} = \frac{\text{measured BMD} - \text{young adult mean BMD}}{\text{young adult standard deviation}} \qquad (10)$$

A recent World Health Organization (WHO) technical report[41,84] advocated an interpretation of bone densitometry measurements based on T-score values in which subjects are divided into the following four categories (Fig. 20-23):

1. *Normal*: A value of BMD not more than 1 SD below the young adult mean value ($T > -1.0$).

2. *Osteopenia*: A BMD value that lies between 1 and 2.5 SD below the young adult mean ($-1.0 > T > -2.5$). Such individuals include those in whom the prevention of bone loss would be most useful.

3. *Osteoporosis*: A BMD value more than 2.5 SD below the young adult mean value ($T < -2.5$).

4. *Established osteoporosis*: A BMD value more than 2.5 SD below the young adult mean value ($T < -2.5$) in the presence of one or more fragility fractures.

The WHO definitions of osteopenia and osteoporosis are useful because they bear an immediate relationship to the fracture threshold which is approximately 2 SD below the young normal mean ($T = -2$).[68] In addition, T-score values are useful when interpreting the results of young adults and perimenopausal women because they indicate how the subject compares with her peers before the effects of age and the menopause. However, caution may be needed in the interpretation of T-score values in the older-age population, when due to normal age-related bone loss, even the mean BMD values may be below the -2.5 SD limit of the young adult normal range (Fig. 20-23). For women over the age of 75 years, the use of Z-scores is probably more appropriate.

Bone Density and Bone Strength

The organic matrix of bone is impregnated with mineral salts that give the skeleton its properties of hardness and rigidity. In vitro data show that the breaking strength of bone is related to its mineral content,[2] and thus it is reasonable to assume that individuals who have greater bone density are less likely to experience fracture. Although any individual can sustain a fracture depend-

ing on the severity of the trauma, and although in osteopenic individuals other factors such as the frequency of falls may be important, nevertheless the amount of bone present is the single most important factor determining the likelihood of fracture. There are now several prospective studies that confirm that bone mass measurements can predict fractures.* Results of studies are presented either in terms of the variation in the fracture incidence in the four quartiles of BMD of the study population or of the increased fracture risk for each 1 SD decrease in BMD. In a recent study of hip fracture incidence in 9700 white women from four cities in the United States, Cummings et al[17] found that women in the lowest quartile of femoral neck BMD were 8.5 times more likely to sustain a hip fracture than those in the highest quartile, and that each SD decrease in BMD increased fracture risk 2.6 times.

Clinical Indications for Bone Density Measurements

Over the years many studies have identified factors that may affect bone mass or fracture risk[13,22,69] and that may be used as indicators for bone densitometry measurements. For most of these indications, however, the routine clinical use of BMD measurements is not justified since the correlations are either too weak or the results are unlikely to influence patient or clinician behavior.

A report issued by the Scientific Advisory Board of the National Osteoporosis Foundation[37] has identified a number of clinical indications thought to justify bone densitometry (Box 20-1). These include scans of perimenopausal and postmenopausal women where a low BMD result might influence the decision to commence hormone replacement therapy, women who are estrogen deficient due to an early menopause, amenorrhea, or anorexia, and patients who have suffered fractures after relatively minor trauma, have been on long-term steroid therapy, or in whom a recent radiograph suggests osteopenia.

The use of repeat BMD measurements to monitor the rate of bone loss or the response of patients commencing

*References 4, 16, 17, 26, 36, 82.

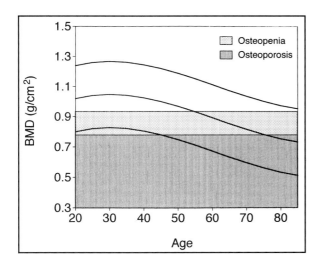

Fig. 20-23. The normal female reference curves for lumbar spine BMD shown in Fig. 20-22 plotted to include the WHO definitions of osteopenia and osteoporosis.[41,84] The lighter stippled area denotes women with osteopenia ($-1.0 > T > -2.5$), and the darker shaded area women with osteoporosis ($T < -2.5$).

BOX 20-1. Clincial Indications for Bone Mass Measurements

1. Menopausal women in whom result will influence treatment (e.g., with estrogen replacement therapy)
2. Estrogen-deficient women (e.g., early menopause, amenorrhea, anorexia nervosa)
3. Radiograph indicates osteopenia or vertebral deformity
4. Fracture after minor trauma
5. Steroid therapy (e.g., >5 mg prednisolone/day)
6. Diseases such as rheumatoid arthritis or primary hyperparathyroidism where result may influence treatment
7. To monitor response to treatment for osteoporosis

treatment needs careful consideration. The sensitivity of bone densitometry measurements for these purposes is limited by the natural slow rates of loss and the long-term precision of the technique as previously discussed in relation to the CFT. This is the time required to determine whether an individual has successfully responded to treatment (i.e., BMD is no longer falling) or is still losing bone at the average rate (−1.5%/year in the early postmenopausal years). It is equally the time to distinguish whether an individual is losing at the average rate or at twice that rate (i.e., could be considered as a fast loser). For DXA or QCT scans of the lumbar spine, this period is about 3 years.[29] Only larger rates of gain or loss can be detected in a shorter period, a factor that limits the value of repeating scans after too short an interval.

Prevention of Osteoporosis

Osteoporosis is a major health care issue. Although the average life expectancy of individuals is increasing, the age of women at the menopause has remained essentially static at about 51 years. Thus the women of the 1990s will spend a longer period in the postmenopausal part of their lives than any previous generation. Unless prophylactic measures are introduced, the incidence of osteoporotic fractures will continue to rise and the need for therapeutic measures increase.

It is likely that future advances in the health care of postmenopausal women will relate to the prevention of fractures rather than the treatment of patients who have already sustained an osteoporotic fracture. Established disease is difficult to treat, whereas prevention of the bone loss that precedes osteoporosis may be practical. Population-based approaches should be considered, and through education (e.g., relating to exercise and diet) it is possible that major benefits could be achieved. However, these measures, while sensible, are not of proven benefit, since long-term studies are not yet available. Problems may also arise in altering the life-styles of teenagers. This is an important aspect, since if these measures are to be successful it is likely they would have their greatest impact on the growing skeleton.

An alternative approach is selective screening—that is, targeting those individuals who are at greatest risk of developing osteoporosis in later life. A typical description of a woman perceived to be at risk might be blonde, thin, small, having an early menopause, and who smokes and drinks. There is now an extensive literature relating to clinical risk factors.[13,22,69] However, while an early menopause must be considered a major risk factor, many of the others correlate only weakly with osteoporosis. Since as many as one in three women will suffer an osteoporotic fracture, such weak associations are of little practical value.

With the introduction of DXA, however, there is now available a technique that allows for routine, reliable, and accurate measurements of bone density in the setting of a speciality bone or menopausal clinic, a physician's office or a screening program. Thus one of the most important applications of bone densitometry measurements is to identify perimenopausal and post-menopausal women with low bone density who can be advised to take preventative therapy (Fig. 20-22). Such patients may receive follow-up scans after 2 or 3 years to

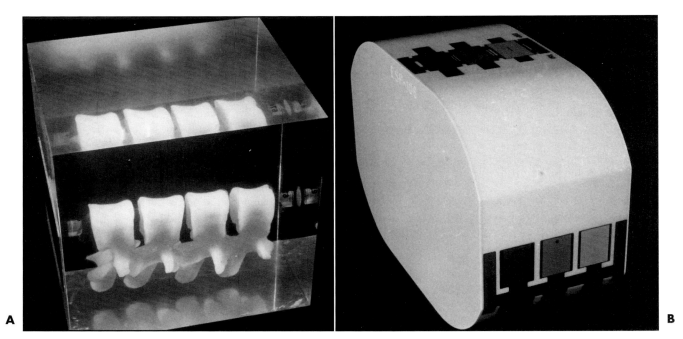

A　　　　　　　　　　　　　　　　　　　　　　　　B

Fig. 20-24. Daily scans of phantoms such as the Hologic spine phantom (**A**) and the European spine phantom (**B**) are an essential part of the quality control of all bone densitometry equipment.

monitor their response and it is important that measurements are performed at sites where response can be reliably measured after a short interval. With its good precision and rapid response to change, a DXA scan of PA lumbar spine BMD is the ideal measurement for many purposes.

Clinical Trials

Because of the high precision and long-term stability of calibration, DXA is widely used for prospective clinical trials of therapies to prevent bone loss in postmenopausal women.[59] High precision is an important factor for clinical trials because it determines the smallest change in bone density that can be detected and thus can influence the size and cost of studies. In longitudinal studies particular care is needed both in the performance of scans and their analysis if optimum precision is to be achieved.[55] Attention to the training of radiographers and consistency in their approach to scanning and analysis are essential. Care is needed in patient positioning so that the spine is straight and central in the area imaged. Vigilance is needed to ensure that items of clothing or jewelry do not introduce artifacts into the scan. For the hip the radiographer must ensure that the angles of internal rotation of the foot and abduction of the leg remain unchanged on follow-up scans.[85] Images from previous studies should be available at the time of scanning to ensure that the best match with past studies is obtained. The use of scout scan facilities such as the 5 s turbo scan on the QDR-2000 is a significant aid to patient positioning.

During scan analysis the compare function is used to ensure that an analysis region identical in size and location to that previously used is employed. To ensure optimum use of the compare function, each follow-up scan is matched directly with the original baseline scan. Greatest care is needed in analysis of the proximal femur where small differences in the positioning of the femoral neck box and Ward's triangle can lead to significant changes in the BMD measurements. Where interactive hip analysis software is provided, this can be used to ensure that regions in the hip reproduce as closely as possible those on the baseline scan.

Repeat scanning of anthropomorphic spine phantoms over several years has demonstrated the stability of calibration of DXA bone densitometers.[59] Nevertheless, daily scanning of a phantom (Fig. 20-24) is an essential quality assurance procedure for all users of DXA equipment.[28] The large number of phantom studies accumulated in this way allow even small drifts in calibration to be detected and are important for ensuring the integrity of data in the event of equipment failure. Suitable phantoms should be constructed of hydroxyapatite and a water equivalent epoxy resin. Ideally they should enable the BMD to be monitored over a range of values so that the linearity of the BMD scale can be regularly verified.[39]

In major clinical trials it is now usual for an experienced international center to coordinate quality assurance for bone densitometry studies.[28] Initial training is given to radiographers, and scans are analyzed at a central laboratory. This ensures a consistent approach to analysis and ensures that both patient and doctor remain blinded to whether the subject is taking the active drug or placebo. A set of master phantoms is passed between participating centers to cross-calibrate DXA systems. Results of daily phantom QC scans at individual sites are regularly reviewed to verify that systems are functioning within specifications and may be used to correct clinical scan data in the event of drifts in system calibration. Particular problems may arise if there is a need to replace a DXA scanner during the course of a study. Because studies may last for 5 years or longer, it is inevitable that some centers will upgrade their scanner during the course of a study, whether due to aging of equipment or to take advantage of advances in technology. In this situation the new scanner should be cross-calibrated with the old, using phantoms recommended by the manufacturer. However, phantoms are not perfect representations of the human body, and it is particularly important that in vivo cross-calibration studies are performed to verify the phantom studies. Typically scans of about 20 subjects are required to cross-calibrate in vivo with an accuracy of 1%.

REFERENCES

1. Baran DT, Kelly AM, Karellas A, et al: Ultrasound attenuation of the os calcis in women with osteoporosis and hip fractures. *Calcif Tissue Int* 1988; 43:138.
2. Bartley MH, Arnold JS, Haslam RK, et al: The relationship of bone strength and bone quantity in health, disease and aging. *J Gerontol* 1966; 21:517.
3. Black DM, Cummings SR, Stone K, et al: A new approach to defining normal vertebral dimensions. *J Bone Miner Res* 1991; 6:883.
4. Black D, Cummings SR, Genant HK, et al: Axial and appendicular bone density predict fractures in older women. *J Bone Miner Res* 1992; 7:633.
5. Blake GM, Tong CM, Fogelman I: Intersite comparison of the Hologic QDR-1000 dual energy X-ray bone densitometer. *Br J Radiol* 1991; 64:440.
6. Blake GM, McKeeney DB, Chhaya SC, et al: Dual energy x-ray absorptiometry: The effects of beam hardening on bone density measurements. *Med Phys* 1992; 19:459.
7. Blake GM, Parker JC, Buxton FMA, Fogelman I: Dual x-ray absorptiometry: A comparison between fan beam and pencil beam scans. *Br J Radiol* 1993; 66:902.
8. Blake GM, Jagathesan T, Herd RJM, Fogelman I: Dual x-ray absorptiometry of the lumbar spine: The precision of paired anteriorposterior/lateral studies. *Br J Radiol* 1994; 67:624.
9. Butz S, Wüster C, Scheidt-Nave, et al: Forearm BMD as measured by peripheral quantitative computed tomography (pQCT) in a German reference population. *Osteoporos Int* 1994; 4:179.
10. Buxton FMA, Blake GM, Parker JC, Fogelman I: Spinal bone density measured with a 5 second scan. *Br J Radiol* 1993; 66:275.
11. Cann CE, Genant HK: Precise measurement of vertebral bone mineral content using computed tomography. *J Comput Assist Tomogr* 1980; 4:493.
12. Cann CE: Quantitative CT for determination of bone mineral density: A review. *Radiology* 1988; 166:509.

13. Cohn AJ, Vaswani AN, Yeh JK, et al: Risk factors for post-menopausal osteoporosis. *Am J Med* 1985; 78:95.

14. Cosman F, Herrington B, Himmelstein S, et al: Radiographic absorptiometry: A simple method for determination of bone mass. *Osteoporos Int* 1991; 2:34.

15. Cullum ID, Ell PJ, Ryder JP: X-ray dual photon absorptiometry: A new method for the measurement of bone density. *Br J Radiol* 1989; 62:587.

16. Cummings SR, Black DM, Nevitt MC, et al: Appendicular bone density and age predict hip fracture in women. *JAMA* 1990; 263:665.

17. Cummings SR, Black DM, Nevitt MC, et al: Bone density at various sites for prediction of hip fractures. *Lancet* 1993; 341:72.

18. Eastell R, Cedel SL, Wahner HW, et al: Classification of vertebral fractures. *J Bone Miner Res* 1991; 6:207.

19. Edmonston SJ, Singer KP, Price RI, Breidahl PD: Accuracy of lateral dual energy x-ray absorptiometry for the determination of bone mineral content in the thoracic and lumbar spine: An in vitro study. *Br J Radiol* 1993; 66:309.

20. Eiken P, Bärenholdt O, Bjorn Jensen L, et al: Switching from DXA pencil-beam to fan-beam. I: Studies in-vitro in four centers. *Bone* 1994; 15:667.

21. Eiken P, Kolthoff N, Bärenholdt O, et al: Switching from DXA pencil-beam to fan-beam. II: Studies in-vivo. *Bone* 1994; 15:671.

22. Elders PJM, Netelenbos JC, Lips P, et al: Perimenopausal bone mass and risk factors. *Bone Miner* 1989; 7:289.

23. Erikson S, Isberg B, Lindgren U: Vertebral bone mineral measurement using dual photon absorptiometry and computed tomography. *Acta Radiol* 1988; 29:89.

24. Faulkner KG, Glüer C-C, Estillo M, Genant HK. Cross-calibration of DXA equipment: Upgrading from a Hologic QDR-1000/W to a QDR-2000. *Calcif Tissue Int* 1993; 52:79.

25. Faulkner KG, McClung MR, Schmeer MS, et al: Densitometry of the radius using single and dual energy absorptiometry. *Calcif Tissue Int* 1994; 54:208.

26. Gardsell P, Johnell O, Nilsson BE: Predicting fractures in women by using forearm bone densitometry. *Calcif Tissue Int* 1989; 44:235.

27. Genant HK, Wu CY, van Kuijk C, Nevitt M: Vertebral fracture assessment using a semi-quantitative technique. *J Bone Miner Res* 1993; 8:1137.

28. Glüer C-C, Faulkner KG, Estilo MJ, et al: Quality assurance for bone densitometry research studies: Concept and impact. *Osteoporos Int* 1993; 3:227.

29. Glüer C-C, Blunt B, Engelke M, et al: Characteristic follow-up time: A new concept for standardized characterization of a technique's ability to monitor longitudinal changes. *Bone Miner* 1994; 25(suppl 2):S40.

30. Gotfredsen A, Podenphant J, Norgaard H, et al: Accuracy of lumbar spine bone mineral content by dual photon absorptiometry. *J Nucl Med* 1988; 29:248.

31. Grampp S, Jergas M, Glüer C-C, et al: Radiological diagnosis of osteoporosis: Current methods and perpectives. *Radiol Clin North Am* 1993; 31:1133.

32. Harper KD, Lobaugh B, King ST, Drezner MK: Upgrading dual energy x-ray absorptiometry scanners: Do new models provide equivalent results? *J Bone Miner Res* 1992; 7(Suppl):S191.

33. Herd RJM, Blake GM, Parker JC, et al: Total body studies in normal British women using dual x-ray absorptiometry. *Br J Radiol* 1993; 66:303.

34. Herd RJM, Blake GM, Ramalingam T, et al: Measurements of postmenopausal bone loss with a new contact ultrasound system. *Calcif Tissue Int* 1993; 53:153.

35. Ho CP, Kim RW, Schaffler MB, Sartoris DJ: Accuracy of dual-energy radiographic absorptiometry of the lumbar spine: A cadaver study. *Radiology* 1990; 176:171.

36. Hui SL, Slemenda CW, Johnston CC: Baseline measurement of bone mass predicts fracture in white women. *Ann Intern Med* 1989; 111:355.

37. Johnston CC, Melton LJ, Lindsay R, et al: Clinical indications for bone mass measurements. A report from the Scientific Advisory Board of the National Osteoporosis Foundation. *J Bone Miner Res* 1989; 4(suppl 2):1.

38. Jones CD, Laval-Jeantet AM, Laval-Jeantet MH, Genant HK: Importance of measurement of spongious vertebral bone mineral density in the assessment of osteoporosis. *Bone* 1987; 8:201.

39. Kalender W: A phantom for standardization and quality control in spinal bone mineral measurements by QCT and DXA: Design considerations and specifications. *Med Phys* 1992; 19:583.

40. Kalender WA: Effective dose values in bone mineral measurements by photon absorptiometry and computed tomography. *Osteoporosis Int* 1992; 2:82.

41. Kanis JA, Melton LJ, Christiansen C, et al: The diagnosis of osteoporosis. *J Bone Miner Res* 1994; 9:1137.

42. Kelly TL, Slovik DM, Schoenfeld DA, Neer RM: Quantitative digital radiography versus dual photon absorptiometry of the lumbar spine. *J Clin Endocrinol Metab* 1988; 67:839.

43. Kelly TL, Crane G, Baran DT: Single x-ray absorptiometry of the forearm: Precision, correlation and reference data. *Calcif Tissue Int* 1994; 54:212.

44. Langton C, Palmer SB, Porter RW: Measurement of broadband ultrasonic attenuation in cancellous bone. *Eng Med* 1984; 13:89.

45. Larnach TA, Boyd SJ, Smart RC, et al: Reproducibility of lateral spine scans using dual energy x-ray absorptiometry. *Calcif Tissue Int* 1992; 51:255.

46. LeBoff MS, El-Hajj A, Fuleihan G, et al: Dual-energy x-ray absorptiometry of the forearm: Reproducibility and correlation with single photon absorptiometry. *J Bone Miner Res* 1992; 7:841.

47. Lehmann R, Wapniarz M, Kvasnicka HM, et al: Reproduzierbarkeit von knochendichtemessungen am distalen radius mit einem hochauflösenden spezialscanner für periphere quantitative computertomographie (single energy pQCT). *Radiologe* 1992; 32:177.

48. Lewis MK, Blake GM, Fogelman I: Patient dose in dual x-ray absorptiometry. *Osteoporos Int* 1994; 4:11.

49. Lewis MK, Blake GM: Patient dose in morphometric x-ray absorptiometry. *Osteoporos Int* 1995; 5:181.

50. Lilly J, Eyre S, Walters B, et al: An investigation of spinal bone mineral density measured laterally: A normal range for UK women. *Br J Radiol* 1994; 67:157.

51. Mazess R, Collick B, Trempe J, Barden H, Hanson J: Performance evaluation of a dual-energy x-ray bone densitometer. *Calcif Tissue Int* 1989; 44:228.

52. McCloskey EV, Murray SA, Miller C, et al: Broadband ultrasonic attenuation in the os calcis: Relationship to bone mineral at other skeletal sites. *Clin Sci* 1990; 78:227.

53. McCloskey EV, Spector TD, Eyres KS, et al: The assessment of vertebral deformity: A method for use in population studies and clinical trials. *Osteoporos Int* 1993; 3:138.

54. Miller CG, Herd RJM, Ramalingam T, et al: Ultrasonic velocity measurements through the calcaneus: Which velocity should be measured? *Osteoporos Int* 1993; 3:31.

55. Miller CG: Bone density measurements in clinical trials: The challenge of ensuring optimal data. *Br J Clin Res* 1993; 4:113.

56. Nord RH, Payne RK: Body composition by DXA: A review of the technology. *Asia Pac J Clin Nutr* 1995; 4:167.

57. Nord RH, Payne RK: DXA vs underwater weighing: Comparison of strengths and weaknesses. *Asia Pac J Clin Nutr* 1995; 4:173.

58. Nord RH, Payne RK: A new equation set for converting body density to percent body fat. *Asia Pac J Clin Nutr* 1995; 4:177.

59. Orwell ES, Oviatt SK, and the Nafarelin bone study group: Longitudinal precision of dual-energy x-ray absorptiometry in a multicenter study. *J Bone Miner Res* 1991; 6:191.

60. Pacifici R, Rupich R, Griffin M, et al: Dual energy radiography versus quantitative computer tomography for the diagnosis of osteoporosis. *J Clin Endocrinol Metab* 1990; 70:705.

61. Pommet R, Chambellan D, Reverchon P, et al: Array multidetector bone densitometer for supine lateral vertebral measurement in lateral projection. *Osteoporos Int* 1991; 1:190.

62. Porter RW, Miller CG, Grainger D, Palmer SB: Prediction of hip fracture in elderly women: A prospective study. *Br Med J* 1990; 301:638.

63. Pye DW, Hannan WJ, Hesp R: Effective dose equivalent in dual x-ray absorptiometry. *Br J Radiol* 1990; 63:149.

64. Ramalingam T, Herd RJM, Lees B, et al: A comparison of three commercial bone ultrasound scanners. *Calcif Tissue Int* 1993; 52:170.

65. Richmond BJ, Eberle RW, Stulberg BN, Deal CL: DEXA measurement of peri-prosthetic bone mineral density in total hip arthroplasty. *Osteoporos Int* 1991; 1:191.

66. Ryan PJ, Blake GM, Fogelman I: Measurement of forearm bone mineral density in normal women by dual energy X-ray absorptiometry. *Br J Radiol* 1992; 65:127.

67. Ryan PJ, Blake GM, Fogelman I: Postmenopausal screening for osteopenia. *Br J Rheumatol* 1992; 31:823.

68. Ryan PJ, Blake GM, Fogelman I: Fracture thresholds in osteoporosis: Implications for hormone replacement therapy. *Ann Rheum Dis* 1992; 51:1063.

69. Slemenda CW, Hui SL, Longcope C, et al: Predictors of bone mass in perimenopausal women. *Ann Intern Med* 1990; 112:96.

70. Slosman DO, Rizzoli R, Donath A, Bonjour J-P: Vertebral bone mineral density measured laterally by dual energy x-ray absorptiometry. *Osteoporos Int* 1990; 1:23.

71. Snead DB, Birge SJ, Kohrt WM: Age related differences in body composition by hydrodensitometry and dual-energy x-ray absorptiometry. *J Appl Physiol* 1993; 74:770.

72. Sorenson JA, Duke PR, Smith SW: Simulation studies of dual-energy X-ray absorptiometry. *Med Phys* 1989; 16:75.

73. Steiger P, von Stetten E, Weiss H, Stein JA: Paired AP and lateral supine dual x-ray absorptiometry of the spine: Initial results with a 32 detector system. *Osteoporos Int* 1991; 1:190.

74. Steiger P, Cummings SR, Genant HK, Weiss H: Morphometric x-ray absorptiometry: Correlation in vivo with morphometric radiography. *Osteoporos Int* 1994; 4:238.

75. Stein JA, Lazewatsky JL, Hochberg AM: Dual-energy x-ray absorptiometry incorporating an internal reference source. *Radiology* 1987; 166(Suppl):313.

76. Tothill P: Methods of bone mineral measurement. *Phys Med Biol* 1989; 34:543.

77. Trevisan C, Cherubini R, Ulivieri FM, et al: Dual energy x-ray absorptiometry in the evaluation of periprosthetic bone mineral status: Analysis protocols and reproducibility. *Osteoporos Int* 1991; 1:191.

78. Uebelhart D, Duboeuf F, Meunier PJ, Delmas PD: Lateral dual photon absorptiometry: A new technique to measure the bone mineral density at the lumbar spine. *J Bone Min Res* 1990; 5:525.

79. Wahner HW, Dunn WL, Mazess RB, et al: Dual-photon absorptiometry of bone. *Radiology* 1985; 156:203.

80. Wahner HW, Dunn WL, Brown ML, et al: Comparison of dual-energy X-ray absorptiometry and dual photon absorptiometry for bone mineral measurements of the lumbar spine. *Mayo Clin Proc* 1988; 63:1075.

81. Wahner HW, Fogelman I: The evaluation of osteoporosis: dual energy x-ray absorptiometry, in *Clinical Practice*, Martin Dunitz, London, 1994.

82. Wasnich RD, Ross PD, Heilbrun LK, Vogel JM: Selection of the optimal site for fracture risk prediction. *Clin Othop* 1987; 216:262.

83. Weinstein RS, New KD, Sappington LJ: Dual-energy x-ray absorptiometry versus single photon absorptiometry of the radius. *Calcif Tissue Int* 1991; 49:313.

84. WHO: WHO Technical Report Series 843. *Assessment of Fracture Risk and Its Application to Screening for Postmenopausal Osteoporosis*. World Health Organization, Geneva, 1994.

85. Wilson CR, Fogelman I, Blake GM, Rodin A: The effect of positioning on dual energy x-ray densitometry of the proximal femur. *Bone Miner* 1991; 13:69.

CHAPTER 21

TREATMENT OF THE PAIN OF BONE METASTASES

Edward B. Silberstein

The prevalence of pain in all patients with cancer, especially in advanced disease, ranges between 60% to 90% in several recent estimates.[9] Although many approaches yielding adequate pain relief are available, there are data indicating these are underutilized.[2] Narcotic-induced analgesia is associated with sedation and constipation and every effort should be made to use supplementary alternative modalities.[23] Radiation therapy is not only an important approach for the noninvasive control of bone pain due to metastatic cancer, but also can improve functional status and even prevent or delay the onset of new painful metastases.[15,17]

Teletherapy, the use of external beam radiation to control pain, is quite efficacious,[4,16] but may be difficult to employ when multiple sites require treatment. Teletherapy is the treatment of choice for impending pathologic fracture, pain from epidural metastasis with cord compression, or pressure on bone from a large soft-tissue mass. Radiation-sensitive tissue such as the lungs, kidneys, or spinal cord may also limit the application of teletherapy in a patient with multiple painful rib or vertebral metastases. Hemibody radiation can also be helpful in such patients, with responses of 70% to 80%, but this modality is not without significant hematologic and gastrointestinal toxicity.[18]

Another radiotherapeutic approach to the treatment of pain from metastatic carcinoma of bone metastases is the intravenous injection of bone-seeking radiopharmaceuticals that emit beta particles or conversion electrons. Beta particles originate from the atomic nucleus and are emitted during some forms of radioactive decay. They have a wide range of energies. The radiopharmaceuticals listed in Table 21-1 have mean energies (measured as MeV, or million electron volts) permitting penetration into soft tissues of 0.2 to 3 mm on average, so that tumor in and around bone can be radiated once the radiopharmaceutical carrying the beta-emitting atom is taken up by reactive bone at the site of metastatic disease. Alpha particles and Auger electrons emitted during radioactive decay have very short ranges in tissues, which are probably inadequate to radiate inhomogeneously distributed intraosseous metastases.

Radiopharmaceuticals that have significant affinity for bone chemically adsorb (chemisorb), or react with, the atoms comprising molecular hydroxyapatite on the surface of bone. Reactive bone formation initially produces smaller hydroxyapatite moieties with a greater surface area than in older bone. Also blood flow is often increased to the involved site as well. These characteristics permit accumulation of bone-seeking agents to a sig-

TABLE 21-1
Beta-Emitting Radiopharmaceuticals for Therapy of Painful Bone Metastases

Radiopharmaceutical	Physical Half-Life (days)	Mean Beta or Electron Energy (MeV)	Mean Beta Path in Soft Tissue (mm)	Gamma Photopeak Energy (percent of decays yielding gammas)(MeV)
Phosphorus-32 as orthophosphate	14.3	0.7	2.5	(No Gamma)
Rhenium-186 as HEDP chelate	3.8	0.35	1.1	0.137 (9%)
Samarium-153 as EDTMP chelate	1.9	0.22	0.8	0.103 (28%)
				0.410 (49%)
Strontium-89 as chloride salt	50.5	0.58	2.4	0.910 (0.01%)
Tin-117m as DTPA chelate	13.6	0.16, 0.13	0.29, 0.21	0.161 (86%)

nificantly greater degree than surrounding normal bone, so that abnormal-to-normal-bone ratios of radiopharmaceutical uptake may range from 3:1 to 15:1. Both Sr-89 and Re-186 HEDP are retained at the site of the osteoblastic response to tumor significantly longer than on normal bone, further increasing the radiation dose to tumor within bone relative to normal marrow in unaffected bone.[5]

The chosen radionuclide that is incorporated in the bone-seeking radiopharmaceutical must have a physical half-life long enough to allow distribution to hospitals from the site of production. The biologic half-life of the radiopharmaceutical must be long enough so that there is time to react with involved bone and radiate adjacent tumor before significant excretion occurs. All of these have significant renal excretion, and renal dysfunction will lead to increased skeletal retention and a greater dose to soft tissues.

Two of the five radiopharmaceuticals that fulfill these criteria (P-32 as orthophosphate; strontium-89 as the chloride) have been approved in many countries for use in patients with bone pain from metastatic carcinoma, whereas the other three (rhenium-186 etidronate, samarium-153 EDTMP [ethylenediamine tetramethylene phosphonate], both phosphonate chelates, and tin-117m DTPA [diethylenetriamene pentaacetic acid], another chelate) are undergoing active investigational new drug (IND) clinical studies in the United States. The relevant characteristics of these radiopharmaceuticals appear in Table 21-1. The radiopharmaceuticals that emit gamma rays do not provide any advantage, since a Tc-99m bisphosphonate bone scan must be performed before administration of any of these expensive agents to document increased uptake in a nonfractured site.

The mechanism of pain relief is not entirely clear, since a decrease in intramedullary pressure alone[6] cannot explain the prompt reduction in pain that may occur in a few days, when the radiation dose that has been delivered has not yet killed a significant percent of the tumor present, and tumor shrinkage has not occurred. In fact,

BOX 21-1. Possible Target Cells for Osseous Pain Reduction

- Lymphocyte
- Macrophage
- Mast cell
- Neuron nociceptors
- Osteoblast
- Osteoclast
- Tumor cell
- Vascular endothelium

BOX 21-2. Potential Intramedullary Pain Mediators

- ATP
- Bradykinin or its metabolites
- Calcitonin
- Histamine
- Interleukins 1 and 2
- Leukotrienes
- Lipidic acids
- Prostaglandins
- Serotonin
- Substance P

with radiation-induced tumor necrosis, there may be swelling of the tissues involved. A variety of local humoral mechanisms for pain modulation, including the action of cytokines,[6] also may be affected by radiation. Possible other cellular targets for these beta particles are listed in Box 21-1 and a list of potential pain mediators appears in Box 21-2. Relatively low radiation levels could have an early lethal effect on radiosensitive cells which produce these cytokines.

Published dosimetry for all these radiopharmaceuticals is probably not very accurate, since the bone marrow models for microdosimetry are being reevaluated. The marked inhomogeneity in distribution of tumor, marrow, and trabecular bone within a site of increased uptake on bone scan remains a major dosimetric challenge.

Since some myelosuppression can occur from marrow radiation by bone that has chemisorbed these agents, patients eligible for treatment should not have severe leukopenia (leukocytes less than 2500 to 4000/μl) or thrombocytopenia (platelets less than 60,000 to 100,000/μl). Concurrent chemotherapy or wide-field external beam radiotherapy can cause significant pancytopenia. These agents are excreted in the urine, so that special handling of contaminated clothing and sheets is required if the patient is incontinent.

These radiopharmaceuticals should be administered only when the painful site or sites show increased osteoblastic activity as documented by an abnormal bone scan. They have no clear analgesic effect when the pain is due to peripheral nerve or spinal cord involvement or to pathologic fracture. Besides myelosuppression, these agents can lead to a brief increase in pain, or flare response, in about 10% of patients.

PHOSPHORUS-32

Of the radiopharmaceuticals currently in active use, phosphorus-32 (P-32), as sodium orthophosphate, has been the most widely studied, with at least 30 articles in the medical literature concerning its efficacy.[19] The clinical evaluative tools employed in the study of the recipients of P-32, most with prostate and breast carcinoma, were not always at the sophisticated level currently in use, but the data on efficacy of P-32 are remarkably consistent in indicating pain reduction in approximately 80% of patients treated.

Based on incomplete data reported in a single abstract, androgen therapy has been employed for many years, usually over a week preceding administration of P-32, in the hope that bone uptake of orthophosphate would be stimulated. Parathyroid hormone has been similarly utilized. There is, however, no evidence that these manipulations provide any therapeutic advantage over simple intravenous administration, without patient preparation, of P-32 as sodium orthophosphate.[19]

Eighty percent to eighty-five percent of injected P-32 is taken up by the hydroxyapatite in bone, with 20% excreted in the urine within a week. Since the phosphate moiety is part of the backbone of nucleic acids, and is intimately involved in the cellular process of energy storage and release and other reactions involving phosphorylation, there is uptake by all viable tissue, especially rapidly dividing tissue like marrow. Thus not only will bone marrow be radiated from radiophosphate-containing bone surrounding and supporting it, but also from the marrow itself.[21]

Many treatment schedules have been employed for administration of P-32 as orthophosphate, including single injection or orally with activities of 6 to 12 mCi, as well as in multiple dosages over a month, totaling as much as 24 mCi. There are no randomized comparative studies to indicate the optimum schedule for P-32 administration (e.g., two or more "split" doses versus a single intravenous dose). The oral route has given results comparable to intravenous P-32. The overall efficacy for pain reduction, about 80%, is independent of the total activity of P-32 given, as long as 8 mCi or more is administered. An analgesic effect is seen after 1 to 4 weeks, lasting several months. No careful dose escalation study has ever been performed, however. Skeletal radiographic or scintigraphic improvement has been noted in 11% to 80% of cases in different series,[19] but this does not correlate with pain reduction (Fig. 21-1).

Myelosuppression occurs between 3 and 8 weeks following therapy but is rarely severe, with only one death reported as being related to marrow depression after multiple P-32 doses totaling 20 mCi.[22] The radiation dose to normal bone has been estimated at between 20 to 63 rad/mCi, depending on the dosimetric assumptions employed. The flare phenomenon, a worsening of pain 3 to 14 days postinjection, lasting another 2 to 4 days, occurs in about 10% of patients receiving any of the radiopharmaceuticals in Table 21-1. If androgens are given to prostate carcinoma patients for a week before P-32 injection, an increase in pain occurs in up to 50%. Nausea has occurred with P-32 therapy only when androgens have been administered.

STRONTIUM-89

Strontium-89 (Sr-89), which substitutes for calcium in the hydroxyapatite molecule, was first suggested for a therapeutic role in the palliation of bone pain from metastatic disease in 1942,[13] actually preceding the earliest reports of P-32 for this purpose (although P-32 had been used for the therapy of hematologic disorders since 1936). The biological half-life of Sr-89 deposited in the reactive bone adjacent to the metastases is greater than 50 days, whereas in normal bone it is about 14 days. This difference in regional kinetics permits delivery of useful doses of beta radiation to the lesions with relative sparing of healthy bone and bone marrow. Bone marrow in the vicinity of metastatic lesions receive a radiation dose which exceeds that of marrow in normal bone by a factor of ten.[5] Excretion of Sr-89 is about 80% renal and 20% fecal. The radiation dose to tumor from a 4-mCi injection of Sr-89 averages 3,000 to 3,500 rads (30 to 35 Gy) with tumor doses up to four times as high reported. The bone marrow dose is about 150 to 300 rads (1.5 to 3 Gy), which commonly causes mild to moderate myelosuppression with leukocyte and platelet counts decreasing to approximately 30 to 80% of the pretreatment levels. The nadir occurs at 4 to 8 weeks with recovery by 10 to 16 weeks.[12]

Pain reduction occurs in 65 to 80% with complete relief in 5 to 20% of these responders. These responses occur within a few days to 4 weeks after intravenous injection, with a median duration of benefit lasting 3 to

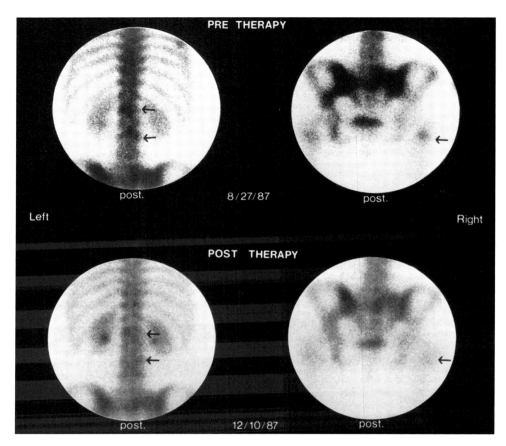

Fig. 21-1. This patient with prostate adenocarcinoma and multiple painful osseous metastases was treated with Re-186 HEDP. The lesions noted with arrows on the Tc-99m MDP bone scan of 8/28/87 have reduced uptake on the subsequent scan of 12/10/87 3 months post-therapy. The bilateral sacroiliac lesions also appear better on the second scan. The patient responded clinically as well.

6 months.[1] Retreatment for responders is possible at approximately 3-month intervals, with a 50% response rate noted to the second treatment. Above a threshold of 20 to 30 µCi/kg most researchers do not find an increase in the probability of pain relief with an increase of strontium activity administered (i.e., the dose-response curve has a slope of zero).[1] The usual dose is between 40 to 60 µCi/kg. Double-blind studies with Sr-89 have shown that this radiopharmaceutical also reduces the occurrence of new painful sites. Two studies have shown that Sr-89, as compared with teletherapy, not only delays the return of pain for a longer time but reduces the incidence of new painful sites. The activities employed were 5.4 and 10.8 mCi.[15,17] There is no evidence that Sr-89, or any other of these radiopharmaceuticals, prolongs life, however.

Sr-89 injection should be performed over 60 to 120 seconds since the patient will experience a warm flushing sensation from a rapid bolus injection.

RHENIUM-186 DIPHOSPHONATE

Diphosphonates such as etidronate were labeled with technetium-99m for bone imaging in the early 1970s. Phosphonates possess a carbon-to-phosphorus bond that is not hydrolyzed by phosphatases and so are quite stable in vivo.

The phosphate moiety of diphosphonates chemisorbs to calcium atoms in bone hydroxyapatite. Since rhenium and technetium both belong to Group VIIA of the Periodic Table, it was a logical step to label etidronate with the beta- and gamma-emitting rhenium-186.[14] The gamma ray from Re-186 can be used to image osteoblastic metastases to confirm localization and potentially do lesion dosimetry, but this approach is far more expensive than employing a technetium-labeled diphosphonate for tumor imaging in bone and has not yet been shown to offer any advantage. The distribution of Re-186 etidronate and diagnostic bone imaging agents is identical. About 70% of the administered activity is excreted in the urine by 72 hours. Therapeutically useful bone-seeking rhenium-186 (Re-186) etidronate has been developed and is now in an extensive phase III study.

The tumor dose from an average of 33.5 mCi of Re-186 HEDP given intravenously is approximately 3,500 rad (35 Gy) but has been measured as high as 14,000 rad (140 Gy) with a mean marrow dose estimated at 120 rad (1.2 Gy). Larger administered activities have not yielded a higher response rate. Clinically significant pain relief has been described in about 80% of patients within 1 to 3 weeks. Ten percent of patients had a brief "flare" or worsening of pain, followed by a clinical response.[11] Both the administered activity-response relationship with rhenium-186 etidronate and the median duration of response are still under investigation, but some patients have maintained an analgesic response for months. About 50% of patients who responded to the first treatment will have pain reduction with the second or even third injection of Re-186 etidronate.

SAMARIUM-153 EDTMP

Samarium-153 (Sm-153) is a beta-emitting radionuclide with a shorter half-life (46.3 hours) than rhenium-186 (90.6 hours), which, like rhenium, has been chelated with bone-seeking polyphosphonates. The best combination of high bone uptake with low nonosseous uptake and rapid blood clearance was found to be a samarium chelate with ethylenediaminetetramethylenephosphonate (EDTMP).[10] Sm-153 EDTMP clears more rapidly from the blood than the bone imaging agent Tc-99m MDP, while providing identical scintigraphic and bone-to-bone-marrow ratios. One half to two thirds of injected Sm-153 EDTMP is taken up by bone, with higher levels of retention in the presence of osteoblastic metastases. One third to one half of Sm-153 EDTMP is excreted in the urine within 8 hours.[20]

Samarium-153 EDTMP, given at an optimal activity of 1.0 mCi/kg, leads to pain reduction in 65% to 73% of evaluable patients, beginning in 1 to 4 weeks and lasting for periods of 1 to 11 months following intravenous administration.[7,8] If pain recurs, it responds to retreatment in half to three fourths of patients. No activity-response relationship has been observed with samarium-153 EDTMP, similar to the other radiopharmaceuticals in Table 21-1. Myelotoxicity is seen with both rhenium-186 etidronate and samarium-153 EDTMP, with reduction in leukocyte and platelet counts of 10 to 70% and a recovery time of 6 to 8 weeks.[8]

TIN-117m DTPA

This chelate delivers Sn-117m to bone surfaces where a tin atom probably forms an oxide with available hydroxyl moieties of hydroxyapatite. Despite very low electron energies and a resultant mean path in soft tissue of only 0.2 to 0.3 mm, recent data indicate clinical efficacy with little myelotoxicity,[3] but more data will be required before it is known if Sn-117m DTPA produces less myelosuppression than other radiopharmaceuticals.

ADMINISTRATION OF BETA/ELECTRON-EMITTING RADIOPHARMACEUTICALS

The recommended criteria for the selection of patients for teletherapy or beta/electron-emitting radiopharmaceuticals are listed in Box 21-3 and Box 21-4. The painful site must correspond to an abnormal area of increased uptake on bone scan. If the bone scan shows no lesion in the site of pain, the radiopharmaceutical should not be administered since pain from this source will not be ameliorated. Pathologic fracture must be excluded. The patient should not have significant pancytopenia; full marrow recovery must have occurred from any chemotherapy, and no such therapy should be given during the 2 to 4 months of potential or actual marrow suppression from the radiopharmaceutical. Injecting these radiopharmaceuticals through a preexisting intravenous line reduces the radiation dose to the therapist's hands and also prevents infiltration of the dose. Beta emitters produce bremsstrahlung proportional to the atomic number of material with which the beta interacts, so a plastic syringe shield, not lead, should be employed. Injection should take place over about 60 seconds to avoid side effects from either the chelator or ionic moieties of these radiopharmaceuticals. Box 21-5 summarizes a recommended method of administering these unsealed sources.

BOX 21-3. When to Treat Painful Bone Metastases with Teletherapy

- Only one or two focal painful metastases
- Cord compression from tumor
- Prophylaxis or treatment of pathologic fracture
- Pain results from soft-tissue tumor extending to bone

BOX 21-4. When to Treat Painful Bone Metastases with Beta-Emitting Radiopharmaceuticals

- Multiple painful bony metastases in the presence of a bone scan showing increased uptake in the painful sites
- Painful solitary vertebral lesion when the spinal cord has received 40 to 45 Gy

---

BOX 21-5. Administered Unsealed Beta Emitters

- The painful site must correspond to an area positive on a recent bone scan.
- Platelet and leukocyte counts must be adequate.
- Informed consent should be obtained and documented.
- Inject through running intravenous line.
- The physician should use a finger dosimeter.
- Inject the radiopharmaceutical over about 1 minute.
- A plastic syringe shield is suggested.

BOX 21-6. Predictive Factors for Pancytopenia Following Therapy with Unsealed Sources

- Degree of marrow infiltration
- Previous chemotherapy
- Previous radiotherapy
- Presence of disseminated intravascular coagulation

CONCLUSION

These five beta-emitting radiopharmaceuticals with high bone affinity—phosphorus-32, strontium-89, rhenium-186 etidronate, samarium-153 EDTMP, and tin-117m DTPA—all have the capability of reducing pain due to osseous metastases in about 65% to 80% of patients. Before such a patient is treated, one must be certain that direct tumor involvement is causing the bone pain and that the diagnostic bone scan shows abnormally increased uptake in that area to ensure similarly enhanced concentration of the therapeutic beta-emitting radiopharmaceutical at a painful site. A complete response to the radiopharmaceutical is far less common than a partial response, but a reduction in the amount of opiate required to control bone pain is usually accomplished. This leads to enhancement of the patient's quality of life by reducing sedation, confusion, and constipation. Responding patients must have an abnormal bone scan in a painful site of metastasis that is not fractured. Responders to treatment cannot be distinguished from nonresponders by any other clinical criteria examined to date.

All these beta-emitting radiopharmaceuticals will produce varying degrees of pancytopenia, depending on the factors listed in Box 21-6.

REFERENCES

1. Ackery D, Yardley J: Radionuclide-targeted therapy for the management of metastatic bone pain. *Semin Oncol* 1993; 20:27.
2. Ad Hoc Committee on Cancer Pain of the American Society of Clinical Oncology. Cancer pain assessment and treatment curriculum guidelines. *J Clin Oncol* 1992; 10:1976.
3. Atkins HL, Mausner LF, Srivastava SC, et al: Tin-117m(4+)-DTPA for palliation of pain from osseous metastases: A pilot study. *J Nucl Med* 1995; 36:725.
4. Bates T, Yarnold JR, Blitzer P, et al: Bone metastasis consensus statement. *Int J Radiat Oncol Biol Phys* 1992; 23:215.
5. Blake GM, Zivanovic MA, McEwan AJ, et al: Sr-89 therapy: Strontium kinetics in disseminated carcinoma of the prostate. *Eur J Nucl Med* 1986; 12:447.
6. Campa JA, Payne R: The management of intractable bone pain: A clinician's perspective. *Semin Nucl Med* 1992; 22:3.
7. Collins C, Eary JF, Donaldson G, et al: Samarium-153-EDTMP in bone metastases of hormone refractory prostate carcinoma: A Phase I/II Trial. *J Nucl Med* 1993; 34:1839.
8. Farhangi M, Holmes RA, Volkert WA, et al: Samarium-153-EDTMP: Pharmacokinetics, toxicity and pain response using an escalating dose schedule in treatment of metastatic bone cancer. *J Nucl Med* 1992; 33:1451.
9. Foley KM: The treatment of cancer pain. *N Engl J Med* 1985; 313:84.
10. Goeckeler WF, Edwards B, Bokert WA, et al: Skeletal localization of Sm-153 chelates: Potential therapeutic bone agents. *J Nucl Med* 1987; 28:495.
11. Maxon HR, Schroder LE, Thomas SR, et al: Re-186(Sn)HEDP for treatment of painful osseous metastases: Initial clinical experience in 20 patients with hormone-resistant prostate cancer. *Radiology* 1992; 176:155.
12. McEwan AJB, Porter AT, Venner PM, et al: An evaluation of the safety and efficacy of treatment with strontium-89 in patients who have previously received wide field radiotherapy. *Antibody Immunoconjugates Radiopharm* 1990; 3:91.
13. Pecher C: Biological investigations with radioactive strontium and calcium: Preliminary report on the use of radioactive strontium in the treatment of bone cancer. *Univ Calif Publ Pharmacol* 1942; 11:117.
14. Pinkerton TC, Heineman WR, Deutsch EA: Separation of technetium hydroxyethylidene diphosphonate complexes by anion-exchange high performance liquid chromatography. *Ann Chem* 1980; 52:1106.
15. Porter AT, McEwan AJM, Powe JE, et al: Results of a randomized phase III trial to evaluate the efficacy of strontium-89 adjuvant to local field external beam irradiation in the management of endocrine resistant metastatic prostate cancer. *Int J Radiat Oncol Biol Phys* 1993; 25:805.
16. Poulson HS, Nielson OS, Klee M, et al: Palliative irradiation of bone metastases. *Cancer Treat Rev* 1989; 16:41.
17. Quilty DM, Kirk D, Bolger JJ, et al: A comparison of the palliative effects of strontium-89 and external beam radiotherapy in metastatic prostate cancer. *Radiother Oncol* 1994; 31:33.
18. Salazar OM, Rubin P, Hendrickson PR, et al: Single dose half-body irradiation for palliation of multiple bone metastases from solid tumors. Final Radiation Therapy Oncology Group Report. *Cancer* 1986; 58:29.
19. Silberstein EB: The treatment of painful osseous metastases with phosphorus-32-labeled phosphates. *Semin Oncol* 1993; 20(suppl 2):10.
20. Singh A, Holmes RA, Farhangi M, et al: Human pharmacokinetics of [153]Sm-EDTMP in metastatic cancer. *J Nucl Med* 1989; 30:1814.
21. Spiers FW, Beddoe AH, King SD, et al: The absorbed dose to bone marrow in the treatment of polycythemia by [32]P. *Br J Radiol* 1976; 49:133.
22. Tong ECK, Finkelstein P: The treatment of prostatic bone metastases with parathormone and radioactive phosphorus. *J Urol* 1973; 109:71.
23. Wilkie DJ: Pharmacologic management of cancer pain: Summary of the science. *J Natl Cancer Inst* 1993; 85:1117.